Reproductive Surgery

Steven R. Lindheim • John C. Petrozza
Editors

Reproductive Surgery

Current Techniques to Optimize Fertility

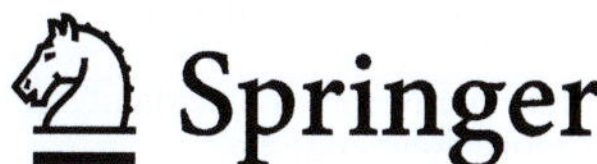 Springer

Editors
Steven R. Lindheim
Department of Obstetrics
and Gynecology
Wright State University
Dayton, OH, USA

John C. Petrozza
Department of Obstetrics
and Gynecology
Massachusetts General Hospital
Boston, MA, USA

ISBN 978-3-031-05242-2   ISBN 978-3-031-05240-8   (eBook)
https://doi.org/10.1007/978-3-031-05240-8

This Springer imprint is published by the registered company Springer Nature Switzerland AG
The registered company address is: Gewerbestrasse 11, 6330 Cham, Switzerland

Foreword

Performed for other than trauma, congenital defects and cosmetics, 'surgery' represents the failure of medicine; failure of elucidating the etiology of the disease and developing specific and effective preventive and therapeutic measures. – Victor Gomel, 2019 [1]

We are still very far from achieving this level of success; hence we must continue to train skilled surgeons to properly treat women with reproductive problems.

Gynecologic practice, like medicine, continues to evolve. The gynecological surgeon of the twenty-first century is typically different from many of those of the other surgical specialties. They must function as both the "internist" and the "surgeon" for women with reproductive disorders. In addition, scientific developments and technical inventions are permitting treatment of many conditions medically, avoiding procedures, including traditional surgery altogether.

The transition of gynecological surgical practice from laparotomy, to largely hysteroscopic and laparoscopically directed procedures, has been both dramatic and uneven. Complicating this transition, specialty training programs are inconsistent. Furthermore, the development of laparoscopic technique has eroded training in vaginal surgery, the original minimally invasive technique, and hysterectomy in particular [2]. While these advances contribute to an overall reduction in the number of gynecologic surgical procedures per population, the complexity of the surgical procedures performed is increasing [3]. Indeed, there is already evidence that complication rates associated with hysterectomy are on the rise [4, 5].

Duration of specialty training is another approach that could result in surgeons who are better prepared to provide the spectrum of minimally invasive approaches. Although training programs in the USA are only 4 years long, those in other developed countries are frequently 5–7 years in duration, or, in some, even based on competency, with no established program duration. The addition of sub specialization to the "core" residency training programs in obstetrics and gynecology clearly prolongs the duration of training. It has been suggested that a solution would be the separation of obstetrics and gynecology, a process that to an extent is already occurring [6].

Reproductive surgery requires very special skills, beyond that of the typical minimally invasive gynecologic surgeon, where reproductive surgeons encounter many unique cases. Most often, the surgery is not intended to remove a reproductive organ but instead to remove the pathology while trying to maintain optimal reproductive function. Often, this can be handled with a minimally invasive approach; however, there are times when this must be handled via a traditional laparotomy. Thus, the approach to surgery is often not as critical as ensuring an optimal outcome for reproductive health. The content of the book *Reproductive Surgery* would certainly support this.

The Book

The book, with its 24 interesting richly illustrated chapters, has a national and international authorship, each recognized in their own fields of expertise.

Chapter 1. Double Uterus with Obstructed Hemi Vagina and Ipsilateral Renal Anomaly (OHVIRA)

This first chapter commences with an interesting embryologic anomaly – a uterine didelphis, an oblique or transverse septum causing an obstructed semi vagina, and an ipsilateral renal anomaly (OHVIRA). The chapter covers the vaginal and abdominal surgical approaches.

Chapter 2: Surgical Techniques for Vaginal Agenesis With and Without a Functioning Uterus

Mullerian anomalies: The chapter commences with embryology and classification. Treatment of vaginal agenesis, with or without a functional uterus, is discussed extensively following evaluation and diagnosis. In addition, non-surgical and various surgical approaches and alternative options have been discussed in great detail.

Chapter 3. Overcoming the Challenging Cervix

A patent cervical canal is essential for normal physiologic function and for reproductive procedures that require access to the uterus. The chapter reviews the various anomalies, several benign and malignant pathologies that create cervical stenosis, and covers the management options.

Chapter 4. Septate Uterus: Diagnosis and Management

A well-illustrated chapter that describes the developmental formation of uterine septums and their classification. It reviews the available methods and techniques for their correction.

Chapter 5. Intrauterine Adhesions

This chapter reviews the etiology, clinical presentation, classification, and the diagnosis of uterine adhesions. Surgical considerations are discussed along with post-operative management and outcomes.

Chapter 6. Intraoperative Management of FIGO Type 2 Fibroids

This chapter provides a classification of fibroids, and discusses their effects on fertility and preoperative considerations starting with imaging and including the use of GnRH and Misoprostol. It explains the hysteroscopic surgical approach in detail and discusses post-operative complications.

Chapter 7. Proximal Tubal Obstruction

Addresses the pathophysiology of cornual tubal occlusion and the necessary measures to achieve a diagnosis. Describes the surgical techniques including microsurgical tubal anastomosis to achieve the best outcome for the patient.

Chapter 8. Diagnosis and Surgical Management of Adenomyosis

This well-illustrated chapter reviews the array of fertility-sparing surgical management options for diffuse adenomyosis and localized adenomyoma and explores the impact on future fertility.

Chapter 9. Hydrosalpinges: Repair or Excise

This chapter discusses hydrosalpinges: their etiology, diagnostic techniques, and the place of salpingostomy for fertility. It also reviews the impact of hydrosalpinx on IVF and the various treatment options.

Chapter 10. Cesarean Scar Defects

In 2018, 31.9% of all deliveries in the USA were cesarean deliveries. As the absolute number of cesarean deliveries increases, the sequelae of cesarean delivery are also expected to increase. Cesarean scar defects are increasingly recognized as the cause of various symptoms including irregular vaginal bleeding, dysmenorrhea, and infertility.

Chapter 11. Fertility Enhancing Ovarian Cystectomy

This chapter describes effectively and in minute detail the evaluation of ovarian cysts and the surgical approach and technique of the benign cysts. The text also includes several colored illustrations of the procedures.

Chapter 12. Ovarian Transposition

This chapter commences with the radiation effects, indications, and preoperative considerations. Reviews a detailed surgical technique, which is followed by ovarian function and pregnancy outcomes after transposition.

Chapter 13. Imaging Modalities to Pre-operatively Detect Fibroid Location

This well-illustrated chapter reviews the imaging modalities that may be used to accurately assess fibroid number, size, position, and site prior to surgery. While pelvic ultrasound may be sufficient in simple, uncomplicated cases, pelvic MRI is the problem-solving tool in complex cases.

Chapter 14. Image-Based Surgery: Treating Fibroids You Can't See

Improvements in imaging technologies supplement surgical techniques in enhancing surgical outcomes. Laparoscopic ultrasound has provided a unique opportunity to find and remove intramural fibroids that would have either been missed or forced the surgeon to commit to an open approach. The use of fluorescent dye creates improved contrast between normal and abnormal tissue and opens a whole new arena for tagged particles that can attach to distinct pathologies of interest to help in its removal. As MRI technology continues to evolve, opportunities for creating 3D models for pre-operative surgical practice and improved pre-operative guidance will continue to prepare the surgeon in providing an individualized approach to their patient.

Chapter 15. Cervical Fibroids

While less common (approximately 5% occurring in the cervix), cervical fibroids present additional challenges due to their proximity to the bladder, ureters, rectum, and the major vascular supply for the uterus. Evidence supporting the use of various surgical techniques to address cervical fibroids is limited, likely due to their relative infrequency compared to fibroids arising from the uterine corpus. This chapter reviews the available literature and discusses some of the various pre-, intra-, and postoperative considerations involved in the management of these challenging lesions. Following a review of the literature, the text discusses the available surgical techniques and approaches including robotic.

Chapter 16. Adeno-myomectomy by the Triple-Flap Method

This is an excellent chapter by Professor Osada that demonstrates his recognized technique of triple flap adeno-myomectomy with clear illustrations. The author presents results and discusses the surgery to pregnancy intervals.

Chapter 17. Uterine Transposition

Uterine transposition is an experimental evolving technique to preserve fertility in young women with pelvic malignancies that require radiation. The goal is to keep the uterus and adnexa outside of the radiotherapy field, with the view to preserve their function. The text includes indications and contraindications and the detailed surgical techniques supported with multiple illustrations of both the initial and second repositioning surgery.

Chapter 18. Recognition and Management of Iatrogenic Injury to the Genitourinary System

This chapter reviews iatrogenic injury to genitourinary system starting with the bladder. The diagnosis and treatment are discussed and demonstrated in great detail with appropriate illustrations.

Chapter 19. Retroperitoneal Dissection

This obviously requires knowledge of anatomy, expertise, and meticulous microsurgical technique. The ability to go peritoneal and dissect the structures within the retroperitoneum is an essential skill for the gynecologic surgeon. This is an important chapter, and it explains this procedure very well with proper illustrations.

Chapter 20. Deep Infiltrating Endometriosis: Diagnosis and Fertility-Sparing Management in the ART Patient

In this chapter, the characteristics and diagnosis of deep infiltrating endometriosis (DIE) and its implications on fertility outcomes are discussed. DIE can be assessed clinically and via imaging (ultrasound, MRI), although definitive diagnosis is via surgical evaluation and pathology. DIE can cause debilitating pelvic pain as well as other symptoms (i.e., urinary, gastrointestinal) that correlate to the location of lesions. Although DIE has not conclusively been shown to cause infertility, it is believed to affect fertility outcomes. Surgical management and excision of lesions has been shown to improve both spontaneous pregnancy rates and success rates of assisted reproductive technologies (ART). Fertility-sparing surgical approaches for management of DIE based on anatomical locations are discussed, including rectovaginal, gastrointestinal tract, genitourinary, and diaphragm. Advanced operative techniques reviewed in this section include shaving, discoid resection, and segmental resection.

The book ends with four interesting chapters.

Chapter 21. Crisis Management in the Office Setting

Crises management will always have importance in both office and operating room settings for the reproductive surgeon. This is an interesting chapter that includes case reports discussed extensively, including their prevention. It offers strategies to optimize patient safety.

Chapter 22. Risk Mitigation Strategies for Physicians

This is an extensive chapter the commences with historical origins of medical malpractice, reviews legal elements related to medical malpractice. It discusses the current litigation landscape (particularly obstetrics and gynecology), explores the driving forces behind litigation, and covers strategies for mitigating legal risk and preserving wellness in the event a lawsuit is filed.

Chapter 23. Complications of Oocyte Retrieval

The chapter commences with a brief history of oocyte retrieval techniques. It then reviews complications starting from bleeding, urinary tract injuries, infections, and pain and anesthesia complications. It presents statistics and suggests what to do to minimize complications in each group.

Chapter 24. Reproductive Surgery in Austere Settings

Multiple elements that feed into optimal healthcare are usually lacking in resource-limited settings. This often results into lack of health services to poor populations. Minimally invasive reproductive surgery is such an example in African countries.

I commend the editors and authors for the comprehensive and detailed writings to these unique clinical scenarios that the reproductive surgeon may encounter. I would argue, as this book suggests, that reproductive surgery is not a dying art in the era of assisted reproduction but rather a needed skill to augment outcomes for all infertile couples.

Professor Emeritus, Former Head Victor Gomel
Department of Obstetrics and Gynecology
University of British Columbia
Vancouver, BC, Canada

References

1. Gomel V. Introduction; reconstructive and reproductive surgery in gynecology. 2nd ed. CRC Press Taylor and Francis; 2019.
2. Barnhart KT, Nakajima ST, Puscheck E, Price TM, Baker VL, Segars J. Practice patterns, satisfaction, and demographics of reproductive endocrinologists: results of the 2014 Society for Reproductive Endocrinology and Infertility Workforce Survey. Fertil Steril. 2016;105(5):1281–6. Munro M, Gomel V. Reconstructive and reproductive surgery in gynecology. 2nd ed. CRC Press Taylor and Francis; 2019.
3. Rayburn WF, Tracy EE. Changes in the practice of obstetrics and gynecology. Obstet Gynecol Surv. 2016;71(1):43–50. Fingar KR, Stocks C, Weiss AJ, Steiner CA. Most frequent operating room procedures performed in U.S. hospitals, 2003–2012: statistical brief #186. Healthcare cost and utilization project (HCUP) statistical briefs. Rockville; 2006.
4. Hilton P, Cromwell DA. The risk of vesicovaginal and urethrovaginal fistula after hysterectomy performed in the English National Health Service--a retrospective cohort study examining patterns of care between 2000 and 2008. BJOG. 2012;119(12):1447–54.
5. Kiran A, Hilton P, Cromwell DA. The risk of ureteric injury associated with hysterectomy: a 10-year retrospective cohort study. BJOG. 2016;123(7):1184–91.
6. Munro M, Gomel V. Reconstructive and reproductive surgery in gynecology. 2nd ed. CRC Press Taylor and Francis; 2019.

Contents

Contributors

Shadain Akhavan, MD EVMS Jones Institute for Reproductive Medicine, Norfolk, VA, USA

Bala Bhagavath, MD Department of OBGYN, University of Wisconsin-Madison, Madison, WI, USA

Rachel Booth, DO Wright State University Boonshoft School of Medicine, Dayton, OH, USA

Pietro Bortoletto, MD, MSc The Ronald O. Perelman and Claudia Cohen Center for Reproductive Medicine, Weill Cornell Medical Center, New York, NY, USA

Audrey O. Chang, MD Department of Obstetrics and Gynecology, Division of Reproductive Endocrinology and Infertility, University of North Carolina Hospitals, Chapel Hill, NC, USA

Mindy S. Christianson, MD, MBA Department of Gynecology and Obstetrics, Johns Hopkins University School of Medicine, Baltimore, MD, USA

Kathryn Coyne, MD, MS University Hospitals Fertility Center, Beachwood, OH, USA

Rony T. Elias, MD The Ronald O. Perelman and Claudia Cohen Center for Reproductive Medicine, Weill Cornell Medical Center, New York, NY, USA

Erin Fee, DO Department of Obstetrics & Gynecology, Division of Pediatric Adolescent Gynecology, Tufts Medical Center & Tufts Children's Hospital, Boston, MA, USA

Joseph Findley, MD Division of Reproductive Endocrinology and Infertility, University Hospitals Cleveland Medical Center, Cleveland, OH, USA

Victoria W. Fitz, MD Division of Reproductive Endocrinology and Infertility, Massachusetts General Fertility Center, Boston, MA, USA

Rebecca Flyckt, MD University Hospitals Fertility Center, Beachwood, OH, USA

Jeffrey M. Goldberg, MD The Cleveland Clinic, Women's Health Institute, Cleveland, OH, USA

Linnea R. Goodman, MD Department of Obstetrics and Gynecology, Division of Reproductive Endocrinology and Infertility, University of North Carolina Hospitals, Chapel Hill, NC, USA

Megan Gornet, MD Department of Gynecology and Obstetrics, Johns Hopkins University School of Medicine, Baltimore, MD, USA

Maria Alejandra Hincapie, MD Nezhat Medical Center, Atlanta Center for Minimally Invasive Surgery and Reproductive Medicine, Atlanta, GA, USA

Leigh A. Humphries, MD Department of Obstetrics and Gynecology, University of Pennsylvania, Philadelphia, PA, USA

Hospital of the University of Pennsylvania, Philadelphia, PA, USA

Nezhat Medical Center, Atlanta Center for Minimally Invasive Surgery and Reproductive Medicine, Atlanta, GA, USA

Christine Hur, MD The Cleveland Clinic, Women's Health Institute, Cleveland, OH, USA

Kathleen Hwang, MD Department of Urology, University of Pittsburgh School of Medicine, Pittsburgh, PA, USA

Victoria S. Jiang Department of Obstetrics and Gynecology, Division of Reproductive Endocrinology and Infertility, Massachusetts General Hospital, Harvard Medical School, Boston, MA, USA

Zaraq Khan, MBBS, MCR, FACOG Division Chair, Reproductive Endocrinology & Infertility, Consultant, Division of Minimally Invasive Gynecologic Surgery, Mayo Clinic, Rochester, MN, USA

Anne E. Kim, MD Department of Obstetrics and Gynecology, University of Pennsylvania, Philadelphia, PA, USA

Mario M. Leitao Jr, MD Department of Surgery, Memorial Sloan-Kettering Cancer Center, New York, NY, USA

Jerry A. Lindheim, JD Lindheim Law, Cherry Hill, NJ, USA

Steven R. Lindheim, MD, MMM Wright State University Boonshoft School of Medicine, Dayton, OH, USA

Center for Reproductive Medicine, Ren Ji Hospital, School of Medicine, Shanghai Jiao Tong University, Shanghai, People's Republic of China

Xiaohong Liu, MD EVMS Jones Institute for Reproductive Medicine, Norfolk, VA, USA

Natalia C. Llarena, MD The Cleveland Clinic, Women's Health Institute, Cleveland, OH, USA

Jody Lyneé Madeira, JD Locks Law Firm, Bloomington, IN, USA

Indiana University Maurer School of Law, Bloomington, IN, USA

David Miller, MD Department of Urology, University of Pittsburgh School of Medicine, Pittsburgh, PA, USA

Alfred Murage, MD, FRCOG Harley Street Fertility Centre, Nairobi, Kenya

Susan Nasab, MD Department of Gynecology and Obstetrics, Johns Hopkins University School of Medicine, Baltimore, MD, USA

Ceana H. Nezhat, MD Nezhat Medical Center, Atlanta Center for Minimally Invasive Surgery and Reproductive Medicine, Atlanta, GA, USA

Joseph Njagi, MD, MMed Department of Obstetrics and Gynecology, PCEA Tumutumu Hospital, Nyeri, Kenya

Timona Obura, MD, MMed Department of Obstetrics and Gynecology, Aga Khan University Hospital, Nairobi, Kenya

Hisao Osada, MD, PhD Natural ART Clinic Nihonbashi, Chuo-ku, Tokyo, Japan

Johannes Ott, MD University of Vienna, Vienna, Austria

J. Preston Parry, MD, MPH Parryscope and Positive Steps Fertility, Madison, MS, USA

Nigel Pereira, MD The Ronald O. Perelman and Claudia Cohen Center for Reproductive Medicine, Weill Cornell Medical College, New York, NY, USA

John C. Petrozza, MD Department of Obstetrics and Gynecology, Division of Reproductive Endocrinology and Infertility, Massachusetts General Hospital, Harvard Medical School, Boston, MA, USA

Samantha M. Pfeifer The Ronald O. Perelman and Claudia Cohen Center for Reproductive Medicine, Weill Cornell Medical Center, New York, NY, USA

Callum Potts, MBBS Division of Reproductive Endocrinology and Infertility, University of Vermont Medical Center, Burlington, VT, USA

Jenna M. Rehmer, MD The Cleveland Clinic, Women's Health Institute, Cleveland, OH, USA

Reitan Ribeiro, MD Department of Surgical Oncology, Erasto Gaertner Hospital, Curitiba, PR, Brazil

Carey Camille Roberts, MD Weill Cornell Medicine, Department of Anesthesiology, New York, NY, USA

Robert A. Roman, MD Medical College of Georgia at Augusta University, Section of Reproductive Endocrinology, Infertility, and Genetics, Augusta, GA, USA

Phillip A. Romanski The Ronald O. Perelman and Claudia Cohen Center for Reproductive Medicine, Weill Cornell Medical Center, New York, NY, USA

Salomeh Salari, MD, MS University Hospitals Fertility Center, Beachwood, OH, USA

Divya K. Shah, MD, MME Division of Reproductive Endocrinology, Department of Obstetrics and Gynecology, University of Pennsylvania, Philadelphia, PA, USA

Laurel Stadtmauer, MD, PhD EVMS Jones Institute for Reproductive Medicine, Norfolk, VA, USA

Matthew K. Wagar, MD Department of OBGYN, University of Wisconsin-Madison, Madison, WI, USA

Thomas Winter, MD TCW, Abdominal Imaging Division, Department of Radiology and Imaging Science, University of Utah Health Sciences, Salt Lake City, UT, USA

Andrea Zuckerman, MD Department of Obstetrics & Gynecology, Division of Pediatric Adolescent Gynecology, Tufts Medical Center & Tufts Children's Hospital, Boston, MA, USA

Double Uterus with Obstructed Hemivagina and Ipsilateral Renal Anomaly (OHVIRA)

Phillip A. Romanski, Pietro Bortoletto, and Samantha M. Pfeifer

Introduction

Double uterus with obstructed hemivagina and ipsilateral renal anomaly, better known as OHVIRA, is a unique Müllerian anomaly in that it involves a constellation of anatomic abnormalities and therefore meets criteria to be considered a syndrome. This syndrome is also known as Herlyn-Werner-Wunderlich syndrome, named after those who were some of the first to describe the associated findings, though the name OHVIRA syndrome has become the more commonly used terminology today [1, 2]. This syndrome is classically characterized by a triad of a uterus didelphys, an oblique or transverse vaginal septum causing an obstructed hemivagina, and renal agenesis ipsilateral to the obstructed hemivagina, though variations do occur (Fig. 1.1).

Development

Central to successful management of OHVIRA syndrome is an understanding of the embryologic origins of urogenital organs. Up until the 5th week of embryonic life, the genital system remains largely undifferentiated with bipotential

P. A. Romanski (✉) · P. Bortoletto · S. M. Pfeifer
The Ronald O. Perelman and Claudia Cohen Center for Reproductive Medicine, Weill Cornell Medical Center, New York, NY, USA
e-mail: Par9114@med.cornell.edu

gonads before mesonephric and paramesonephric ducts develop.

The mesonephric duct first arises from mesodermal tissue and elongates to form the epididymis, vas deferens, and seminal vesicles in males. In females, the mesonephric duct will regress but not before it outpouches to form a diverticulum that will mature into a ureteric bud that migrates cephalad & induces metanephric tissue to form the metanephros (i.e., kidneys). By the 7th week of development, in the absence of anti-Müllerian hormone and SRY genes being expressed, paramesonephric ducts will originate lateral to the upper poles of mesonephros and descend caudally into the pelvis crossing anteriorly to the mesonephric ducts to form the uterus. The paramesonephric ducts undergo fusion at the midline and resorption of the median septum to form a uterine cavity as well as cervix, upper third of the vagina and proximal fallopian tubes.

Classically, the upper third of the vagina is thought to arise from paramesonephric tissue with the lower two-thirds originating from the urogenital sinus. However, OHVIRA syndrome challenges this assumption. In 1992, Spanish gynecologist Paul Acién postulated that the upper vagina is derived from the mesonephric ducts with paramesonephric tissue contributing to the vaginal epithelium [3]. As a result, when the mesonephric duct develops abnormally it causes a lateralization of the ipsilateral Müllerian duct away from the urogenital sinus,

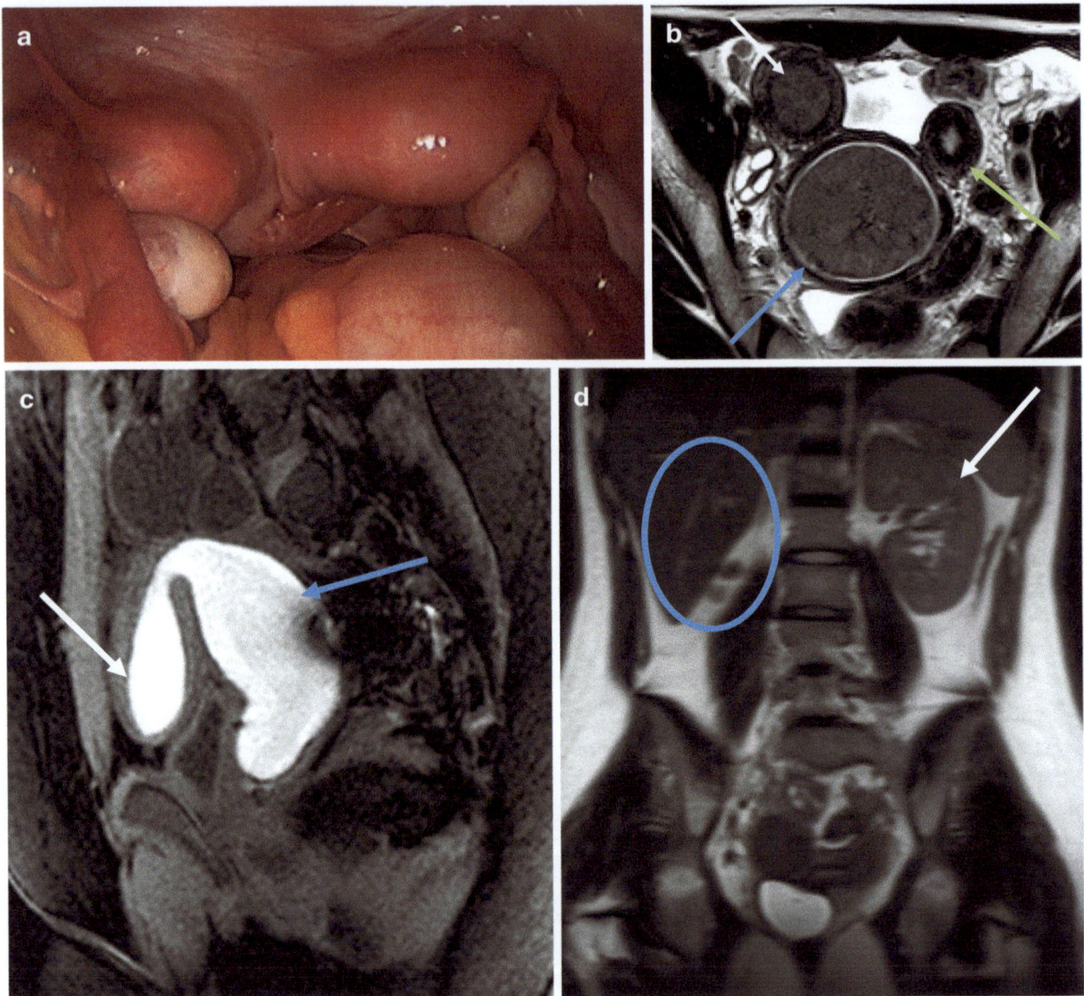

Fig. 1.1 Classic OHVIRA triad of findings. (**a**) Laparoscopic view of a didelphic uterus (**b**) Axial MRI image of obstructed hemivagina with hematocolpos (blue arrow) and a didelphic uterus. The obstructed right hemiuterus can be seen with hematometra (white arrow) as well as the patent left hemiuterus with a normal appear-ing endometrial cavity (green arrow) (**c**) Sagittal MRI image of an obstructed right hemivagina with hematocolpos (blue arrow) and hematometra (white arrow) (**d**) Coronal abdominal MRI image of a patient with OHVIRA demonstrating right renal agenesis (blue circle) and left kidney in typical location (white arrow)

causing the formation of a blind pouch that develops into the obstructed hemivagina. The distal portion of the vagina is unaffected as it arises from the urogenital sinus. Furthermore, given the influence of the mesonephros, which is under developmental control from the meso-nephric duct, on development and fusion of the paramesonephric tissue this hypothesis may fur-ther explain the concurrent uterine didelphys seen in OHVIRA syndrome [4].

Classification

OHVIRA is most classically defined by a uterus didelphys, an oblique vaginal septum causing an obstructed hemivagina, and an ipsilateral renal anomaly. Müllerian anomalies are classified by the American Society of Reproductive Medicine primarily based on the uterine malformation involved. Because cases of OHVIRA classically contain a didelphic uterus, this syndrome has often been considered to be a subcategory of the uterus didelphys [5]. However, many variations of the uterine malformation, point of obstruction, and type of renal anomaly have been reported and it is not uncommon for a patient to present with a variation on the classical syndrome [6, 7].

One series of 87 patients reported that about one in four patients with OHVIRA will present with a non-classic variant [7]. Some uterine variations that may occur are depicted in Fig. 1.2 and include a bicornuate bicollis uterus or a complete septate uterus with duplicated cervix and an oblique obstructing vaginal septum and ipsilateral renal anomaly [7]. Another described presentation includes a didelphic uterus with unilateral cervical atresia as the cause of the obstruction. The most common renal anomaly to occur with OHVIRA is ipsilateral renal agenesis, however other reported ipsilateral renal anomalies to occur include duplicated ureter, renal dysplasia, polycystic kidney, or even the absence of any renal anomaly [6]. Given the many variations that can occur with each component of this syndrome, the definition of OHVIRA syndrome frequently varies in the literature. It is important to recognize that all of these unilateral anomalies represent a continuum that frequently involves ipsilateral renal anomalies. Therefore, while the term OHVIRA is used in this chapter and throughout the literature as a general term to describe this syndrome, individual cases should be described by the type of uterine anomaly and level of obstruction, as is demonstrated in Fig. 1.2, and should also include a description of the renal anomaly when present. For example, if instead of a didelphic uterus there is a complete septate uterus with an obstructed hemivagina and ipsilateral renal agenesis, the anomaly should be described as a complete septate uterus with an obstructed hemivagina and ipsilateral renal agenesis rather than the less specific term OHVIRA (Fig. 1.2b). Note that if the obstruction is due to cervical atresia instead of an obstructed hemivagina, the anomaly should be described by the type of uterine anomaly with cervical atresia such as a didelphic uterus with unilateral cervical atresia (Fig. 1.2d), rather than using the less specific and in this case incorrect term OHVIRA.

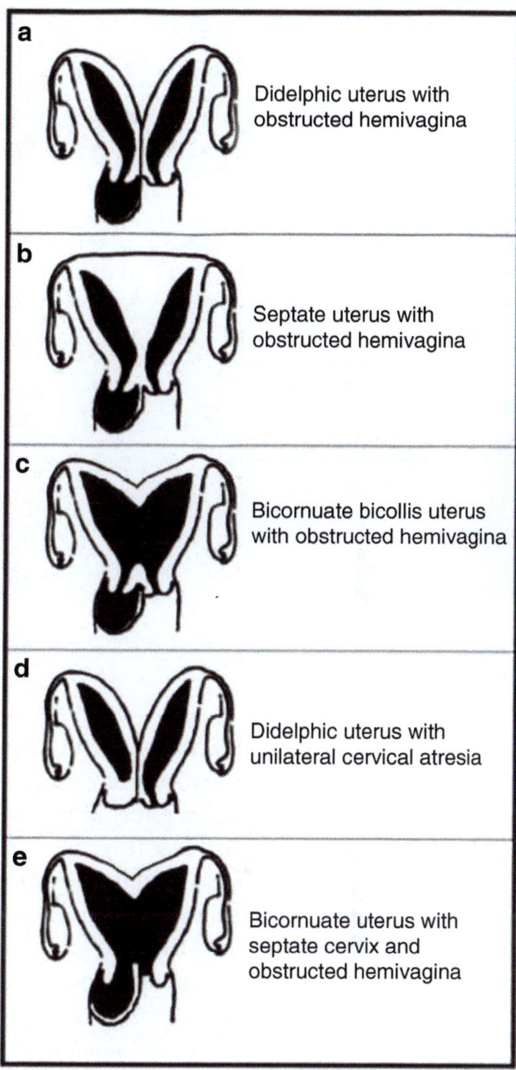

Fig. 1.2 (**a**) Didelphic uterus with obstructed hemivagina. (**b**) Septate uterus with obstructed hemivagina. (**c**) Bicornuate bicollis uterus with obstructed hemivagina. (**d**) Didelphic uterus with unilateral cervical atresia. (**e**) Bicornuate uterus with septate cervix and obstructed hemivagina. (Figure from Fedele et al. [7]. Permission to use this figure was granted by Oxford University Press)

Presentation

As with many Müllerian anomalies, the time from onset of symptoms to diagnosis is fraught with delays and challenges. Typically, patients with OHVIRA present with worsening dysmenorrhea around the time of the onset of menses [8].

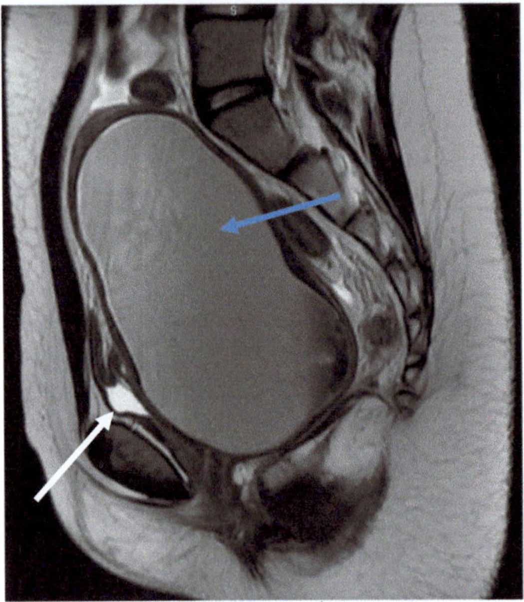

Fig. 1.3 Large volume hematocolpos (blue arrow) with bladder compression (white arrow)

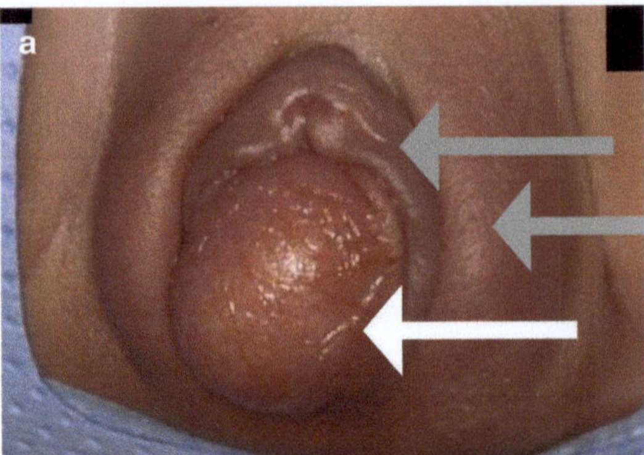

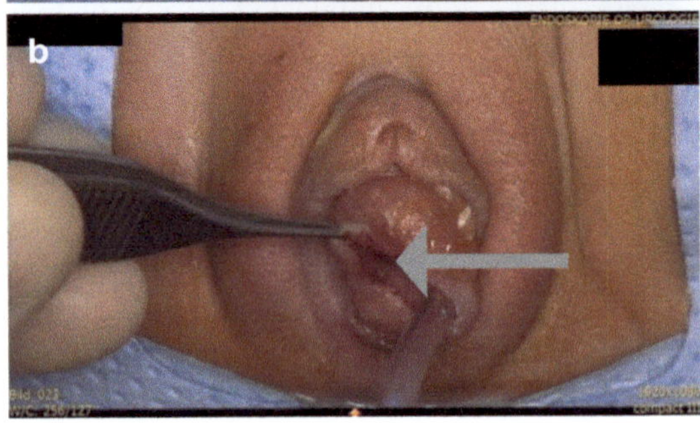

Fig. 1.4 Left obstructed hemivagina in a newborn presenting as a vaginal mass. (Figure from Kueppers et al. [10]. Permission to use this figure was granted by Elsevier). (**a**) Left oblique vaginal septum in a newborn causing mucocolpos and a protruding vaginal mass (white arrow). Gray arrows point to normal appearing labia. (**b**) Incision through the oblique vaginal septum reveals the opening to the left hemivagina (gray arrow)

Patients may also present with bulk symptoms such as urinary frequency and urgency or even urinary retention from the mass effect of the distended hemivagina on the bladder (Fig. 1.3) [9]. Less commonly, a pelvic mass may be identified in newborns antenatally via ultrasonography or in the neonatal period (Fig. 1.4) [10].

In adolescents, initial presentation can sometimes be complicated by a super-infection of the hematocolpos which requires urgent antibiotic treatment and drainage [6, 11]. The infection may be preceded by an inciting event and this risk may be increased in patients that are sexually active or have a microperforation of the vaginal septum (Fig. 1.5) or cervix by increasing the risk of ascending bacteria. Patients with a microperforation may present with persistent intermenstrual spotting and/or malodorous vaginal discharge from pyocolpos.

Unfortunately, the length of time from symptom onset to diagnosis is on average 37.8 weeks with the vast majority of patients being misdiagnosed initially [12]. During this period, obstruction of menstrual bleeding outflow can result in hematometra and retrograde menstruation – both of which contribute to cyclic pain, adhesions, and even infertility. Efficient and accurate

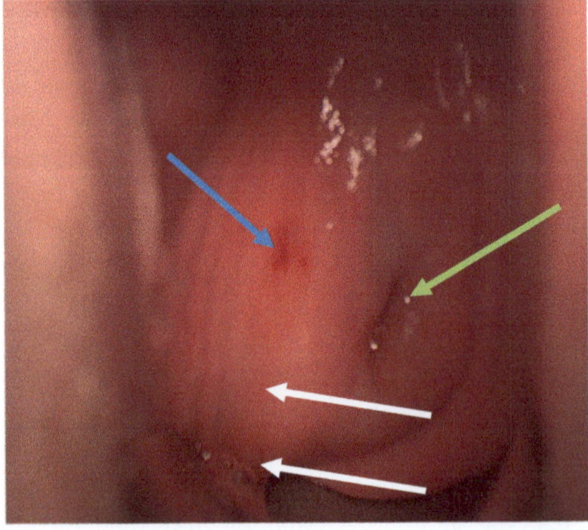

Fig. 1.5 Microperforation of a right oblique vaginal septum (blue arrow) in a patient that presented with pyocolpos and was found to have OHVIRA syndrome. Drainage of the pyocolpos from the microperforation can be seen (white arrows). The left cervix can also be seen adjacent to the oblique vaginal septum (gray arrow)

diagnostic work-up is essential as it may allow for symptom relief as well as prevention of long-term sequelae.

Diagnosis

Magnetic resonance imaging (MRI) is considered the gold-standard assessment in patients with suspected Müllerian anomalies with accuracy approaching 100% in some studies [13]. MRI not only provides excellent characterization of the external uterine contour but also the uterine zonal anatomy, allowing for differentiation between a hypoplastic, nonfunctional hemiuterus and a non-communicating hemiuterus with functional endometrium, information which may be beneficial for surgical planning and counseling. Additionally, MRI allows for image capture outside of the pelvis which will identify renal anomalies as well as lower urinary tract pathology.

MRI for the purpose of diagnosis should be performed when the patient is menstruating as this allows for distention of uterine cavity as well as the proximal upper vagina maximizing potential for careful delineation of the anatomy in what are otherwise collapsed tissues (Fig. 1.6). This step often requires discontinuation of oral contraceptives which are commonly prescribed to manage dysmenorrhea and abnormal uterine bleeding. It is important to counsel patients that discontinuation may potentiate acute exacerbation of pelvic pain and make plans for alternative pain management during this window. In some patients, depending on their age and pain tolerance, sedation may be recommended to facilitate the diagnostic study.

Pre-study planning with a radiologist who is experienced in pelvic imaging may be particularly beneficial in the evaluation of suspected OHVIRA as specific imaging sequences may further help delineate these anomalies. For example, T2-weighted sequences obtained without fat suppression provide soft-tissue contrast that is useful in evaluating uterine zonal anatomy, identifying rudimentary uteri, as well as for assessment of the vaginal canal. When hematometra is sus-

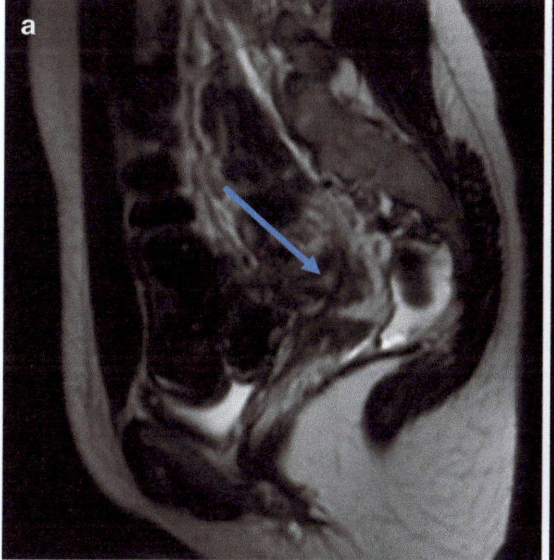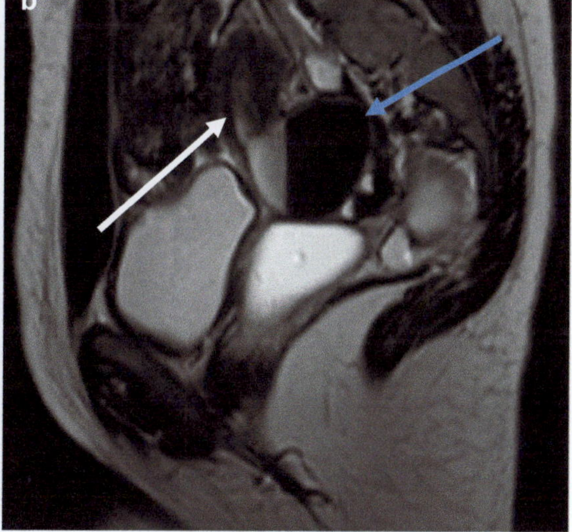

Fig. 1.6 Sagittal pelvic MRI image from a patient with OHVIRA before and after cessation of hormonal suppression to allow for the development of hematocolpos. (**a**) Obstructed right hemivagina (blue arrow) in a patient with OHVIRA syndrome on hormonal suppression resulting in no hematocolpos. Note the difficulty in discerning the vaginal anatomy and the relationship to adjacent pelvic organs (**b**) Obstructed right hemivagina (blue arrow) in the same patient with OHVIRA syndrome after 1 month off hormonal suppression. Note the presence of hematocolpos and clear anatomical borders of the hemivagina and right uterus (white arrow)

pected, T1-weighted images with and without fat suppression are essential as they allow for differentiation between fat and blood products [13].

When delineation of the vaginal anomaly is inadequate, contrast dye or ultrasound gel may be instilled into the vagina to improve visualization (Fig. 1.7) [14, 15]. This is typically done using IV tubing or a small Foley catheter placed at the introitus immediately before the MRI images are collected. Contrast gel may be superior to contrast dye given its viscosity and likelihood of remaining within the vaginal canal.

Even though MRI remains the preferred imaging modality to confirm the diagnosis of OHVIRA, most patients that present with pelvic pain will first receive a pelvic ultrasound because it is quicker and more affordable compared to MRI. For patients with OHVIRA, two-

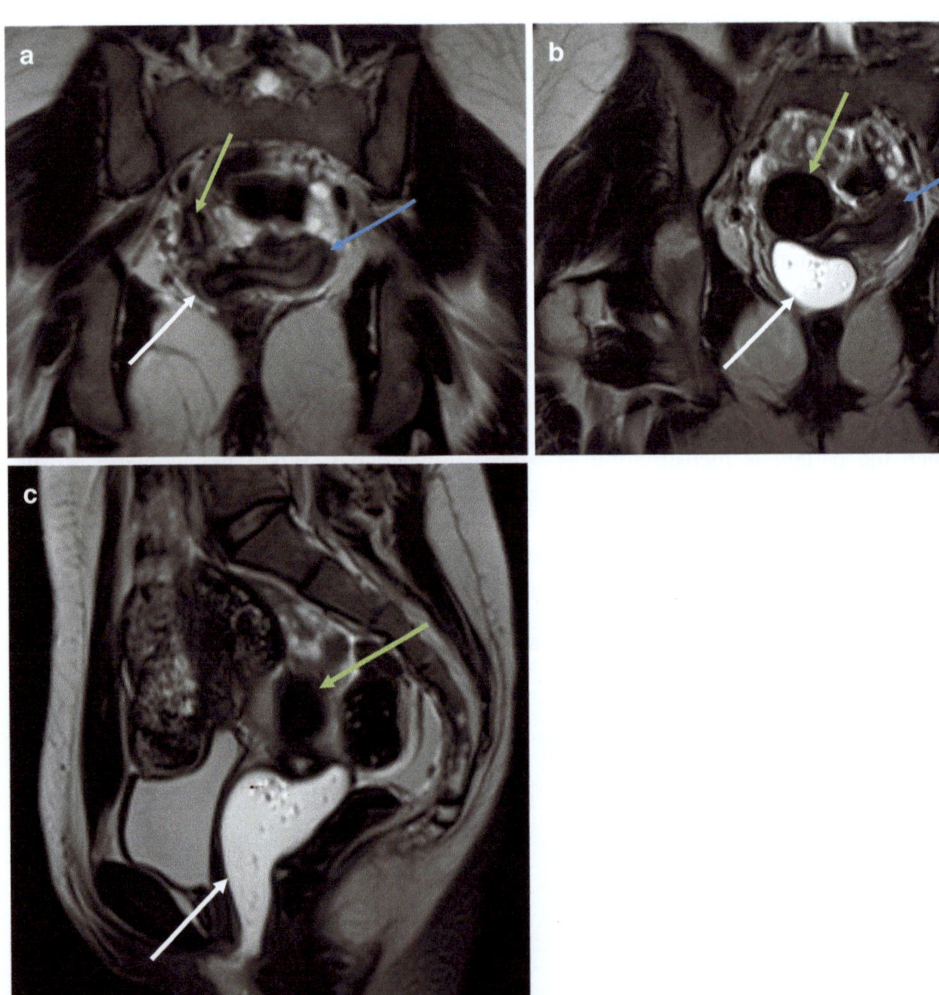

Fig. 1.7 Pelvic MRI images from a patient with OHVIRA with an obstructed right hemivagina before and after the addition of aqueous vaginal contrast gel. (**a**) Prior to the addition of aqueous vaginal contrast gel, the left uterus (blue arrow) can be seen adjacent to a patent compressed left hemivagina (white arrow). The cervix of the obstructed right uterus can also be seen in this image (green arrow). (**b**) After the addition of aqueous vaginal contrast gel, the left uterus (blue arrow) and patent left hemivagina (white arrow) are clearly seen in relationship to the hematocolpos of the obstructed right hemivagina (green arrow). (**c**) A sagittal pelvic MRI image from the same patient with the patent left hemivagina (white arrow) filled with aqueous vaginal contrast gel. The hematocolpos of the obstructed right hemivagina (green arrow) can also be seen in this image

dimensional ultrasound can identify the uterine malformation, hematocolpos or hematometra, and a renal anomaly if it is present [16]. Three-dimensional ultrasound can help to improve the diagnostic accuracy by depicting both the endometrial cavity and the serosal surface of the uterus so that the uterine shape and malformation can be accurately described [17]. When performed by an experienced radiologist, three-dimensional ultrasound has even been shown to have a sensitivity and specificity comparable to MRI for the diagnosis of Müllerian anomalies [17]. It is important to recognize that the accuracy of ultrasound is highly operator dependent and the reported sensitivity and specificity in most studies comes from highly experienced centers and is likely lower when performed by less experienced radiologists. In addition, MRI allows for a more thorough evaluation of the urinary tract and vaginal canal compared to ultrasound which is an important part of the evaluation in patients with suspected OHVIRA syndrome. Therefore, when OHVIRA syndrome is suspected based on ultrasound imaging, an MRI of the abdomen and pelvis should be performed to confirm the diagnosis and help with surgical planning.

Management Objectives

Management of OHVIRA can be divided into the acute and definitive phases. The presenting symptom for most cases of OHVIRA is dysmenorrhea secondary to the obstructed hemivagina. This pain is often severe and can be debilitating. The acute phase of treatment should focus on pain control and menstrual suppression in order to stabilize the patient until a definitive treatment plan can be made.

First-line pain management should be with acetaminophen and ketorolac or ibuprofen in patients with normal renal function. Intravenous or oral opioids may be additionally needed for episodes of acutely worsening pain. Longer term, pain control can usually be achieved through menstrual suppression with oral contraceptive pills dosed continuously. Oral contraceptive pills should be initiated as soon as possible in order to decrease menstruation and limit the distension of the hematocolpos. In rare cases in which the above regimen is unable to adequately control the dysmenorrhea and there is not an available surgeon to perform definitive surgical management of the obstructed hemivagina, drainage of the hematocolpos can be performed as a temporizing measure either vaginally with an incision through the obstructing septum, laparoscopically with a small uterine incision, or percutaneously by an interventional radiologist.

Importantly, the symptoms and complications that occur with OHVIRA are due to the obstructing oblique vaginal septum, thus definitive management can only be accomplished with removal of the obstruction. An ideal time to perform resection of the vaginal septum in patients with OHVIRA is at the time of initial presentation when the vaginal tissue and septum are expanded by hematocolpos because this improves the identification of the obstruction and helps to delineate septum from normal vaginal tissue. However, there are multiple reasons why surgical management may not be appropriate at the time of initial presentation including uncertainty about the diagnosis, a lack of an available surgeon with expertise in Müllerian anomalies, or a patient that is not yet mentally prepared to undergo a vaginal procedure. In these cases, definitive surgical management should be delayed until a more appropriate time and oral contraceptives should be used in the interim for menstrual suppression to prevent dysmenorrhea. If at any time a superimposed infection of the hematocolpos is suspected, surgical management must be performed urgently in order to evacuate the infection and preserve the gynecologic organs. While uncommon, the development of septic shock has been reported arising from an infection of the pelvic organs and removal of one or both fallopian tubes and possibly the uterus may ultimately be necessary to adequately resolve the infection [18].

Operative Approach

Definitive management of OHVIRA can only be accomplished by the surgical resection of the obstructing vaginal septum with preservation of reproductive function. When the obstructed cervix and vagina are parallel or near-parallel with the patent cervix and vagina, the oblique vaginal septum can most easily be accessed vaginally and in these cases, speculoscopic or vaginoscopic resection of the septum is the preferred approach [19]. In rare cases where the obstructed cervix and vagina are located too far cephalad to safely resect vaginally, or the distended vaginal cavity is extremely small, an alternative surgical approach is a laparoscopic hemihysterectomy with ipsilateral vaginectomy of the obstructed side [14, 20]. Finally, diagnostic laparoscopy should be considered in complex presentations where direct visualization of the abdominal cavity may help to determine the anatomy.

Procedural Steps

Vaginal Approach

Under general anesthesia, a careful pelvic exam should be performed to palpate the location of the obstructed uterus, cervix, and hemivagina and its relationship to the patent uterus and cervix. Careful evaluation of the remainder of the vagina and external genitalia should be performed to determine whether any additional anatomic variations are present. Next, the location of the bladder and the rectum and their proximity to the vaginal septum should be noted and carefully monitored throughout the resection to avoid injury to these structures. If needed at any point during the procedure, a rectal exam or retrograde saline distension of the bladder can be performed to better delineate these structures.

A key step in this procedure is the identification of the oblique vaginal septum and determination of where the incision should be made [21]. If a large bulge is present in the vagina from the hematocolpos, the location of the septum is clear (Fig. 1.8) [22]. If the location of the septum is not

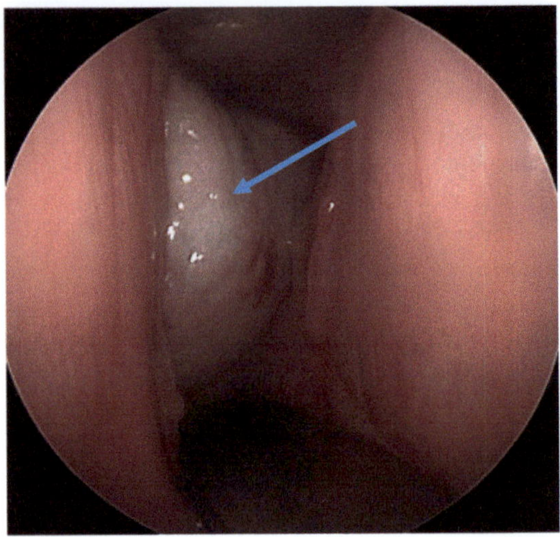

Fig. 1.8 Oblique vaginal septum bulging into patent vagina due to pressure from hematocolpos (blue arrow). (Figure from Cosgrove et al. [22]. Permission to use this figure was granted by Elsevier)

clear on visual inspection, transabdominal or transrectal ultrasound can be used to help identify the correct location of the septum. If the patient has been on menstrual suppression prior to the surgery resulting in minimal or no hematocolpos, the oral contraceptive should be discontinued 1–2 months prior to surgery to allow hematocolpos to develop to help with both the direct visualization and ultrasound-guided visualization of the septum. Once the oblique vaginal septum has been identified, resection can be performed under direct visualization via either speculoscopy or hysteroscopy and simultaneous ultrasound-guidance should be used [23].

Speculoscopy Following speculum placement, the planned site of the incision on the oblique vaginal septum should be injected with a local anesthetic that contains epinephrine in order to minimize blood loss from the incision site to improve visualization throughout the procedure. Next, a cruciate incision should be made at the center of the septum using a long monopolar electrocautery needle. The length of the incision may vary depending on the anatomy and size of the septum; generally, an approximately 3 cm incision is sufficient to adequately drain the

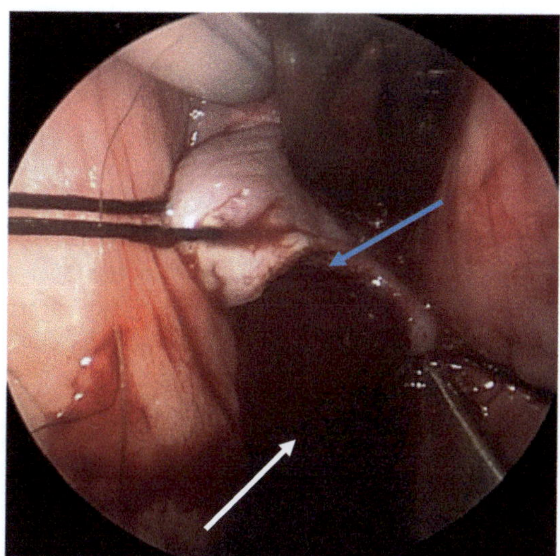

Fig. 1.9 Incised oblique vaginal septum (blue arrow) with draining hematocolpos (white arrow). (Figure from Cosgrove et al. [22]. Permission to use this figure was granted by Elsevier)

hematocolpos and prevent stenosis of the vaginal tissue (Fig. 1.9). Once the hematocolpos has been drained with suction and irrigation, the vaginal septum may be completely resected taking care to avoid injury to adjacent bowel and bladder. The edges may then be marsupialized using interrupted stitches of 2–0 or 3–0 vicryl to create a functional connection and decrease the risk of stenosis at the site of resection. Stenosis at the site of resection occurs in generally <5% of cases. The surgeon should also keep in mind that the opening should ideally be large enough to prevent dyspareunia in the future and so that the cervix can be clearly visualized for cervical cancer screening. The cervix behind the resected septum should then be visualized either directly or with vaginoscopy. Some advocate a diagnostic hysteroscope can then be inserted into both cervices to visually inspect the endometrial cavities and to confirm no other cervical or uterine anomalies are present. However, if the pre-operative imaging is accurate, the added benefit of hysteroscopy is debatable and can potentially increase post-operative infection risk. In OHVIRA cases with a septate uterus, concomitant incision of the uterine septum at the time of the oblique vaginal septum resection is not advised because the uterine

cavity may be distorted from the hematometra. In these cases, if a uterine septum incision is indicated, it is best to perform this as a separate procedure after the oblique vaginal septum resection has healed.

Vaginoscopy The size and location of the oblique vaginal septum can often be in a location that is difficult to easily reach or directly visualize and operative vaginoscopy has been used as an alternative option to resect the vaginal septum [23]. Vaginoscopy can also be used as an approach to help ensure the hymen remains intact throughout the procedure. The same steps that are described above should be followed, except that the septum incision is made vaginoscopically with an electrocautery knife. After suction and irrigation, the cervix behind the incised septum should be visualized and the remaining edges of the septum can be resected with a resectoscope. Video depictions of the vaginoscopic technique have been published by Ludwin et al. [23] and Xu et al. [24].

Abdominal Approach

While a vaginal approach to remove the oblique vaginal septum is the preferred surgical route in most OHVIRA cases, in some cases of OHVIRA the obstructed uterus, cervix, and vagina are located too far cephalad to safely access vaginally. In these cases, resection of the obstructed uterus, cervix, and vagina should be considered as an alternative approach to remove the obstruction while preserving the reproductive potential of the remaining hemiuterus [25].

This surgery can be completed laparoscopically in the majority of cases; however, a laparotomy may be necessary in cases of severe pelvic adhesions due to endometriosis or prior surgery [20]. The obstructed uterus, fallopian tube, and cervix should be dissected from the pelvic sidewall, carefully identifying and sealing all vessels leading to the hemiuterus. Often, a single uterine artery will not be identified as in cases of normal uterine anatomy, but instead an unpredictable dispersion of small arteries and veins. In addition, in cases that involve ipsilateral renal agenesis, there is no concern for ureteral injury during the retroperitoneal dissection. Once the dissection reaches the obstructed vagina, the vaginal wall should be grasped and similarly carefully dissected away from the pelvic sidewall [14]. It is important to ensure that the obstructed vagina is resected in its entirety; glandular secretions from vaginal tissue not completely resected may lead to hydrocolpos and recurrent pain. A video depiction of the steps of a laparoscopic resection of an obstructed uterus, cervix, and vagina in a patient with OHVIRA syndrome has been published by Romanski et al. [14].

Reproductive Outcomes

There is a paucity of literature on reproductive outcomes in patients with OHVIRA syndrome. Of the available literature most report favorable reproductive outcomes, both before and after surgical management of the obstructed hemi-vagina.

Tong et al. reviewed their 15-year experience in caring for women with OHVIRA in mainland China [26]. They reported 52 pregnancies among 28 of the 33 women (pregnancy rate = 84.8%) who were actively trying to conceive. Of these 52 pregnancies there were 20 live births, only 1 of which was delivered preterm. They go on to report that pregnancy occurred in the hemiuterus ipsilateral to the hemivagina in 33% of cases and that 8 women experienced separate pregnancies in each hemiuterus. Importantly, 54% of women with live births conceived prior to surgical treatment for obstructed hemivagina.

In a similar sized case series by Haddad et al., 42 patients with OHVIRA were contacted an average of 6.5 years after their surgical treatment regarding their symptoms and reproductive outcomes [27]. Of the 38 patients who responded to the telephone questionnaire, only 11 of them had attempted to conceive. Among these 11 patients, 2 had been trying to conceive for 12 months or less and the other 9 had conceived a total of 20 pregnancies resulting in 13 live births.

Candiani et al. have also retrospectively assessed reproductive outcomes in 36 women with OHVIRA [8]. Of the 15 women who attempted conception they reported a pregnancy rate of 87% and a live birth rate of 77%. A lower pregnancy rate was seen by Heinonen who reviewed 21 Finish women with OHVIRA and reported that 13 of the 21 were able to conceive (pregnancy rate 61.9%). Similar to Tong et al., 77% conceived in the hemiuterus contralateral to the treated obstructed hemivagina [28]. The median interval between surgical treatment and first pregnancy was approximately 10 years. Of the 22 pregnancies recorded, the preterm birth rate was 36% with a cesarean section rate of 67%.

A larger body of literature is available regarding reproductive outcomes in women with uterine didelphys without hemivagina or renal anomalies. One systematic review of women with congenital uterine anomalies reported non-significant differences in conception rate, miscarriage rate, and second trimester miscarriage rate in some with uterine didelphys compared to women with normal uteri [29]. There was however an increased risk of preterm labor (RR: 3.58, 95% CI: 2.00–6.40) and malpresentation (RR: 3.7, 95% CI: 2.04–6.70), which was comparable to those seen in other unification defects such as bicornuate uterus and unicornuate uterus.

Conclusion

OHVIRA syndrome, despite its classic presentation and triad of findings, is a frequently misdiagnosed syndrome due to its rarity in the general population. Understanding that the anomalies that occur as part of this syndrome can present with many slight variations is central in making the correct diagnosis and developing a treatment plan. Acute treatment should focus on pain management and menstrual suppression, but definitive treatment requires removal of the obstructing tissue. The preferred surgical treatment is a vaginal resection of the oblique septum, however in some cases an abdominal approach to remove the entirety of the obstructed side is necessary.

Regardless, surgical management of OHVIRA should only be performed by a surgeon with experience managing Müllerian anomalies. Reproductive outcomes in patients with OHVIRA are generally quite good, however they are driven by the particular uterine anomaly involved and may differ for patients with a bicornuate or septate uterus.

References

1. Herlyn U, Werner H. Simultaneous occurrence of an open Gartner-duct cyst, a homolateral aplasia of the kidney and a double uterus as a typical syndrome of abnormalities. Geburtshilfe Frauenheilkd. 1971;31:340–7.
2. Wunderlich M. Unusual form of genital malformation with aplasia of the right kidney. Zentralbl Gynakol. 1976;98:559–62.
3. Acién P. Embryological observations on the female genital tract. Hum Reprod. 1992;7:437–45.
4. Aswani Y, Varma R, Choudhary P, Gupta RB. Wolffian origin of vagina unfolds the embryopathogenesis of OHVIRA (Obstructed Hemivagina and Ipsilateral Renal Anomaly) syndrome and places OHVIRA as a female counterpart of Zinner syndrome in males. Pol J Radiol. 2016;81:549–56.
5. The American Fertility Society classifications of adnexal adhesions, distal tubal occlusion, tubal occlusion secondary to tubal ligation, tubal pregnancies, Müllerian anomalies and intrauterine adhesions. Fertil Steril. 1988;49:944–55.
6. Smith NA, Laufer MR. Obstructed hemivagina and ipsilateral renal anomaly (OHVIRA) syndrome: management and follow-up. Fertil Steril. 2007;87:918–22.
7. Fedele L, Motta F, Frontino G, Restelli E, Bianchi S. Double uterus with obstructed hemivagina and ipsilateral renal agenesis: pelvic anatomic variants in 87 cases. Hum Reprod. 2013;28:1580–3.
8. Candiani GB, Fedele L, Candiani M. Double uterus, blind hemivagina, and ipsilateral renal agenesis: 36 cases and long-term follow-up. Obstet Gynecol. 1997;90:26–32.
9. Mandava A, Prabhakar RR, Smitha S. OHVIRA syndrome (obstructed hemivagina and ipsilateral renal anomaly) with uterus didelphys, an unusual presentation. J Pediatr Adolesc Gynecol. 2012;25:e23–5.
10. Kueppers J, Wehrli L, Zundel S, Shavit S, Stahr N, Szavay PO. OHVIRA-syndrome in a newborn. J Pediatr Surg Case Rep. 2021;69:101859.
11. Dhar H, Razek YA, Hamdi I. Uterus didelphys with obstructed right hemivagina, ipsilateral renal agenesis and right pyocolpos: a case report. Oman Med J. 2011;26:447–50.
12. Zurawin RK, Dietrich JE, Heard MJ, Edwards CL. Didelphic uterus and obstructed hemivagina with renal agenesis: case report and review of the literature. J Pediatr Adolesc Gynecol. 2004;17:137–41.
13. Rivas AG, Epelman M, Ellsworth PI, Podberesky DJ, Gould SW. Magnetic resonance imaging of Müllerian anomalies in girls: concepts and controversies. Pediatr Radiol. 2021. https://doi.org/10.1007/s00247-021-05089-6.
14. Romanski PA, Aluko A, Bortoletto P, Troiano RN, Pfeifer SM. Aqueous vaginal contrast and scheduled hematocolpos with magnetic resonance imaging to delineate complex Müllerian anomalies. Fertil Steril. 2022;117(1):221–3.
15. Unlu E, Virarkar M, Rao S, Sun J, Bhosale P. Assessment of the effectiveness of the vaginal contrast media in magnetic resonance imaging for detection of pelvic pathologies: a meta-analysis. J Comput Assist Tomogr. 2020;44:436–42.
16. Mishra N, Ng S. Sonographic diagnosis of obstructed hemivagina and ipsilateral renal anomaly syndrome: a report of two cases. Australas J Ultrasound Med. 2014;17:153–8.
17. Deutch TD, Abuhamad AZ. The role of 3-dimensional ultrasonography and magnetic resonance imaging in the diagnosis of Müllerian duct anomalies. J Ultrasound Med. 2008;27:413–23.
18. Kamio M, Nagata C, Sameshima H, Togami S, Kobayashi H. Obstructed hemivagina and ipsilateral renal anomaly (OHVIRA) syndrome with septic shock: a case report. J Obstet Gynaecol Res. 2018;44:1326–9.
19. Ludwin A, Lindheim SR, Bhagavath B, Martins WP, Ludwin I. Longitudinal vaginal septum: a proposed classification and surgical management. Fertil Steril. 2020. https://doi.org/10.1016/j.fertnstert.2020.06.014.
20. Romanski PA, Bortoletto P, Pfeifer SM. Unilateral obstructed Müllerian anomalies: a series of unusual variants of known anomalies. J Pediatr Adolesc Gynecol. 2021. https://doi.org/10.1016/j.jpag.2021.04.005.
21. Ludwin A, Pfeifer SM. Reproductive surgery for Müllerian anomalies: a review of progress in the last decade. Fertil Steril. 2019;112:408–16.
22. Cosgrove P, Kahlden K, Barr L, Sanchez J. Obstructed hemivagina with ipsilateral renal agenesis (OHVIRA) syndrome with imperforate anus. J Pediatr Surg Case Rep. 2016;12:34–7.
23. Ludwin A, Ludwin I, Bhagavath B, Martins WP, Lindheim SR. Virginity-sparing management of blind hemivagina in obstructed hemivagina and ipsilateral renal anomaly syndrome. Fertil Steril. 2018;110:976–8.
24. Xu B, Xue M, Xu D. Hysteroscopic management of an oblique vaginal septum in a virgin girl with a rare variant of Herlyn-Werner-Wunderlich syndrome. J Minim Invasive Gynecol. 2015;22:7.
25. Gungor Ugurlucan F, Dural O, Yasa C, Kirpinar G, Akhan SE. Diagnosis, management, and outcome of obstructed hemivagina and ipsilateral renal

agenesis (OHVIRA syndrome): is there a correlation between MRI findings and outcome? Clin Imaging. 2020;59:172–8.

26. Tong J, Zhu L, Lang J. Clinical characteristics of 70 patients with Herlyn–Werner–Wunderlich syndrome. Int J Gynecol Obstet. 2013;121:173–5.

27. Haddad B, Barranger E, Paniel BJ. Blind hemivagina: long-term follow-up and reproductive performance in 42 cases. Hum Reprod. 1999;14:1962–4.

28. Heinonen PK. Pregnancies in women with uterine malformation, treated obstruction of hemivagina and ipsilateral renal agenesis. Arch Gynecol Obstet. 2013;287:975–8.

29. Chan YY, Jayaprakasan K, Tan A, Thornton JG, Coomarasamy A, Raine-Fenning NJ. Reproductive outcomes in women with congenital uterine anomalies: a systematic review. Ultrasound Obstet Gynecol. 2011;38:371–82.

Surgical Techniques for Vaginal Agenesis With and Without a Functioning Uterus

Andrea Zuckerman and Erin Fee

Müllerian Anomalies

Background and Terminology

Anomalies of the female urogenital tract vary in structure, etiology, location, and presentation. Müllerian anomalies are defects caused by malformations or dysfunction in Müllerian duct development that occurs during female embryogenesis. Anomalies may have complete underdevelopment of the Müllerian duct system with agenesis or atresia of the vagina, uterus, and/or fallopian tubes. These disorders are referred to as Müllerian agenesis, Müllerian aplasia, Mayer-Rokitansky-Küster-Hauser (MRKH) syndrome, and vaginal agenesis [1]. The incidence of Müllerian or vaginal agenesis is 1 per 4500–5000 females [1], whereas the exact prevalence of all Müllerian anomalies is unknown. Defects in the female reproductive tract development are estimated in 7% of healthy reproductive-aged women [2]. Many abnormalities of the female reproductive tract are likely undiagnosed, but may be seen more frequently in women with miscarriages or infertility [3].

The presentation of a Müllerian anomaly depends on the stage of embryogenesis dysfunction that occurs, the location and structure of the defect, and the presence or absence of obstruction. Obstruction refers to outflow blockage with backup of fluids, especially mucus or menstrual blood, when a uterus or uterine structure with a functioning endometrium is present. This occurs in patients with transverse vaginal septum, distal vaginal atresia, imperforate hymen, or obstructed uterine horn(s). Obstruction does not occur in patients with Müllerian agenesis or MRKH as they lack a uterus unless incomplete Müllerian duct development results in an isolated uterine horn. This is seen in patients with OHVIRA (Obstructed Hemivagina, Ipsilateral Renal Anomaly), or Herlyn-Werner-Wunderlich syndrome, who have complete duplication of the Müllerian duct system comprising of a uterine didelphys and two vaginas. In these patients, one vagina is not patent causing outflow obstruction on that uterine side and a renal anomaly is found on the ipsilateral side.

Terminology regarding Müllerian anomalies is often confusing as multiple names for each diagnosis may be used interchangeably. There is clinical distinction between patients with vaginal agenesis (Müllerian agenesis) who lack a developed uterus, and those with an obstructive Müllerian anomaly such as distal vaginal atresia, or vaginal agenesis involving a normal uterus. Multiple classification systems exist to attempt to

A. Zuckerman (✉) · E. Fee
Department of Obstetrics & Gynecology, Division of
Pediatric Adolescent Gynecology, Tufts Medical
Center & Tufts Children's Hospital,
Boston, MA, USA
e-mail: azuckerman@tuftsmedicalcenter.org;
efee@tuftsmedicalcenter.org

S. R. Lindheim, J. C. Petrozza (eds.), *Reproductive Surgery*,
https://doi.org/10.1007/978-3-031-05240-8_2

categorize the wide variety of these reproductive tract defects and are described in the following sections. The focus of this chapter will be concerning Müllerian anomalies involving abnormal vaginal development. There is distinction between clinical recommendations for patients with Müllerian or vaginal agenesis who lack a uterus, and those with obstructive Müllerian anomalies or vaginal agenesis and a functioning uterus (distal vaginal atresia). Each type of Müllerian anomaly is unique, and patient management should always be individualized.

Embryology

Development of the female reproductive structures begins at 6–7 weeks of gestation and is guided by the presence or absence of the SRY (sex-determining region Y) gene [4]. At approximately 37 days of fertilization, the Müllerian ducts appear lateral to the Wolffian duct system. In the absence of the SRY gene, the Müllerian structures fuse in the midline, and canalize until 14 weeks to caudally join the sinovaginal bulb, or vaginal plate. The Müllerian ducts ultimately develop into the fallopian tube, uterine cavity, cervix, and upper one-third of the vagina. Distal to the vaginal plate, the urogenital sinus, which is derived from the fetal cloaca, fuses with the Müllerian structures and canalizes to form the lower two-thirds of the vagina and the hymen [2, 4]. Defects in female reproductive tract development can occur at any point in fetal development. Failed vertical fusion of the Müllerian duct with the sinovaginal bulb may result in cervical atresia, a transverse vaginal septum, or distal vaginal agenesis. Underdevelopment and/or incomplete canalization of the upper Müllerian duct structures can cause structural uterine anomalies such as a uterine septa, a bicornuate uterus, or a longitudinal vaginal septum.

Classification Systems

There are several different classification systems for Müllerian anomalies. The most widely used system in the United States is proposed by ASRM (The American Society for Reproductive Medicine) and is based on the uterine structure (Fig. 2.1). In Europe, the most widely used classification terminology, also based on uterine shape, is from The European Society of Human Reproduction & The European Society for Gynaecological Endoscopy (ESHRE-ESGE) [5]. Another classification system that may be clinically useful, called the Acién Classification of Genital Tract Anomalies, is based on the type of embryologic dysfunction that occurs during different phases of female urogenital development [5]. The VCUAM (vagina cervix uterus adnexassociated malformation) Classification was developed to simplify the grouping while remaining precise [6]. There are downsides to all of the classification systems available, and most are difficult to apply in routine gynecologic practice. These limitations may include the lack of genetic, syndromic, or ovarian considerations. In addition, most of the existing classification systems may exclude those with hybrid or very rare anomalies. Disorders of the female urogenital tract are diverse and difficult to characterize in a precise way; they exist on a spectrum of structural and developmental issues that occur in embryogenesis. ASRM has published a more comprehensive classification system, ASRM MAC 2021, which describes anomalies involving the uterus, cervix and vagina for clinical application. The focus of this chapter will be regarding ASRM Class 1 Müllerian anomalies from the 1988 classification system and the mullerian agenesis category from the 2021 tool.

Vaginal Agenesis With and Without a Functional Uterus

Differential Diagnosis

A patient presenting with primary amenorrhea and evidence of vaginal or Müllerian agenesis should be evaluated for other reproductive tract anomalies that appear clinically similar and can be misdiagnosed. The differential diagnosis includes imperforate hymen, transverse vaginal septum, androgen insensitivity syndrome, and Swyer's syndrome. In patients with MRKH

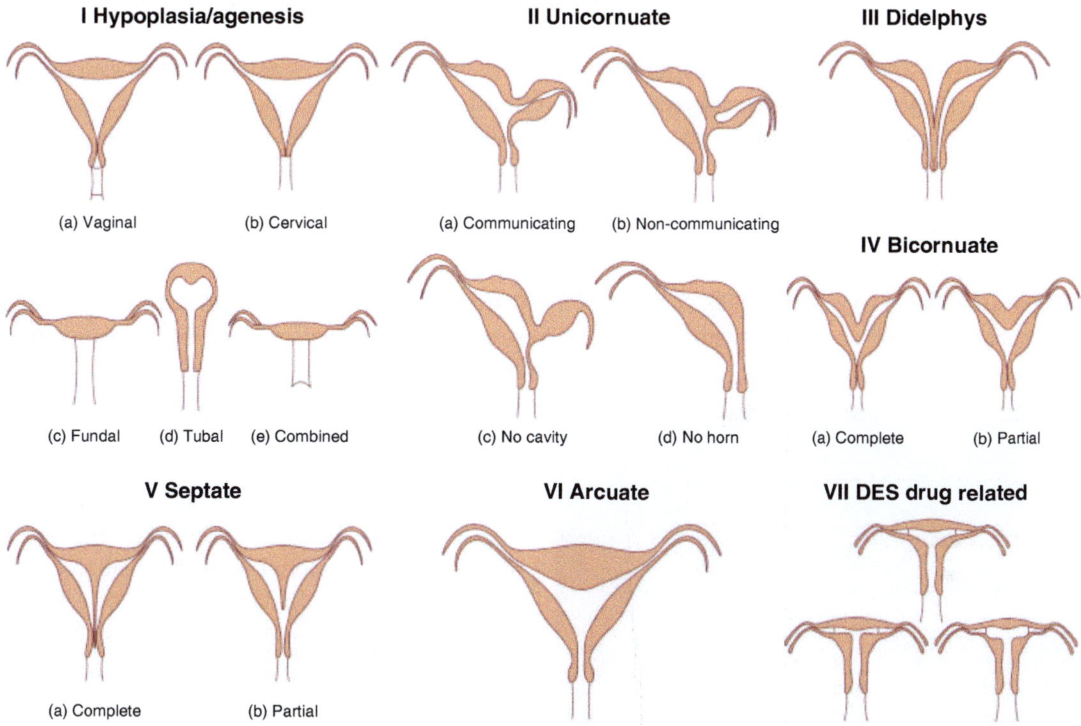

Fig. 2.1 Classification of Müllerian anomalies from The American Fertility Society. (Reprinted from Rackow et al. [67]. Copyright (2017), Elsevier publishing)

(Müllerian agenesis) and partial androgen insensitivity syndrome, physical exam will show normal secondary sexual characteristics, such as full breast development, pubic/axillary hair, and absent vagina. Patient's with Swyer's syndrome present with delayed puberty, absent breast tissue, and a normal functional vagina and uterus. An imperforate hymen and transverse septum may also present with obstruction, primary amenorrhea, and worsening cyclic abdominal pain similar to vaginal agenesis with a functioning uterus (distal vaginal atresia). Prior to puberty, a young girl with labial adhesions seen on physical exam can be mistaken for vaginal or Müllerian agenesis.

Evaluation and Diagnosis

Patients with any type of Müllerian anomaly present at variable points in life depending on the severity of the defect and presence or absence of outflow obstruction. Identifying Müllerian anomalies on a routine pediatric exam is uncommon and diagnosis is often delayed. Neonates with an imperforate hymen or obstructive Müllerian anomaly, such as a transverse vaginal septum or distal vaginal atresia, may present with a protruding vaginal mass caused by obstructed mucus (mucocolpos). These reproductive tract anomalies are ideally diagnosed prior to puberty in order to prevent the anticipated blockage, back-up of menstrual products, and pelvic pain by educating the patient and parents and in some cases surgical correction. Unfortunately, most are diagnosed after puberty with symptoms of an acute outflow obstruction. These patients present with absent menses, abdominal discomfort and/or a pelvic mass caused by painful build-up of menstrual blood in the upper genital tract (hematocolpos). For patients with vaginal agenesis, the diagnosis is often missed until late adolescence as patients are asymptomatic and have normal growth and development.

A thorough physical exam in the office is obligatory for any patient diagnosed with a

Müllerian anomaly. This exam should include an evaluation of the external genitalia and assessing the patient for secondary sex characteristics of breast development and pubic and axillary hair growth. Performing an exam under anesthesia may be necessary if a patient does not tolerate an exam in the office, and imaging is inconclusive. In this operative setting, complete visualization of the anatomy may include vaginoscopy and/or diagnostic laparoscopy especially for complex anomalies and if a vagina with incomplete

Müllerian development is present. Müllerian anomalies are frequently associated with renal, vertebral, anorectal, cardiac, tracheoesophageal and limb anomalies, and assessment of defects involving these organ systems during a patient's evaluation should be considered [7].

Imaging is helpful with both obstructive and nonobstructive Müllerian anomalies; a pelvic ultrasound should be performed early in the evaluation. A pelvic ultrasound assesses uterine structures, identifies masses or hematocolpos, and evaluates the adnexa (Figs. 2.2 and 2.3a, b). Ultrasound is beneficial as the initial imaging modality of choice as it is minimally invasive, low cost, and readily available. However, a normal ultrasound does not rule out the presence of a genital tract anomaly. Magnetic resonance imaging (MRI) is more useful in visualizing urogenital anatomy by looking more closely at soft tissue structures in close proximity (Fig. 2.4). An MRI study can be especially useful in girls with Müllerian agenesis and coexisting urogenital or colorectal anomalies. However, this should not be the initial diagnostic imaging of choice given its high cost, frequent challenges obtaining the study on young children, and overall good reliability of images obtained with ultrasound instead.

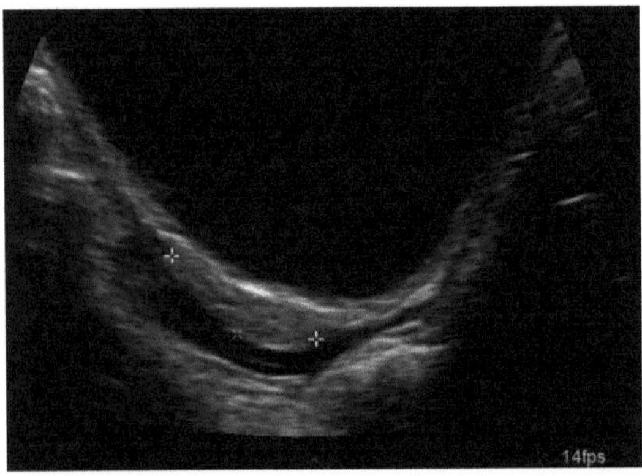

Fig. 2.2 Pelvic ultrasound of a Müllerian anomaly. Example of a pelvic ultrasound showing a hypoplastic uterine structure in Müllerian anomaly work-up of a patient with an absent vagina

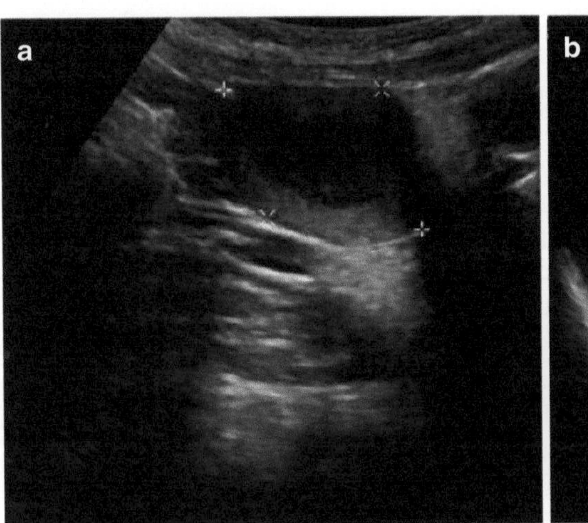

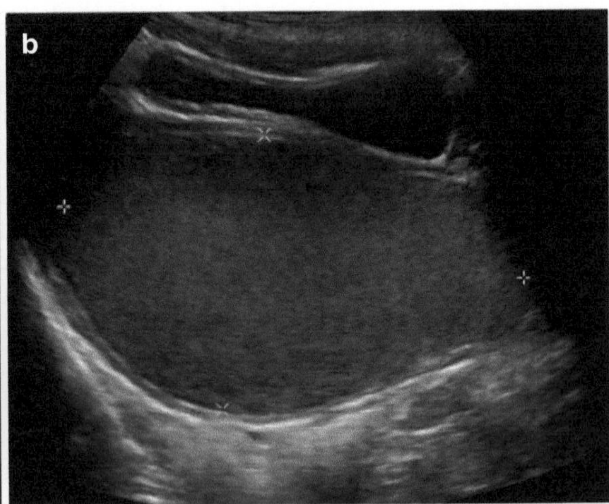

Fig. 2.3 (**a**, **b**) Pelvic ultrasound of an obstructive Müllerian anomaly. Diagnostic ultrasound in a patient with primary amenorrhea and cyclic pelvic pain showing hematometra (**a**) and large distended hematocolpos (**b**).

There are normally developed upper reproductive tract structures, including a uterus and ovaries, but an absent distal vagina (distal vaginal atresia)

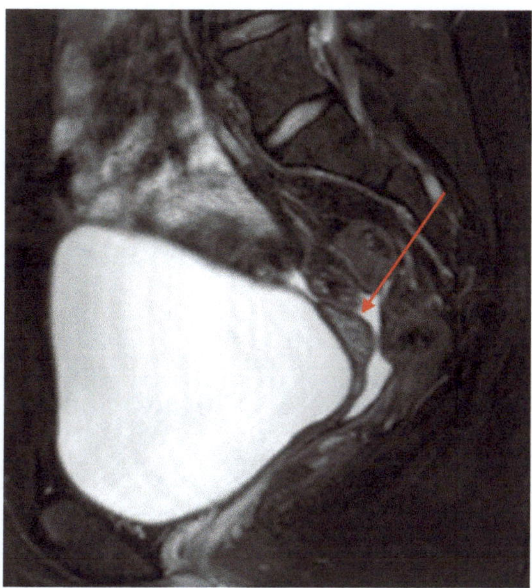

Fig. 2.4 Pelvic MRI of a Müllerian anomaly. T2-weighted magnetic resonance imaging (MRI) of the patient from Fig. 2.2. The hypoplastic uterine structure (red arrow) posterior to the distended bladder does not show an endometrial stripe and there is no vaginal structure

In order to provide appropriate clinical counseling, the complete evaluation (including history, physical, and imaging) should precede disclosure of the final diagnosis. Receiving the diagnosis of a Müllerian anomaly, especially vaginal agenesis, can be emotional with psychosocial implications for patients and families, especially regarding vaginal dilation or vaginal surgery at a young age. Concerns over future reproductive capabilities and sexual functioning are common and deserve adequate counseling throughout care. There should be multiple visits with a multidisciplinary team, including pediatric gynecology or urology, psychology, and reproductive endocrinology, to carefully review the patient's anatomy, management options, and address any emotional or psychologic problems in the process.

Reproductive Considerations

Women with Müllerian tract defects containing a functioning uterine structure can be reassured of favorable reproductive outcomes and fertility. In obstructive anomalies, patients can have normal sexual activity and child-bearing capabilities with surgical correction of the anatomic blockage. In patients with distal vaginal atresia, there is a normal upper vagina, cervix, and uterus. These patients and those with vaginal agenesis involving a cervix and functioning uterus have reproductive success following surgical correction by pull-through vaginoplasty or a similar procedure. These surgical procedures are described in the following sections.

Almost all patients with Müllerian anomalies have normal functioning ovaries as the development of the gonads is separate in embryogenesis. For patients with vaginal agenesis involving uterine atresia, artificial reproductive technology (ART) by oocyte harvesting and in-vitro fertilization can produce biologic offspring with the use of gestational surrogacy [8, 9]. Patients with disorders that lack functioning ovaries, such as Turner syndrome, Gonadal dysgenesis, or androgen insensitivity syndrome, may present similar to those with Müllerian anomalies or Müllerian agenesis; however, counseling and management in these patients are different and will not be discussed here.

In women who cannot carry a pregnancy and are opposed to gestational surrogacy, information should be provided regarding available reproductive options such as adoption or uterine transplantation. The first live birth in a patient with MRKH syndrome after uterine transplantation was reported in 2014 in Gothenburg, Sweden. Since then, there has been rising clinical interest and several US centers have conducted uterine transplantation with successful results [10, 11]. In a survey of women diagnosed with Mayer-Rokitansky-Küster-Hauser (MRKH) syndrome by Chmel et al., 62% expressed interest in uterine transplantation at the time of Vecchietti neovagina creation after being counseled on the risks, benefits, and lack of long-term data on the experimental procedure [12]. There is some debate regarding the ethics with living donors and the recipient patient's risk-to-benefit of elective uterine transplantation as it is a complex, lengthy procedure, and requires postoperative immunosuppression. Reported data on adverse outcomes after transplantation is limited, but few cases of surgical complications include (but are not limited to): graft-vs-host disease, thromboembolisms, hemorrhage, pelvic infections/abscess, graft ischemia, emergency hysterectomy (transplant removal), fistula, cystitis, cuff dehiscence, and vaginal stenosis. However, most (more than half) of uterine transplant procedures performed internationally did not have any reported surgical or medical complications in the postoperative period. This innovative procedure, although complex, will likely continue to increase in success as a surgical option for select patients desiring fertility and pregnancy who have uterine absence.

Vaginal Agenesis with a Functioning Uterus (Distal Vaginal Atresia)

Presentation and Management

Unless diagnosed earlier in childhood, variants of vaginal agenesis with a functioning uterus, also referred to as distal vaginal atresia, present with pain and outflow obstruction at menarche. These anomalies, as well as transverse vaginal septum or imperforate hymen, are considered obstructive Müllerian anomalies and are treated similarly. Management of complex obstructive Müllerian anomalies, such as noncommunicating uterine horns or OHVIRA syndrome, is not discussed here.

Vaginal agenesis with a functioning uterus, imperforate hymen, or transverse vaginal septum will ultimately require surgery to allow for normal female reproductive function and spontaneous passage of menstrual blood. If one of these obstructive anomalies is identified before menarche, surgical management can be performed at an appropriate time to prevent obstruction at puberty. If not diagnosed before spontaneous menses begin, these patients will present with acute obstructive symptoms including abdominal pain, amenorrhea, and a pelvic mass or vaginal bulge caused by a hematocolpos (Fig. 2.5).

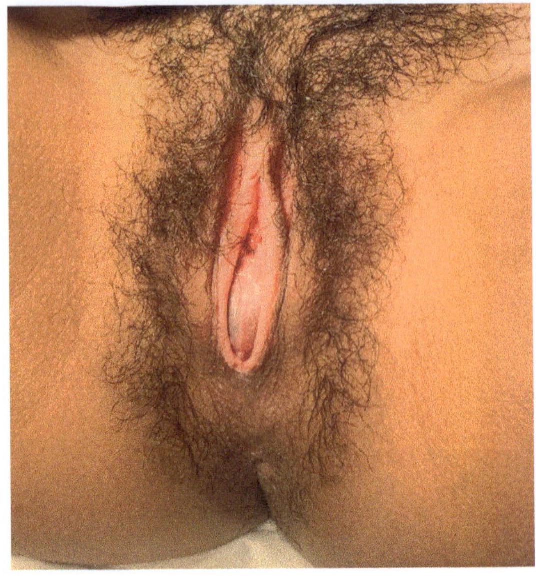

Fig. 2.5 Acute obstruction with bulging hematocolpos. Vaginal bulge from obstructed menses (hematocolpos) in an adolescent with an obstructive Müllerian anomaly. Differential diagnosis includes vaginal agenesis with a functioning uterus (distal vaginal atresia), transverse vaginal septum, and imperforate hymen

In the setting of an acute obstruction at the time of diagnosis, management options include either menstrual suppression to delay surgery or immediate surgical decompression. Delay in surgical management can be considered if pain is well-controlled, the patient is uninfected, and is able to void without issues. This strategy is preferred for young girls who may not be appropriately mature for surgery and possible postoperative vaginal dilator therapy if required. Pursuing immediate surgical management and decompression of an outflow obstruction is often necessary if the patient has uncontrolled pain, voiding difficulty, or evidence of infected hematocolpos.

The surgical procedure performed on patients with vaginal agenesis and a functioning uterus (distal vaginal atresia) is referred to as the pull-through vaginoplasty. Prior to surgery, the diagnosis of a suspected obstructive Müllerian anomaly should be confirmed, and the patient's urogenital anatomy assessed by an external genital exam and imaging. If able, the distance between the leading edge of the upper vagina and the top of the vaginal dimple or lower vagina should be estimated preoperatively. In surgical planning, if there is a large distance between the proximal and distal vaginal ends, vaginal dilation, or use of an interposition graft may be necessary. The guidelines for management for these larger vaginal agenesis or septal defects are described below.

In performing the vaginal pull-through procedure, the visible apex of the lower vagina, or vaginal dimple is incised transversely and sharp dissection is carried toward the upper vagina that may be bulging from acute obstruction. A large hematocolpos can aid in this procedure by pushing the leading edge of upper vagina closer to the introitus and decreasing the thickness of the tissue being incised. Once old menstrual blood products, if present, have been adequately drained at entry into the upper vagina, the initial incision is extended laterally. For adequate diameter of the vaginal opening and to prevent stricture formation, additional small cuts are made at the superolateral and inferolateral aspects of both ends of the transverse incision (at the 1 o'clock, 5 o'clock, 7 o'clock, and 11 o'clock positions respectively). The upper vaginal mucosa should be tagged or grasped as soon as possible in the procedure and ultimately sutured circumferentially to the level of the lower vagina or introitus (Fig. 2.6).

Surgical management of transverse vaginal septum or an imperforate hymen is similar to that of distal vaginal atresia. Excision of a transverse vaginal septum involves surgical removal of the intervening septal tissue and anastomosis of the proximal and distal vagina. This is sometimes accomplished with a Z-plasty technique, involving creation of vaginal flaps sutured superiorly and inferiorly along the vaginal canal in order to increase vaginal length and minimize the risk of stenosis [1].

Larger transverse septal or vaginal atretic defects are those with more than 3–4 cm between the leading edges of the upper and lower vagina. These anomalies are managed differently as they have higher risk for stricture or stenosis. To decrease the risk in these patients, preoperative dilation of the lower vagina to approximate the upper and lower vagina and/or the use of a mucosal skin bridge (such as a buccal graft) at surgery may

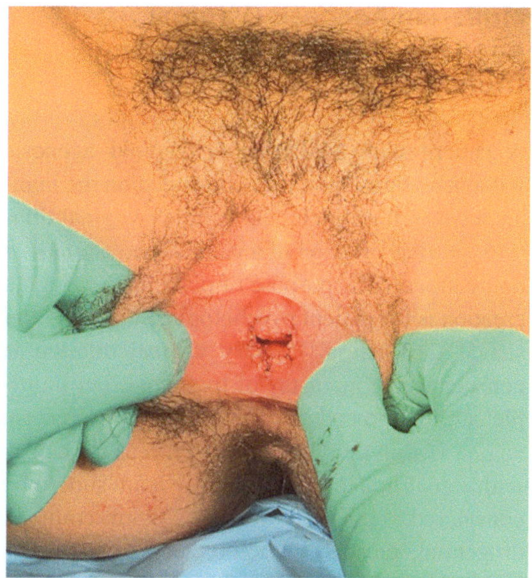

Fig. 2.6 Surgical correction of distal vaginal atresia by pull-through vaginoplasty. Vaginal canal after the pull-through vaginoplasty technique described in this chapter

be useful [7, 13, 14]. Postoperative use of soft or hard dilators to prevent strictures is often recommended after pull-through vaginoplasty, but has not been shown to benefit patients with defects measuring less than 3 cm. In those that vaginal dilator use after surgery is recommended, patients should perform vaginal dilation daily using hard dilators for 10- to 30-minute intervals. Alternatively, soft flexible vaginal dilators can be inserted and remain in place 24 hours-a-day for a week at-a-time with removal only to void. Patients with grafts placed surgically should not initiate dilator therapy until a follow-up exam confirms adequate graft healing and update though will likely need a vaginal mold to help prevent stenosis [1].

Risks and complications of surgical management of distal vaginal atresia, imperforate hymen, transverse vaginal septum, or vaginal agenesis with a functioning uterus include infection, vaginal scar tissue formation, vaginal stenosis or stricture, dyspareunia and need for repeat surgery [15]. Repeat surgeries to manage recurrent obstructions from postoperative vaginal stenosis have increased morbidity. Each subsequent surgery is more challenging with increasing risk of recurrent stenosis and treatment failure.

Müllerian Agenesis (Vaginal Agenesis Without a Functioning Uterus)

A patient with Müllerian or vaginal agenesis without a uterus should be counseled on the management options including primary vaginal dilation, surgical creation of a vagina (neovagina), or no treatment. The purpose of pursuing neovagina creation is for patient psychological wellness and sexual satisfaction. Primary vaginal dilation is considered the mainstay of treatment, but multiple surgical procedures are available to create a vagina if this fails. Referral to a tertiary center with a qualified multidisciplinary team should be considered, especially for girls with complex urogenital, cloacal, or colorectal anomalies, as they may have more favorable outcomes for the management of vaginal agenesis [15].

Nonsurgical Management (Primary Vaginal Dilation)

Vaginal elongation by using dilators is considered the first-line treatment of MRKH, vaginal agenesis, or Müllerian agenesis [16]. Important to the success of dilation is beginning when the patient is ready and committed to spending the time needed to perform dilation. Advantages of nonsurgical elongation of the vagina include the ability for the patient to proceed at her speed, no need for anesthesia, no hospitalization or scarring, and less risk of vaginal stenosis, pain, and expense compared with surgical management [17]. Disadvantages include longer time until successful creation of a neovagina and the need for patient privacy. Possible risks of using dilators to create or elongate the vagina include discomfort during dilation, bleeding from abrasions, and inadvertent dilation of the urethra instead of the vagina. It is necessary to have frequent follow-up visits with a healthcare provider comfortable with counseling and instruction of vaginal dilator use.

Graduated hard dilators come in a wide variety of sizes (Fig. 2.7). A knowledgeable medical professional should be able to select appropriate starting vaginal dilator size and the rate of advancing the diameter used during the dilation process. The usual process in selecting size is to start with the smallest size that is comfortable for the patient but provides appropriate soft tissue pressure and then advance up. Teaching adolescent and adult women how to use the dilators requires educating the patient about their own

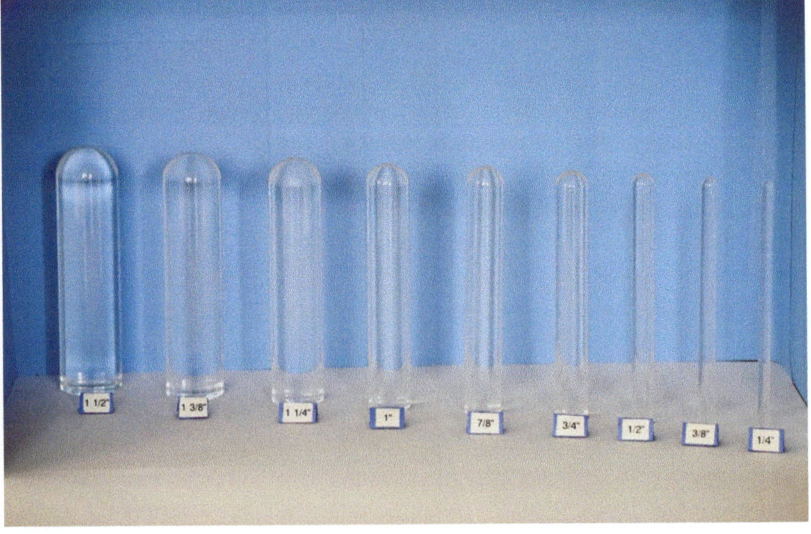

Fig. 2.7 Graduated hard vaginal dilators. Graduated plexiglass vaginal dilators ranging from ¼ inch to 1½ inch. If desired and to assist with dilation using a stationary seat, the length of the dilator may be modified by a carpenter or professional who is comfortable with cutting that specific material qualified company

external anatomy. The use of a mirror and frequent office visits are helpful in the success of patient's vaginal dilator therapy. Historically, vaginal dilation used hard dilators cut down to slightly extend beyond the patient's introitus when placed in the vaginal space and was held in place with spandex underwear [18, 19]. Patients were then instructed to sit on a bicycle seat attached to a firm board in order to apply pressure on the dilator at the perineum in order to perform dilation. Now, patients often find it more comfortable to lie down with hips flexed, retract the labia with their nondominant hand, and hold the lubricated dilator using the dominant hand at the perineum pointing downward toward the sacrum to create pressure on the dilator (Fig. 2.8). Ideally the patient uses the dilator for 10–30 minutes one to three times a day and gradually advances to a larger sized vaginal dilator when appropriate. It is recommended patients empty their bladder before and after dilation sessions. Patients who need to stop or interrupt dilation therapy during the graduated dilator process may need to use a smaller size dilator than previously used when they start-up again.

One study of patients with vaginal agenesis reported 80–92% success in creating a functional vagina using graduated hard dilators [20]. Adequate vaginal length, typically 6–7 cm, is attained once the patient can comfortably have vaginal intercourse. Vaginal dilation can also be achieved by penetrative sexual activity exclusively, or in combination with hard dilators, which has similar success rates [21]. Attention should be given to each patient's self-esteem and mood during the treatment process. Often, patients feel depressed over the need to use dilators, and are especially distressed if this treatment fails.

Surgical Management

Multiple surgical techniques to create a functional vagina (neovagina) in patients with vaginal agenesis have been performed since the early twentieth century. These techniques are secondary to vaginal dilation in management, and are often reserved for those who have failed or are unable to perform dilation [22]. The advantage of surgery over primary dilation is more rapid creation of a functional vagina. No singular technique has been found to be superior in terms of outcomes and patient satisfaction [3]. Each surgery has unique requirements, complications, and outcomes (Table 2.1). Regardless of type of surgery, complication rates are significantly reduced if performed prepuberty (14%) as opposed to postpuberty (58%) [23].

All surgical neovagina methods require close follow-up with a minimum of annual exams for evaluation of sexually transmitted infections, vaginal strictures, and evaluation of rare malignancies that may be associated with certain neovagina epitheliums [1, 24]. Almost all procedures require the use of vaginal dilators or molds after

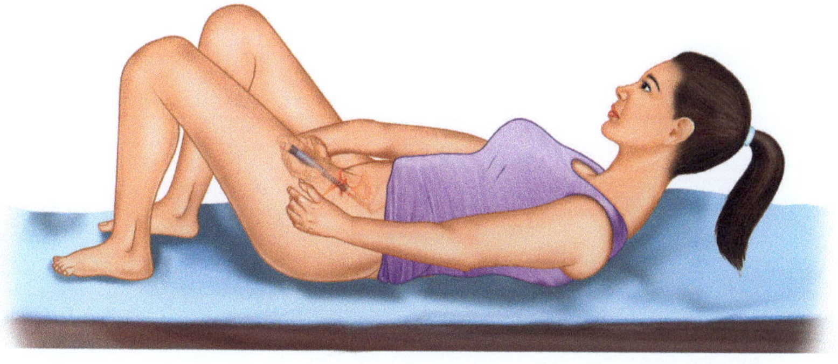

Fig. 2.8 Preferred patient positioning for vaginal dilation. The preferred patient position for vaginal dilation described in the text

Table 2.1 Summary of options for vaginal creation (neovagina) in patients with vaginal agenesis

Procedure	Description	Advantages & outcomes	Disadvantages & complications
Nonsurgical options			
Primary Vaginal Dilation	Patient performs vaginal dilation using graduated hard dilators or coitus *Considered first-line option*	Success in 80–92% Vaginal length 6.7–8.7 cm Avoidance of surgery and hospitalization Ability to perform at patient's preferred speed Decreased risk of stricture, stenosis, or dyspareunia Low-cost	Complication 5–35% Laborious and time consuming to patients Longer time to end result Emotional distress Need for routine privacy Discomfort during dilation Bleeding caused by abrasions Inadvertent urethral dilation Failure of therapy and requiring surgery
Surgical neovagina techniques			

Abbe-McIndoe Vaginoplasty, 1938 Or Modified McIndoe Procedures	Perineal dissection with split-thickness skin grafting performed in two surgeries
	Modified McIndoe techniques use of an alternative (mucosal-like) material grafted into the vaginal space
	Example:
	   Human amnion
	   Autologous buccal mucosa
	   Surgical adhesive barrier
	   Artificial created dermis
		Success in 85%
		Vaginal length 7.4 cm
			Complications 19–65%
			Prolonged hospitalization
			Pain
			Secondary surgery for vaginal mold removal
			Required postoperative dilator use
			Wound infection
			Neovagina stricture or stenosis
			Neovaginal fistula
			Graft failure
			Scarring at graft site
			Complications requiring reoperation

Davydov Procedure, 1974	Autologous pelvic peritoneum is surgically connected to the external vaginal opening	Success in 68–87% Vaginal length 7.8 cm High sexual satisfaction scores	Complications 14% Required postoperative dilator use Surrounding organ injury during procedure Neovaginal fistula Pelvic adhesions Granulation tissue formation Vaginal stricture, vaginismus Complications requiring reoperation
Vecchietti Procedure, 1965	Active perineal dilation by gradual increased tension of a surgically placed device over 1 week followed by a second surgery to remove the apparatus	Success in 80–98% Vaginal length 9.5 cm High sexual satisfaction scores	Complications 11–13% Prolonged hospitalization Secondary surgery for device removal Pain Required postoperative dilator use Urinary tract infection Granulation tissue formation Postoperative fever Vaginal stricture or stenosis Complications requiring reoperation

Table 2.1 (continued)

Procedure	Description	Advantages & outcomes	Disadvantages & complications
Intestinal Vaginoplasty, 1892	Surgical transposition of a closed loop segment of large or small bowel	Success in 73–83% Vaginal length 10 cm Option for surgery before puberty No requirement for postoperative dilation	Complications 7–79% Introital stenosis and subsequent need for dilation Trauma or discomfort with intercourse Excessive malodorous vaginal discharge Mucosal prolapse Small bowel obstruction Fistula formation Complications requiring reoperation
Vulvovaginal Pouch or Williams Procedure, 1964	Full-thickness skin graft and external labial suturing to create a vertical perineal pouch for intercourse	Success in 95% Vaginal length of 10–12 cm Minimally invasive reversible procedure High sexual satisfaction Low complication rates No requirement for postoperative dilation unless vagina is short	Complications unknown to 4% Immediate postoperative hospitalization Bleeding with intercourse Wound infection Hematoma Irritation from graft with hair-bearing skin Disfiguring scars Change in anatomic axis for intercourse Awkward angle of vaginal intercourse Scarring at graft sites Complications requiring reoperation

Complied from data in McIndoe et al. [25], Buss et al. [52], Herlin et al. [38], Højsgaard et al. [53], Klingele et al. [54], Davydov et al. [36], Willemsen et al. [55], Allen et al. [56], Giannesi et al. [57], Borruto et al. [41], Borruto et al. [42], Brucker et al. [43], Rall et al. [58], Baldwin et al. [46], Karateke et al. [47], Carrard et al. [48], Communal et al. [59], Hensle et al. [60], Nowier et al. [61], Burgu et al. [23], Parsons et al. [62], Williams et al. [49], Creatsas et al. [51], and Creatsas et al. [63]

surgery for an extended period of time. With vaginal molds, the device can be created from flexible foam material covered by a condom that the patient wears continuously with removal only to urinate or defecate. Alternatives include intermittent vaginal dilation with hard dilators and/or eventually regular intercourse. The appropriate length of time for postoperative vaginal dilation or mold placements is individualized to the type of surgery, risk of stenosis, patient goals for vaginal length, and if the patient plans to use coitus to maintain patency. Careful consideration should be taken in deciding candidates for a surgical neovagina procedure. The risks of surgery and the postoperative requirements, including dilation and close follow-up, should be disclosed to the patient before surgery. As maturity to per-form these tasks is needed, the provider may consider delaying surgical neovagina surgery until the patient is more ready at an older age.

Techniques for Surgical Vaginal Construction (Neovagina)

Active Dissection of the Perineal Space

The Abbe-McIndoe or McIndoe Vaginoplasty was first described in 1938 [25]. This technique uses a split-thickness graft (0.018–0.022 in) from the buttock to line a surgically created neovaginal space in a two-step surgical technique for girls with vaginal agenesis [25, 26]. Similar to a pull-through procedure described earlier in this chapter, the top of the distal vagina, or vaginal dimple, is incised transversely and midline dissection is carried inward at the sub-urethral level. Once adequate space is obtained, a sterile mold is created using expandable foam material within a condom, covered with affixed split-thickness skin graft, and placed in the surgically created vaginal space. The edges are then sewn to the introitus, and labia are sewn closed to keep the mold in place. The patient remains in the hospital for a week, on bedrest, with a foley catheter and placed on a stool softening bowel regimen before returning to the operating room for mold removal and graft assessment. After surgery, the patient must follow a meticulous regimen using vaginal dilators to maintain vaginal patency and prevent stricture or stenosis while the graft continues to heal. Initially, the patient keeps a mold or flexible dilator in place continuously for minimum of a month; removing only to urinate and defecate. This is followed by insertion of a flexible or hard dilator several times a day for 3–6 months. Eventually, the dilator is used only nightly until the patient can maintain vaginal patency with intercourse alone [26].

Modifications of the McIndoe technique with split-thickness skin grafts are frequently performed and have variable functional outcomes. These modified techniques involve alternative graft materials which are placed on the vaginal mold similar to the initial McIndoe procedure. Tissues that have been successfully used in modified McIndoe procedures include autologous buccal mucosal grafts [27, 28], human amnion [29–31], and artificial adhesion barriers with *Interceed* [32, 33]. Similar to the split-thickness skin graft, these different mucosa-like materials are affixed to the temporary vaginal mold. Postoperative use of vaginal dilators is essential for preventing the vaginal strictures commonly experienced with the classic McIndoe procedure. More recently, the use of an artificially-created dermis by medical recombinant fibroblast growth factor mucosa has been described [34]. Lastly, full-thickness skin grafts obtained by harvesting myocutaneous rectus abdominis skin, gracilis or pudendal fasciocutaneous flaps, or skin taken from the lower abdominal wall by pfannensteil-like excision are reported [35]. These skin grafts can be associated with large disfiguring scars [35]. Full-thickness graft techniques are considered a last surgical option for creation of a neovagina, and are difficult to graft into the surgically created vaginal space [35].

Autologous Pelvic Peritoneum

The Davydov method for surgical vagina creation was initially described in 1974, and has reported outcomes similar to the McIndoe techniques [36–38]. The initial portion of the procedure is identical to the perineal approach of the McIndoe procedure, but pelvic dissection is slightly deeper and directed toward the abdominal peritoneum of the Pouch of Douglas. Then, via laparoscopy, the peritoneum is advanced by "push-down" approach from the pelvis and brought to the level of the introitus [13, 37, 39, 40]. The abdominal portion of the peritoneum is then closed in a purse-string fashion [13, 37, 39, 40]. Complications of this approach can include vaginal stricture or stenosis, as well as potential bladder or ureteral injury, which may in time may lead to vesicovaginal fistula formation [37, 40].

Active Perineal Dilation

The Vecchietti-technique, performed since approximately 1965, utilizes a method of active tension on the perineum for creation of a neovagina, and is the preferred technique used at European centers [41, 42]. A plexiglass olive, or modified dilator, is attached to the vaginal introitus with permanent sutures and secured through the perineum. The sutures are run through the lower abdominal wall to a metal device that allows for increasing tension on the perineum by tightening the sutures externally to stretch the blind vaginal pouch until sufficient vaginal length is achieved [26, 41–44]. This surgery requires a week of hospitalization with parenteral anesthesia for pain, as well as a second short-interval surgery for removal of the tension device and olive when dilation is complete. After removal of the device, the patient is instructed to perform continued vaginal dilation with hard dilators to maintain this newly created space and length [13, 26, 41–44]. A more recent strategy to the Vecchietti is a laparoscopic-assisted balloon vaginoplasty that was introduced in 2007 [45]. The active portion of dilation at the perineum is instead accomplished by feeding a retropubic foley catheter to the introitus and slowly increasing tension on the opposite end of the foley [45].

Intestinal Vaginoplasty

A method often preferred by pediatric surgeons, bowel loop or sigmoid vaginoplasty, is one of the oldest procedures for surgical creation of a vagina. As opposed to the other neovagina methods, bowel vaginoplasty for creation of a vagina can be performed in infancy or childhood [13, 15]. First described in 1892, the procedure was made popular in the United States in the early 1900s, and both small and large bowels have been used [46]. Steps of the procedure include open or laparoscopic mobilization of the bowel to the introitus with end-to-end re-anastomosis to create a blind vaginal pouch [15, 46–48]. Blood supply of the utilized bowel segment is maintained during the procedure.

Labial Skin Flap or Vulvovaginal Pouch

The Williams vulvovaginoplasty is an alternative surgical option to consider in certain patients as the surgery is reversible, minimally invasive, and does not require entry into the pelvis. Good candidates for creation of an artificial vagina by the Williams technique may include those who have failed dilator therapy, are unable to perform vaginal dilation, individuals with extensive urogenital malformations, such as a cloaca, or for patients who are unsuccessful in creating a functional vagina with one of the other described surgeries [13, 15, 49, 50]. This technique may be the preferred option for patients with severe pelvic scarring from prior procedures or pelvic radiation [13, 15, 49, 50]. The Williams vaginoplasty involves the creation of an exterior "kangaroo pouch" horizontal to the perineum. The pouch-space is created by suturing full-thickness skin flaps from the labia in a "U-shaped" configuration [15, 49–51]. Patients must be counseled on the different axis required for intercourse after this procedure, and the need for dilator use or regular intercourse to prevent adhesion formation and maintain the space as a functional vagina.

Complications and Outcomes of Surgical Neovagina Techniques

In studies of surgical techniques for vaginal construction in patients with Müllerian agenesis, no single procedure is superior and each carries unique disadvantages, side effects, or complications (Table 2.1). Although surgical management may produce more rapid results for these patients, surgery is still considered secondary to vaginal dilation in the management of vaginal agenesis due to their surgical risks and potentially morbid complications [22].

Active Dissection of the Perineal Space

Long-term surgical outcomes for the McIndoe procedure have been well-studied and functional success was reported in 85% of girls who underwent this procedure in a study by Buss et al. [52]. Reported complications of this procedure come in a wide range of severity and rates range from 19% to 65% [38, 53]. Disadvantages of this technique include the need for two surgeries, hospitalization, prolonged postoperative dilator, and unique surgical risks including graft failure. Surgical complications include vaginal stenosis, disfiguring scar at donor graft site, wound infection, and fistula formation [52, 54]. The McIndoe techniques involving alternative material grafted into the vaginal space have similar reported outcomes and there is inconclusive evidence demonstrating advantage over the classic split-thickness Abbe-McIndoe procedure.

Autologous Pelvic Peritoneum

In a retrospective cohort study by Willemsen et al., 160 women with vaginal agenesis who underwent neovagina procedure by the Davydov technique were studied for long-term outcomes [55]. Women who underwent the Davydov procedure had a 68–87% success in creating a functional vagina (defined as length greater than 5 cm) with a mean vaginal length of 7.8 cm; the results did not change significantly if the patient performed vaginal dilation prior to surgery [55]. Sexual satisfaction scores after this procedure are shown to be similar for scores in sexual arousal, lubrication, orgasm, and comfort in studies comparing these patients to a random female control population [55, 56]. The rate of adverse outcomes associated with the Davydov peritoneal neovagina is reported at 14% in one study [57]. Complications associated with this procedure include rectal or bladder injury at the time of the procedure, recto-neovaginal fistula, pelvic adhesions, granulation tissue formation, stricture, and vaginismus [55, 56].

Active Perineal Dilation

The laparoscopically assisted neovagina creation by Vecchietti active perineal dilation results in a successful creation of a functional vagina in over 98% [42, 58]. The reported mean length of 9.5 centimeters with sexual satisfaction scores that are similar to female age-matched controls in several studies [43, 58]. Similar to the McIndoe procedure, the Vecchietti method requires postoperative hospitalization and two surgeries 1 week apart. There must be aggressive pain control and close monitoring during the active portion of vaginal dilation. Typical complications of the Vecchietti procedure are postoperative fever, urinary tract infection, granulation tissue formation, vaginal stricture, and rarely, urethral necrosis [43, 58]. Rates of adverse outcomes of either laparoscopic or open approach Vecchietti are 11–13% [41].

Intestinal Vaginoplasty

Bowel vaginoplasty has been performed for over a century with multiple long-term studies of outcomes, complications, and modifications of the procedure. Most studies of this surgery report a 73–83% patient satisfaction with final vaginal length (mean of 10 cm) and good sexual function [48, 59–61]. Advantages of bowel vaginoplasty include the lack of multiple procedures or required postoperative vaginal dilation.

Multiple complications and complaints after bowel vaginoplasty have been reported and the exact rate of all postoperative issues is difficult to know. The biggest disadvantages include the common complaint of copious foul smelling mucus discharge requiring daily pad use or douching, trauma with intercourse (especially if small bowel is used), and an abnormal vaginal length later in life if the surgery is performed in childhood [13, 15, 23, 47, 48, 62]. The occurrence rates of significant complications range from 7% to 79% and include introital stenosis requiring dilation (especially if blood supply is compromised), mucosal prolapse, small bowel obstruction, and fistula formation [23, 47, 62].

Labial Skin Flap or Vulvovaginal Pouch

The Williams vulvovaginoplasty is the most simple, noninvasive neovagina surgical technique and is the only reversible option currently available. First described by Williams 1964, the Williams procedure and other reported surgical modifications demonstrate good results in sexual function and patient satisfaction with final vaginal length [49, 51]. Creatsas et al. found that of 178 patients with MRKH, approximately 95% were successful in obtaining a vaginal length of 10–12 cm and 94% of patients reported satisfactory quality of sexual life after surgery [51]. Data on complication rates is limited as this procedure is rarely performed. In reports by Creatsas et al., specific issues such as wound complications, hematoma formation, or need for dilation each occurred in about 4%. Those requiring dilation (4.5%) had a 7–9 cm neovagina and most reported good sexual function after dilator therapy [51, 63]. Patient complaints after Williams procedure are often of postoperative bleeding, need for initial hospitalization, scarring at the graft site or vulva, different vaginal axis with intercourse, and irritating hair growth within the vagina [51, 63].

Criteria of "success" vary between surgeries and studies. Most cited sources define surgical success by a patient's satisfaction with the neovagina, subsequent sexual function, and/or a final vaginal length of more than 5–6 cm.

"Vaginal length" in centimeters is reported in the referenced studies as mean, range, or an average.

Conclusion

Management of patients with vaginal agenesis, with or without a functional uterus, is complex and clinical recommendations depend on age at diagnosis and the clinical presentation. Disclosing the diagnosis of a reproductive tract anomaly can be distressing especially with anomalies that affect future fertility or in patients that require vaginal dilation or surgery. Frequent counseling visits with the patient and family by a provider familiar with the management of these complex disorders are required. When appropriate, girls and women without a developed uterus should be provided with information on available advanced fertility options and their alternatives if childbearing is desired. Referral to a specialty or tertiary center may be necessary as developmental defects involving other organ systems are frequently encountered in girls with genital tract anomalies and a multidisciplinary approach is preferred.

Patients with vaginal agenesis and their families can be reassured of the favorable outcomes in most by vaginal dilation only. If dilation is not an option or is unsuccessful for these patients, many surgical techniques exist for the creation of a neo-vagina with high success rates and good sexual satisfaction. If a provider is comfortable recommending and performing one of these procedures, the postoperative requirements and unique surgical complications should be carefully reviewed before surgery.

Preventative health care and screening recommendations for women and girls with Müllerian anomalies should not be overlooked. Genital tract anomalies are not contraindications to the human papillomavirus (HPV) vaccine [64]. This vaccine is administered in late childhood and is recommended for all patients regardless of their genital anatomy as it can help decrease virus transmission to sexual partners and prevent HPV-related oropharyngeal or genital tract malignancies [64]. Patients with Müllerian agenesis or cervical atresia do not fall under the USPTF (US Preventative Services Task Force) criteria for routine cervical cancer screening regardless of sexual activity or HPV vaccination status [65]. Those with an identifiable cervix should undergo routine cervical cancer screening starting at age 21 according to current guidelines [65]. Patients with duplicated Müllerian systems require cytology samples of each cervix at each screening. Safe sex counseling and annual screening for sexually transmitted infections, especially

Gonorrhea and Chlamydia, are recommended for all sexually active women younger than 25 years, or older if additional risk factors are present [66]. Lastly, preventative health visits that include an annual pelvic and breast exam by a healthcare provider are recommended for all women regardless of their anatomy.

References

1. Müllerian agenesis: diagnosis, management, and treatment. ACOG Committee Opinion No. 728. American College of Obstetricians and Gynecologists. Obstet Gynecol. 2018;131:e35–42.
2. Breech LL, Laufer MR. Müllerian anomalies. Obstet Gynecol Clin N Am. 2009;36(1):47–68.
3. Skinner B, Quint EH. Nonobstructive reproductive tract anomalies: a review of surgical management. J Minim Invasive Gynecol. 2017;24(6):909–14.
4. Dietrich JE, Millar DM, Quint EH. Obstructive reproductive tract anomalies. J Pediatr Adolesc Gynecol. 2014;27(6):396–402.
5. Acién P, Acién MI. The history of female genital tract malformation classifications and proposal of an updated system. Hum Reprod Update. 2011;17(5):693–705.
6. Oppelt P, Renner SP, Brucker S, Strissel PL, Strick R, Oppelt PG, et al. The VCUAM (Vagina Cervix Uterus Adnex-associated Malformation) classification: a new classification for genital malformations. Fertil Steril. 2005;84(5):1493–7.
7. Management of acute obstructive uterovaginal anomalies: ACOG Committee Opinion, Number 779. Obstet Gynecol. 2019;133(6):e363–71.
8. Friedler S, Grin L, Liberti G, Saar-Ryss B, Rabinson Y, Meltzer S. The reproductive potential of patients with Mayer-Rokitansky-Küster-Hauser syndrome using gestational surrogacy: a systematic review. Reprod Biomed Online. 2016;32(1):54–61.
9. Beski S, Gorgy A, Venkat G, Craft IL, Edmonds K. Gestational surrogacy: a feasible option for patients with Rokitansky syndrome. Hum Reprod. 2000;15(11):2326–8.
10. Brännström M, Johannesson L, Bokström H, Kvarnström N, Mölne J, Dahm-Kähler P, et al. Livebirth after uterus transplantation. Lancet. 2015;385(9968):607–16.
11. Ozkan O, Akar ME, Ozkan O, Erdogan O, Hadimioglu N, Yilmaz M, et al. Preliminary results of the first human uterus transplantation from a multiorgan donor. Fertil Steril. 2013;99(2):470–6.
12. Chmel R, Novackova M, Pastor Z, Fronek J. The interest of women with Mayer–Rokitansky–Küster–Hauser syndrome and laparoscopic Vecchietti neovagina in uterus transplantation. J Pediatr Adolesc Gynecol. 2018;31(5):480–4.

13. Sanfilippo JS, Pokorny SF, Reindollar RH. Pediatric and adolescent gynecology. Curr Probl Obstet Gynecol Fertil. 1990;13:183–222.

14. Mansouri R, Dietrich JE. Postoperative course and complications after pull-through vaginoplaasty for distal vaginal atresia. J Pediatr Adolesc Gynecol. 2015;28(6):433–6.

15. Emans SJ, Laufer MR. Emans, Laufer, Goldstein's pediatric and adolescent gynecology. Philadelphia: Lippincott Williams & Wilkins; 2011.

16. Edmonds DK, Rose GL, Lipton MG, Quek J. Mayer-Rokitansky-Küster-Hauser syndrome: a review of 245 consecutive cases managed by a multidisciplinary approach with vaginal dilators. Fertil Steril. 2012;97(3):686–90.

17. Routh JC, Laufer MR, Cannon GM, Diamond DA, Gargollo PC. Management strategies for Mayer-Rokitansky-Kuster-Hauser related vaginal agenesis: a cost-effectiveness analysis. J Urol. 2010;184(5):2116–22.

18. Frank RT. The formation of an artificial vagina without operation. Am J Obstet Gynecol. 1938;35(6):1053–5.

19. Ingram JM. The bicycle seat stool in the treatment of vaginal agenesis and stenosis: a preliminary report. Am J Obstet Gynecol. 1981;140(8):867–73.

20. Roberts CP, Haber MJ, Rock JA. Vaginal creation for Müllerian agenesis. Am J Obstet Gynecol. 2001;185(6):1349–53.

21. Moen MH. Vaginal agenesis treated by coital dilatation in 20 patients. Int J Gynecol Obstet. 2014;3(125):282–3.

22. Cheikhelard A, Bidet M, Baptiste A, Viaud M, Fagot C, Khen-Dunlop N, Louis-Sylvestre C, Sarnacki S, Touraine P, Elie C, et al. Surgery is not superior to dilation for the management of vaginal agenesis in Mayer-Rokitansky-Küster-Hauser syndrome: A multicenter comparative observational study in 131 patients. Am. J. Obstet. Gynecol. 2018;219:281.e1–281.e9

23. Burgu B, Duffy PG, Cuckow P, Ransley P, Wilcox DT. Long-term outcome of vaginal reconstruction: comparing techniques and timing. J Pediatr Urol. 2007;3(4):316–20.

24. Duckler L. Squamous cell carcinoma developing in an artificial vagina. Obstet Gynecol. 1972;40(1):35–8.

25. McIndoe AH, Banister JB. An operation for the cure of congenital absence of the vagina. BJOG: Int J Obstet Gynaecol. 1938;45(3):490–4.

26. Baggish MS, Karram MM. Atlas of pelvic anatomy and gynecologic surgery. 4th ed. Philadelphia: Elsevier Inc; 2016. p. 779–98.

27. Lin WC, Chang CYY, Shen YY, Tsai HD. Use of autologous buccal mucosa for vaginoplasty: a study of eight cases. Hum Reprod. 2003;18(3):604–7.

28. Chan JL, Levin PJ, Ford BP, Stanton DC, Pfeifer SM. Vaginoplasty with an autologous buccal mucosa fenestrated graft in two patients with vaginal agenesis: a multidisciplinary approach and literature review. J Minim Invasive Gynecol. 2017;24(4):670–6.

29. Ashworth MF, Morton KE, Dewhurst J, Lilford RJ, Bates RG. Vaginoplasty using amnion. Obstet Gynecol. 1986;67(443).

30. Morton KE, Dewhurst CJ. Human amnion in the treatment of vaginal malformations. BJOG: Int J Obstet Gynaecol. 1986;93(1):50–4.

31. Vatsa R, Bharti J, Roy KK, Kumar S, Sharma JB, Singh N, et al. Evaluation of amnion in creation of neovagina in women with Mayer-Rokitansky-Kuster-Hauser syndrome. Fertil Steril. 2017;108(2):341–5.

32. Motoyama S, Laoag-Fernandez JB, Mochizuki S, Yamabe S, Maruo T. Vaginoplasty with Interceed absorbable adhesion barrier for complete squamous epithelialization in vaginal agenesis. Am J Obstet Gynecol. 2003;188(5):1260–4.

33. Jackson ND, Rosenblatt PL. Use of interceed absorbable adhesion barrier for vaginoplasty. Obstet Gynecol. 1994;84(6):1048–50.

34. Noguchi S, Nakatsuka M, Sugiyama Y, Chekir C, Kamada Y, Hiramatsu Y. Use of artificial dermis and recombinant basic fibroblast growth factor for creating a neovagina in a patient with Mayer-Rokitansky-Küster-Hauser syndrome. Hum Reprod. 2004;19(7):1629–32.

35. Miller RJ, Breech LL. Surgical correction of vaginal anomalies. Clin Obstet Gynecol. 2008;51(2):223–36.

36. Davydov SN, Zhvitiashvili OD. Formation of vagina (colpopoiesis) from peritoneum of Douglas pouch. Acta Chir Plast. 1974;16(1):35–41.

37. Dargent D, Marchiol P, Giannesi A, Benchaïb M, Chevret-Masson M, Mathevet P. Laparoscopic Davydov or laparoscopic transposition of the peritoneal colpopoeisis described by Davydov for the treatment of congenital vaginal agenesis: the technique and its evolution. Gynecol Obstet Fertil. 2004;32(12):1023–30.

38. Herlin M, Bay Bjørn AM, Jørgensen LK, Trolle B, Petersen MB. Treatment of vaginal agenesis in Mayer-Rokitansky-Küster-Hauser syndrome in Denmark: a nationwide comparative study of anatomical outcome and complications. Fertil Steril. 2018;110(4):746–53.

39. Ward G, Panda S, Anwar K. Davydov's colpopoeisis: vaginal construction using peritoneum. Curr Obstet Gynaecol. 1998;8(4):224–6.

40. de Sousa Marques H, dos Santos FL, Lopes-Costa PV, dos Santos AR, da Silva BB. Creation of a neovagina in patients with Rokitansky syndrome using peritoneum from the pouch of Douglas: an analysis of 48 cases. Fertil Steril. 2008;90(3):827–32.

41. Borruto F, Chasen ST, Chervenak FA, Fedele L. The Vecchietti procedure for surgical treatment of vaginal agenesis: comparison of laparoscopy and laparotomy. Int J Gynecol Obstet. 1999;64(2):153–8.

42. Borruto F, Camoglio FS, Zampieri N, Fedele L. The laparoscopic Vecchietti technique for vaginal agenesis. Int J Gynecol Obstet. 2007;98(1):15–9.

43. Brucker SY, Gegusch M, Zubke W, Rall K, Gauwerky JF, Wallwiener D. Neovagina creation in vaginal agenesis: development of a new laparoscopic Vecchietti-based procedure and optimized instruments in a

prospective comparative interventional study in 101 patients. Fertil Steril. 2008;90(5):1940–52.

44. Veronikis DK, McClure GB, Nichols DH. The Vecchietti operation for constructing a neovagina: indications, instrumentation, and techniques. Obstet Gynecol. 1997;90(2):301–4.

45. El Saman AM. Retropubic balloon vaginoplasty for management of Mayer-Rokitansky-Küster-Hauser syndrome. Fertil Steril. 2010;93(6):2016–9.

46. Baldwin JF. The formation of an artificial vagina by intestinal transplantation. Ann Surg. 1904;40(3):398–403.

47. Karateke A, Haliloglu B, Parlak O, Cam C, Coksuer H. Intestinal vaginoplasty: seven years' experience of a tertiary center. Fertil Steril. 2010;94(6):2312–5.

48. Carrard C, Chevret-Measson M, Lunel A, Raudrant D. Sexuality after sigmoid vaginoplasty in patients with Mayer-Rokitansky- Küster-Hauser syndrome. Fertil Steril. 2012;97(3):691–6.

49. Williams EA. Congenital absence of the vagina: a simple operation for its relief. J Obstet Gynaecol Br Commonw. 1964;71(4):511–6.

50. Williams EA. Congenital absence of the vagina. BJOG: Int J Obstet Gynaecol. 1972.

51. Creatsas G, Deligeoroglou E, Christopoulos P. Creation of a neovagina after Creatsas modification of Williams vaginoplasty for the treatment of 200 patients with Mayer-Rokitansky-Kuster- Hauser syndrome. Fertil Steril. 2010;94(5):1848–52.

52. Buss JG, Lee RA. McIndoe procedure for vaginal agenesis: results and complications. Mayo Clin Proc. 1989;64:758–61.

53. Højsgaard A, Villadsen I. McIndoe procedure for congenital vaginal agenesis : complications and results. Br J Plast Surg. 1995;48(2):97–102.

54. Klingele CJ, Gebhart JB, Croak AJ, DiMarco CS, Lesnick TG, Lee RA, et al. McIndoe procedure for vaginal agenesis: long-term outcome and effect on quality of life. Am J Obstet Gynecol. 2003;189(6):1569–72.

55. Willemsen WNP, Kluivers KB. Long-term results of vaginal construction with the use of Frank dilation and a peritoneal graft (Davydov procedure) in patients with Mayer-Rokitansky-Küster syndrome. Fertil Steril. 2015;103(1):220–7.

56. Allen LM, Lucco KL, Brown CM, Spitzer RF, Kives S. Psychosexual and functional outcomes after cre-ation of a neovagina with laparoscopic Davydov in patients with vaginal agenesis. Fertil Steril. 2010;94(6):2272–6.

57. Giannesi A, Marchiole P, Benchaib M, Chevret-Measson M, Mathevet P, Dargent D. Sexuality after laparoscopic Davydov in patients affected by congenital complete vaginal agenesis associated with uterine agenesis or hypoplasia. Hum Reprod. 2005;20(10):2954–7.

58. Rall K, Wallwiener D, Brucker S. Laparoscopic-assisted methods for neovaginoplasty. Sex Reprod Menopause. 2010;8(3):15–20.

59. Communal PH, Chevret-Measson M, Golfier F, Raudrant D. Sexuality after sigmoid colpopoiesis in patients with Mayer-Rokitansky-Kuster-Hauser syndrome. Fertil Steril. 2003;80(3):600–6.

60. Hensle TW, Shabsigh A, Shabsigh R, Reiley EA, Meyer-Bahlburg HFL. Sexual function following bowel vaginoplasty. J Urol. 2006;175(6):2283–6.

61. Nowier A, Esmat M, Hamza RT. Surgical and functional outcomes of sigmoid vaginoplasty among patients with variants of disorders of sex development. Int Braz J Urol. 2012;38(3):380–8.

62. Parsons JK, Gearhart SL, Gearhart JP. Vaginal reconstruction utilizing sigmoid colon: complications and long-term results. J Pediatr Surg. 2002;37(4):629–33.

63. Creatsas G, Deligeoroglou E. Creatsas modification of Williams vaginoplasty for reconstruction of the vaginal aplasia in Mayer-Rokitansky-Küster-Hauser syndrome cases. Womens Health. 2010;6(3):367–75.

64. CDC. HPV I Who should get vaccine I Human papillomavirus I CDC. Webpage. 2016.

65. Curry SJ, Krist AH, Owens DK, Barry MJ, Caughey AB, Davidson KW, et al. Screening for cervical cancer us preventive services task force recommendation statement. JAMA - J Am Med Assoc. 2018;320(7):674–86.

66. Workowski KA, Bolan GA. Sexually transmitted diseases treatment guidelines, 2015. MMWR Recomm Rep. 2015;64(RR-03):1.

67. Rackow B, Lobo R, Lentz G, Valea F. Chapter 11: Congenital abnormalities of the female reproductive tract: anomalies of the vagina, cervix, uterus and adnexa. In: Comprehensive gynecology. 7th ed. Philadelphia: Elsevier Publishing; 2017. p. 205–18.

Overcoming the Challenging Cervix

Pietro Bortoletto and Rony T. Elias

Access to the uterine cavity is a prerequisite for the reproductive surgeon. However, ready access can be obstructed by various iatrogenic and cervical pathologies. Within this chapter, we will review the structure and function of the cervix, discuss cervical pathology, and review management options for the challenging cervix.

Development

By approximately the 6–7th week after fertilization, the paired Müllerian ducts fuse to form the early precursors to the uterus, cervix, and upper third of the vagina. However, it is not until between the 13th and 15th week of gestation that endocervical glands begin to form the early rudimentary cervix. The canal of the cervix is lined by glandular columnar epithelium and transitions to squamous epithelium near the vagina. With advancing age, the demarcation line (the squamocolumnar junction) regresses from well beyond the external os in childhood & adolescence to higher in the cervical canal in menopausal women. The columnar epithelium is notably responsive to estrogen and progesterone

P. Bortoletto (✉) · R. T. Elias
The Ronald O. Perelman and Claudia Cohen Center for Reproductive Medicine, Weill Cornell Medical Center, New York, NY, USA
e-mail: rta9002@med.cornell.edu

and is capable of producing a watery, alkaline discharge or thick, acidic mucus, respectively. Additionally, the cervix contains stroma, elastic tissue, and smooth muscle fibers which aid in its reproductive function during childbirth.

At birth, the cervix is twice the length of the uterine body and by the time of the first menstruation the cervix is approximately 1/2 to 1/3 the length of the uterus and can measure up to 5 cm in length. The visible portion of the cervix on exam is known as the *portio vaginalis* and the portion not visible, or the intraabdominal cervix, is known as the supravaginal cervix. The cervix is supported by bilateral uterosacral ligaments and cardinal ligaments and receives its autonomic innervation from the terminal portion of the presacral plexus to form two lateral semicircular plexuses entering from the upper vagina known as the Frankenhauser plexus. The blood supply to the cervix is from the descending branches of the uterine artery and lymphatic drainage extends to the parametria followed by obturator, common iliac, and para-aortic lymph nodes [1].

Failure of appropriate Müllerian duct development may result in cervical anomalies ranging from agenesis to duplications. Cervical agenesis is categorized by the absence of not only the cervix but also the upper vagina given its shared embryologic origin. If the cervix is hypoplastic, the amount visible on exam or imaging can be quite variable however, the upper vagina can be normal. The diagnosis of both cervical hypoplasia and agenesis are often made peri-menarche with teens presenting with primary amenorrhea and cyclic abdominal pain. Pelvic or abdominal ultrasonography and magnetic resonance imaging are essential for accurate diagnosis ahead of any surgical intervention.

In cases where Müllerian ducts fail to fuse appropriately, the cervix may appear to be fused or may appear as two distinct cervices. Classically, the duplicated, two distinct cervix scenario is also accompanied by a duplicated uterus, but not always. The duplication can also arise from a longitudinal uterine septum and careful thought should be taken to differentiate between both prior to any surgical intervention. Surgical intervention is indicated in symptomatic patients with an obstructive lesion from either or both cervices.

Cervical Pathology

By nature of its various structural components, the cervix is able to manifest a wide variety of benign and malignant pathologies. Perhaps the most common benign finding is the Nabothian cyst, or mucinous retention cyst. Nabothian cysts are largely asymptomatic cystic structures that arise from plugged columnar epithelial clefts. While they are usually quite small, they may be dilated to be several centimeters in size. A variant, the mesonephric cyst (remnant of Wolffian ducts within the cervix), may also be encountered and often presents as small Nabothian cyst-like structures and can be managed in a similar fashion. Surgical management is only indicated in cases of vaginal pain, fullness, or if the large cyst interferes with cervical procedures such as endometrial biopsy, intrauterine insemination or embryo transfer. Hysteroscopic, vaginal and laparoscopic approaches have been reported using both excision and ablative techniques [2–4].

Other common benign cervical pathologies that may require advanced surgical intervention include cervical endometriosis, polyps, and fibroids. Superficial endometriosis of the cervix has been reported in reproductive aged women and often masquerades as premalignant or malignant glandular lesions. When encountered, it is typically confined within the superficial aspects of the cervix and amenable to resection and or electrosurgery ablation if patients report dyspareunia, bleeding, or pelvic pain [5]. Cervical polyps usually present with mid cycle or poscoital bleeding and in most cases can be safely managed in an office setting. More commonly they are identified as an incidental finding during the annual gynecologic exam and expectant management is reasonable. Cervical fibroids typically present concurrently with uterine fibroids and can often present as pedunculated uterine fibroids prolapsing out through the cervix. While they are not readily seen on visual inspection, a bimanual exam may reveal areas of tenderness or bulk within the cervical stroma. Vaginal excision is indicated when symptoms are present or if the leiomyoma obstructs routine care such as cervical cytology screening or reproductive procedures. Removal of large cervical fibroids can be complicated due to proximity to bladder, rectum, and ureter. As such, sometimes a laparoscopic approach is utilized to safely develop retroperitoneal spaces and minimize surgical morbidity [6].

Cervical Stenosis

Cervical stenosis is another common benign cervical pathology that is often encountered by reproductive surgeons. Cervical stenosis, defined as a narrowing of the canal preventing insertion of a 2.5 mm dilator, can be multifactorial, resulting from ablative or excisional cervical procedures, prolonged hypoestrogenic milieu such as menopause, infection, and nulliparity. Typically, these patients present with amenorrhea, pelvic pain, and/or infertility but can often be diagnosed during collection of a cervical or uterine specimen in the office. Pelvic sonogram often reveals hematometra or fluid behind the area of stenosis, within the uterine cavity. Bettochi et al. have proposed a classification system for cervical stenosis based on the localization of stenosis as follows: stenosis of external cervical ostium (ECO; type I); stenosis of distal third of cervical canal and the internal cervical ostium (ICO; type II);

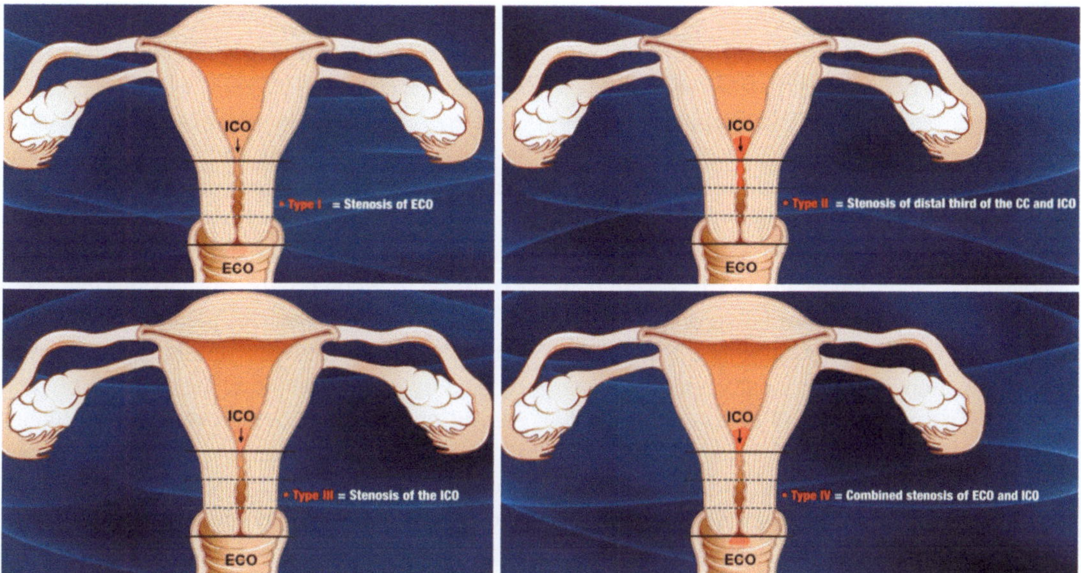

Fig. 3.1 Bettochi et al. classification system for cervical stenosis

stenosis of the ICO (type III), and combined stenosis of ECO and ICO (type IV) [7] (see Fig. 3.1).

Preoperative Management

The management of cervical stenosis depends on the clinical scenario. In the case of women whose pap smear, endometrial biopsy, or hysteroscopy are complicated by the stenosis, pre-treatment with vaginal misoprostol or vaginal estrogen is recommended. Typically 200–400 mcg of vaginal misoprostol 12–24 h prior to procedure has been shown to facilitate cervical dilation while minimizing lacerations or false tracks [8]. Rectal administration is associated with slower time to onset while sublingual administration may afford fastest onset time. Intracervical laminaria dilators, which work via osmosis-induced dilation, have also been shown to be effective alternatives to vaginal misoprostol but require an additional office visit, cost, and discomfort [9–11]. In postmenopausal women, the addition of 25 mcg vaginal estradiol daily for 14 days to vaginal misoprostol is often utilized in cases where a hypoestrogenic source of stenosis is suspected [12]. Mifepristone, an antiprogesterone, pre-treatment 48 h ahead of dilation & curettage in postmenopausal women has been shown to increase mean preoperative dilation and decrease the subjective amount of force required to dilate the cervical canal [13].

Intraoperative Management

Cervical stenosis is encountered in approximately 10% of postmenopausal women undergoing outpatient hysteroscopy and 6% of women after a loop electrocautery excision procedure [14, 15]. For patients whose cervical stenosis is diagnosed intraoperatively, several technical options are available to facilitate safe dilation. First, a "no touch" vaginoscopy technique has shown to be useful in identifying the pinpoint/invisible external cervical os when location of the os is in question due to the enhanced digital magnification afforded by the hysteroscope [16]. Second, ensure adequate analgesia as further and more invasive surgical manipulation is forthcoming. While most women are able to tolerate biopsy and pap smear without analgesia, diagnostic and operative hysteroscopy frequently require paracervical blocks or IV sedation. In post-menopausal women, the use of a 3.5 mm hysteroscope without anesthesia was associated with significantly less pain than those undergoing hysteroscopy with a 5 mm hysteroscopy, despite use of a paracervical block [14]. However, when stenosis is encountered intraoperatively or expected preoperatively, and the patient is not anesthetized, we recommend the addition of a paracervical block as they have been shown to decrease pain with dilation, pain with uterine interventions, and reduces the risk of severe pain [17]. Paracervical block can be accomplished by injecting 10 cc of 1% lidocaine into the 8 and 4 o'clock position of the cervical vaginal junction using a spinal needle. In all cases, we strongly recommend the concomitant use of transvaginal and/or abdominal ultrasound with back-filled bladder by an experienced assistant to help guide the cervical dilators.

With appropriate analgesia, several additional interventions can be considered. First, lacrimal dilators, utilized for lacrimal duct dilation by ophthalmologists, can often be requested and come in sizes as small as 0.5 mm. The dilators, when used serially, may help to facilitate initial cannulation of the stenosed external os but also run the risk of creating false tracts and perforation if not used judiciously. Their use with intraoperative transabdominal ultrasound may help to lessen this risk as the operator can receive real-time guidance. A full bladder, or retrograde bladder distention, is essential for optimal visualization of the lower uterine segment. Infiltration of the cervix with sterile saline or water may help to further delineate the cervical canal when ultrasound guidance is being utilized. Lindheim et al. have reported on the use of a 5.7F coaxial catheter with an outer echogenic sheath and inter guidewire with coude tip that can be utilized under ultrasound guidance to gain entry to the uterine cavity [18]. When these dilators or instruments are not available, one can consider the use of the single tip of an Adson surgical forceps, with progression to both tips, and eventually gentle spreading to delineate the external cervical os. A disposable skin biopsy punch has also been reported for recanalization in patients with external cervical occlusion after conization procedures [19]. Lastly, surgical devices such as the Definity by Hologic have been brought to market to facilitate cannulation of stenotic or tortuous cervices by utilizing a ballon to slowly distend the cervix.

If these maneuvers prove successful, more invasive incisional and excisional procedures can be explored. A cruciate incision at the level of the external os using an 11-blade may facilitate the opening of a distal stenotic site. The expulsion of blood products or mucous can often be indicators of successful identification of the cervical canal. This can similarly be accomplished by hysteroscopic scissors in a slow and careful manner. In extreme cases, where cannulation is absolutely necessary, excisional options such as a conization or even loop electrocautery excision procedure may be considered. Laser vaporization of scar tissue using a CO_2 laser has also been described in symptomatic cervical stenosis following excisional cervical procedures but requires specialized training and machinery for unexpected intraoperative use [20]. Finally, a hysteroscopic morcellator technique has been described to where you both shave and remove tissue within the cervical canal to gain entry to the uterine cavity [21].

Post-procedure Prevention Strategies

There are several post-procedure interventions that have been described to avoid re-stenosis of the cervix and to facilitate further transcervical procedures. In 1990, Luesley et al. developed a high-density plastic disposable stent that was hollow funnel in shape and fit into the cervical canal [22]. Their study of 33 patients with a history of cold knife conization treated with this novel stent for 14 days demonstrated a stenosis rate of 6% at 6-month follow-up. Grund et al. have described the use of a self-expanding, nitinol-coated stent, typically used for the stenting of large blood vessels, in a patient with recurrent cervical stenosis from conization procedure. The stent was left in place for 9 months to allow for normal menstruation. Two months after the removal of the stent, the patient became spontaneously pregnant [23]. Polyurethane-covered tracheobronchial stents (Alveolus, Inc., Charlotte, NC), used in stenting of large airways, have been described in the management of patients with Müllerian anomalies, cervical stenosis, and vaginal agenesis as have the use of a Petit-Le Four tube, a silver-plated tube used primarily in Europe in the 1960s, post-trachelectomy [24, 25]. Recently, Nasu et al. have described the use of an intrauterine device tied up with nylon threads for treatment of cervical stenosis after conization in symptomatic patients. Using a commercially available intrauterine device (Multiload Cu 250, Multilan AG, Dublin, Ireland) they tied up with three 3–0 nylon threads to the existing nylon thread and left the device in-situ for 3 months prior to removal with complete relief of symptoms and no evidence of long-term restenosis [26]. Lastly, post-procedure placement of around 2 cm of intercede (Interceed; Gynecare, Ethicon, Somerville, NJ), an absorbable adhesion barrier, in the cervical canal has also been described as a successful re-stenosis prevention strategy [27]. Regardless of what kind of transcervical device is used, the concern for infection exists with any prolonged indwelling device and those that artificially keep the cervix patent, potentiating an ascending infection. Care should be given to patient selection, duration of treatment, and antibiotic prophylaxis when considering any of these novel interventions.

Post-procedure Medical Management

An additional consideration for the management of the challenging cervix is the promotion of regular menstruation. The regular egress of blood products through a cervix is thought to help minimize early adhesion formation following surgical intervention and to help proliferation of the cervical lining. Additionally, regular menses provides additional reassurance to patients and clinicians alike that the canal is patent to some degree. The conversion from regular menses to scant or absent menses should be an early warning sign of cervical re-stenosis, warranting further investigation. In the immediate postoperative period after an

initial cervical procedure with risk for stenosis, the use of oral or transdermal estrogens can be considered to avoid a hypoestrogenic environment followed by a progesterone-induced withdrawal bleed to ensure early canal patency.

Cervical Stenosis in the Infertile Population

Management of stenosis in patients undergoing ART procedures poses new and unique challenges. Abusheikha et al. retrospectively reviewed their experience of 57 patients with a history of previous failed embryo transfer attempts whose transfer was classified as "difficult" [28]. In the GnRH agonist downregulation phase of an upcoming stimulation cycle, they performed cervical dilation under general anesthesia and found that 31.6% of women achieved a clinical pregnancy in their subsequent cycle and two-thirds of women had their subsequent transfer rated as "easy". Higher pregnancy rates were reported when the transfer was rated as "easy" compared to difficult (40 versus 11.8%).

Groutz et al. and Visser et al. have previously described a strategy of cervical dilation performed under anesthesia at the time of transvaginal oocyte retrieval, 48 h prior to embryo transfer [29, 30]. Unfortunately, both studies reported exceedingly low implantation rates and the authors have speculated that trauma to the endometrial lining and presence of blood may be to blame. The use of laminaria tents 24 h prior to embryo transfer has also been reported by others [31].

When attempts at dilation and pre-treatment have failed, groups have attempted transmyometrial transfer of embryos to bypass cervical stenosis. Kato et al. reported on ultrasound-guided transmyometrial puncture for embryo transfer in 104 patients with a history of difficult transfers due to cervical abnormalities [32]. Thirty-eight patients conceived for a clinical pregnancy rate of 36.5% per attempt. However, similar studies comparing to transcervical transfer in patients with cervical stenosis or in patients with at least three fresh transfers have failed to show benefit to the transmyometrial approach [33].

Noyes et al. described a technique of hysteroscopic shaving of the cervical canal of a patient with extremely tortuous cervix and challenging embryo transfer [34]. Following hysteroscopic shaving, an intrauterine foley balloon was placed for 14 days. Subsequent embryo transfers were noted to be significantly easier and the patient went on to deliver at 36 weeks without evidence of cervical insufficiency. Placement of transcervical catheters and stents has also been described in various case reports and series. Since then, commercially available catheters and stents have been used and reported on. Yanushpolsky et al. described the placement of a transcervical Malecot catheter for an average of 10 days following hysteroscopic evaluation and/or correction of the endocervix [35]. They reported that in 32 out of the 36 patients treated, subsequent intrauterine inseminations, embryo transfers, or endometrial biopsies were significantly easier after treatment with the Malecot catheter.

Conclusion

A patent cervical canal is essential for normal physiologic function as well as for reproductive procedures that require access to the uterus. Given its unique composition and function, the cervix can be the source of both benign and malignant pathologies that may result in a "challenging cervix" for both patients and clinicians. Restoring access to the uterus requires a thoughtful approach that draws from a mixture of evidence-based and novel strategies. Preoperative planning is essential when the diagnosis is known; however, there are multiple intraoperative steps that can be taken to facilitate completion of the planned procedure. More attention and research are needed to stenosis prevention strategies to minimize surgical and reproductive morbidity from cervical pathology and treatment.

References

1. Jones HW, Rock JA. Te Linde's operative gynecology. 10th ed. Philadelphia: Wolters Kluwer; 2015.
2. Chen F, Duan H, Zhang Y, Liu Y, Wang X, Guo Y. A giant nabothian cyst with massive abnormal uterine bleeding: a case report. Clin Exp Obstet Gynecol. 2017;44(2):326–8.
3. Frega A, Verrone A, Schimberni M, Manzara F, Ralli E, Catalano A, et al. Feasibility of office CO2 laser surgery in patients affected by benign pathologies and congenital malformations of female lower genital tract. Eur Rev Med Pharmacol Sci. 2015;19(14):2528–36.
4. Vural F, Sanverdi I, Coskun ADE, Kusgöz A, Temel O. Large nabothian cyst obstructing labour passage. J Clin Diagn Res. 2015;9(10):QD06–7.
5. Baker PM, Clement PB, Bell DA, Young RH. Superficial endometriosis of the uterine cervix: a report of 20 cases of a process that may be confused with endocervical glandular dysplasia or adenocarcinoma in situ. Int J Gynecol Pathol. 1999;18(3):198–205.
6. Matsuoka S, Kikuchi I, Kitade M, Kumakiri J, Kuroda K, Tokita S, et al. Strategy for laparoscopic cervical myomectomy. J Minim Invasive Gynecol. 2010;17(3):301–5.
7. Bettocchi S, Bramante S, Bifulco G, Spinelli M, Ceci O, Fascilla FD, et al. Challenging the cervix: strategies to overcome the anatomic impediments to hysteroscopy: analysis of 31,052 office hysteroscopies. Fertil Steril. 2016;105(5):e16–7.
8. Al-Fozan H, Firwana B, Al Kadri H, Hassan S, Tulandi T. Preoperative ripening of the cervix before operative hysteroscopy. Cochrane Database Syst Rev. 2015;(4):CD005998.
9. Darwish AM, Ahmad AM, Mohammad AM. Cervical priming prior to operative hysteroscopy: a randomized comparison of laminaria versus misoprostol. Hum Reprod. 2004;19(10):2391–4.
10. Karakus S, Akkar OB, Yildiz C, Yenicesu GI, Cetin M, Cetin A. Comparison of effectiveness of laminaria versus vaginal misoprostol for cervical preparation before operative hysteroscopy in women of reproductive age: a prospective randomized trial. J Minim Invasive Gynecol. 2016;23(1):46–52.
11. Lin Y-H, Hwang J-L, Seow K-M, Huang L-W, Chen H-J, Hsieh B-C. Laminaria tent vs misoprostol for cervical priming before hysteroscopy: randomized study. J Minim Invasive Gynecol. 2009;16(6):708–12.
12. Oppegaard KS, Lieng M, Berg A, Istre O, Qvigstad E, Nesheim B-I. A combination of misoprostol and estradiol for preoperative cervical ripening in postmenopausal women: a randomised controlled trial. BJOG Int J Obstet Gynaecol. 2010;117(1):53–61.
13. Gupta JK, Johnson N. Effect of mifepristone on dilatation of the pregnant and non-pregnant cervix. Lancet. 1990;335(8700):1238–40.
14. Giorda G, Scarabelli C, Franceschi S, Campagnutta E. Feasibility and pain control in outpatient hysteroscopy in postmenopausal women: a randomized trial. Acta Obstet Gynecol Scand. 2000;79(7):593–7.
15. Suh-Burgmann EJ, Whall-Strojwas D, Chang Y, Hundley D, Goodman A. Risk factors for cervical

stenosis after loop electrocautery excision procedure. Obstet Gynecol. 2000;96(5 Pt 1):657–60.

16. Di Spiezio SA, Giampaolino P, Manzi A, De Angelis MC, Zizolfi B, Alonso L, et al. The invisible external cervical os. Tips and tricks to overcome this challenge during in-office hysteroscopy. J Minim Invasive Gynecol. 2021;28(2):172–3.

17. Tangsiriwatthana T, Sangkomkamhang US, Lumbiganon P, Laopaiboon M. Paracervical local anaesthesia for cervical dilatation and uterine intervention. Cochrane Database Syst Rev. 2013;(9):CD005056.

18. Lindheim SR. Echosight patton coaxial catheter-guided hysteroscopy. J Am Assoc Gynecol Laparosc. 2001;8(2):307–11.

19. Funada R, Adachi K, Yamamoto Y, Nakamichi I. Usefulness of disposable skin biopsy punch for cervical occlusion after cervical conization. Gynecol Minim Invasive Ther. 2020;9(2):95–7.

20. Luesley DM, Williams DR, Gee H, Chan KK, Jordan JA. Management of postconization cervical stenosis by laser vaporization. Obstet Gynecol. 1986;67(1):126–8.

21. Salari BW, Bhagavath B, Galloway ML, Findley AD, Yaklic JL, Lindheim SR. Hysteroscopic morcellator to overcome cervical stenosis. Fertil Steril. 2016;106(6):e12–3. https://doi.org/10.1016/j.fertnstert.2016.07.1091. Epub 2016 Aug 16. PMID: 27542706.

22. Luesley DM, Redman CWE, Buxton EJ, Lawton FG, Williams DR. Prevention of post-cone biopsy cervical stenosis using a temporary cervical stent. BJOG Int J Obstet Gynaecol. 1990;97(4):334–7.

23. Grund D, Köhler C, Krauel H, Schneider A. A new approach to preserve fertility by using a coated nitinol stent in a patient with recurrent cervical stenosis. Fertil Steril. 2007;87(5):1212.e13–6.

24. Babayev SN, Reed B, Wilson EE. Novel use of tracheobronchial stents in cervical stenosis and mullerian anomalies. Fertil Steril. 2015;104(3):e180–1.

25. Palaia I, Perniola G, Arrivi C, Sansone M, Pastore M, Calcagno M, et al. Persistent posttrachelectomy cervical stenosis treated with Petit-Le Four pessary in early cervical cancer patients: a report of two cases. Fertil Steril. 2007;88(6):1677.e5–7.

26. Nasu K, Narahara H. Management of severe cervical stenosis after conization by detention of nylon threads tied up to intrauterine contraceptive device. Arch Gynecol Obstet. 2010;281(5):887–9.

27. Gudipudi D, Montemarano N, Priore GD. Alternative approaches to cervical stenosis. Fertil Steril. 2007;88(3):763–4.

28. Abusheikha N, Lass A, Burnley A, Brinsden P. In vitro fertilization cycles converted to intrauterine insemination because of poor follicular response have low success rates. Fertil Steril. 2001;75(3):634–5.

29. Visser DS, Fourie FL, Kruger HF. Multiple attempts at embryo transfer: effect on pregnancy outcome in an in vitro fertilization and embryo transfer program. J Assist Reprod Genet. 1993;10(1):37–43.

30. Groutz A, Lessing JB, Wolf Y, Yovel I, Azem F, Amit A. Cervical dilatation during ovum pick-up in patients with cervical stenosis: effect on pregnancy outcome in an in vitro fertilization-embryo transfer program. Fertil Steril. 1997;67(5):909–11.

31. Glatstein IZ, Pang SC, McShane PM. Successful pregnancies with the use of laminaria tents before embryo transfer for refractory cervical stenosis. Fertil Steril. 1997;67(6):1172–4.

32. Kato O, Takatsuka R, Asch RH. Transvaginal-transmyometrial embryo transfer: the Towako method; experiences of 104 cases. Fertil Steril. 1993;59(1):51–3.

33. Groutz A, Lessing JB, Wolf Y, Azem F, Yovel I, Amit A. Comparison of transmyometrial and transcervical embryo transfer in patients with previously failed in vitro fertilization-embryo transfer cycles and/or cervical stenosis. Fertil Steril. 1997;67(6):1073–6.

34. Noyes N. Hysteroscopic cervical canal shaving: a new therapy for cervical stenosis before embryo transfer in patients undergoing in vitro fertilization. Fertil Steril. 1999;71(5):965–6.

35. Yanushpolsky EH, Ginsburg ES, Fox JH, Stewart EA. Transcervical placement of a Malecot catheter after hysteroscopic evaluation provides for easier entry into the endometrial cavity for women with histories of difficult intrauterine inseminations and/or embryo transfers: a prospective case series. Fertil Steril. 2000;73(2):402–5.

Septate Uterus: Diagnosis and Management

4

Phillip A. Romanski and Samantha M. Pfeifer

Objectives

- Describe the developmental formation of a uterine septum and review different variations that can occur
- Explain the classification systems used to define a uterine septum and the imaging modalities available to identify and diagnose this anomaly
- Discuss the literature evaluating the prevalence of this anomaly and the potential impact on reproductive outcomes
- Review the available methods and techniques used for uterine septum incision

Introduction

A septate uterus is a müllerian anomaly that is commonly encountered during an evaluation for infertility or adverse pregnancy outcome. This anomaly is the most common of the müllerian anomalies, though the true prevalence is unknown

Supplementary Information The online version contains supplementary material available at [https://doi.org/10.1007/978-3-031-05240-8_4].

P. A. Romanski · S. M. Pfeifer (✉)
The Ronald O. Perelman and Claudia Cohen Center for Reproductive Medicine, Weill Cornell Medical Center, New York, NY, USA
e-mail: par9114@med.cornell.edu;
SPfeifer@med.cornell.edu

because in many women, this anomaly is asymptomatic. Many aspects of the diagnosis and treatment of septate uteri are debated among experts including what defines a uterine septum, whether the septum causes abnormal reproductive outcomes, whether surgical treatment of the septum improves reproductive outcomes, and what technique is best for septum correction. In this chapter, these topics will be reviewed to provide a foundation for how to diagnose and manage patients with a uterine septum.

Development

A uterine septum occurs when there is incomplete uterine septum resorption during fetal development. In female fetuses, by the tenth week of gestation, the two müllerian ducts fuse in the midline to create a Y-shaped luminal structure that is destined to become the fallopian tubes, uterine cavity, cervical cavity, and upper third of the vagina [1]. The midline fusion creates a thick septum, composed of fibromuscular tissue, attached to the upper pole of the uterus which resolves by the twentieth week of gestation in normal development [2, 3].

Alternatively, the uterine septum will persist if resorption fails or is incomplete. There is great variability in the structure and appearance of septate uteri. This relates to the developmental stage of the uterus achieved during organogenesis prior to cessation of septum resorption. Developmental variations may be viewed as a continuum. The feature that distinguishes a uterine septum from other müllerian anomalies is the presence of a single fundus with normal external contour and internal fundal indentation. The etiology of this anomaly is not well understood and is most likely multifactorial. There are no consistently reported gene mutations or epigenetic alterations that lead to the formation of a uterine septum [3].

Septate uteri have been classified as either partial or complete. Partial septate uterus refers to a single outer uterine body with an indentation in the endometrial cavity. There is a spectrum of length and width that can occur ranging from a small internal indentation at the fundus to a thick septum from the fundus that extends down to the level of the external cervical os. A septum is considered partial if it extends towards but does not reach the internal cervical os (Fig. 4.1).

A complete septate uterus refers to a single external uterine cavity with an internal septum that extends through the cervical canal resulting in a septate cervix or duplicated cervices often seen in association with a longitudinal vaginal septum (Fig. 4.2). It is important to differentiate a

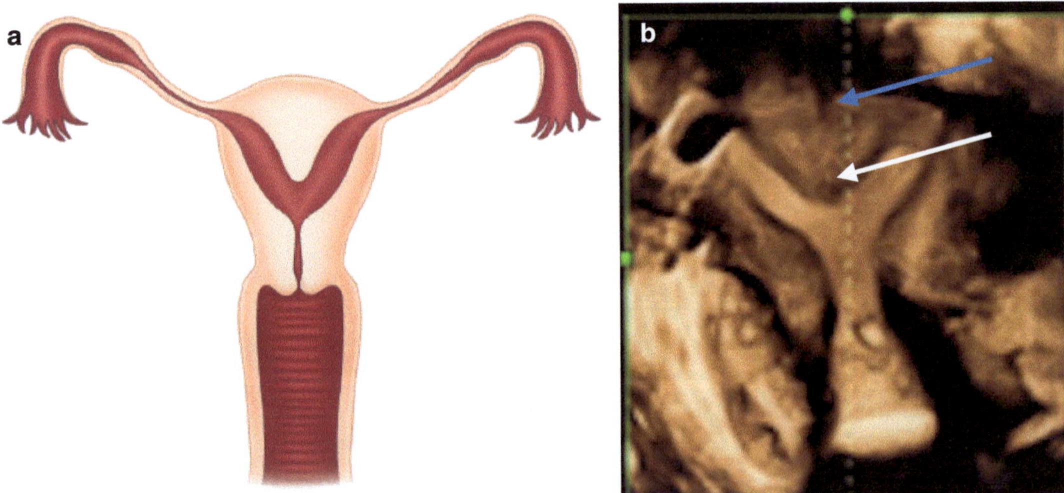

Fig. 4.1 Partial uterine septum. (**a**) Depiction of partial uterine septum. (**b**) 3D ultrasound image of partial uterine septum (Blue arrow: Normal fundal uterine contour) (White arrow: Partial uterine septum)

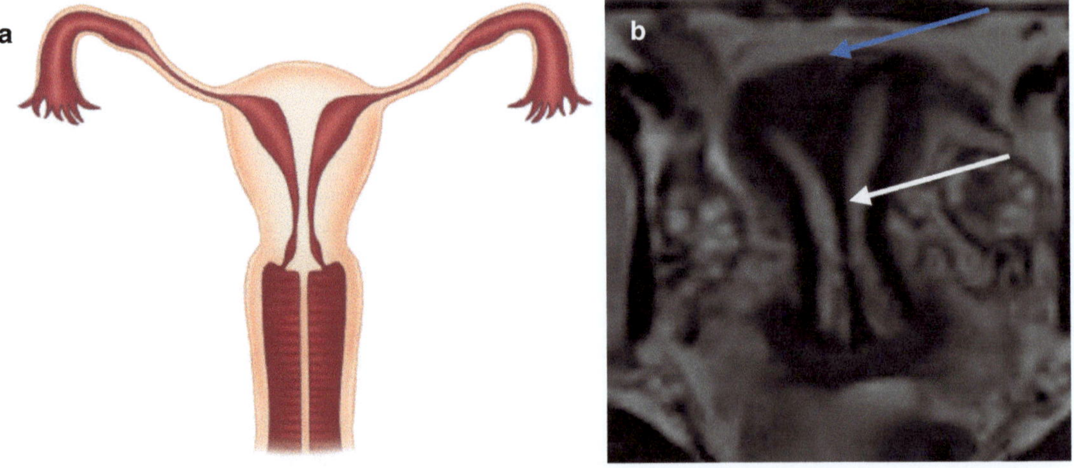

Fig. 4.2 Complete uterine septum. (**a**) Depiction of complete uterine septum. (**b**) MRI of complete uterine septum (Blue arrow: Normal fundal uterine contour) (White arrow: Complete uterine septum)

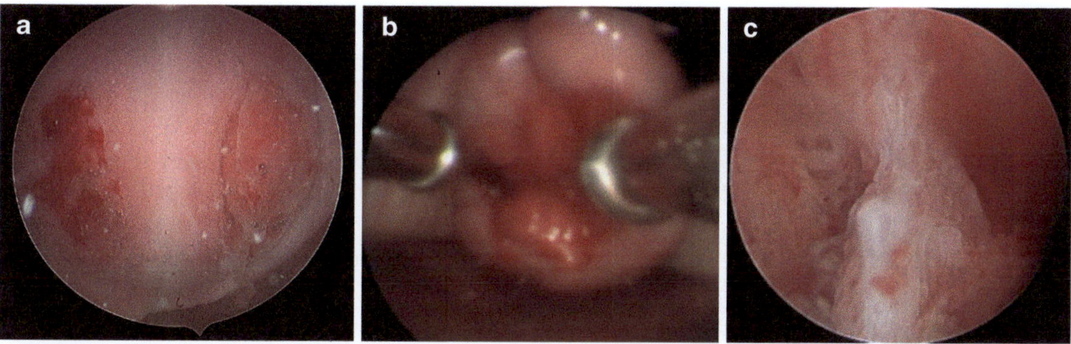

Fig. 4.3 (**a**) Cervical septum seen at vaginoscopy. (**b**) Cervical septum – dilator in each external os. (**c**) Cervical septum seen at hysteroscopy. Cervical mucosa easily identified. (Photos permission of Samantha Pfeifer MD)

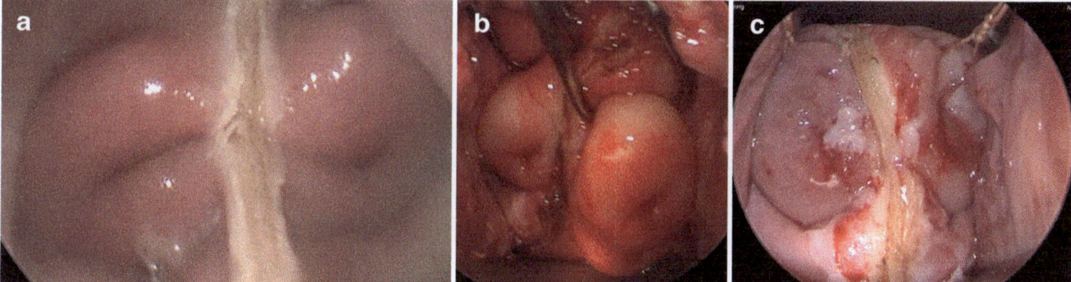

Fig. 4.4 (**a**) Two well-defined cervices see following resection of longitudinal vaginal septum. (**b**) Two separate cervices associated with complete septate uterus. Right cervix smaller and higher in vagina, left cervix larger and inferior. (**c**) Duplicated cervix showing placement of stitches on anterior lip of cervix for traction rather that Allis clamps. (Photos permission of Samantha Pfeifer MD)

cervical septum from a double cervix as surgical management may differ. A cervical septum appears as a single cervix or widened cervical body with a septum typically in the midline dividing the cervical canal into two parts (Fig. 4.3). In contrast, a double cervix has two distinct ectocervices which are separated by an intercervical cleft (Fig. 4.4) [4]. Both of these anomalies are often seen in combination with a longitudinal vaginal septum. A complete septum is also not always contiguous from fundus to cervix and may be observed to have been resorbed in the lower uterine segment creating a connection between the septum [5]. A complete septate uterus is often mistaken as a uterus didelphys by both clinicians and radiologists that are not familiar with the differences between these two anomalies.

When a uterine septum is identified, a thorough evaluation of the vagina, cervix, and fallopian tubes should be done to determine whether any additional anomalies are present. While other müllerian anomalies are associated with renal anomalies in 30% of cases, this association is not observed with septate uteri, and therefore a renal evaluation is not necessary in these patients [6, 7]. The structure of the septum has been demonstrated to be primarily muscle fibers and less fibrous tissue as assessed by MRI and biopsy specimens [8, 9].

The true prevalence of septate uteri in the general population is unknown because many patients with a uterine septum are asymptomatic and therefore never have this anomaly diagnosed. One study that evaluated uterine shape in nearly 700 patients at the time of tubal ligation followed by a hysterosalpingogram reported a prevalence of müllerian anomalies of 3.2% in women who desire sterilization [10]. Septate uteri are one of the more commonly identified müllerian anomalies, accounting for 35–90% of diagnosed anomalies [10, 11]. The prevalence of septate uteri is increased in patients with a history of miscarriage (5%) and in patients with a history of both miscarriage and infertility (15%) [12]. Current data do not support an association between septate uteri and primary infertility; however, it is associated with first- and second-trimester miscarriage [11]. It should be recognized that the observed prevalence varies widely between studies. This is both due to the baseline prevalence in the study population (i.e., general population, infertile population, recurrent miscarriage population) as well as the fact that multiple classification systems to define a uterine septum exist and the prevalence depends on which definition is utilized in the study design.

Classification

The variability in shape and appearance of the septate uterus has led to difficulty in developing a universally accepted classification system. The American Society for Reproductive Medicine (ASRM) defines a uterine septum as a uterus with normal external contour or with an external fundal indentation of less than 1.0 cm and an internal fundal indentation that is greater than 1.0 cm in length measured from the interstitial line (a straight line drawn to connect the interstitial openings) to the tip and has an angle of indentation that is less than 90 degrees [13].

An arcuate uterus is defined as a fundal indentation that is less than or equal to 1.0 cm in length and has an angle of indentation that is greater than 90 degrees (Fig. 4.5) [13]. The arcuate uterus is thought to occur similarly due to an incomplete septum resorption during organogenesis. However, it is clinically important to distinguish an arcuate uterus because it is not associated with adverse reproductive outcomes and is thus considered a normal anatomic variant [7, 14]. Notably, the ASRM classification system was developed based on the current literature evaluating reproductive outcomes and the measurements were selected to differentiate between a septum that may cause adverse clinical outcomes and an indentation that is a normal variant.

The European Society of Human Reproduction and Embryology (ESHRE) and the European Society for Gynaecological Endoscopy (ESGE) jointly developed an alternative classification system that is more objective and leaves less room for clinical interpretation. ESHRE/ESGE defines a uterine septum as a uterus with normal external contour or that is indented less than 50% of the width of the uterine wall and with a fundal internal indentation with a length that measures greater than 50% of the width of the uterine wall, when measured from the interstitial line to the tip of the indentation (Fig. 4.6) [15]. The ESHRE/ESGE definition of septate uterus by 3D imaging was developed without any input of clinical outcomes associated with this definition. In addition, the ESHRE classification system does not include a separate definition for arcuate uteri and many uteri that would be classified as arcuate and a normal anatomic variant by ASRM criteria meet the definition of a uterine septum when using the ESHRE classification system [16].

The difference between the two classification systems was evaluated in a cohort of 44 patients with a uterine septum as defined by ESHRE criteria. In that cohort, 16 patients (36.4%) had an internal indentation less than 1 cm and would be classified as arcuate based on ASRM criteria [16]. Clinically, the importance in correctly differentiating a uterine septum from an arcuate uterus is that an arcuate uterus is considered a normal variant and does not require corrective surgery compared to the septate uterus that is associated with adverse reproductive outcomes. As there is no universally accepted standard definition of septate uterus, differences among the available definitions may lead to variability in diagnostic classifications with correspondingly increased or decreased incidence of surgery performed to correct these anomalies. Thus, there is concern that defining a septate uterus by ESHRE/ESGE criteria would lead to potential unnecessary surgery to correct an anomaly that is not associated with adverse reproductive outcomes.

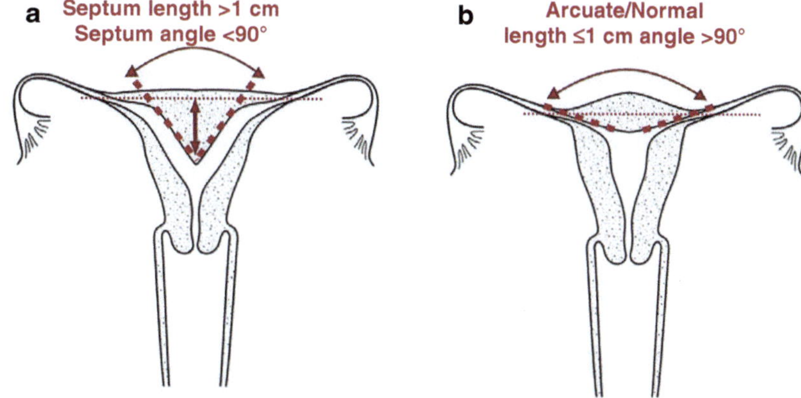

Fig. 4.5 ASRM Mullerian anomalies classification 2021 depicting the specific measurements of depth and angle of indentation to define partial septate and arcuate/normal uterus

Fig. 4.6 ESHRE/ESGE definition of partial and complete septate uterus

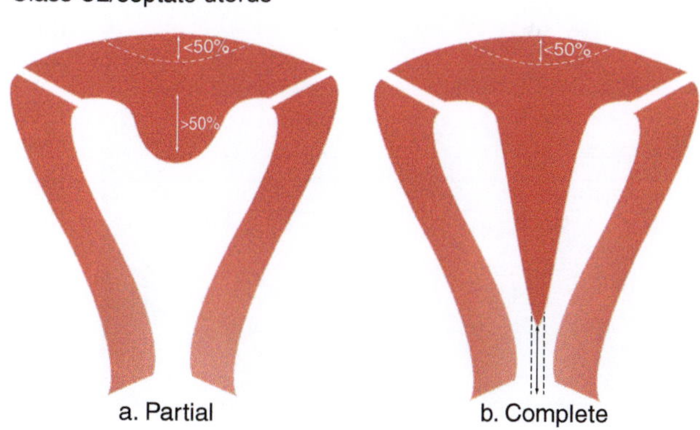

Diagnosis

The most important point to understand when diagnosing a uterine septum is that both the internal and external uterine contour must be adequately visualized in order to distinguish a uterine septum from a bicornuate uterus. The internal indentation may appear the same in both types of müllerian anomalies; however, in a bicornuate uterus, the external fundus will also be indented greater than 1 cm per the ASRM definition [13]. If a uterine septum is incorrectly diagnosed in a patient with a bicornuate uterus, the risk of uterine perforation during "septum" incision is very high.

Accordingly, the imaging modality utilized to diagnose a uterine septum must be able to assess both the internal and external shape of the uterus. The gold standard has traditionally been direct visualization with combined hysteroscopy and laparoscopy. However, with the advent of improved imaging modalities, the diagnosis can almost always be made with less invasive radiologic imaging techniques. Evidence supports that the two best methods to use are either magnetic resonance imaging (MRI) or three-dimensional ultrasonography (3D) with or without saline infusion sonohysterography (SIS). Hysterosalpingography may also be a helpful adjunct to initially identify the presence of a müllerian anomaly; however, because this method is unable to assess the external contour of the uterus, it alone cannot distinguish between a uterine septum and a bicornuate uterus.

All studies that evaluate the sensitivity and specificity of imaging modalities to accurately diagnose uterine septum are limited by their small sample size and sometimes lack a gold standard for comparison due to the invasive nature of surgical diagnosis. The sensitivity and specificity of MRI have been reported as high as 100% due to the ability to clearly delineate both the external and internal shape of the uterus [9]. Another study showed the diagnostic agreement between MRI and final clinical diagnosis (based on history, pelvic exam, complete imaging studies, surgery, and clinical follow-up) to be 70%; however, a clear measurement cutoff to distinguish a septum from an arcuate uterus was not utilized, and this represents a good example of the clinical ambiguity that can occur when evaluating the uterine shape without objective guidelines to distinguish between the different types of müllerian anomalies [17].

Transvaginal ultrasound is another excellent modality that can be used to accurately diagnose a uterine septum as it has comparable predictive value compared to MRI and it is readily available in many outpatient office settings. Both 3D transvaginal ultrasound (Fig. 4.7) and 2D-SIS (Fig. 4.8) have a diagnostic accuracy greater than 90%. When 3D transvaginal ultrasound is performed in combination with SIS, the sensitivity and specificity have been reported as high as 100% and can distinguish a septum from an arcuate uterus with high precision [18]. When considering radiologic imaging accuracy, it is important to remember that the test results are operator dependent and most studies that evaluate test accuracy are performed at high volume centers with gynecologic imaging experts. Therefore, the diagnostic accuracy of each imaging test is dependent on the evaluators experience with both the imaging modality and the diagnosis of uterine malformations.

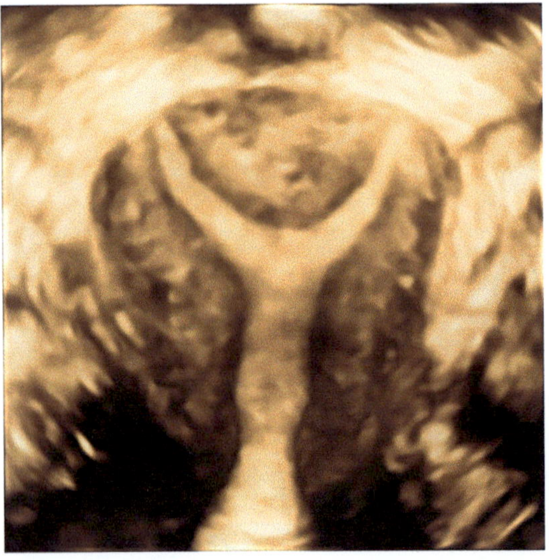

Fig. 4.7 3D-ultrasound coronal view of a uterus with partial septum

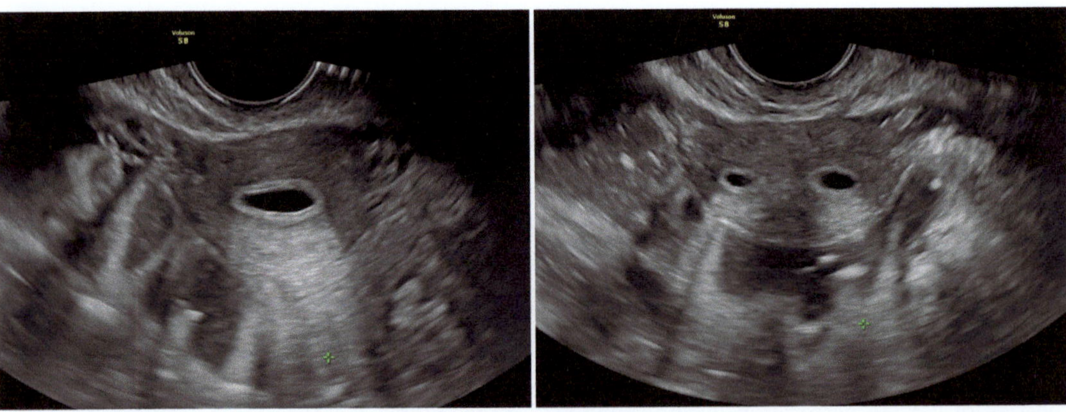

Fig. 4.8 2D-SIS axial view of a uterus with partial septum. (**a**) Lower uterine segment. (**b**) Superiorly located view (compared to Fig. 4.6a) with partial septum visualized

Impact on Fertility and Obstetric Outcomes

As mentioned previously, many women with a septate uterus will not have any difficulty achieving a pregnancy or experience any adverse obstetric events. Yet, there is a correlation between the occurrence of a uterine septum and history of miscarriage or preterm delivery. Most available literature evaluating this association is observational. Further, many studies are limited by a lack of a comparison group or by a paucity of delivery outcomes. In addition, many studies do not differentiate size, shape of septum or distinguish between partial and complete septum. The current management and counseling of patients with a uterine septum are mainly based on these descriptive and observational studies as well as expert opinion.

A uterine septum may often go unnoticed until a patient undergoes a uterine evaluation. This diagnosis will often occur at the time of an infertility evaluation because all of these patients undergo a thorough uterine evaluation regardless of their obstetric history. This leads to an increased prevalence of septate uteri diagnosed in patients with infertility, but it is not clear if the septum is causal for infertility or if it is an incidental finding [19, 20]. Small studies aimed to evaluate this association have failed to identify a significant relationship [21–23]. A systematic review on the topic concluded that there is a significant gap in the literature of high-quality evidence; based on the current literature, it cannot be concluded that there is an association between infertility and septate uteri [7, 24].

However, when a patient presents with infertility and is diagnosed with a uterine septum, study results are mixed regarding whether septum incision will improve infertility treatment outcomes. The only randomized controlled trial to evaluate this question enrolled 80 women with a uterine septum and a history of either infertility, one or more miscarriages before 24 weeks, or a history of preterm delivery and randomized participants to septum incision or expectant management [25]. The outcomes of live birth, pregnancy loss, and preterm delivery were similar between groups. While this study provides the best prospective data on the use of septum incision in this population, it was only powered to detect an absolute improvement in live birth of 35% and is limited by the heterogenous population enrolled and the 9-year enrollment period.

In contrast, multiple retrospective studies have provided evidence that septum incision in infertile patients will improve infertility treatment outcomes [7]. Many otherwise good prognosis patients with infertility and a uterine septum are able to conceive spontaneously after septum incision [26]. In the largest study to evaluate the association between septum incision and embryo transfer outcomes, the authors observed that patients with a uterine septum have significantly lower odds of achieving pregnancy and live birth following embryo transfer compared to a matched control group, but that patients that are treated with uterine septum incision have similar odds of achieving pregnancy and live birth following embryo transfer compared to a matched control group (20).

In patients with a septum that achieve a pregnancy, many will go on to have an uncomplicated term gestation delivery. In a retrospective study of a heterogenous group of women who selected uterine septum incision compared to women who selected expectant management, uterine septum incision did not affect miscarriage, preterm delivery, or live birth outcomes [27]. Still, observational and descriptive studies that have assessed the impact of septate uteri on adverse pregnancy outcomes report an association with miscarriage and preterm delivery. Retrospective studies have reported that in women with a septate uterus, first-trimester miscarriage was observed in 36–42% compared to a 9–12% occurrence in patients with a normal uterine cavity [22, 28, 29]. A meta-analysis that evaluated obstetric outcomes similarly reported a higher risk of first trimester miscarriage in patients with a septate uterus (RR 2.65, 95% CI 1.39–5.06). This analysis also reported that pregnant patients with a septate uterus have an increased risk for preterm delivery (RR 2.11, 95% CI 1.51–2.94), malpresentation (RR 4.35, 95% CI 2.52–7.50), intrauterine growth restriction (RR 2.54, 95% CI 1.04–6.23), and perinatal mortality (RR 2.43, 95% CI 1.10–5.36) [24].

Based on these data, pregnant patients with a uterine septum should be counseled on the risks of adverse obstetric outcomes, but that the absolute risk of these outcomes remains low. When a uterine septum incision is performed in patients with a history of infertility, miscarriage, or recurrent pregnancy loss, two meta-analyses report that miscarriage risk and live birth outcomes are improved [24, 30]. Again, it is important to understand that the published data on this topic is retrospective and some studies lack a comparison group and is therefore at risk of selection bias.

The size and shape should not be taken into consideration when determining whether to incise a uterine septum. Given the wide variability in septum presentation in both length and thickness, most studies do not stratify patients by septum size. Studies that do stratify patients by either septum length, thickness, or both to assess the effect of septum size on obstetric outcomes have not observed an association between adverse reproductive outcomes (including miscarriage, preterm delivery, and live birth outcomes) and septum length or thickness [31–33].

Therefore, patients should be counseled to undergo uterine septum incision if they have a history of miscarriage, preterm delivery, and/or recurrent pregnancy loss. The effect of a uterine septum on implantation is still unclear because the data evaluating this association are limited. However, in patients that present with a history of infertility and a diagnosis of a uterine septum, incision should be offered to improve treatment outcomes. Finally, in a patient that desires fertility with an incidentally diagnosed uterine septum but no history of infertility or adverse obstetric outcome, septum incision can be considered after a discussion regarding the risks, benefits, and alternatives discussed above. In a patient that does not desire fertility with an incidentally diagnosed uterine septum, there is no role for septum incision.

Operative Technique

Uterine septum incision is most commonly performed via the hysteroscopic route. Before the advent of hysteroscopy, septum resection was done via laparotomy using either the Jones metroplasty or modified Tompkins metroplasty techniques (Fig. 4.9). The Jones metroplasty is essentially a wedge resection of the septum and overlying myometrium and uterine serosa followed by closure of the remaining myometrium. The Tompkins metroplasty differs in that no myometrium is removed. Instead, an incision is made through the fundal myometrium, anterior to posterior, and continues through the middle of the septum in order to divide it in half. A second incision is made perpendicular to the first incision, but through the septum only in order to incise it on each side. The myometrial and serosal layers are then closed. These invasive techniques now mostly serve as historical perspective.

In current practice, operative hysteroscopy is a less invasive option that produces effective results and is the standard of care for treatment of uterine septum. While the procedure is commonly referred to as septum resection, the procedure most often utilized is actually septum incision or transection. This procedure can be safely performed in either the office setting or in an operating room under anesthesia. There are a few hysteroscopic instruments that are commonly used for septum incision including hysteroscopic scissors, monopolar or bipolar electrocautery, or laser. Each technique has theoretical advantages, but no large well-designed studies have been performed to compare techniques [7]. All methods are considered to generally produce comparable clinical results, and the choice is determined by surgeon preference. The primary questions to consider to ultimately determine the best technique to use include the following:

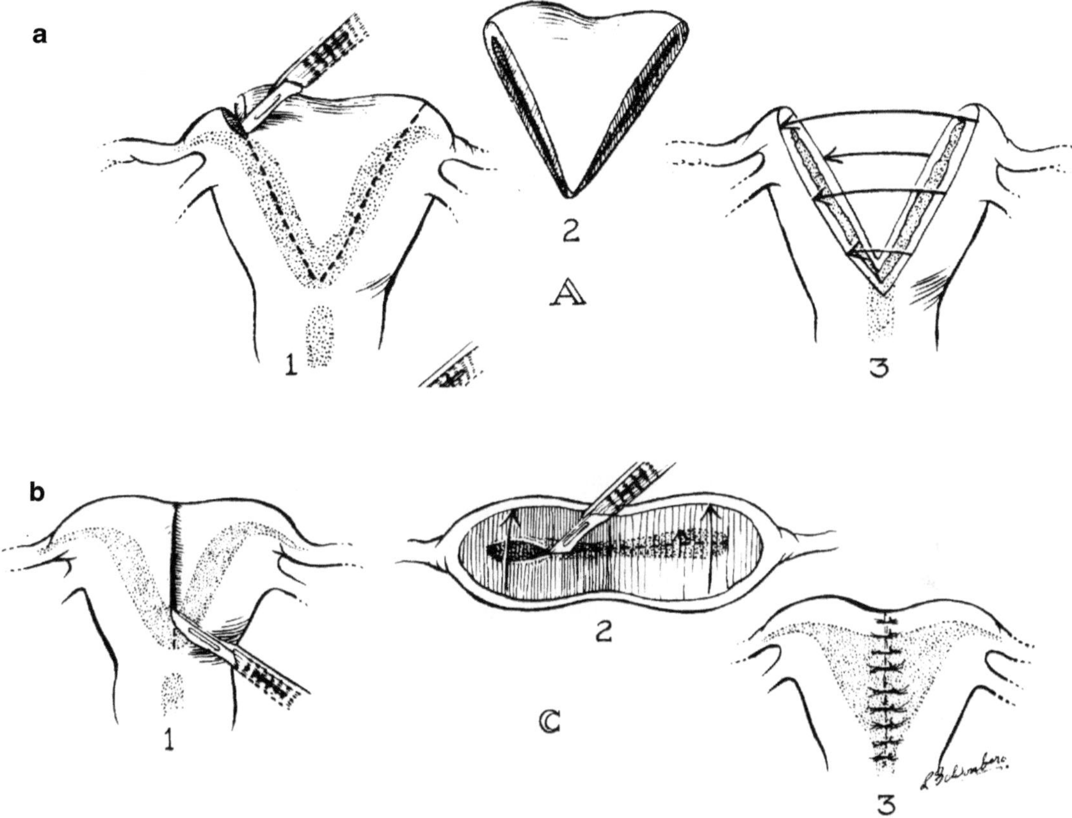

Fig. 4.9 Depiction of abdominal metroplasty techniques. (a) Jones metroplasty. (b) Tompkins metroplasty. (Figure from Rock and Jones [33]. Permission to use this figure was granted by Elsevier)

1. Will the procedure be performed in the office or operating room?
2. Does cervical dilation need to be avoided?
3. Should energy sources be avoided?
4. How does cost vary between instruments?
5. How complex is the instrument to set-up or to operate?
6. What distension media options are available?

Hysteroscopic cold scissors require the least amount of equipment and therefore are a cost-effective option and are ideal for use in the office setting. Hysteroscopes with an outer diameter as small as 5 millimeters have been made to accommodate the scissors, and cervical dilation is often not necessary when using a hysteroscope of this size. Additionally, some clinicians prefer to use scissors in order to avoid the use of energy sources in the endometrial cavity that may increase the risk of postoperative intrauterine adhesions or endometrial injury. Some difficulties encountered include poor visibility if the scissors pass through the inflow channel as this reduces flow of distending fluid and clearing of blood. The true risk reduction to endometrial damage with the use of cold scissors for septum incision has not been well studied and remains more of a theoretical concern.

Many hysteroscopic electrocautery devices have been developed that can also be used for septum incision. These options include hooks, loops, and various pointed tip electrodes. Some of these options are designed to be used with larger diameter hysteroscopes (22 or 26 French) and cervical dilation may be required. When using electrocautery, surgeons must always be aware of the thermal spread from the contact surface of the instrument, which varies depending on the instrument type, power setting, and the application time. In general, bipolar devices result in less thermal spread compared to monopolar devices, with thermal spread up to 2–6 mm recorded for bipolar instruments and thermal spread of greater than 10 mm recorded for monopolar instruments [34, 35]. This risk is important to be aware of when operating within the endometrial cavity as myometrial damage may occur, but also if uterine perforation occurs due to the injury that can then occur to intra-abdominal organs.

If uterine perforation occurs, the surgeon must decide whether to end the procedure and expectantly manage the patient or whether abdominal exploration to evaluate for injury should be performed. This decision should be made based on the risk of intra-abdominal injury at the time of perforation taking into consideration the risk of potential bladder, bowel, or vascular injury depending on the location of injury and causal instrument. Generally, if perforation occurs with a blunt instrument and no electrocautery, expectant management can be considered if there are no other signs of vascular or visceral organ injury. If perforation occurs with the use of electrocautery or if the surgeon is concerned for possible intra-abdominal injury based on the type and location of perforation, abdominal exploration should be performed. The hysteroscopic surgeon should be aware and capable of performing management of uterine perforation.

The hysteroscopic use of laser (argon, KTP [potassium titanyl phosphate], and Neodymium-YAG) has also been described as a successful method for uterine septum incision [36, 37]. While effective, the use of laser is generally more expensive, more dangerous for the operating room staff, and leads to longer operating times when compared to incision with scissors [38]. Thus, this method is less commonly utilized than the other techniques previously described.

The choice of distension media to us depends on the time of operative instrument chosen for incision [39]. Both electrolyte-free and electrolyte-rich media can be used. Electrolyte-free media such as 3% sorbitol, 1.5% glycine, and 5% mannitol are commonly used with monopolar devices. The greatest risks that can occur when using these solutions is electrolyte imbalance such as hyponatremia, which has been observed when high amounts of solution are absorbed into the systemic circulation. Maximum absorption of electrolyte-free media is 1000 ml [39, 40]. When using electrolyte-free solutions, the surgeon must always be aware of the operating fluid deficit and institutional procedures and guidelines used to mitigate the risks of fluid overload and electrolyte imbalance. High amounts of distension media absorption are more likely to occur with prolonged procedures. However, uterine septum incision procedures are generally completed in under 30 minutes and therefore high fluid deficits are rarely observed with this procedure.

When using bipolar instruments, an electrolyte-rich media, such as normal saline, must be used for distention. This media is advantageous because it is isotonic and contains physiologic electrolytes, thus, mitigating the risk of electrolyte imbalances like hyponatremia making it the preferred choice by many surgeons, especially for cases with an expected longer operating time. The maximum fluid deficit with normal saline is far greater than with glycine and approaches 2000–2500 [39, 40]. However, high fluid deficits with normal saline can still cause fluid overload and the surgeon must always pay close attention to fluid management during any hysteroscopic procedure.

Procedural Steps

Partial Septate Uterus

Regardless of the hysteroscopic instrument chosen for septum incision, the principles of the procedure remain the same. Once the hysteroscope is in the uterine cavity, the surgeon should perform a careful survey of the cavity and identify the location of both tubal ostia. It is easy to become disoriented within the endometrial cavity during hysteroscopic septum incision if the surgeon is not constantly monitoring these landmarks. Two techniques can be utilized: shortening and thinning (Fig. 4.10 and Video 4.1). Shortening involves incising the septum starting at the leading edge and continuing toward the fundal region. The septum is incised horizontally typically starting at one side moving across to the other side, parallel to the anterior and posterior uterine walls and in the same plane defined by the tubal ostia. If the incision begins to deviate toward the anterior and posterior walls, this trajectory could eventually lead to uterine perforation if not recognized and corrected. Thinning technique involves incising the septum along the lateral edges of the septum on both sides to reduce the width of the septum. The shortening technique can then be facilitated as the septum will be smaller. Another benefit of this technique is it helps to keep the surgeon in the intended plane throughout the procedure as these incisions are placed in the correct plane midline between anterior and posterior uterine walls and in the

plane of the tubal ostia. In practice, it is often helpful to use a combination of these two techniques depending on the size and shape of the septum to be incised.

If scissors are utilized, small incisions are made at the leading edge allowing the septal fibers to separate (Video 4.2). Blood vessels if visualized may be avoided to minimize bleeding. If using electrocautery, a combination of a brief incision with energy followed by gentle blunt dissection without energy can be used to safely incise the septum with the least amount of applied thermal energy. As the incision progresses, the surgeon must constantly be aware of the incisional plane and the uterine orientation by monitoring the location of the tubal ostia in relation to the incision (Fig. 4.11). It is usually not possible to keep the ostia continuously visible during the procedure due to the proximity that must be maintained between the operating instrument and the surface of the septum. Thus, the surgeon must frequently move the camera from the incision to the ostium to ensure the orientation of the uterus has not been lost. If this occurs, there is a high risk of perforation as the surgeon will no longer be incising the correct plane.

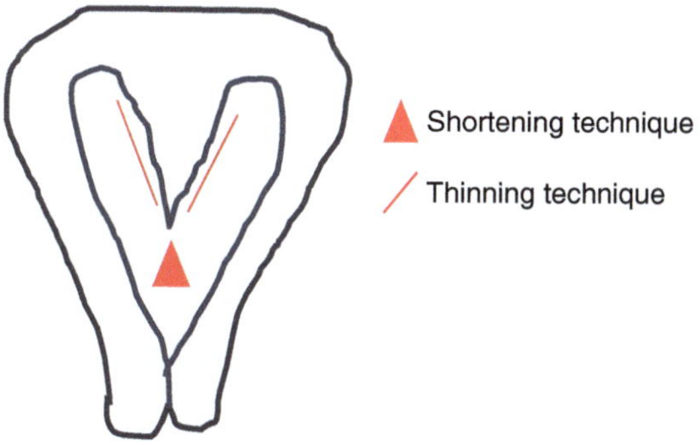

Fig. 4.10 Depiction of incision techniques: shortening and thinning

Complete Septate Uterus

With a complete septate uterus, there is debate regarding whether the cervical septum should be incised as part of the uterine septum incision or left intact. The concern with cervical septum incision is that it could compromise the remaining cervical tissue leading to cervical insufficiency in pregnancy. However, there are no high-quality studies that evaluate pregnancy outcomes after cervical septum incision and results

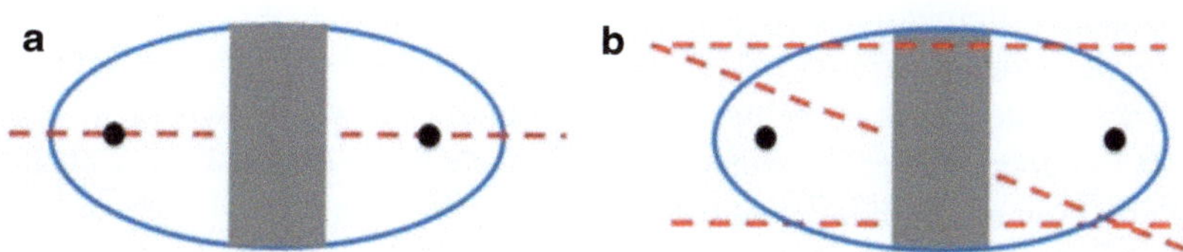

Fig. 4.11 (**a**) Correct plane of incision (red dashed line) – same plane as ostia (black dots). (**b**) Incorrect planes – can lead to damage to myometrium and possible perforation

are conflicting. Nor do these studies clearly define a cervical septum or differentiate it from a duplicated cervix. A cervical septum appears as a single thickened outer rim with a band that may be thin or thick dividing the cervix (Fig. 4.3). This band is typically continuous with the uterine septum and longitudinal vaginal septum when present. With a duplicated cervix, there are two distinct cervical entities, and the cervical ostia are separated by a large distance or may even be in different planes (Fig. 4.4).

Incising the cervical septum along with the uterine septum for a complete septate uterus has been advocated as this procedure has been shown to be significantly shorter, associated with less fluid absorption, less bleeding, and easier when compared to preservation of the cervical septum [41, 42]. Techniques described include cutting the cervical septum with Metzenbaum scissors [41], or cutting the cervical septum with scissors after first dilating each cervical canal to 10 mm [43, 44]. In lieu of scissors, a 5-mm hand-held tissue sealing device can be used to transect the cervical septum with minimal bleeding. Others have reported using the hysteroscopic resectoscope [42]. In these studies, the uterine septum was incised with hysteroscope and either scissors or bipolar or monopolar cautery independent of the technique to remove the cervical septum. All these techniques have been shown to be performed immediately following resection of longitudinal vaginal septum. The cervical septum was observed to recur following incision in 3 of 10 patients in one observational study [44]. Cervical incompetence following incision of cervical septum is a concern with incidence of cerclage in studies ranging from 9% to 24% [42, 43]. However, in a randomized controlled trial of 28 patients comparing cervical septum incision versus preservation, rates of cerclage placement were not significantly different nor were preterm delivery rates between the two groups [41].

For a complete septate uterus with duplicated cervix, there are a couple of effective techniques to incise the uterine septum without compromising the cervical septum. The main strategy is to make an opening in the septum just above the level of the internal cervical os, to create a lead-ing edge of the uterine septum that can be incised hysteroscopically. The challenge is to identify a thin portion of uterine septum in the correct location and the correct plane to create this opening. One approach is to make a blind entry across at the presumed correct location, but this risks deviating the incision toward the anterior or posterior wall especially if the uterus is rotated thereby increasing the risk of perforation. A safer option is to identify where to incise the septum by placing an instrument in the contralateral side to tent the septum where the incision should be made (Fig. 4.12). Instruments that have been used include a foley balloon, a uterine sound, or a thin curved clamp in the endocervical/uterine canal with the hysteroscope in the adjacent canal. The septum may then be incised over the area demarcated by these instruments using scissors, or any hysteroscopic tools used for uterine septum incision. When using a balloon, once it is beyond the cervix, it can be slowly inflated and the incision can be made through the septum above the cervix, using the balloon to delineate the location for the incision and the prevent the instrument from perforating through the contralateral uterine wall. Although the foley is effective, it can distort the anatomy and make it difficult to pass the hysteroscope. A thin long curved clamp can overcome these issues (Fig. 4.12a and Video 4.3). Once inserted through the contralateral side of the cervix and beyond the cervix, the surgeon can angle the tip of the clamp into the septum and then open the clamp to delineate a clear area where the incision can safely be made to incise the cervix in the lower uterine segment without perforating through the contralateral wall.

Once the septum has been crossed, the hysteroscopic distending media will egress through the adjacent cervical canal and uterine distension may be difficult. When this occurs, occlusion of the second cervical opening can be helpful. This can be done by placing a figure-of-eight stitch around the cervical opening, using an Allis clamp to occlude the external cervical os, or by placing a foley balloon through the cervix, slightly inflating the balloon, and then pulling back on the foley catheter until the second cervical opening is occluded. Interestingly, incidence of cesarean

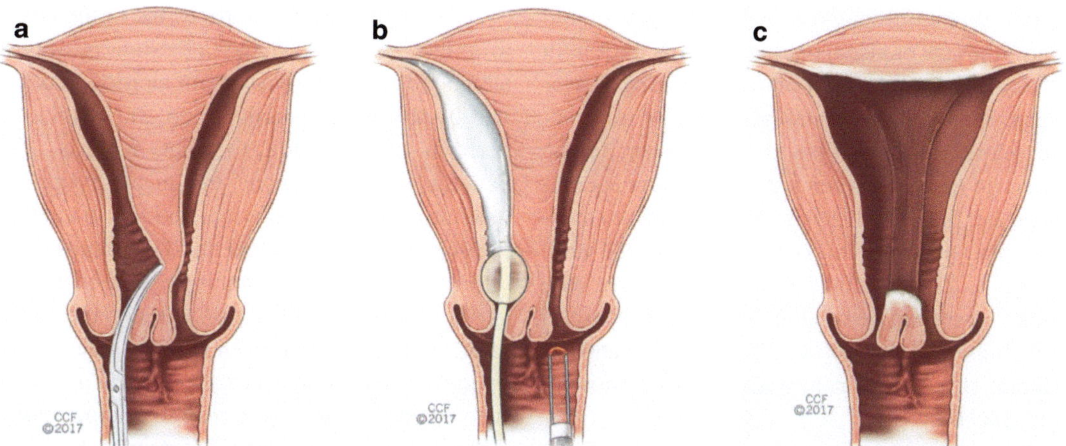

Fig. 4.12 Technique for complete uterine septum incision while preserving cervical septum. (**a**) Using a fine long curved clamp to identify where to cross lower uterine septum. (**b**) Use of foley balloon catheter to mark where to cross lower uterine septum. (**c**) Complete septate uterus following incision of uterine septum while preserving cervical septum. (Figure from Jeff Goldberg MD, Cleveland Clinic Foundation)

section following preservation of the cervical septum was higher, 7% versus 2% ($P < 0.05$) in one randomized study [41]. However, vaginal delivery is not impeded with an intact cervical septum or complete duplicated cervix post hysteroscopic septum as the fetal head displaces the cervix or cervical septum to one side as it descends [44].

Septate uteri can also be associated with the presence of a longitudinal vaginal septum. In one retrospective study of patients with longitudinal vaginal septum, a septate uterus was present nearly 2/3 of cases [45]. The decision to resect a longitudinal vaginal septum and the available techniques are beyond the scope of this chapter, but it is possible to resect the vaginal septum at the time of cervical septum surgery. When these procedures are done together, it is usually best to first resect the vaginal septum to allow for easier vaginal wall retraction and visualization during the cervical septum incision.

Once the uterine septum is incised, the procedure is complete. However, deciding when enough of the septum has been incised is a crucial step. If the septum is incised too far resulting in thinning of the fundal myometrial wall, there is a risk for uterine rupture to occur in future pregnancies. Eighteen cases of uterine rupture in

subsequent pregnancy have been reported following septum incision seen in association with excessive septum excision/incision, penetration of myometrium, uterine wall perforation, or excessive use of cautery or laser energy [30]. This risk can seemingly be mitigated by a careful surgical approach and appropriate knowledge for when to stop the incision. Ending the procedure once the septum has been incised down to one centimeter away from the interstitial line is a safe distance as this ensures that the myometrial wall remains intact and is a length of indentation that does not affect pregnancy outcomes [14].

Clues that the incision is nearing the interstitial line can be gathered from visual signs, direct measurement, and external monitoring with laparoscopy or ultrasound imaging. Visually, the myometrial wall is often much more vascular than the septum. When bleeding begins to occur at the level of the incision, this is a sign that myometrium is near and the remaining length of the septum should be reassessed. It is important to remember that the septum can contain muscle and vessels which may also cause bleeding during incision and this approach may lead to a large residual septum. Length of the residual septum may also be assessed by placing the extended operating instrument and directly measuring the depth. When utilizing this technique, one should know the size of visual markers such as the length of scissors or insulation on the operating instrument. Simultaneous transabdominal or transrectal ultrasonography has been shown to be effective to assess when septum incision is complete and has the advantage of being able to measure the remaining thickness of the uterine wall. Direct external visualization of the uterus with laparoscopy can be used; however, transabdominal ultrasound monitoring is less invasive and has similar efficacy and safety when used to monitor the procedure [46].

Assessing for Adequacy of Septum Incision and Adhesion Formation

After uterine septum incision is complete, it can take weeks for endometrial growth to cover the anterior and posterior walls of the uterine cavity where the septum was previously located. In the interim, these opposing edges remain at risk for adhesion formation and distortion of the uterine cavity. Adhesion formation after septum incision has been reported to occur in 5.3–24.1% of cases [47–49]. Hormonal and barrier methods have been proposed to decrease the risk of postoperative adhesion formation; however, studies evaluating the use of these methods are small. Barrier methods create a physical separation between the uterine walls to prevent adhesion formation during the period of endometrial growth, and hormonal methods may help to facilitate and expedite recovering of the incised uterine will with normal endometrium.

One study of 100 women treated with uterine septum incision was randomized to four groups: no adhesion prevention, estradiol plus norgestrel daily for 2 months, copper IUD, and a combination of estradiol plus norgestrel plus copper IUD. Patients underwent cavity evaluation 2 months postoperatively and adhesions were present in 5.3% of control group, 0% of the hormone treatment group, 12% of the copper IUD group, and 10.5% of the hormone plus copper IUD group with no statistical significance in any treatment group compared to the control group

[47]. Even though this study is one of the largest to prospectively evaluate adhesion prevention techniques after uterine septum incision, it is limited by the small patient cohort and a failure to perform an intention to treat analysis. Five patients in the hormone treatment group self-discontinued the medication, and four patients in the copper IUD group had the IUD removed.

Despite a lack of conclusive data, many surgeons recommend the use of adhesion prevention after septum incision given the high rate of postoperative adhesion formation. When barrier methods are used, a barrier with a large enough surface area to prevent the uterine walls from touching should be used. Therefore, a foley balloon or a balloon specially shaped to fit into the uterine cavity are likely to be more effective than a T-shaped IUD device. When hormone therapy is used by itself or in combination to a barrier method, a physiologic dosing schedule should be chosen by administering estradiol at physiologic doses for 21–28 days with the addition of a progestin around days 10–14.

Another method used to manage postoperative adhesions is a second-look office hysteroscopy with incision of any adhesions at that time. In one study that used this method, adhesions were observed in 25.6% of patients at 1 month postoperatively [48]. The majority of adhesions were filmy and were able to be incised with the tip of the hysteroscope or scissors. At repeat hysteroscopy performed at 3 months postoperatively, adhesions were observed in only 1.7% of patients.

Due to the risk of adhesion formation or incomplete septum incision, all septum incision procedures should be followed up with a cavity evaluation to ensure that the septum has been adequately incised and that no intrauterine adhesions are present. Office hysteroscopy, as described above, is an effective option because it can be both diagnostic and therapeutic. Other options include imaging techniques that are able to evaluate the cavity for both adhesions and residual septum with a high sensitivity and specificity – either hysterosalpingography or a 3D-SIS. If a residual septum or intrauterine adhesions are identified, a second procedure to restore the cavity should be performed.

Attempting Pregnancy Following Septum Incision

Once a uterine septum has been incised, patients should wait to conceive until a follow-up evaluation confirms a normal uterine cavity and the endometrium has sufficiently covered the entirety of the uterine cavity. Data from second-look hysteroscopies have described the length of time that it takes for endometrium to cover the area of septum incision. One study of 19 patients was designed to specifically evaluate the endometrial repair that occurs after septum incision. Hysteroscopy was performed 1, 2, 4, and 8 weeks following septum incision with hysteroscopic scissors [38]. At 1 week postoperatively, the incised area was still very clearly visualized on hysteroscopy with an absence of epithelial cells on histological examination. At 2 weeks postoperatively, the incised area was still depressed with areas still lacking endometrial covering with simple epithelium without stromal tissue observed on histology. Four weeks postoperatively, the incised areas remained depressed in comparison to the adjacent endometrium, but these were completely covered by a thin epithelium. Proliferative endometrium with epithelium and stroma was observed on histology. At 8 weeks postoperatively, the endometrial cavity and histology appeared normal, with only a slight depression at the incised area identified in three patients. Other studies that include second-look hysteroscopies have similarly reported that the endometrial lining appears normal in most patients after 2–3 months [49, 50]. Therefore, it is reasonable to wait for 2 months after uterine septum incision prior to attempting pregnancy, either naturally or with infertility treatment [7].

Conclusion

Septate uterus may be asymptomatic or lead to poor reproductive outcomes. Septum may be partial or complete. Diagnosis may be confirmed by 3D ultrasound, SIS, MRI, or HSG or hysteroscopy in conjunction with ultrasound confirmation of external uterine contour. Septum incision is indicated following poor reproductive outcome or for those individuals with infertility. Septum incision may also be performed for asymptomatic individuals to decrease potential for poor reproductive outcome following counseling of the risks and benefits. Many techniques have been described and none have been proven superior. Care should be taken to avoid damage to the fundal myometrium by either excessive septum incision or cautery. Reproductive outcomes following septum incision have been shown to improve.

References

1. Taylor H, Pal L, Emre S. Speroff's clinical gynecologic endocrinology and infertility. 9th ed. Lippincott Williams & Wilkins; 2019.
2. Hoffman B, Schorge J, Bradshaw K, Halvorson L, Schaffer J, Corton MM. Williams Gynecology. 2nd ed. McGraw-Hill; 2012.
3. Rikken JFW, Leeuwis-Fedorovich NE, Letteboer S, Emanuel MH, Limpens J, Veen F van der, et al. The pathophysiology of the septate uterus: a systematic review. BJOG Int J Obstet Gynaecol. 2019;126(10):1192–9.
4. Ludwin A, Ludwin I, Pityński K, Banas T, Jach R. Differentiating between a double cervix or cervical duplication and a complete septate uterus with longitudinal vaginal septum. Taiwan J Obstet Gynecol. 2013;52(2):308–10.
5. Acién P, Acién M, Sánchez-Ferrer ML. Müllerian anomalies "without a classification": from the didelphys-unicollis uterus to the bicervical uterus with or without septate vagina. Fertil Steril. 2009;91(6):2369–75.
6. Oppelt P, von Have M, Paulsen M, Strissel PL, Strick R, Brucker S, et al. Female genital malformations and their associated abnormalities. Fertil Steril. 2007;87(2):335–42.
7. Uterine septum: a guideline. Fertil Steril. 2016;106(3):530–40.
8. Dabirashrafi H, Bahadori M, Mohammad K, Alavi M, Moghadami-Tabrizi N, Zandinejad K, et al. Septate uterus: new idea on the histologic features of the septum in this abnormal uterus. Am J Obstet Gynecol. 1995;172(1, Part 1):105–7.
9. Pellerito JS, McCarthy SM, Doyle MB, Glickman MG, DeCherney AH. Diagnosis of uterine anomalies: relative accuracy of MR imaging, endovaginal sonography, and hysterosalpingography. Radiology. 1992;183(3):795–800.
10. Simón C, Martinez L, Pardo F, Tortajada M, Pellicer A. Müllerian defects in women with normal reproductive outcome. Fertil Steril. 1991;56(6):1192–3.

11. Grimbizis GF, Camus M, Tarlatzis BC, Bontis JN, Devroey P. Clinical implications of uterine malformations and hysteroscopic treatment results. Hum Reprod Update. 2001;7(2):161–74.

12. Chan YY, Jayaprakasan K, Zamora J, Thornton JG, Raine-Fenning N, Coomarasamy A. The prevalence of congenital uterine anomalies in unselected and high-risk populations: a systematic review. Hum Reprod Update. 2011;17(6):761–71.

13. Pfeifer SM, Attaran M, Goldstein J, Lindheim S, Petrozza J, Rackow B, Zuckerman A, Siegelman E, Troiano R, Winters T, Ramaiah SD. ASRM Mullerian anomalies classification 2021. Fertil Steril. 2021;116:1238–52.

14. The American Fertility Society classifications of adnexal adhesions. distal tubal occlusion, tubal occlusion secondary to tubal ligation, tubal pregnancies, Müllerian anomalies and intrauterine adhesions. Fertil Steril. 1988;49(6):944–55.

15. Grimbizis GF, Gordts S, Di Spiezio SA, Brucker S, De Angelis C, Gergolet M, et al. The ESHRE/ESGE consensus on the classification of female genital tract congenital anomalies. Hum Reprod Oxf Engl. 2013;28(8):2032–44.

16. Ludwin A, Ludwin I. Comparison of the ESHRE–ESGE and ASRM classifications of Müllerian duct anomalies in everyday practice. Hum Reprod. 2015;30(3):569–80.

17. Mueller GC, Hussain HK, Smith YR, Quint EH, Carlos RC, Johnson TD, et al. Müllerian duct anomalies: comparison of MRI diagnosis and clinical diagnosis. Am J Roentgenol. 2007;189(6):1294–302.

18. Ludwin A, Pityński K, Ludwin I, Banas T, Knafel A. Two- and three-dimensional ultrasonography and Sonohysterography versus hysteroscopy with laparoscopy in the differential diagnosis of septate, Bicornuate, and arcuate uteri. J Minim Invasive Gynecol. 2013;20(1):90–9.

19. Raga F, Bauset C, Remohi J, Bonilla-Musoles F, Simón C, Pellicer A. Reproductive impact of congenital Müllerian anomalies. Hum Reprod. 1997;12(10):2277–81.

20. Tomaževič T, Ban-Frangež H, Virant-Klun I, Verdenik I, Požlep B, Vrtačnik-Bokal E. Septate, subseptate and arcuate uterus decrease pregnancy and live birth rates in IVF/ICSI. Reprod Biomed Online. 2010;21(5):700–5.

21. Maneschi F, Zupi E, Marconi D, Valli E, Romanini C, Mancuso S. Hysteroscopically detected asymptomatic müllerian anomalies. Prevalence and reproductive implications. J Reprod Med. 1995;40(10):684–8.

22. Shuiqing M, Xuming B, Jinghe L. Pregnancy and its outcome in women with malformed uterus. Chin Med Sci J Chung-Kuo Hsueh Ko Hsueh Tsa Chih. 2002;17(4):242–5.

23. Demir B, Dilbaz B, Karadag B, Duraker R, Akkurt O, Kocak M, et al. Coexistence of endometriosis and uterine septum in patients with abortion or infertility. J Obstet Gynaecol Res. 2011;37(11):1596–600.

24. Venetis CA, Papadopoulos SP, Campo R, Gordts S, Tarlatzis BC, Grimbizis GF. Clinical implications of congenital uterine anomalies: a meta-analysis of comparative studies. Reprod Biomed Online. 2014;29(6):665–83.

25. Rikken JFW, Kowalik CR, Emanuel MH, Bongers MY, Spinder T, Jansen FW, et al. Septum resection versus expectant management in women with a septate uterus: an international multicentre open-label randomized controlled trial. Hum Reprod [Internet] 2021 [cited 2021 Apr 7];(deab037). Available from: https://doi.org/10.1093/humrep/deab037.

26. Shokeir T, Abdelshaheed M, El-Shafie M, Sherif L, Badawy A. Determinants of fertility and reproductive success after hysteroscopic septoplasty for women with unexplained primary infertility: a prospective analysis of 88 cases. Eur J Obstet Gynecol Reprod Biol. 2011;155(1):54–7.

27. Rikken J, Verhostert K, Emanuel M, Bongers M, Spinder T, Kuchenbecker W, et al. Septum resection in women with a septate uterus: a cohort study. Hum Reprod. 2020;35(7):1578–88.

28. Woelfer B, Salim R, Banerjee S, Elson J, Regan L, Jurkovic D. Reproductive outcomes in women with congenital uterine anomalies detected by three-dimensional ultrasound screening. Obstet Gynecol. 2001;98(6):1099–103.

29. Kupešić S, Kurjak A, Skenderovic S, Bjelos D. Screening for uterine abnormalities by three-dimensional ultrasound improves perinatal outcome. J Perinat Med. 2002;30(1):9–17.

30. Valle RF, Ekpo GE. Hysteroscopic Metroplasty for the septate uterus: review and meta-analysis. J Minim Invasive Gynecol. 2013;20(1):22–42.

31. Zlopaša G, Škrablin S, Kalafatić D, Banović V, Lešin J. Uterine anomalies and pregnancy outcome following resectoscope metroplasty. Int J Gynecol Obstet. 2007;98(2):129–33.

32. Kupesic S, Kurjak A. Septate uterus: detection and prediction of obstetrical complications by different forms of ultrasonography. J Ultrasound Med. 1998;17(10):631–6.

33. Tomaževič T, Ban-Frangež H, Ribič-Pucelj M, Premru-Sršen T, Verdenik I. Small uterine septum is an important risk variable for preterm birth. Eur J Obstet Gynecol Reprod Biol. 2007;135(2):154–7.

34. Moore O, Haimovich S. Energy sources in hysteroscopy [Internet]. In: Tandulwadkar S, Pal B, editors. Hysteroscopy simplified by masters. Singapore: Springer; 2021 [cited 2021 Apr 7]. p. 11–20. Available from: https://doi.org/10.1007/978-981-15-2505-6_3.

35. Sutton PA, Awad S, Perkins AC, Lobo DN. Comparison of lateral thermal spread using monopolar and bipolar diathermy, the Harmonic Scalpel™ and the Ligasure™. Br J Surg. 2010;97(3):428–33.

36. Daniell JF, Osher S, Miller W. Hysteroscopic resection of uterine Septi with visible light laser energy. J Gynecol Surg. 1987;3(4):217–20.

37. Choe JK, Baggish MS. Hysteroscopic treatment of septate uterus with Neodymium-YAG laser. Fertil Steril. 1992;57(1):81–4.
38. Candiani GB, Vercellini P, Fedele L, Carinelli SG, Merlo D, Arcaini L. Repair of the uterine cavity after hysteroscopic septal incision. Fertil Steril. 1990;54(6):991–4.
39. AAGL Practice Report. Practice guidelines for the management of hysteroscopic distending media. J Minim Invasive Gynecol. 2013;20(2):137–48.
40. The use of hysteroscopy for the diagnosis and treatment of intrauterine pathology: ACOG Committee Opinion, Number 800. Obstet Gynecol 2020;135(3):e138.
41. Parsanezhad ME, Alborzi S, Zarei A, Dehbashi S, Shirazi LG, Rajaeefard A, et al. Hysteroscopic metroplasty of the complete uterine septum, duplicate cervix, and vaginal septum. Fertil Steril. 2006;85(5):1473–7.
42. Darwish AM, ElSaman AM. Extended resectoscopic versus sequential cold knife–resectoscopic excision of the unclassified complete uterocervicovaginal septum: a randomized trial. Fertil Steril. 2009;92(2):722–6.
43. Grynberg M, Gervaise A, Faivre E, Deffieux X, Frydman R, Fernandez H. Treatment of twenty-two patients with complete uterine and vaginal septum. J Minim Invasive Gynecol. 2012;19(1):34–9.
44. Vercellini P, De Giorgi O, Cortesi I, Aimi G, Mazza P, Crosignani PG. Metroplasty for the complete septate uterus: does cervical sparing matter? J Am Assoc Gynecol Laparosc. 1996;3(4):509–14.
45. Haddad B, Louis-Sylvestre C, Poitout P, Paniel B-J. Longitudinal vaginal septum: a retrospective study of 202 cases. Eur J Obstet Gynecol Reprod Biol. 1997;74(2):197–9.
46. Coccia ME, Becattini C, Bracco GL, Bargelli G, Scarselli G. Intraoperative ultrasound guidance for operative hysteroscopy. A prospective study. J Reprod Med. 2000;45(5):413–8.
47. Tonguc EA, Var T, Yilmaz N, Batioglu S. Intrauterine device or estrogen treatment after hysteroscopic uterine septum resection. Int J Gynecol Obstet. 2010;109(3):226–9.
48. Yu X, Yuhan L, Dongmei S, Enlan X, Tinchiu L. The incidence of post-operative adhesion following transection of uterine septum: a cohort study comparing three different adjuvant therapies. Eur J Obstet Gynecol Reprod Biol. 2016;201:61–4.
49. Yang J-H, Chen M-J, Chen C-D, Chen S-U, Ho H-N, Yang Y-S. Optimal waiting period for subsequent fertility treatment after various hysteroscopic surgeries. Fertil Steril. 2013;99(7):2092–2096.e3.
50. Wang S, Shi X, Hua X, Gu X, Yang D. Hysteroscopic transcervical resection of uterine septum. JSLS. 2013;17(4):517–20.

Intrauterine Adhesions

J. Preston Parry and Johannes Ott

Background

Intrauterine adhesions (IUA) have been recognized as a source for reproductive dysfunction for over a century. The condition was first described in 1894 by Henrich Fritsch for a woman who underwent curettage 24 days postpartum for bleeding, and then she subsequently became amenorrheic [1]. A more comprehensive description of the condition was published by Israeli gynecologist Joseph Asherman 54 years later in his landmark paper "Amenorrhoea traumatica (atretica)" [2]. Of note, this initial article by Dr. Asherman emphasized cervical adhesive disease. His article "Traumatic intrauterine adhesions," 2 years later gave greater emphasis to the more common finding of intrauterine disease [3].

The condition is often still referred to through terms relating to Joseph Asherman and his article titles, including Asherman's syndrome, traumatic uterine atrophy, and uterine atresia, as well as endometrial sclerosis. When initially published and described as Asherman's syndrome, there was emphasis on hematometra with associated pain. Intrauterine adhesions has come to be the preferred term, as it includes circumstances without pain and covering the full spectrum of disease.

Etiology

Setting aside deliberate creation of IUA through endometrial ablation, 90% of IUA or more can relate to curettage [4–6], consistent with how it was first described by Fritsch [1]. A study with hysteroscopy 8–10 weeks after dilation and curettage (D&C) saw a 31% incidence of post-D&C intrauterine adhesion formation [7]. Non-curettage surgeries can also contribute to IUA, including myomectomies (hysteroscopic, laparoscopic, and abdominal) (Fig. 5.1), metroplasty, and compressive uterine suturing post-partum, as well as inflammatory environments such as with an embedded IUD (Fig. 5.2) [8]. As a more general principle, the greater the number of procedures that can traumatize the endometrium, the greater the risk for intrauterine adhesions [9].

The reason surgery is often a driving force for IUA is that it can cause trauma to the stratum basalis, when damage to the stratum functionale can frequently be sloughed with menses. For this reason, it is uncommon to see IUA associated with ascending infections such as PID, unless there is concurrent surgery, such as with curettage for septic abortion. Similarly, when chronic endometritis is found at hysteroscopic adhesioly-

J. P. Parry (✉)
Parryscope and Positive Steps Fertility,
Madison, MS, USA
e-mail: fertility@parryscope.com

J. Ott
University of Vienna, Vienna, Austria
e-mail: johannes.ott@meduniwien.ac.at

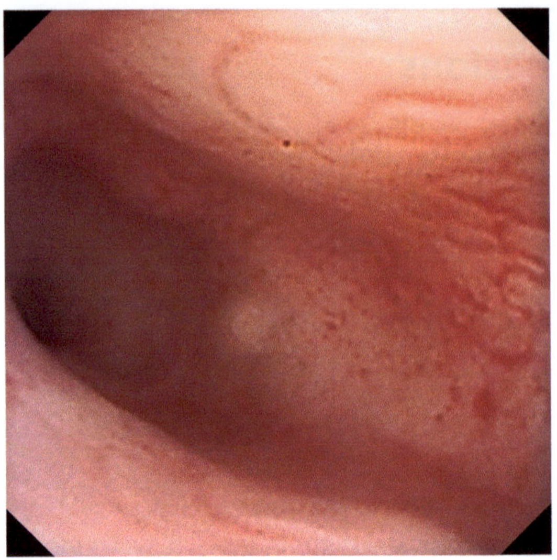

Fig. 5.1 Complete obliteration of the left portion of the endometrial cavity after open myomectomy

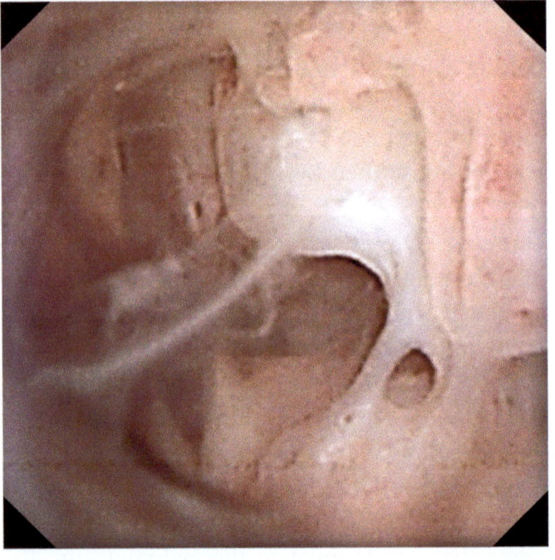

Fig. 5.2 Thick and filmy adhesions after removal of an embedded IUD

sis, there is a higher rate of IUA recurrence (44.8% vs 20.8%) [10]. Uterine tuberculosis (and arguably schistosomiasis) seems to be among the rare non-iatrogenic causes and can result in meaningful IUA [6, 11]. Also of note, etiology can influence distribution of IUA. Curettage-associated adhesions are often midline with lower rates of loss of the ostial landmarks. However,

IUA deriving from infection may be less likely to follow this pattern and appear more random in their distribution. IUAs after septal incision tend to be in the location of the transected septum and myomectomy-associated IUAs tend to be in the site of the previous myoma(s). Also notably, as a general surgical principle, juxtaposed traumatized surfaces are more likely to result in adhesions than when distant from each other, which is part of why laparoscopy results in fewer adhesions than laparotomy. For IUA, curettage often traumatizes both the anterior and posterior stratum basale. Similarly, hysteroscopic myomectomy for a single fibroid is less likely to result in adhesions than resection of anterior and posterior "kissing" fibroids [12].

Estimates of the extent attributable to obstetrical curettage (elective termination, miscarriage, and postpartum indications) vary widely. One summary suggested that misoprostol-induced expulsion of pregnancy led to negligible rates of IUA, while it was 15–20% after D&C and 20–40% after curettage for postpartum hemorrhage [13]. Variation in estimates can relate to indications, instrumentation (sharp vs. suction curettage), and visualization (blind vs. ultrasound guided). Postpartum curettage may have IUA exacerbated by lactational amenorrhea hindering endometrial proliferation. It has been proposed that hysteroscopic management of retained products of conception may decrease IUA risk [14].

Pathophysiology

Intrauterine adhesions at the microscopic level can be characterized by loss of ribosomes and mitochondria, as well as cellular hypoxia [15]. Correction of hypoxia relates to successful correction of IUA, where patients with higher VEGF levels and microvessel density appear more likely to redevelop the endometrium after surgical management [15]. Histology can be myometrial, endometrial, or connective tissue and may relate to etiology. Fibromuscular bands are the most common finding and these sometimes contain endometrial tissue [16].

Clinical Presentation

IUA are considered rare, with Orphanet estimating the prevalence at 1–5/10,000 people. (Orpha:137686, [17]) Paradoxically, Orphanet also estimates the prevalence in subfertile populations from 2.8% to 46%, when subfertility affects one in eight couples. Regardless, the true incidence of IUA is likely underreported. If only 10% of the uterine cavity is annealed and 90% is normal, some women may not notice a 10% reduction in menstrual volume. Also, when IUA are more extensive, many women do not seek gynecologic care to assess lighter menstrual flow. A recent study saw a trend toward lighter menses with increasing severity of IUA, where for mild disease 57.4% of women had light or absent menses, for moderate 69.6%, and severe 90% (9/10), but this trend was not statistically significant [18].

Additionally, though IUA may be recognizable to experienced sonographers, some are more attuned to finding masses than they are to endometrial thinning or loss of the border delineating anterior from posterior endometrium. Because it is difficult to find what one is not looking for, IUA-associated absences on sonography can require insight similar to that in Sherlock Holmes's recognition of a "dog that didn't bark." Wider use of office hysteroscopy will likely lead to increased estimates in the prevalence of IUA.

Acknowledging that the most common presentation for IUA may be an absence of symptoms, menstrual disturbance is likely the most common complaint resulting from IUA. A large study from four decades ago noted in women with IUA a 37% rate of amenorrhea and 31% reporting hypomenorrhea [4]. A more recent study in a subfertility population observed 14.6% and 46.3% rates respectively [19]. Symptoms do not clearly correlate with the extent of adhesions [20].

If amenorrhea and hypomenorrhea relate to the extent of endometrial loss, then dysmenorrhea and pelvic pain are proportionate to menstrual entrapment. In this setting, it is easier for pain-associated symptoms to derive from cervical adhesive disease than uterine. The reason is that it takes an extended area of adhesions within the uterus to fully obstruct outflow from a small area (and with proportionate reduction in menstrual flow for that adherent region). However, adhesions only a few millimeters wide in the cervix may be sufficient to completely block outflow. Tubal occlusion can further exacerbate dysmenorrhea and pelvic pain from intrauterine and intracervical adhesions when menses are obstructed, similar to that seen with iatrogenically induced adhesions found in post-ablation tubal sterilization syndrome (PATSS).

IUA can also contribute to subfertility and recurrent pregnancy loss. IUA don't have overlying endometrium favorable to implantation and typically lack vascularity that would help sustain a developing pregnancy. Though up to half of women with IUA can have difficulties conceiving and sustaining a pregnancy, this may be an overestimate influenced by detection bias [21, 22].

Diagnosis of Intrauterine Adhesions

Multiple approaches are used to identify IUA, including hysterosalpingography (HSG), sonography, saline infusion sonography (SIS), 3D sonohysterography (including 3D power Doppler), and MRI. HSG seems to have a particularly high rate of false positives and negatives for IUA relative to SIS, with relative accuracies of 26.9% and 63.2% respectively [23]. Hysteroscopy remains the gold standard and can identify up to a third more IUA than 3D sonohysterography [24], but not all studies find a clear advantage [25]. Not only can saline infusion sonography be used for preoperative visualization of IUA, but catheter placement and balloon inflation can even offer some development of the cavity. However, beyond detection of adhesions, there are multiple advantages to office hysteroscopy relative to other approaches prior to surgical intervention. First, office hysteroscopy is the best proxy for intraoperative conditions. Knowing whether there are visible intraoperative landmarks has important implications when addressing the balance of risk and benefit for informed consent, including expectations for the number of procedures required for more extensive disease. Second, office hysteroscopy facilitates better preparation, such as whether intraoperative sonography would be advantageous. Third, office hysteroscopy allows for a degree of see and treat, where with gentle sweeping of filmy adhesions, one can better develop the cavity, better delineating surgical planes.

For detecting IUA, all estimates of accuracy through sonography should be interpreted in the light of the year of the study, the timing within the menstrual cycle, the nature of image analysis, and the type of IUA being identified. The earlier the study, the greater the risk for lower resolution which negatively affects sensitivity and specificity. Within the menstrual cycle, the luteal phase allows for easier delineation of intracavitary structures that contrast with the robust endometrium. The greater the use of iatrogenic contrast or 3D, the greater the amount of information, which enhances accuracy. Finally, the more prevalent hematometra are in studies, the easier it is to identify IUA due to contrasting intracavitary blood.

Intracervical adhesions often present sonographically as an echogenic line that can be traced from the cervix to a point where the line dissipates. Depending on where the patient is in the menstrual cycle, a cervical mucocele or hematocele should prompt suspicion for adhesions or stricture in the lower cervix. These may fill the upper cervix due to difficult egression, with difficulty identifying the lower path to the outer cervical os on sonography. When MRI is used due to cervical adhesions hindering SIS, T2-weighted images will visualize IUA as having low signal intensity within the uterine cavity.

When using sonography for intracavitary evaluation, intrauterine adhesions may present more as heterogeneous opacity, where there is homogeneous echogenicity across measurements of endometrial thickness, excepting portions where an interface between the anterior and posterior can be segmentally identified. The less the interface can be visualized, the greater the potential for thicker adhesions. Saline and other contrast, such as fluids, foams, and gels, can further help delineate points of fusion between the anterior and posterior endometrium. Hematometra may present as low-level homogeneous echoes, though this will be dependent on where the patient is in the menstrual cycle and the duration the hematometra has been present.

Classification of Intrauterine Adhesions

In 1978, March proposed a hysteroscopic classification system for intrauterine adhesions that remains in wide use due to its simplicity [26]. It is broken into three categories: minimal (Fig. 5.3), moderate (Fig. 5.4), and severe (Fig. 5.5). This approximately correlates with the American Fertility Society classifications of I, II, and III respectively [27]. Though these classification systems are easy to understand and communicate, their ability to predict subsequent menstrual function and fecundity are limited. However, more advanced classification systems, such as those proposed by the European Society for Hysteroscopy [28], Nasr [29], and others have had less widespread use (Table 5.1). Moreover, heterogeneity in IUA etiology, presentation, severity, and management (both technique and surgical skill) will hinder the predictive value for any model.

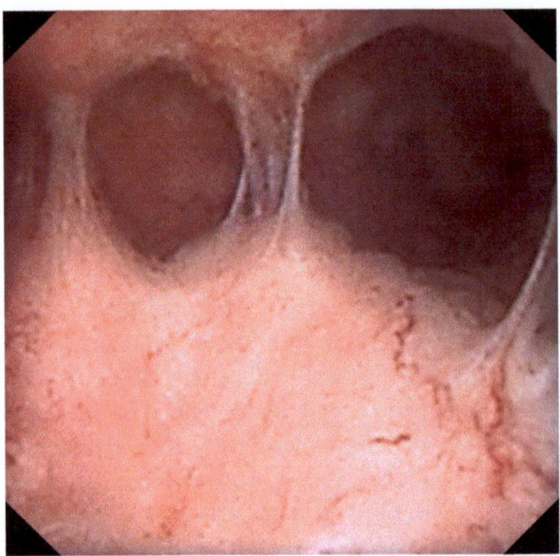

Fig. 5.3 Minimal adhesions after dilation and curettage for endometrial hyperplasia, followed by Megace treatment

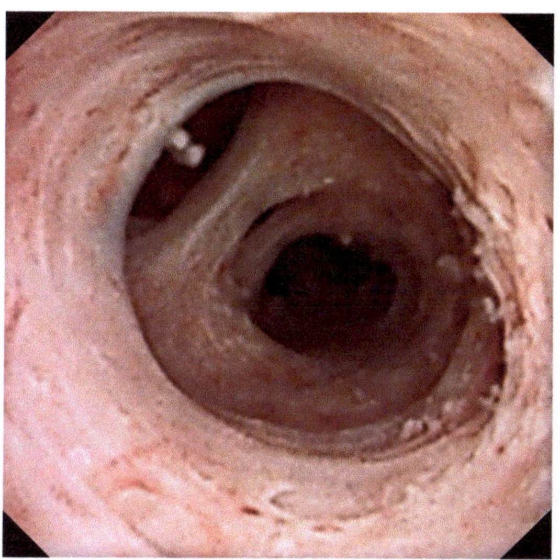

Fig. 5.4 Moderate adhesions after dilation and curettage for first-trimester miscarriage

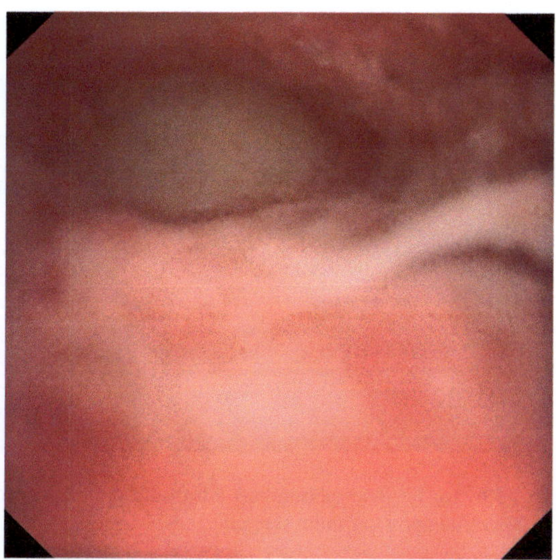

Fig. 5.5 Severe adhesions, with almost complete intra-cavitary obliteration after dilation and curettage to remove a polyp (rather than directed visualization and resection). Central and fundal location of the hysteroscope was confirmed with concurrent sonography

Table 5.1 Classification systems for intrauterine adhesions

References	Findings at assessment	Diagnosis	Symptoms
March et al. 1978 [26]	Minimal, moderate, and severe stratified by extent of obliteration (<1/4, 1/4–3/4, >3/4), agglutination, and visualization of landmarks	Hysteroscopic	N/A
Hamous et al. 1983 [30]	Stratified by location (isthmic, marginal, central) and severity	Hysteroscopic	N/A
American Fertility Society 1988 [27]	Mild, moderate, and severe stratified by extent of obliteration and adhesion quality	Hysteroscopic, HSG, and clinical	Menstrual
Valle and Sciarra 1988 [31]	Mild, moderate, and severe stratified by partial or total obliteration at HSG	Hysteroscopic and HSG	Menstrual
Wamsteker and DeBlok (European Society for Hysteroscopy) 1989 [28]	Grades I–V stratified by the number and quality of adhesions, with subtypes	Hysteroscopic, HSG, and clinical	Menstrual
Donnez and Nisolle 1994 [32]	Grades I–III based on location (central, marginal, complete obliteration), with subtypes. Emphasis is on anticipated postoperative fecundity.	Hysteroscopic or HSG	N/A
Nasr et al. 2000 [29]	Prognostic scoring system based on adhesion location and density	Hysteroscopic and clinical	Menstrual and obstetrical history

Surgical Considerations

In 1950, Joseph Asherman described the management of IUA through hysterotomy and sweeping his finger to lyse adhesions [3]. With advancements in intraoperative imaging and hysteroscopy, such an approach should be rarely utilized for modern surgical management. Surgical planning to correct IUA focuses on patients wishing to preserve fertility, as hysterectomy and uterine artery embolization are less depending on the extent of intracavitary disease.

Under March's classification system, mild and moderate diseases have lateral landmarks, which

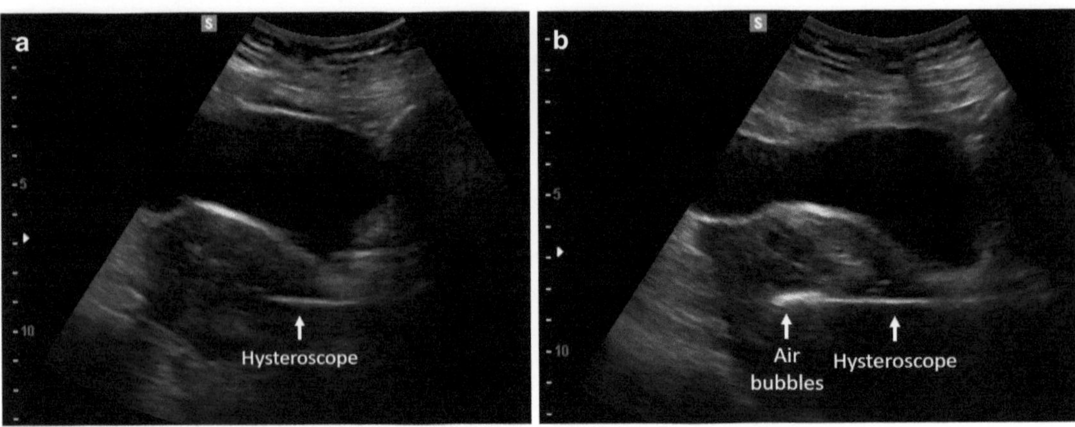

Fig. 5.6 (**a**, **b**). Transabdominal ultrasound-guided resection of intrauterine adhesions, where the distance from the endometrial apex to fundal serosa is less clear in **a**, but more clear after addition of air bubbles in **b**

would typically allow them to be managed as a single hysteroscopic surgery, whether in the office or in the operating room. Severe disease often should be managed in the operating room owing to the degree of risk for uterine perforation. Two preoperative steps have high value in facilitating surgery prior to the actual event. First, preoperative estrogen (2 mg estradiol BID or TID for 4–8 weeks) driving endometrial proliferation may help visualize the endometrium when intraoperative sonography is used (particularly if adhesions prevent saline-associated delineation of the uterine cavity), as well as contribute to postoperative healing. Second, preoperative mapping within the office may enhance planes and efficiency within the operating room. Care is needed to avoid false tracts and patient analgesia must be considered if using sonographically guided dilators or small caliber office hysteroscopy. However, sweeping filmy adhesions to define landmarks and more dense adhesions, coupled with a degree of healing preoperatively, can facilitate efficient use of time within the operating room, as well as guide expectations for outcomes. This preoperative approach parallels McComb and Wagner's operative technique with laparoscopic observation of transcervical exploration with 13 French Pratt dilators, followed by hysteroscopic resection of residual bands [33].

For surgical technique, there is significant debate among gynecologists regarding the use of scissors relative to energy (or laser), such as with a resectoscope or needle point cautery. Proponents of a cold scissors approach note that the use of cautery can hinder endometrial regrowth and perforation when energy has been used poses greater risk of meaningful bowel injury than when this occurs through mechanical means [34]. However, when adhesions have strictured the cervix and a cruciate incision for expansion is planned or when myometrial scoring is used to expand the uterine cavity, cautery can reduce bleeding that might otherwise lead to early cessation of the procedure [35, 36].

Intraoperatively, concurrent sonographic imaging can enhance confidence for location when surgical boundaries are obscured. Particularly in obese patients, transrectal sonography may offer greater clarity through improved proximity to the anatomy. If transabdominal visualization of the remaining distance to the fundal serosa is suboptimal, a few air bubbles can be added and may be more readily visible due to their echogenicity (Fig. 5.6a, b).

Postoperative Management

The need for postoperative adhesion prevention is proportionate to the extent of disease. One study did not observe adhesion reformation for mild disease, but it occurred in a sixth with moderate disease and in 42% of those with severe disease [37]. There are three core approaches to preventing adhesion recurrence postoperatively: hormonal therapy, barrier placement, and office hysteroscopy with lysis of newly forming adhesions. All approaches appear beneficial in preventing reformation of adhesions and there isn't clear or convincing evidence that use in combination improves outcomes. However, this may also be a function of limited statistical power to assess such differences. Though estrogen is known to improve endometrial proliferation, it may not be able to cause regeneration over scarred and devascularized tissue. Of note, sildenafil has been used for endometrial proliferation after IUA, but this was a case report with only two patients [38].

IUDs have been used as barriers, but copper IUDs can be inflammatory. Though one trial showed improved menses with copper IUD use [39], another study showed worse outcomes than not using any postoperative treatment [40]. Similarly, progesterone containing IUDs can thin endometrium, when the goal is for endometrial proliferation. Inflating the balloon for a pediatric foley catheter is particularly good for midline disease and one study showed superior outcomes relative to the use of an IUD (33.9% vs 27.5% subsequent conception) [41]. However, when using this approach, one should avoid overinflation, as this can lead to significant discomfort. There are balloon stents designed for placement after hysteroscopic adhesiolysis, but these can be difficult to place and remove.

Though not shown to be superior for outcomes, arguably second look office hysteroscopy should be the gold standard. The reason is that it is not only effective in treating recurring adhesions, but will also validate the efficacy of the initial surgery [12, 42]. Cost in some settings can be an obstacle, and as such may be more appropriate for patients with moderate to severe IUA, where recurrence is more probable. Alternatively, pressure lavage under ultrasound guidance (PLUG) can be performed, where overdistention of the uterus can lead to lysis of filmy adhesions through separation of the anterior and posterior walls [43]. However, without direct visualization there may be a greater risk for missing lateral adhesion reformation. Additionally, though in the initial publication only 43% (three out of seven)

patients reported moderate discomfort, procedures that overdistend the uterus are inherently more likely to be uncomfortable than those that do not.

Regarding emerging approaches to prevent postoperative IUA recurrence, antibiotics do not appear to improve outcomes before or after surgical management of IUA [9]. The use of barriers derived from hyaluronic acid and freeze-dried amnion applied to a Foley balloon seem to have potential according to a meta-analysis of randomized controlled trials [44]. However, the challenge in interpreting results relating to dissolvable barrier therapy is that few centers have published data relating to their use, leading to debate for external validity. The most supportive data seem to relate to alginate hyaluronate–carboxymethylcellulose use and to polyethylene oxide with sodium carboxymethyl cellulose. However comparative effectiveness, as well as cost-effectiveness, relative to approaches such as postoperative estrogen and second-look hysteroscopy need to be better addressed before there is wider uptake. There has been a case report of successful stem cell use after bone marrow biopsy (coupled with estrogen therapy and subsequent IVF with donor eggs), but without additional data, this is likely best left to research settings at this time [45]. Similarly, aspirin, nitroglycerin, and sildenafil have been used for enhancing myometrial and endometrial perfusion, but additional studies are needed to have confidence in recommendations.

Postoperative Outcomes

The more severe the presence of adhesions, the greater the likelihood for needing additional surgery. Patients with limited endometrium preoperatively are less likely to have a satisfactory postoperative outcome [46]. (Fig. 5.7) Minimal disease is almost always manageable with a single procedure. For moderate IUA, 78% of women require a single surgery for completion, and 50% with severe IUA [31, 47]. Moreover, for severe disease, 26% may require three to four surgeries

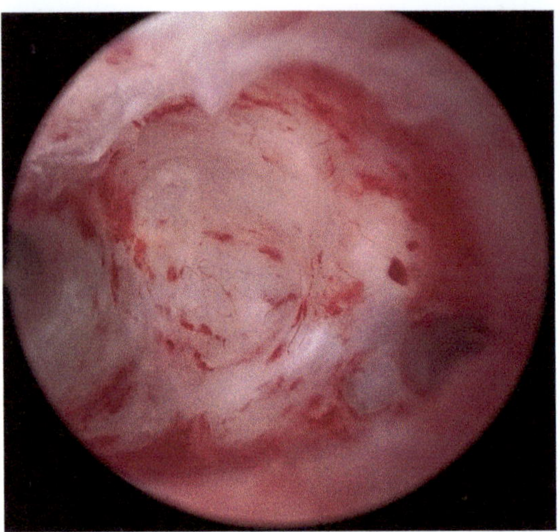

Fig. 5.7 Partially reconstructed uterine cavity after endometrial ablation

[47]. Additionally, Adhesion recurrence is highly dependent on the extent of initial disease. One large series with hysteroscopic reassessment 8–10 weeks postoperatively in 683 women saw a 28.7% rate of IUA recurrence [6]. Favorable outcomes seem linked not only to preexisting pathology, but also the age of the patient and adhesions being more in the uterus than the cervix [48].

Postoperative success is not simply surgical completion, or restoration of the uterine cavity—for women with procreative goals, success is defined through conception leading to a live birth. Approximately half of women having adhesiolysis for IUA will subsequently conceive [49]. For good prognosis women, pregnancy rates can be as high as 79% with a 63.7% chance of live birth [5]. Of note, for these good prognosis women, two-thirds of them conceived spontaneously. Practically all of these conceptions were within the first year when followed as far as 5 years postoperatively. However, for women with severe IUA, only 27–32% may successfully have a live birth [20, 47, 50]. A recent large retrospective study via phone survey saw 54.3% (38/70) of women with mild adhesions able to have a term or pre-term delivery or ongoing pregnancy and 70.9% (51/72) of those with moderate adhesions [18]. However, for those with severe disease, only 28.8% (2/7) had a term, pre-term, or ongo-ing pregnancy. Similarly, a large retrospective study from China's largest women's hospital showed subsequent conception rates of 60.7% for mild disease, 53.4% for moderate disease, and 25% for severe disease [51].

Patients with severe disease should know that a quarter to a third of pregnancies may result in first- or second-trimester loss and 10.1% of live births may be associated with placenta accreta [5, 49]. The recent large retrospective study previously cited saw 45.7% of those with mild disease having spontaneous loss, termination, or ectopic pregnancy [18]. This was only 29.2% of those with moderate disease but 71.4% (5/7) of those with severe disease. Another large study detailing obstetrical outcomes saw 17.6% with abnormal placentation, 4.7% with postpartum hysterectomy, and 29.4% with prematurity [5].

Conclusions

Intrauterine adhesions are a meaningful source of reproductive dysfunction. Causing hypomenorrhea, dysmenorrhea, pelvic pain, and subfertility, correction can improve reproductive outcomes. Imaging or hysteroscopic visualization coupled with an appropriate index of suspicion are central to diagnosis. Multiple treatment options exist, but limitations of sample size for many established approaches and single or a few centers having expertise for emerging approaches need to be considered when considering overall validity. However, many women after treatment, particularly with minimal or moderate disease, will successfully conceive without need for a gestational carrier. Core research opportunities include not only better understanding of the molecular mechanisms behind IUA, but also surgical technique and postoperative treatments to minimize recurrence.

References

1. Fritsch H. Ein fall von volligem schwaund der gebor-mutterhohle nach auskratzung. Zentralbl Gynaekol. 1894;18:1337–42.

2. Asherman JG. Amenorrhoea traumatica (atretica). J Obstet Gynaecol Br Emp. 1948;55:23–30.
3. Asherman JG. Traumatic intrauterine adhesions. J Obstet Gynaecol Br Emp. 1950;57:892–6.
4. Schenker JG, Margalioth EJ. Intrauterine adhesions: an updated appraisal. Fertil Steril. 1982;37(5):593–610.
5. Deans R, Vancaillie T, Ledger W, Liu J, Abbott JA. Live birth rate and obstetric complications following the hysteroscopic management of intrauterine adhesions including Asherman syndrome. Hum Reprod. 2018;33(10):1847–53.
6. Hanstede MM, Van Der Meij E, Goedemans L, Emanuel MH. Results of centralized Asherman surgery, 2003–2013. Fertil Steril. 2015;104(6):1561–8.
7. Hooker AB, de Leeuw RA, Twisk JW, Brölmann HA, Huirne JA. Reproductive performance of women with and without intrauterine adhesions following recurrent dilatation and curettage for miscarriage: long-term follow-up of a randomized controlled trial. Hum Reprod. 2021;36:70–81.
8. Ibrahim MI, Raafat TA, Ellaithy MI, Aly RT. Risk of postpartum uterine synechiae following uterine compression suturing during postpartum haemorrhage. Aust N Z J Obstet Gynaecol. 2013;53(1):37–45.
9. Deans R, Abbott J. Review of intrauterine adhesions. J Minim Invasive Gynecol. 2010;17:555–69.
10. Chen Y, Liu L, Luo Y, Chen M, Huan Y, Fang R. Prevalence and impact of chronic endometritis in patients with intrauterine adhesions: a prospective cohort study. J Minim Invasive Gynecol. 2017;24:74–9.
11. Krolikowski A, Janowski K, Larsen JV. Asherman syndrome caused by schistosomiasis. Obstet Gynecol. 1995;85:898–9.
12. Taskin O, Sadik S, Onoglu A, Gokdeniz R, Erturan E, Burak K, Wheeler JM. Role of endometrial suppression on the frequency of intrauterine adhesions after resectoscopic surgery. J Am Assoc Gynecol Laparosc. 2000;7(3):351–4.
13. Hooker AB, Lemmers M, Thurkow AL, Heymans MW, Opmeer BC, Brolmann HA, Mol BW, Huirne JA. Systematic review and meta-analysis of intrauterine adhesions after miscarriage: prevalence, risk factors and long-term reproductive outcome. Hum Reprod Update. 2013;20:262–78.
14. Vitale SG, Parry JP, Carugno J, Chokeri-Singh A, Della Corte L, Cianci S, Schiattarella A, Riemma G, De Franciscis P. Surgical and reproductive outcomes after hysteroscopic removal of retained products of conception: a systematic review and meta-analysis. J Minim Invasive Gynecol. 2021;28(2):204–17.
15. Chen Y, Chang Y, Yao S. Role of angiogenesis in endometrial repair of patients with severe intrauterine adhesion. Int J Clin Exp Pathol. 2013;15:1343–50.
16. Dmowski WP, Greenblatt RB. Asherman's syndrome and risk of placenta accreta. Obstet Gynecol. 1969;34:288–99.
17. https://www.orpha.net/consor/cgi-bin/Disease_Search.php?lng=EN&data_id=16708&Disease_Disease_Search_diseaseGroup=asherman-syndrome&Disease_Disease_Search_diseaseType=Pat&Disease(s)/group%20of%20diseases=Asherman-syndrome&title=Asherman%20syndrome&search=Disease_Search_Simple. Accessed on 13 Apr 21.
18. Morales B, Movilla P, Wang J, Wang J, Williams A, Chen T, Reddy H, Tavcar J, Loring M, Morris S, Isaacson K. Patient reported menstrual and obstetrical outcomes following hysteroscopic adhesiolysis for Asherman syndrome. F S Rep. 2021;2:118–25.
19. Baradwan S, Baradwan A, Al-Jaroudi D. The association between menstrual cycle pattern and hysteroscopic March classification with endometrial thickness among infertile women with Asherman syndrome. Medicine. 2018;97(27):1–4.
20. March CM. Intrauterine adhesions. Obstet Gynecol Clin N Am. 1995;22:491–505.
21. Schenker JG. Etiology of a therapeutic approach to synechia uteri. Eur J Obstet Gynecol Reprod Biol. 1996;65:109–13.
22. Practice Committee of the American Society for Reproductive Medicine. Evaluation and treatment of recurrent pregnancy loss: a committee opinion. Fertil Steril. 2012;98(5):1103–11.
23. Acholonu UC Jr, Silberzweig J, Stein DE, Keltz M. Hysterosalpingography versus sonohysterography for intrauterine abnormalities. JSLS. 2011;15(4):471–4.
24. Makris N, Kalmantis K, Skartados N, et al. Three-dimensional hysterosonography versus hysteroscopy for the detection of intracavitary uterine abnormalities. Int J Gynecol Obstet. 2007;97:6–9.
25. Abou-Salem N, Elmazny A, El-Sherbiny W. Value of 3-dimensional sonohysterography for detection of intrauterine lesions in women with abnormal uterine bleeding. J Minim Invasive Gynecol. 2010;17:200–4.
26. March C, Israel R, March A. Hysteroscopic managment of intrauterine adhesions. Am J Obstet Gynecol. 1978;130:653–7.
27. American Fertility Society classifications of adnexal adhesions, distal tubal occlusion, tubal occlusion secondary to tubal ligation, tubal pregnancies, Mullerian anomalies and intrauterine adhesions. Fertil Steril. 1988;49:944–55.
28. Wamsteker K, DeBlok SJ. Diagnostic hysteroscopy: technique and documentation. In: Sutton C, Diamond M, editors. Endoscopic surgery for gynecologists. New York: Lippincott Williams & Wilkins Publishers; 1995. p. 263–76.
29. Nasr AL, Al-Inany HG, Thabet SM, Aboulghar MA. A clinicohysteroscopic scoring system of intrauterine adhesions. Gynecol Obstet Investig. 2000;50:178–81.
30. Hamou J, Salat-Baroux J, Siegler A. Diagnosis and treatment of intrauterine adhesions by microhysteroscopy. Fertil Steril. 1983;39:321–6.
31. Valle RF, Sciarra JJ. Intrauterine adhesions: hysteroscopic diagnosis classification, treatment, and reproductive outcome. Am J Obstet Gynecol. 1988;158:1459–70.

32. Donnez J, Nisolle M. Hysteroscopic adheisolysis of intrauterine adhesions (Asherman syndrome). In: Donnez J, editor. An atlas of laser operative laparoscopy and hysteroscopy. London: Parthenon Publishing Group; 1994.

33. McComb PF, Wagner BL. Simplified therapy for Asherman's syndrome. Fertil Steril. 1997;68:1047–50.

34. March CM, Miller C. Hysteroscopic lysis of intrauterine adhesions. Obs Gynecol News. 2006;41:36–7.

35. Wood MA, Kerrigan KL, Burns MK, Glenn TL, Ludwin A, Christianson MS, Bhagavath B, Lindheim SR. Overcoming the challenging cervix: identification and techniques to access the uterine cavity. Obstet Gynecol Surv. 2018;73(11):641–9.

36. Protopapas A, Shushan A, Magos A. Myometrial scoring: a new technique for the management of severe Asherman's syndrome. Fertil Steril. 1998;69:860–4.

37. Yu D, Tin-Chiu L, Xia E, et al. Factors affecting reproductive outcome of hysteroscopic adhesiolysis for Asherman's syndrome. Fertil Steril. 2008;89(3):715–22.

38. Zinger M, Liu JH, Thomas MA. Successful use of vaginal sildenafil citrate in two infertility patients with Asherman's syndrome. J Women's Health. 2006;15:442–4.

39. Vesce F, Jorizzo G, Bianciotto A, Gotti G. Use of the copper intrauterine device in the management of secondary amenorrhea. Fertil Steril. 2000;73:162–5.

40. Acunzo G, Guida M, Pellicano M, et al. Effectiveness of auto-crosslinked hyaluronic acid gel in the prevention of intrauterine adhesions after hysteroscopic adhesiolysis: a prospective, randomized, controlled study. Hum Reprod. 2003;18:1918–21.

41. Orhue AA, Aziken ME, Igbefoh JO. A comparison of two adjunctive treatments for intrauterine adhesions following lysis. Int J Gynaecol Obstet. 2003;82:49–56.

42. Robinson JK, Colimon LM, Isaacson KB. Postoperative adhesiolysis therapy for intrauterine adhesions (Asherman's syndrome). Fertil Steril. 2008;90(2):409–14.

43. Coccia ME, Becattini C, Bracco GL, Pampaloni F, Bargelli G, Scarselli G. Pressure lavage under ultrasound guidance: a new approach for outpatient treatment of intrauterine adhesions. Fertil Steril. 2001;75(3):601–6.

44. Yan Y, Xu D. The effect of adjuvant treatment to prevent and treat intrauterine adhesions: a network meta-analysis of randomized controlled trials. J Minim Invasive Gynecol. 2018;25(4):589–99.

45. Nagori CB, Panchal SY, Patel H. Endometrial regeneration using autologous adult stem cells followed by conception by in vitro fertilization in a patient of severe Asherman's syndrome. J Hum Reprod Sci. 2011;4:43–8.

46. Schlaff WD, Hurst BS. Preoperative sonographic measurement of endometrial pattern predicts outcome of surgical repair in patients with severe Asherman's syndrome. Fertil Steril. 1995;63:410–3.

47. Capella-Allouc S, Morsad F, Rongieres-Bertrand C, et al. Hysteroscopic treatment of severe Asherman's syndrome and subsequent fertility. Hum Reprod. 1999;14(5):1230–3.

48. Chen L, Xiao S, He S, Tian Q, Xue M. Factors that impact fertility after hysteroscopic adhesiolysis for intrauterine adhesions and amenorrhea: a retrospective cohort study. J Minim Invasive Gynecol. 2020;27:54–9.

49. Guo EJ, Chung JP, Poon LC, Li TC. Reproductive outcomes after surgical treatment of Asherman syndrome: a systematic review. Best Pract Res Clin Obstet Gynaecol. 2019;59:98–114.

50. Fernandez H, Peyrelevade S, Legendre G, et al. Total adhesions treated by hysteroscopy: must we stop at two procedures? Fertil Steril. 2012;98(4):980–5.

51. Chen L, Zhang H, Wang Q, Xie F, Gao S, Song Y, Dong J, Feng H, Xie K, Sui L. Reproductive outcomes in patients with intrauterine adhesions following hysteroscopic adhesiolysis: experience from the largest women's hospital in China. J Minim Invasive Gynecol. 2017;24:299–304.

Zaraq Khan

Leiomyoma/myomas or commonly referred to as fibroids are benign uterine tumors that are present in up to 70–80% of premenopausal women by age 50 [1]. The prevalence in symptom-free women is as high as 40% in white and more than 60% in black patients of the same age group [1]. Even though 1 out of 3 women in the United States have a hysterectomy by age 60, more than 90% of these are performed for non-life-threatening indications [2]. The most common indication for hysterectomy in the United States remains leiomyoma at around 40% [3]. Most common symptoms caused by fibroids include abnormal uterine bleeding (AUB) – specifically heavy menstrual bleeding, bulk related symptoms due to the mass effect of the lesion, and an association with sub/infertility.

Approximately 40% of premenopausal women who seek evaluation for heavy menstrual bleeding are found to have intracavitary lesions like polyps or fibroids [4]. Submucosal fibroids are more likely to cause issues with AUB and are primarily lesions that have the potential to impair fertility. For these intracavitary lesions, myomectomy is more often recommended – especially for women seeking fertility in the future, and a hysteroscopic myomectomy is considered the gold standard for women who have symptomatic submucosal disease burden [5].

Classification

Categorization of fibroids is very useful when evaluating the need to intervene in an otherwise asymptomatic patient with infertility. Location of the lesion within the uterus is most useful in such cases. It is also paramount when considering therapeutic options and surgical approach for patients with symptoms. There are primarily three different systems used to classify fibroids.

The ESGE (European Society of Gynecologic Endoscopists) classifies fibroids based on its location in relation to its location in one of the three basic layers of the uterus: the endometrium (submucosal fibroids), the myometrium (intramural fibroids), and the visceral peritoneum or serosa (subserosal fibroids). The submucosal fibroids are further divided into type 0, 1, and 2 [6, 7] (Fig. 6.1a) (Table 6.1).

The FIGO (International Federation of Gynecology and Obstetrics) utilizes the same classification for submucosal fibroids but adds several other categories (type 3–7) [8]. The FIGO classification system provides information on the myoma's outer boundary within the uterine wall/serosa. This is much needed information for a surgeon planning route of surgery. For example, a fibroid that has 20% cavitary component is

Z. Khan (✉)
Division Chair, Reproductive Endocrinology & Infertility, Consultant, Division of Minimally Invasive Gynecologic Surgery, Mayo Clinic, Rochester, MN, USA
e-mail: khan.zaraq@mayo.edu

© The Author(s), under exclusive license to Springer Nature Switzerland AG 2022
S. R. Lindheim, J. C. Petrozza (eds.), *Reproductive Surgery*,
https://doi.org/10.1007/978-3-031-05240-8_6

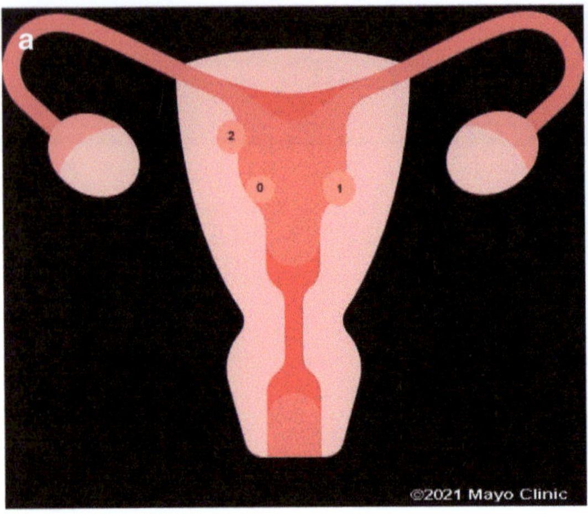
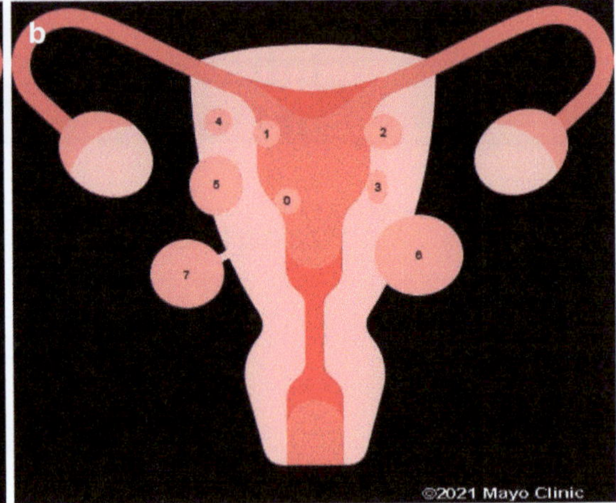

Fig. 6.1 Classification of uterine fibroids based on location is key for preoperative planning. Two most widely accepted classifications systems are shown (**a**) European Society for Gynecological Endoscopy (ESGE) classification of uterine fibroids. (**b**) International Federation of Gynecology and Obstetrics (FIGO) classification of uterine fibroids

Table 6.1 ESGE classification of submucosal fibroids

Type	Entirely within the endometrial cavity
0	No myometrial extension (pedunculated)
Type	<50% myometrial extension
1	<90° angle of myoma surface to uterine wall
Type	≥50% myometrial extension
2	≥90° angle of myoma surface to the uterine wall

classified as a type 2 fibroid by both ESGE and FIGO classification systems. If this fibroid however is large enough to occupy the entirety of the uterine wall and has a subserosal portion as well, it will still be a type 2 fibroid on ESGE system where as it would be a type 2–5 lesion per FIGO classification and therefore not a candidate for hysteroscopic surgery (Fig. 6.1b).

Lasmar classification of submucosal myomas addresses many limitations in the previous two systems and takes into account: (a) the penetration of the myoma into the myometrium (same as ESGE/FIGO submucosal lesion classification), (b) the size of the largest myoma, (c) proportion of the endometrial surface area occupied by the base of the myoma, and (d) topography of the lesion – the location of the myoma with the uterus (upper, middle, or lower body and whether it is present in lateral walls as opposed to anterior or posterior uterine wall) [9]. The classification system provides a point system to calculate a score. The final score can predict the likelihood of completing a hysteroscopic myomectomy and the amount of fluid deficit during the procedure. The system was however not analyzed for its prediction of other important outcomes like successful treatment of AUB or fertility.

Fibroids and Fertility

The impact of fibroids on fertility is not well understood and is not without significant controversy. Whether removal of myomas in asymptomatic women improves fertility remains unknown and overall, there is insufficient evidence that uterine fibroids (all types) reduce the likelihood of pregnancy [10]. Data evaluating reproductive outcomes related to fibroids are generated from observational studies with many biases. Most studies have a heterogenous study design, insufficient patient recruitment and follow-up as well as lack of ideal controls (women without fibroids). Most reports have no means to control for size and location of the fibroids, have inappropriate primary outcomes (clinical pregnancy rates rather than live birth rates) and there is no accounting for major confounders for fertility like age in most studies [10].

However, there is consensus to intervene when there is presence of cavity-distorting myomas for women with sub/infertility [11]. Pritts and colleagues observed lower fertility in women with cavity distorting fibroids and noted improvements in fertility after removal of these lesions [12]. The American Society of Reproductive Medicine (ASRM) committee opinion also states that there is fair evidence that hysteroscopic myomectomy for submucosal fibroids improves clinical pregnancy rates [10]. This improvement in pregnancy rates is, however, not seen after removal of subserosal or intramural fibroids that are not distorting the uterine cavity [10, 12, 13].

It is widely accepted that type 2 fibroids up to 4 cm in diameter and type 0–1 fibroids up to 5 cm in diameter can be safely excised with hysteroscopic approach [5]. Prior to proceeding with hysteroscopic surgery, there are several preoperative issues to keep in mind.

Preoperative Considerations

Imaging

Even though a thorough history and physical examination is the first step in evaluation of any patient, the importance of preoperative imaging especially in women with submucosal fibroids cannot be overemphasized. The three most important things to consider are (a) location, (b) size, and (c) number of fibroids present. Imaging can hence dictate the route of surgery (abdominal vs. laparoscopic vs. hysteroscopic myomectomy). Additionally, imaging will help determine if asymptomatic patients need a myomectomy for enhancement/optimization of fertility. An asymptomatic patient with a type 1 myoma may require hysteroscopic surgery for fertility enhancement compared to an asymptomatic patient with a type 4 myoma that otherwise does not distort the cavity. Likewise, a patient with multiple (>10), large (largest >18 cm) fibroids that range from type 2–6 might require an abdominal approach compared to a patient with a solitary type 2 myoma

who would benefit from hysteroscopic excision. Likewise, women with larger type 2 myomas may need a multi-step hysteroscopic resection (mostly because of fluid deficit limits being hit in these cases with larger lesions) versus a single laparoscopic myomectomy, An individualized discussion with the patient and weighing risk and benefits of hysteroscopy versus laparoscopy is necessary.

Ultrasonographic evaluation is typically the first imaging modality used in most patients however, ultrasound imaging has operator-dependent variability, limited field of view (especially when evaluating large myomas), and can have difficulty in accurately classifying a submucosal fibroid [3]. Other imaging modalities include 3D-ultrasonography, saline sonohysterography, magnetic resonance imaging (MRI) and office hysteroscopy [2] (Fig. 6.2a–d).

Imaging of submucosal myomas can also help predict the likelihood of completing a hysteroscopic myomectomy in one sitting based on the Lasmar classification system [9]. Additionally, depth of penetrance of submucosal fibroids in the wall of uterus and myoma size can help guide a surgeon in picking appropriate hysteroscopic instruments as well as help counsel the patient for the need of preoperative therapy to help reduce myoma volume and size for optimal surgical conditions. Finally, imaging with gadolinium-enhanced MRI in combination with elevated lactate dehydrogenase isoenzyme-3 may be helpful in preoperatively diagnosing leiomyosarcoma and may help appropriate management [14].

Evaluation of Hemoglobin/Iron Stores and Other Possible Causes of Heavy Menstrual Bleeding

Screening for anemia and assessment of iron stores prior to surgical intervention is critical in women who present with heavy menstrual bleeding. A complete blood count and ferritin levels might be useful prior to surgery in patients with long-standing heavy menstrual bleeding. Although most hysteroscopic myomectomy procedures have limited blood loss, normalizing

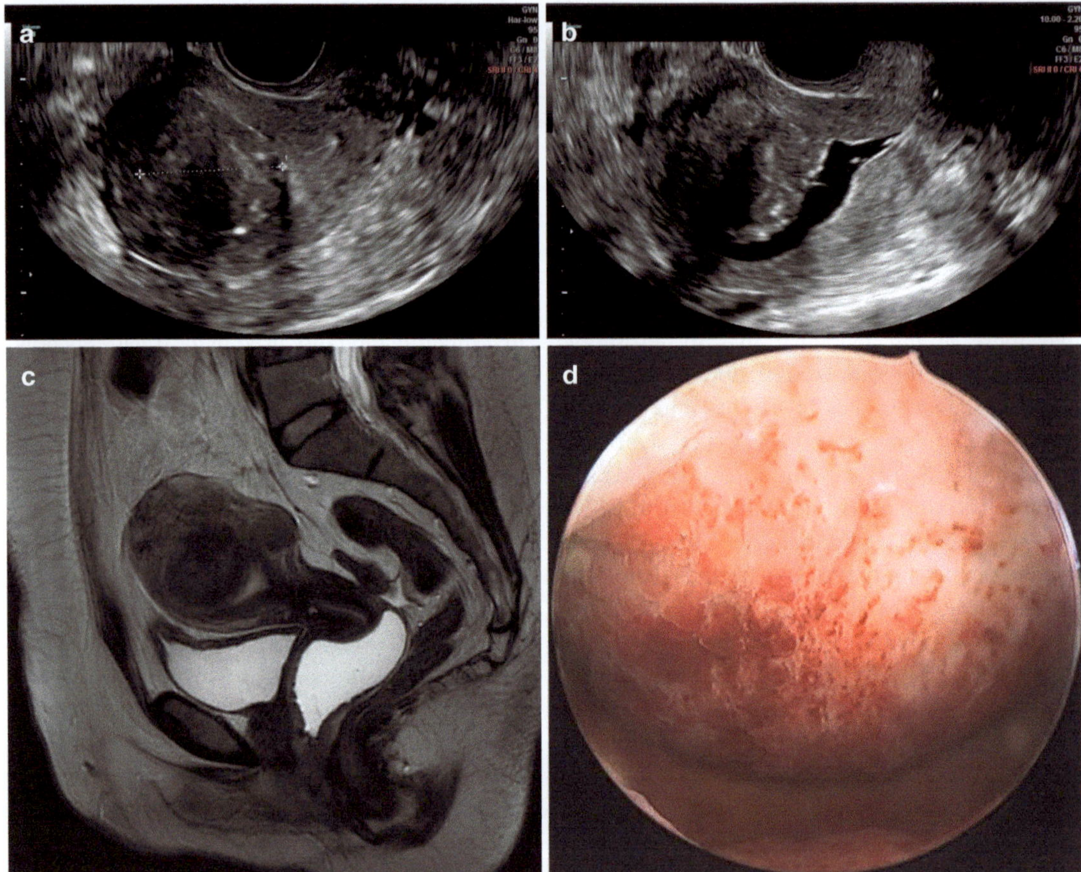

Fig. 6.2 Imaging for submucosal fibroid of the same patient with different techniques. (**a**) Ultrasonography is the most used imaging modality for the diagnosis of uterine fibroids. A sagittal view of the uterus is shown here with a fundal submucosal myoma. (**b**) Saline sonohysterography can further highlight the boundaries of the myoma. After saline infusion the myoma can be classified as FIGO type 1 as more than 50% of it is seen in the endometrial cavity. (**c**) Magnetic resonance imaging (MRI) is another accurate way to assess a uterine fibroid. Here a sagittal T2-weighted image is shown of the same patient where the myoma can be classified as FIGO type 1 as more than 50% of it is seen in the endometrial cavity. (**d**) A hysteroscopy can help identify submucosal lesions as shown in this image. An anterior wall FIGO type 1 myoma is noted consistent with sonohysterogram and MRI

hemoglobin and iron stores prior to surgery reduces overall risk and can prevent unnecessary post-operative blood transfusions that can otherwise lead to morbidity after myomectomy [15]. Oral, and intravenous iron, epoetin (a recombinant form of erythropoietin) and gonadotropin releasing hormone (GnRH) analogs and antagonists have all been used for improving hemoglobin and iron stores in otherwise anemic patients [16–18]. In general, the author utilizes oral iron therapy as first line and offers intravenous iron and GnRH analogs to induce amenorrhea if anemia is not corrected with first line measures.

Assessing other common metabolic causes for heavy bleeding like thyroid dysfunction and abnormalities in prolactin is essential to rule out causes of abnormal bleeding other than the myoma.

Use of Gonadotropin Releasing Hormone (GnRH) Analogs and Antagonists

The use of GnRH analogs is adopted by many to reduce myoma size prior to surgery. Typically, submucosal myomas >4 or 5 cm could benefit from size reduction so the lesion could be amenable to hysteroscopic removal in a single sitting. The use of GnRH analogs does make dissection of the myoma from its bed harder and the author in his practice prefers not to use this. The data supports the use of GnRH analogs for 3–4 months prior to surgery to decrease fibroid size, uterine volume, and postoperative anemia; however, its use has not been shown to improve rates of complete myoma removal [19–21]. Most recently GnRH antagonist use has shown to reduce heavy bleeding in women with fibroids [49]; however, the specific use of GnRH antagonists in the perioperative period is still understudied.

Use of Cervical Ripening Agents

Most complications during hysteroscopy occur with entry of the hysteroscope [22]. Cervical ripening with the use of prostaglandin E1 analog (Misoprostol 200–400 µg) taken vaginally or orally 12–24 h before surgery may facilitate cervical dilation, reducing the risk cervical lacerations and uterine perforations with stenotic cervices. A Cochrane review supports the routine use of ripening agents which lead to reduction in cervical lacerations and creation of false cervical passages [23]. Some intracavitary lesions can prolapse further into the cavity due to uterine contractions following administration of Misoprostol making them more amenable to hysteroscopic excision [2].

Timing of Hysteroscopic Surgery

Timing of hysteroscopic surgery in relation to the menstrual cycle is key for adequate visualization. Most surgeons perform hysteroscopic procedures in the mid proliferative phase of the menstrual cycle after cessation of menses. A thin endometrial lining can be beneficial in adequate intracavitary visualization. Alternatively, patients can be placed on combined oral contraceptives or GnRH analogs to induce amenorrhea to allow for scheduling surgery.

Intraoperative Considerations

Use of Preoperative Antibiotics

The overall risk of an infection after hysteroscopy is very low (0.01–1.42%) [24, 25]. The role of preoperative antibiotics in this scenario has not been well established. Given the low risk of infection the author does not use preoperative antibiotics, an approach that is supported by the American College of Obstetricians and Gynecologists [26]. An exception to the rule includes resectoscopic surgery in women with a history of pelvic inflammatory disease (PID) [27].

Choice of Distension Medium for Hysteroscopy

The uterine cavity is a potential dead space that needs to be distended by a medium for visualization during surgery. Classically the distension medium used has either been carbon dioxide or some form of fluid [28]. The former is only used for diagnostic hysteroscopy and the latter for operative procedures. While distension of the cavity is key for surgical visualization, it also causes a common issue of fluid deficit in hysteroscopic procedures. Absorption of large volumes of fluid can occur during hysteroscopy leading to serious complications arising from fluid overload [29]. Distension fluids are characterized by viscosity and osmolality. The type of distension medium used for operative hysteroscopy is mainly dependent on surgeon preference and is dictated by the type of surgical instrument being used. (Table 6.2).

High Viscosity Distension Medium

Dextran 32% is an example of high viscosity solution. This fluid produces excellent visualization, especially in cases of bleeding as the solution is immiscible with blood, however, can cause anaphylactic reactions and also lead to crystallization within the hysteroscope [30]. The use of high viscosity fluids is hence not common at all. The recommended fluid deficit with high viscosity medium is as low as 300–500 mL [31].

Table 6.2 Details of common distension media and their applicability in operative hysteroscopy

Distension medium	Classification	Osmolality (mOSm/L)- normal plasma 285 mOsm/L	Electrolyte free	Compatibility of energy source
Glycine 1.5%	Hypotonic	200	Yes	Monopolar
Sorbitol 3%	Hypotonic	165	Yes	Monopolar
Mannitol 5%	Isotonic	274	Yes	Monopolar
Normal saline	Isotonic	285	No	Bipolar
Ringer's lactate	Isotonic	279	No	Bipolar

Low Viscosity Distension Medium

Low viscosity distension media can be divided into isotonic or hypotonic solutions in relation to the osmolality of plasma which is typically around 285 mOsm/L. (Table 6.2).

Hypotonic Distension Medium

Low viscosity hypotonic solutions can be used when utilizing monopolar energy devices during operative hysteroscopy. Common examples are: Glycine 1.5%, Sorbitol 3%, and Dextrose 5%. When the fluid deficit reaches 750 mL, the entire team including the anesthesiologist and nurse should be aware and surgery may be continued with caution. Strong consideration should be given to stopping the procedure when a fluid deficit of 1000 mL is reached. Going over the recommended deficit can lead to serious complications that include hypervolemia, hyponatremia, and in severe cases cerebral edema and increased intracranial pressure [29]. Excessive absorption of sorbitol can lead to hyperglycemia and hypocalcemia [32].

Isotonic Distension Medium

Isotonic solutions may contain electrolytes such as normal saline solution and Ringer's lactate solution, whereas some may be electrolyte free like mannitol 5% solution. Isotonic solutions containing electrolytes are used when bipolar energy devices are available. The use of isotonic fluid is considered safer as fluid absorption causes volume overload but not hyponatremia. When the fluid deficit reaches 1500 mL, the entire team including the anesthesiologist and nurse should be aware and surgery may be continued with caution. Strong consideration should be given to stopping the procedure when a fluid deficit of 2500 mL is reached. Complications of fluid overload include flash pulmonary edema, which can usually be reversed with careful use of diuretics [29].

The ideal distension solution should be isotonic, nontoxic, cheap, readily available, hypoallergenic, and should be able to be rapidly cleared by the body. For these reasons the author supports the use of normal saline or lactated Ringers solution for almost all operative hysteroscopies, provided bipolar instruments are available.

Choice of Hysteroscopic Surgical Instruments

The first description of hysteroscopic myomectomy utilized a urologic monopolar energy resectoscope [33]. Since then major advancements have been made in the field and these days gynecologic surgeons have a list of instruments to pick and choose from. As a rule, hypotonic fluid with electrolytes is utilized when monopolar energy devices are used, whereas isotonic electrolyte fluid with bipolar energy devices [29].

Overall surgeons have a choice of the following three types of devices for hysteroscopic myomectomy:

A. Hysteroscopic resectoscope (monopolar or bipolar)
B. Tissue retrieval systems/hysteroscopic morcellators
C. Hysteroscopic vaporization probes

A. *Hysteroscopic Resectoscope*

This technique requires a wire loop that can resect almost all type 0 and 1 and selected type 2 fibroids. The cutting current for monopolar devices is generally sufficient between 60 and 80 Watts; however, denser and calcified fibroids might require higher energy in the range of 120 Watts. Bipolar devices use a default setting for both cutting and hemostasis [2]. Resectoscopes have an added advantage of being able to excise myomas with more uterine wall penetration when compared to morcellators. These devices are also more helpful than morcellators when bleeding is encountered at the time of myomectomy. Bleeding typically obscures visualization (especially when using isotonic fluid). Loop resectoscope devices are helpful in the cauterization of a bleeding vessel which not only helps visualization but can also decrease fluid deficit. Briefly, the electrode is activated with low voltage current to allow repetitive creation of strips of the myoma. The loop should only be activated when target tissue is in contact and once all landmarks within the cavity (both tubal ostia)

are assessed to confirm correct placement of the scope within the uterine cavity (rather than a false passage). There is periodic interruption needed for removal of tissue fragments, which can be removed one at a time or all at once [6] (Fig. 6.3a–c).

The use of loop resectoscope requires surgical skill and experience. The risk of perforation can be high with deeper myometrial penetration [34]. Moreover, the risk of formation of intrauterine scar tissue is higher with use of electrocautery especially if energy is was used on opposing surfaces within the endometrial cavity. When targeting deeply seated type 1 (>40% in wall of the uterus) and type 2 fibroids, the author finds loop resectoscopes to be most useful for a hysteroscopic approach. Several techniques can be used to enucleate deeply seated type 1 and type 2 myomas (see tips and tricks below).

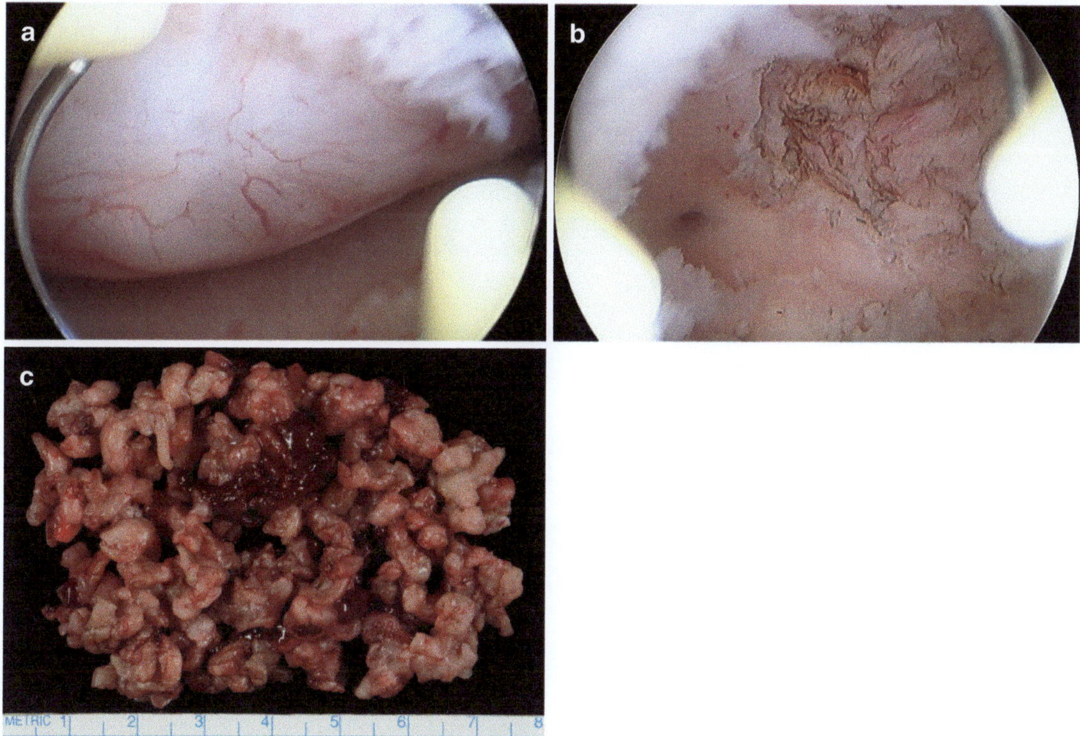

Fig. 6.3 Hysteroscopic myomectomy utilizing loop resectoscope. The loop resectoscope is helpful in removal of deeply seated myomas within the uterine wall. (**a**) Image of myoma prior to resection with the loop resectoscope. (**b**) The myoma bed can be seen after completion of the myomectomy. All myoma fragments were removed hysteroscopically. (**c**) Gross pathology picture of myoma fragments removed at the time of hysteroscopic myomectomy. Large amounts of tissue can be removed efficiently with loop resectoscopic devices as shown here

B. *Tissue Retrieval Systems/Hysteroscopic Morcellators*

Newer techniques have utilized a tissue retrieval system which mechanically shaves and suctions out tissue into a trap or "sock" permitting adequate removal and histologic evaluation. The hand piece of a hysteroscopic morcellator has a window at the tip to feed target tissue into and a rotary-style morcellator that is housed within the window. As the window is opened, the tissue is suctioned into it due to negative pressure. The rotary-style morcellator is then able to shave the tissue as it is being fed into the window, with the tissue fragments being suctioned into the trap or sock [2, 3, 6, 35] (Fig. 6.4a–c).

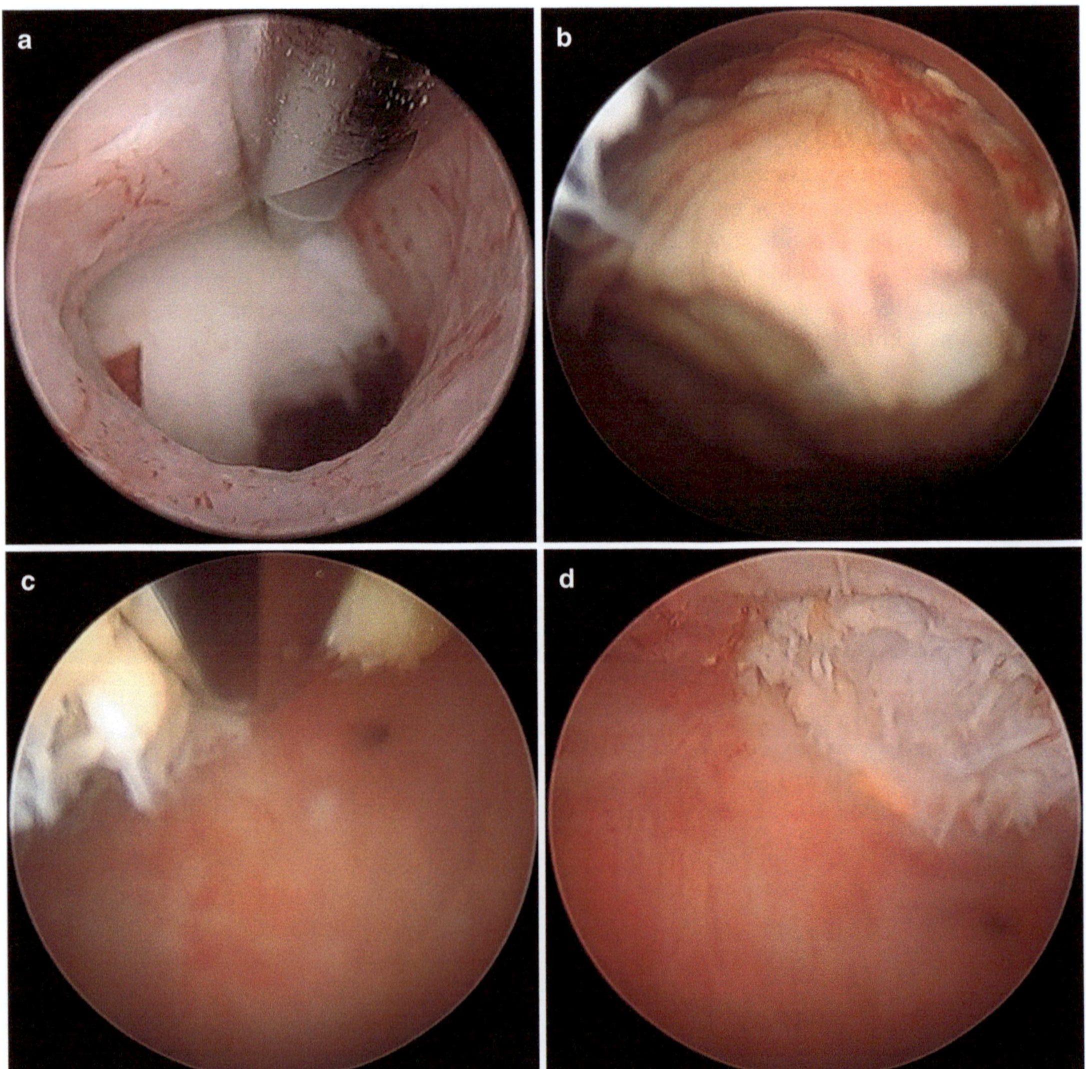

Fig. 6.4 Hysteroscopic morcellator can be used for FIGO type 0 and type 1 myomas that are not deeply seated within the wall of the uterus. In these images, a case of a previously incomplete resected type 2 myoma with loop resectoscope is shown. Most of the myoma had extruded into the cavity and for the second surgery a hysteroscopic morcellator was used. (**a**) This image shows the end of the morcellator with the window and blade within the window noted just above the black mark. (**b**) The previously partially resected myoma can be seen with the lesion extruded into the uterine cavity- changing it from a FIGO type 2 to a FIGO type 0 myoma. (**c**) The specimen is fed into this window. Activation of the morcellator creates a suction and causes the blade to rotate within this window, resulting in shaving of the lesion. (**d**) The myoma bed can be appreciated after completion of myomectomy with a morcellator

Hysteroscopic morcellators are user-friendly and several reports have described fewer complications and less risk of intra-uterine scar tissue. New trainees acquire adept skills quicker than with the resecto-scope [2]. Conversely, these devices tend to work mostly for type 0 and type 1 lesions where a significant amount of the fibroids is within the endometrial cavity. Compared to loop resectoscopes these devices also don't work as well when fibroids are hard and cal-cified based on pre-operative imaging. Finally, any bleeding during the procedure makes it much harder to visualize as the device does not have the ability to pin-point cauterize a bleeding vessel. The author uti-lizes hysteroscopic morcellation for all endometrial polyps and type 0 fibroids as well as type 1 myomas with <40% wall encroachment.

C. *Hysteroscopic Vaporization Probes*

A multiple edge density electrode can be used to desiccate larger leiomyomas hystero-scopically. Vaporizing electrodes are avail-able for mono and bipolar hysteroscopic devices [2]. This technique is beneficial for larger myomas that are not deeply seated in the uterine wall. Vaporization of the tissue makes it smaller and more amenable to removal with loop resectoscope. Although this technique has its advantages, its use pre-cludes tissue for histopathology.

This technique should specifically be avoided at the cornua and isthmus since these anatomical areas are the thinnest and at high-est risk of perforation and intraperitoneal injuries.

Many reports have compared outcomes from hysteroscopic morcellation to hystero-scopic resectoscope use for myomas [5] (Table 6.3). Generally the deeper the extent of the lesion the lower the success rate of complete excision with both morcellation and loop resectoscope; however, a systematic review concluded that both modalities had similar resection rate [36]. Long-term out-comes are also seen to be very similar between the two modalities [5].

Table 6.3 Comparison of hysteroscopic resectoscope to tissue retrieval systems/hysteroscopic morcellator

Hysteroscopic loop resectoscope	Tissue retrieval systems/ hysteroscopic morcellator
Utilizes electric energy (mono or bipolar devices)	Utilizes mechanical force of rotary blade
Suited of deeply seated lesions (deep type 1 and type 2 myomas)	Ideal for type 0 and most type 1 myomas
Has capacity to coagulate bleeding vessels	Visualization can sometimes be more challenging
Requires surgical expertise and skill	Can be easily adopted by newer trainees
Risk of formation of postop scar tissue is higher	Lower risk for scar tissue formation
Specimen pathology is preserved	Specimen pathology is preserved

Miscellaneous Tips and Tricks for Deeply Seated Type 1, and Type 2 Fibroids

It is recommended that deeply seated type 1 and type 2 submucosal fibroids be addressed by expert and experienced surgeons as the excision of these fibroids is technically difficult and these procedures are associated with higher risk of complications. Conventionally type 1 fibroids should not exceed 5–6 cm, whereas a safe proposed cut off for type 2 fibroids is 4–5 cm for hysteroscopic excision [37]. Several techniques have been described that can assist with safe removal of deeply seated myomas. The common shared objective for all hystero-scopic resectoscope techniques is to expose the fibroid capsule as to extrude as much of the fibroid tissue into the cavity so it can be safely excised without mechanical or thermal injury to adjacent endometrium. Some of these tips and tricks are:

- *Cold Loop Technique*

  This technique is carried out by repeated and progressive passage of the loop electrode resectoscope up to the capsule of the fibroid. Once the plane between the fibroid and myometrial bed is identified, a suitable cold blunt loop is used to roll the fibroid and mobilize it from surrounding myometrial by traction and counter-traction rather than energy. Once a significant portion of the fibroid has delivered to the cavity, a loop resectoscope can be used to enucleate any remaining disease [38] (Fig. 6.5a–e).

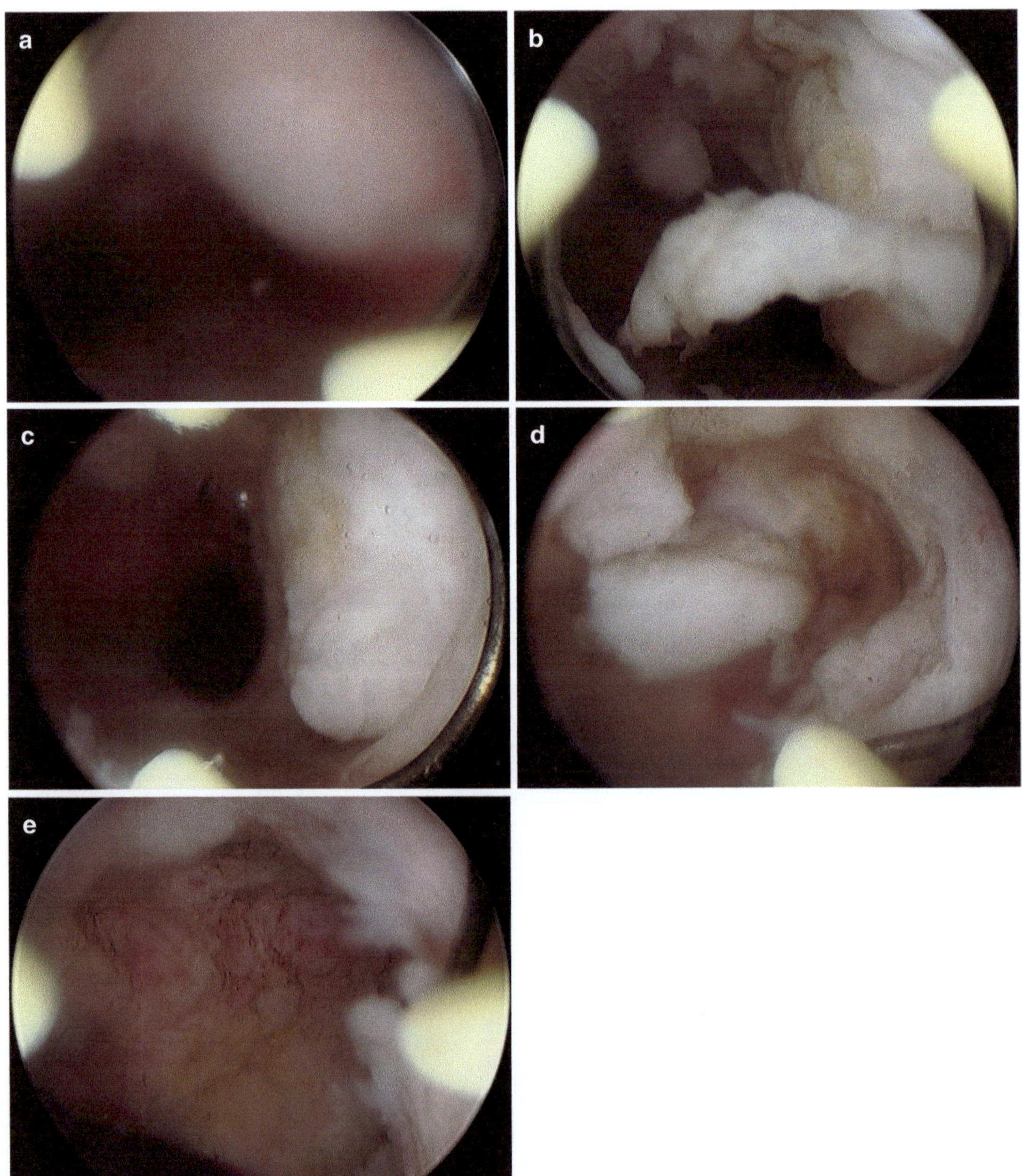

Fig. 6.5 Hysteroscopic removal of difficult, deeply seated submucosal fibroid. (**a**) A deeply seated lateral wall FIGO type 2 myoma is noted on hysteroscopy. (**b**) The loop resectoscope is used to enter the myoma capsule as shown. This allows for some of the myoma to be extruded into the uterine cavity. (**c**) The plane between the myoma and the myometrium is identified, and a cold loop is used to roll the fibroid from the surrounding myoma bed as is seen. (**d**) Once most of the myoma is mobilized from the myometrial bed, the loop resectoscope is used to excise the extruded portion of the lesion. This process is repeated until the entire lesion is successfully excised. (**e**) The large, deep myoma bed is noted here after complete removal of a large type 2 fibroid

- *Enucleation* in Toto (*Litta's Technique*)

  This method utilized a 90° Collins electrode to make an elliptical incision on the endometrial mucosa that covers the fibroid. The incision is continued till the plane between the myoma and surrounding myometrium is noted. Connecting tissue between the fibroid and myometrium is taken down with electrocautery. This maneuver leads to extrusion of the myoma into the cavity, which can then be excised in the traditional method with loop resectoscope [39].

- *Lasmar Technique*

  Very similar to Litta's technique where the Collins electrode is used to make an "L" shaped incision (instead of an elliptical) to get into the myoma capsule [9].

- *Hydromassage*

  Reducing intracavitary fluid pressure aids the myoma to be extruded toward the cavity. This principle was first explored by Hamou, who was the first to propose a rapid cyclic change in intrauterine pressures using an electronically controlled irrigation and suction device [40]. This "hydromassage" could help the partially resected myoma to further deliver toward the endometrial cavity for conventional excision with loop resectoscope.

- *Manual Massage*

  A manual massage of the uterus has also been proposed to help a partially resected myoma in the uterine wall [41].

- *Circumferential Incision into the Capsule*

  A circumferential incision around the protrusion of a deeply seated myoma can also be another way of entering the capsule from all sides and allowing the myoma to deliver more toward the endometrial cavity [42].

- *Use of Pharmacologic Agents*

  Most hysteroscopic procedures are terminated primarily for safety and to reduce excessive fluid deficit. Intracervical injection of dilute vasopressin at 3 and 9 0'clock can help with vasoconstriction of endometrial vessels. This helps with reduced fluid deficit and allows for better visualization as bleeding can be minimized [3].

Intracervical (at hysteroscopy) or intramyometrial injection (at laparoscopy) of Carboprost (a methyl analog of prostaglandin F (PGF) 2α) can cause uterine contractions and facilitate in excision of deeply seated lesions [43, 44].

Finally, as described previously, GnRH analogs can be used to reduce the size of the myoma and could help in reducing the risk of incomplete removal of a deeply seated myoma [19].

- *Safely Completing the Procedure in Two Sittings*

  While the goal should always be to completely excise a myoma, some patients with larger, deep lesions can reach the fluid deficit safety sooner than later. In these cases, it might be best to schedule a second procedure 20–30 days after the initial surgery. The observation of rapid migration of residual disease toward the endometrium with parallel increase in myometrial thickness at the time of hysteroscopic resection clarifies that once the myoma capsule is breached, it will typically deliver toward the cavity [45, 46]. An interval procedure will allow for more of this migration to occur, which could allow complete excision at the second surgery.

- *Convert to a Laparoscopic Approach*

  If the myoma is much larger than anticipated and completing the surgery in one sitting is key, the procedure could be converted to a laparoscopic myomectomy which can facilitate the removal of the deeply seated lesion. Having surgical expertise and laparoscopic suturing skills are essential in being successful.

Intra- and Postoperative Complications

Hysteroscopic myomectomy is generally considered a safe outpatient procedure with overall low complication rates at 0.1–5% [2]. A few common complications from the procedure are listed below:

Uterine Perforation

The most reported complication during hysteroscopy is uterine perforation. This commonly occurs at the time of entry into the cavity or occasionally with uterine sounding. A sudden loss of visualization or drop in intrauterine pressure and a rapidly rising fluid deficit are some signs of perforation. If perforation occurs the procedure must be terminated. If increased bleeding is noted or if perforation occurred with a sharp object or with cautery, a laparoscopy is recommended [6].

Acute Bleeding/Cervical Trauma

Bleeding is rare but occurs more frequently after hysteroscopic myomectomy than other hysteroscopic procedures. Localizing the site of bleeding is most important. If a cervical laceration or trauma is noted, it should be addressed with pressure, chemical cauterization with silver nitrate or suturing. If bleeding is from within the cavity and perforation has been ruled out, a hysteroscopic evaluation may be beneficial. A bleeding vessel can be cauterized with pin-point cautery. If bleeding continues, an intrauterine foley bulb can be placed to tamponade bleeding. Pharmacologic agents that aid in uterine contraction like prostaglandin E1, PGF 2α, methergine, etc., can be used as well to aid with hemostasis [2, 3, 6].

Air/Gas Embolism

Air embolism during a hysteroscopic excision of a myoma can occur secondary to absorption of room air or gas generated during the procedure. Trendelenburg favors gas absorption, most likely due to the pressure difference in operating field and right atrium [31]. A sudden decrease in end-tidal carbon dioxide is typically the first sign of gas embolism. Avoiding excessive cervical dilation, minimizing Trendelenburg position, and purging gas from fluid tubing can be helpful in prevention of this complication.

Fluid Overload

Fluid overload is a common complication of large myomas that are deeply seated in the uterine wall. Having an objective assessment of the fluid deficit is hence critical for operative hysteroscopy. This can be achieved using a closed loop/circuit fluid management system that can accurately determine the amount of fluid given to the patient through the hysteroscope and the amount of fluid returned.

Fluid overload can have serious health consequences especially when it results in hypervolemic hyponatremia as has been described earlier. Knowing the fluid deficit limits for each type of distention fluid (high vs. low viscosity and isotonic vs. hypotonic) is important. For high viscosity and low viscosity hypotonic media, the author recommends stopping the procedure at a deficit of 500 and 1000 mL respectively. When using isotonic solution like normal saline the fluid deficit should not exceed 2500 mL, unless the surgeon, anesthesia team, and nurse are aware. In certain select cases when the patient is young and has robust cardiovascular system, the author does exceed that amount only if the procedure is close to completion. In these scenarios the author will typically insert a foley catheter to record output closely and provide gentle diuresis with Lasix (10–20 mg).

Postoperative Intrauterine Adhesions

Formation of intrauterine adhesions has been reported specifically after hysteroscopic myomectomy that utilized the loop resectoscope and electrocautery. The rate of scar tissue was around 1.5% in women who underwent a single leiomyoma excision, compared to 78% in those who underwent resection of apposing lesions [47]. Multiple methods have been described to reduce the chance of formation of scar tissue. These include the use of postoperative hormone therapy with high dose estrogen for 1 month followed by progestin-induced withdrawal bleed, use of physical barriers like intrauterine stents, intrauterine devices, etc. Overall, none of these methods have shown superiority when compared with one another [48].

While the risk of postoperative scar tissue is low, liberal approach to an early "second" look hysteroscopy has been proposed by some which may help in reducing the formation of postop intrauterine scar tissue [31].

Summary

Hysteroscopy overall and hysteroscopic myomectomy in particular has made great advances in gynecologic surgery. Approaching submucosal fibroids is key as most of these lesions result in heavy menstrual bleeding and have an impact on fertility. Classification of these lesions is extremely important to select a surgical route. Preoperating imaging is essential in developing a surgical plan. Surgeons should be well versed with the various forms of distension media for hysteroscopy and different types of surgical instruments. Deeply seated myomas (some type 1 and all type 2 lesions) require surgical experience and expertise and in most cases, the use of loop resectoscope. Certain tips and tricks have been described in the literature to facilitate the excision of these tricky lesions. Finally, to safely perform surgery, one must be aware of the common complications that can occur during and after hysteroscopic myomectomy.

References

1. Baird DD, Dunson DB, Hill MC, Cousins D, Schectman JM. High cumulative incidence of uterine leiomyoma in black and white women: ultrasound evidence. Am J Obstet Gynecol. 2003;188(1):100–7.
2. Valentine LN, Bradley LD. Hysteroscopy for abnormal uterine bleeding and fibroids. Clin Obstet Gynecol. 2017;60(2):231–44.
3. Falcone T, Parker WH. Surgical management of leiomyomas for fertility or uterine preservation. Obstet Gynecol. 2013;121(4):856–68.
4. Maheux-Lacroix S, Mennen J, Arnold A, Budden A, Nesbitt-Hawes E, Won H, et al. The need for further surgical intervention following primary hysteroscopic morcellation of submucosal leiomyomas in women with abnormal uterine bleeding. Aust N Z J Obstet Gynaecol. 2018;58(5):570–5.
5. Friedman JA, Wong JMK, Chaudhari A, Tsai S, Milad MP. Hysteroscopic myomectomy: a comparison of techniques and review of current evidence in the management of abnormal uterine bleeding. Curr Opin Obstet Gynecol. 2018;30(4):243–51.
6. American Association of Gynecologic Laparoscopists: Advancing Minimally Invasive Gynecology W. AAGL practice report: practice guidelines for the diagnosis and management of submucous leiomyomas. J Minim Invasive Gynecol. 2012;19(2):152–71.
7. Wamsteker K, Emanuel MH, de Kruif JH. Transcervical hysteroscopic resection of submucous fibroids for abnormal uterine bleeding: results regarding the degree of intramural extension. Obstet Gynecol. 1993;82(5):736–40.
8. Munro MG, Critchley HOD, Fraser IS, Committee FMD. The two FIGO systems for normal and abnormal uterine bleeding symptoms and classification of causes of abnormal uterine bleeding in the reproductive years: 2018 revisions. Int J Gynaecol Obstet. 2018;143(3):393–408.
9. Lasmar RB, Barrozo PR, Dias R, Oliveira MA. Submucous myomas: a new presurgical classification to evaluate the viability of hysteroscopic surgical treatment--preliminary report. J Minim Invasive Gynecol. 2005;12(4):308–11.
10. Practice Committee of the American Society for Reproductive Medicine. Electronic address Aao, Practice Committee of the American Society for Reproductive M. Removal of myomas in asymptomatic patients to improve fertility and/or reduce miscarriage rate: a guideline. Fertil Steril. 2017;108(3):416–25.
11. Bosteels J, van Wessel S, Weyers S, Broekmans FJ, D'Hooghe TM, Bongers MY, et al. Hysteroscopy for treating subfertility associated with suspected major uterine cavity abnormalities. Cochrane Database Syst Rev. 2018;12(12):CD009461.
12. Pritts EA, Parker WH, Olive DL. Fibroids and infertility: an updated systematic review of the evidence. Fertil Steril. 2009;91(4):1215–23.
13. Casini ML, Rossi F, Agostini R, Unfer V. Effects of the position of fibroids on fertility. Gynecol Endocrinol. 2006;22(2):106–9.
14. Goto A, Takeuchi S, Sugimura K, Maruo T. Usefulness of Gd-DTPA contrast-enhanced dynamic MRI and serum determination of LDH and its isozymes in the differential diagnosis of leiomyosarcoma from degenerated leiomyoma of the uterus. Int J Gynecol Cancer. 2002;12(4):354–61.
15. Kim T, Purdy MP, Kendall-Rauchfuss L, Habermann EB, Bews KA, Glasgow AE, et al. Myomectomy associated blood transfusion risk and morbidity after surgery. Fertil Steril. 2020;114(1):175–84.
16. Kim YH, Chung HH, Kang SB, Kim SC, Kim YT. Safety and usefulness of intravenous iron

sucrose in the management of preoperative anemia in patients with menorrhagia: a phase IV, open-label, prospective, randomized study. Acta Haematol. 2009;121(1):37–41.

17. Wurnig C, Schatz K, Noske H, Hemon Y, Dahlberg G, Josefsson G, et al. Subcutaneous low-dose epoetin beta for the avoidance of transfusion in patients scheduled for elective surgery not eligible for autologous blood donation. Eur Surg Res. 2001;33(5–6):303–10.

18. Stovall TG, Muneyyirci-Delale O, Summitt RL Jr, Scialli AR. GnRH agonist and iron versus placebo and iron in the anemic patient before surgery for leiomyomas: a randomized controlled trial. Leuprolide Acetate Study Group. Obstet Gynecol. 1995;86(1):65–71.

19. Lethaby A, Puscasiu L, Vollenhoven B. Preoperative medical therapy before surgery for uterine fibroids. Cochrane Database Syst Rev. 2017;11(11):CD000547.

20. Favilli A, Mazzon I, Grasso M, Horvath S, Bini V, Di Renzo GC, et al. Intraoperative effect of preoperative gonadotropin-releasing hormone analogue administration in women undergoing cold loop hysteroscopic myomectomy: a randomized controlled trial. J Minim Invasive Gynecol. 2018;25(4):706–14.

21. Kamath MS, Kalampokas EE, Kalampokas TE. Use of GnRH analogues pre-operatively for hysteroscopic resection of submucous fibroids: a systematic review and meta-analysis. Eur J Obstet Gynecol Reprod Biol. 2014;177:11–8.

22. Bradley LD. Complications in hysteroscopy: prevention, treatment and legal risk. Curr Opin Obstet Gynecol. 2002;14(4):409–15.

23. Al-Fozan H, Firwana B, Al Kadri H, Hassan S, Tulandi T. Preoperative ripening of the cervix before operative hysteroscopy. Cochrane Database Syst Rev. 2015;(4):CD005998.

24. Aydeniz B, Gruber IV, Schauf B, Kurek R, Meyer A, Wallwiener D. A multicenter survey of complications associated with 21,676 operative hysteroscopies. Eur J Obstet Gynecol Reprod Biol. 2002;104(2):160–4.

25. Agostini A, Cravello L, Shojai R, Ronda I, Roger V, Blanc B. Postoperative infection and surgical hysteroscopy. Fertil Steril. 2002;77(4):766–8.

26. ACOG Practice Bulletin No. 195: prevention of infection after gynecologic procedures. Obstet Gynecol. 2018;131(6):e172–e89.

27. McCausland VM, Fields GA, McCausland AM, Townsend DE. Tuboovarian abscesses after operative hysteroscopy. J Reprod Med. 1993;38(3):198–200.

28. Brusco GF, Arena S, Angelini A. Use of carbon dioxide versus normal saline for diagnostic hysteroscopy. Fertil Steril. 2003;79(4):993–7.

29. Umranikar S, Clark TJ, Saridogan E, Miligkos D, Arambage K, Torbe E, et al. BSGE/ESGE guideline on management of fluid distension media in operative hysteroscopy. Gynecol Surg. 2016;13(4):289–303.

30. Witz CA, Silverberg KM, Burns WN, Schenken RS, Olive DL. Complications associated with the absorption of hysteroscopic fluid media. Fertil Steril. 1993;60(5):745–56.

31. Munro MG, Christianson LA. Complications of hysteroscopic and uterine resectoscopic surgery. Clin Obstet Gynecol. 2015;58(4):765–97.

32. Lee GY, Han JI, Heo HJ. Severe hypocalcemia caused by absorption of sorbitol-mannitol solution during hysteroscopy. J Korean Med Sci. 2009;24(3):532–4.

33. Neuwirth RS, Amin HK. Excision of submucus fibroids with hysteroscopic control. Am J Obstet Gynecol. 1976;126(1):95–9.

34. Murakami T, Hayasaka S, Terada Y, Yuki H, Tamura M, Yokomizo R, et al. Predicting outcome of one-step total hysteroscopic resection of sessile submucous myoma. J Minim Invasive Gynecol. 2008;15(1):74–7.

35. Emanuel MH, Wamsteker K. The intra uterine morcellator: a new hysteroscopic operating technique to remove intrauterine polyps and myomas. J Minim Invasive Gynecol. 2005;12(1):62–6.

36. Hamidouche A, Vincienne M, Thubert T, Trichot C, Demoulin G, Nazac A, et al. Operative hysteroscopy for myoma removal: morcellation versus bipolar loop resection. J Gynecol Obstet Biol Reprod (Paris). 2015;44(7):658–64.

37. Di Spiezio SA, Mazzon I, Bramante S, Bettocchi S, Bifulco G, Guida M, et al. Hysteroscopic myomectomy: a comprehensive review of surgical techniques. Hum Reprod Update. 2008;14(2):101–19.

38. Osorio W, Posada N, Cano J, Tamayo S, Giraldo J. Hysteroscopic myomectomy for submucosal type 2 fibroids with cold enucleation technique and complete fibroid extraction using a double-lumen intracervical cannula. Fertil Steril. 2021;115(2):522–4.

39. Litta P, Vasile C, Merlin F, Pozzan C, Sacco G, Gravila P, et al. A new technique of hysteroscopic myomectomy with enucleation in toto. J Am Assoc Gynecol Laparosc. 2003;10(2):263–70.

40. JH. Electroresection of fibroids. In: Sutton C, DM, editors. London: WB Saunders; 1993.

41. Hallez JP. Single-stage total hysteroscopic myomectomies: indications, techniques, and results. Fertil Steril. 1995;63(4):703–8.

42. Munro MG. Hysteroscopic myomectomy of FIGO type 2 leiomyomas under local anesthesia: bipolar radiofrequency needle-based release followed by electromechanical morcellation. J Minim Invasive Gynecol. 2016;23(1):12–3.

43. Murakami T, Tamura M, Ozawa Y, Suzuki H, Terada Y, Okamura K. Safe techniques in surgery for hysteroscopic myomectomy. J Obstet Gynaecol Res. 2005;31(3):216–23.

44. Indman PD. Use of carboprost to facilitate hysteroscopic resection of submucous myomas. J Am Assoc Gynecol Laparosc. 2004;11(1):68–72.

45. Loffer FD. Removal of large symptomatic intrauterine growths by the hysteroscopic resectoscope. Obstet Gynecol. 1990;76(5 Pt 1):836–40.
46. Yang JH, Lin BL. Changes in myometrial thickness during hysteroscopic resection of deeply invasive submucous myomas. J Am Assoc Gynecol Laparosc. 2001;8(4):501–5.
47. Yang JH, Chen MJ, Wu MY, Chao KH, Ho HN, Yang YS. Office hysteroscopic early lysis of intrauterine adhesion after transcervical resection of multiple apposing submucous myomas. Fertil Steril. 2008;89(5):1254–9.
48. Khan Z, Goldberg JM. Hysteroscopic management of Asherman's syndrome. J Minim Invasive Gynecol. 2018;25(2):218–28.
49. Schlaff WD, Ackerman RT, Al-Hendy A, Archer DF, Barnhart KT, Bradley LD, Carr BR, et al. Elagolix for heavy menstrual bleeding in women with uterine fibroids. N Engl J Med. 2020;382(4):328–40. https://doi.org/10.1056/NEJMoa1904351.

Proximal Tubal Obstruction

Xiaohong Liu, Shadain Akhavan,
and Laurel Stadtmauer

Pathophysiology

Tubal disease is responsible for around 25–35% of female infertility cases of which proximal tubal disease accounts for 10–25% [1, 2] Proximal tubal disease is categorized into obstructions, which are reversible and occlusion, which are true anatomic blockage. Most common causes of obstruction are spasm of proximal tubal, mucus plug, or amorphous debris. Tubal occlusion is mainly due to pathological changes in the tube caused by disease processes leading to inflammation and scarring and fibrosis. This is commonly caused by salpingitis isthmica nodosa (SIN), acute and chronic salpingitis, cornual fibroids, intratubal endometriosis, pelvic adhesive disease, prior ectopic pregnancy, polypoid lesions, and adenomyosis.

The oviduct which averages 10–12 cm is a seromuscular organ consisting of outer serous coat, middle muscular myosalpinx, and inner mucus coated endosalpinx with ciliated and secretory cells [3]. The muscularis layer consists of two smooth muscle layers, an inner circular or spiral and outer longitudinal muscle fibers. The most proximal portion of the fallopian tube, the intramural segment is 1.5–2.5 cm in length, its luminal diameter is 100 μm, and its route to fundus may be tortuous (about 70% of the tubes), straight (about 20% of tubes), and curved (about 10% of tubes) [4]. There is a muscular and vascular loop around the distal intramural segment, which, in addition to the commonly found tortuous course and the narrowing of the intramural duct, is thought to be prone to build up of uterine content and eventually blockage or obstruction [5, 6].

Occlusion

Salpingitis

Infection of the upper genital tract in women may lead to acute salpingitis, causing epithelial destruction, luminal obliteration, and fibrosis. The cornual and the fimbriae are the two most common sites of occlusion. The rate of tubal blockage is 12.8% after first infection, 35.5% after two infection, and 75% after three or more infections [7, 8].

Salpingitis Isthmica Nodosa (SIN)

Salpingitis isthmica nodosa is found in about 35% of cases of tubal occlusion. It is often described as a progressive progress with uncertain etiology, but likely inflammatory or acquired.

X. Liu · S. Akhavan · L. Stadtmauer (✉)
EVMS Jones Institute for Reproductive Medicine,
Norfolk, VA, USA
e-mail: liux@evms.edu; shadain.akhavan@Inova.org;
stadtmla@evms.edu

S. R. Lindheim, J. C. Petrozza (eds.), *Reproductive Surgery*,
https://doi.org/10.1007/978-3-031-05240-8_7

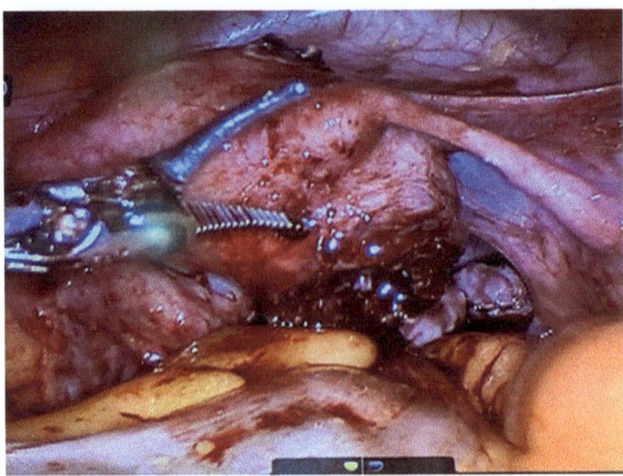

Fig. 7.1 Salpingitis isthmica nodosum associated with proximal tubal blockage and uterine fibroids and tubal infertility noted during Da Vinci assisted laparoscopic myomectomy

SIN can be identified on HSG. Radiographic findings are significant for diverticula that extend from the intramural/isthmic lumens. On laparoscopy, a proximal tubal nodule can be observed (Fig. 7.1). Definitive diagnosis is confirmed with histology. Selective salpingography or tubal cannulation should not be attempted once SIN is diagnosed [9].

Endometriosis

The pathophysiology of attachment and implantation of endometrial glands and stroma in the fallopian tube is still controversial but theories such as retrograde menstruation, hematogenous or lymphatic transport, bone marrow stem cell origin, and coelomic metaplasia have found popularity [10]. Prevalence of endometriosis is about 6–10% of which one-third demonstrates tubal endometriosis [11, 12]. Tubal endometriosis is found more often in the left fallopian tube than the right based on histology from unilateral and bilateral salpingectomies. Pathologic examination has identified the mucosa of the proximal tubes as the most likely location [12]. Risk factors for tubal endometriosis include abnormal uterine bleeding, previous endometriosis surgery, and tubal ligation.

Obstruction

Mucus Plugs

Mucus plugs are a frequently unrecognized cause of unexplained infertility and generally are thought to form as a response to inflammation or tissue injury. Histological examinations have shown cast of debris containing aggregates of histiocytic-like cells of endometrial stromal or mesothelial origin, as well as white to yellow mucus-like fragments [13]. Mucus plugs are known to be one of the most common causes of reversible proximal tubal obstruction possibly and are often dislodged during a hysterosalpingogram (HSG). About two-thirds of all proximal blockages found on initial HSG are due to mucus plug or uterotubal spams and will be patent on a subsequent HSG [14].

Uterotubal Spasms

The spasm and transient closure of the tube is a functional anomaly that can mimic a mechanical tubal occlusion. Most common site of spasm is at the cornual portion of the fallopian tube where the tube is encased by the smooth muscle of the uterus [15]. Therefore, the tubal spasm is a physiological response to uterine distention during diagnostic procedures and is a normal function of the uterotubal junction [16]. Delayed radiography may help to differentiate tubal spasm from other true causes of tubal occlusion.

Diagnosis

Proximal tubal blockage often refers to the failure of contrast dye to enter the intramural or isthmic portion of the fallopian tube using the most commonly available imaging modality, hysterosalpingography (HSG). There are many readily available approaches to the diagnosis of proximal tubal blockage, including HSG, sonohysterosalpingography, and salpingoscopy, but laparoscopic chromopertubation still remains the gold standard for investigating tubal blockage and patency [17].

HSG

HSG has demonstrated a sensitivity of 65% and specificity of 83% when compared to diagnostic laparoscopy with chromopertubation [17]. Its inability to detect peritubal adhesions and false-positive diagnosis in presence of tubal spasms adds to its lower sensitivity as a diagnostic test. Although the use of spasmolytic agents to combat such high false-positive rates has been proposed in some literature, their efficacy has not yet been shown [18]. Rotation of the hips placing the obstructed tube more inferior has shown resolution of tubal patency in 63% of unilaterally obstructed HSG cases [19]. When proximal tubal blockage is found on initial HSG, a second HSG or laparoscopy is needed for confirmation [20].

Sonohysterosalpingography (HyCoSy)

Although the quality of sonographic images may be inferior, sonohysterosalpingography with saline or contrast medium can be a great alternative to HSG for detecting tubal blockage. With sensitivity and specificity of 100% and 96% for abdominal ultrasound and 89% and 100% for vaginal ultrasound, sonohysterosalpingography is comparable in accuracy to laparoscopic chromopertubation [21, 22]. Gel installation uses hydroxyethylcellulose gel instead of saline, which has a more stable filling of the cavity and proximal tube, making it easier to see [23]. Other alternatives for contrast include ExFoam. HyCoSy is advantageous as it does not involve the use of ionizing radiation, can be considered in women with iodine allergy, and can be performed by the reproductive specialist.

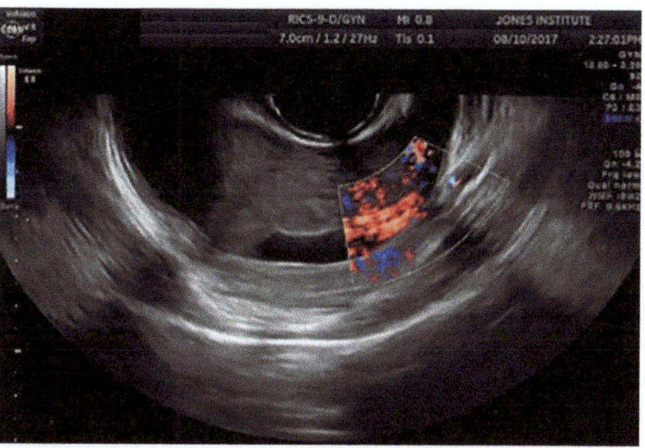

Fig. 7.2 Diagnosis of proximal tubal occlusion with HyCoSy

Air-Contrast Sonohysterography (SHG)

With the use of air and saline mix (agitated saline) to assess the passage of air bubbles through fallopian tubes, SHG has shown sensitivity of 85% and specificity of 87% while detecting tubal blockage accurately, 79.4% when compared to laparoscopic chromopertubation [24]. SHG allows for identification of uterine anomalies but does not allow assessment of the morphology of the fallopian tubes. It is a cheaper exam to use saline instead of contrast. The use of B flow or color Doppler can be used to improve visualization of the agitated saline. Figure 7.2 shows a coronal view of the uterus after sonohysterography showing proximal tubal blockage using Doppler in color flow. Free fill into the peritoneal cavity is not seen.

Surgical Treatment of Proximal Tubal Blockage

Treatment of proximal tubal obstruction historically included macrosurgical tubouterine implantation and progressed to microsurgical techniques with tubocornual anastomosis. Tubouterine implantation was performed in occlusions that spanned the entire intramural tubal segment. Pregnancy rates achieved through macrosurgical tubouterine implantation were reported between 34% and 39% [25, 26]. Pregnancy rates achieved through microsurgical techniques have been reported to be between 53.8% and 69% [20, 27, 28]. It is imperative to establish true cornual occlusion diagnosis prior to pursuing microsurgical anastomosis as false-positive results from HSG have been reported to be as high as 50%. Recently, transcervical cannulation of the oviduct using fluoroscopic or hysteroscopic guidance has been performed, which allows for diagnostic and therapeutic measures. Selective salpingography or tubal cannulation may be performed, unless proximal blockage appears to be due to SIN on HSG [29].

The exact effectiveness of these methods is difficult to establish because many patients have co-existing abnormalities.

Microsurgical Anastomosis Technique

Microsurgical anastomosis is described in 1977 by Dr. Gomel [27]. Delicate tissue handling, and meticulous technique are important to achieving successful anastomosis of tubes. The surgery is optimally conducted with an operating microscope or surgical loupes. A uterine manipulator is placed to allow for uterine manipulation and chromopertubation. Once entry into the peritoneal cavity has been made, the uterus and adnexa are identified and elevated with surgical lap sponges. The occluded end of the fallopian tube is resected, and damaged tube is cut back with microsurgical scissors until healthy patent tubes are reached. Hemostasis is achieved with microelectrode. Methylene blue is injected into the uterine cavity and through the fimbriated end to observe patency from the proximal and distal tubal segment, respectively. A cannula is passed through the fimbriated end through the distal end brought to the proximal end and into the uterine cavity to allow for approximation of the tubes. A 4-0 Vicryl suture is placed in the mesosalpinx to bring together and relieve tension off the two

tubal segments. End-to-end anastomosis is then performed in two layers first with approximation of the muscularis followed by approximation of the serosa. Four interrupted 8-0 sutures are placed through the muscularis at the 12, 3, 6, and 9 o'clock positions. After placement and the proximal and distal tubes are brought together in proper alignment, the 4 sutures are tied. The second layer is closed with 4 interrupted sutures through the serosa using 8-0 suture.

Throughout the procedure, heparinized Lactate Ringers solution is used for tissue irrigation. Lactate Ringers helps to eliminate tubal edema and the heparin reduces fibrin deposition and subsequent adhesion formation [30].

Radiographic Selective Salpingography

Fluoroscopic tubal cannulation has the advantage of being performed at the same time as HSG if cornual occlusion is diagnosed. Radiation exposure risk is also minimal. Thurmond et al. in 1987 described the technique, which uses a coaxial catheter system. Upon visualization of the cervix, an occlusive cannula or intrauterine balloon that allows for passage of a 5-French catheter is placed within the cervix. Under fluoroscopic guidance, the 5-F catheter, advanced over a guidewire, is directed toward the tubal ostium. Contrast agent is then gently injected to identify patency of the tube. If selective salpingography identifies tubal obstruction, a 3-F catheter, with a guidewire threaded within, is then gently directed through the tubal ostium and through the obstruction via the cornual catheter. Figure 7.3a, b shows proximal tubal blockage and successful cannulation of the fallopian tubes under fluoroscopy.

Successful tubal recanalization was achieved in 71–92% of recanalizations. Of the patients who failed to achieve pregnancy in 6–12 months after successful recanalization, only 62% of tubes remained patent [31].

Tubal perforation has been reported in 2% of cases without adverse sequelae. Ectopic pregnancies were reported in 3% of patients [31].

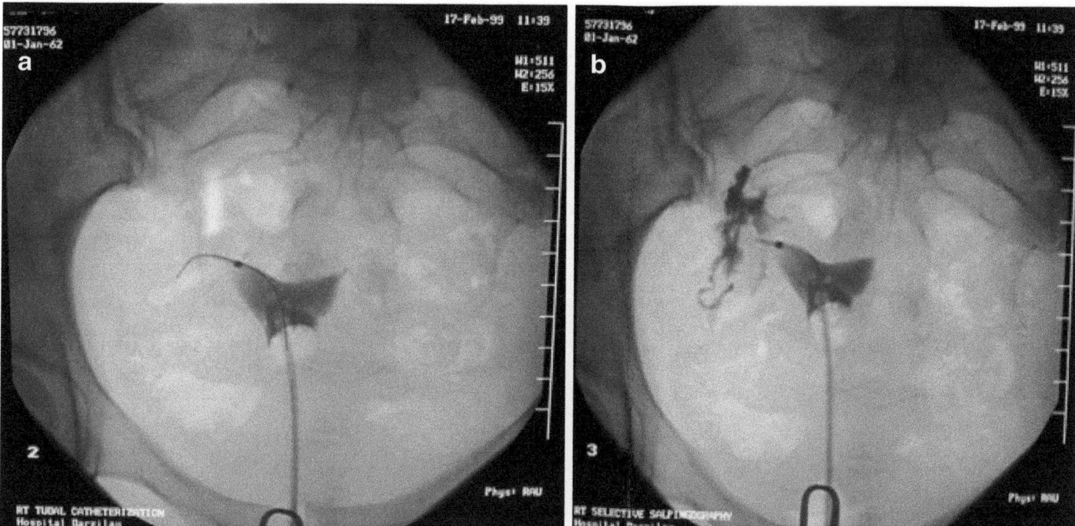

Fig. 7.3 (**a, b**) demonstrates fluoroscopic tubal cannulation performed at the same time as HSG after tubal blockage is diagnosed. Successful tubal canalization was achieved after a catheter with guidewire is threaded through the tubal ostium, opening the obstruction

Laparoscopy with Hysteroscopic Tubal Cannulation

In tubal catheterization, a fine catheter, balloon, or guidewire is inserted into the fallopian tube from the tubal ostium. The tubal catheter is placed under hysteroscopic-laparoscopic or fluoroscopic guidance. Novy et al. in 1988 described transcervical cannulation of the proximal oviduct using a 3-French Teflon catheter [32]. A 5.5-French outer cannula is placed through the operative hysteroscope and directed toward the tubal ostium. The 3-French catheter, through which a stainless-steel guidewire is threaded, is then directed toward the internal ostium and introduced within the tube. Laparoscopy is used to identify the cannula within the fallopian tube and help to manipulate the tube to facilitate cannulation. Chromopertubation using methylene blue is performed after cannulation to document tubal patency. This approach also offers the opportunity to survey the pelvis and identify and potentially treat any further tubal disease. Successful cannulation rate is 70% with pregnancy rate of 33% and live birth rate of 26% [33]. Figure 7.4a–c show cannulation of the right fallopian tube at the time of hysteroscopy/laparoscopy with a double set-up—Fig. 7.4a, b are via hysteroscopy and Fig. 7.4c laparoscopy.

Pregnancy Rates

A systematic review performed by De Silva et al. in 2017 combined all studies regarding reproductive outcome after proximal tubal catheterization. The review included 27 studies and 1556 patients and reported a pooled clinical pregnancy rate of 27% (95% CI 25–30%) after tubal catheterization for unilateral or bilateral proximal tubal obstruction. Pooled clinical pregnancy rate was 27% (95% CI 23–32%) for patients with bilateral obstruction. Pooled live birth rate from 14 studies (551 patients) was 22% (95% CI 1–26%). The pooled ectopic pregnancy rate was 4% (95% CI 3–5%) and pooled miscarriage rate was 6% (95% CI 4–8%). Comparing hysteroscopic versus fluoroscopic approaches, the pooled pregnancy rates were 31% versus 26%, respectively, which was not significantly different ($P = 0.596$) [34].

Studies examining pregnancy outcomes after surgical treatment of proximal tubal

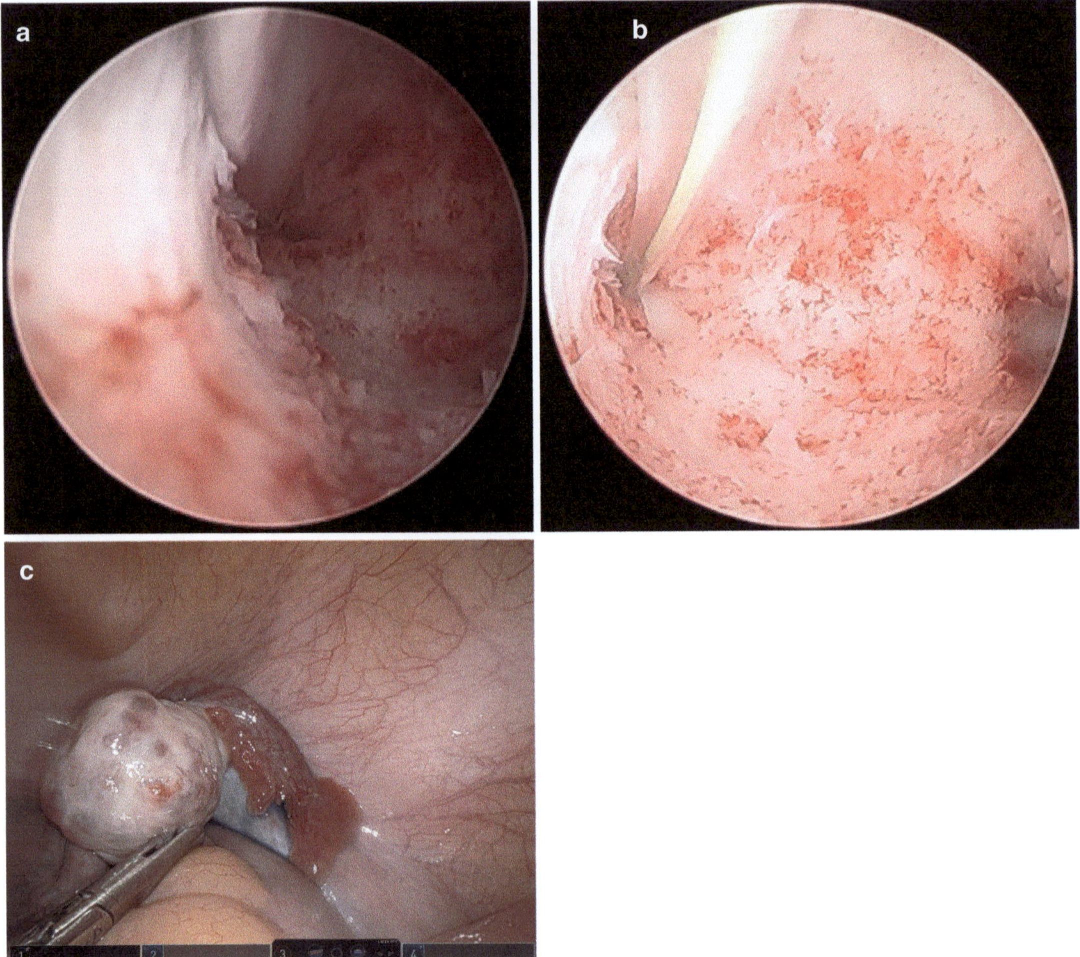

Fig. 7.4 (**a**) Hysteroscopic placement of Novy catheter through the tubal ostium. (**b**) After placement of the outer sheathe of the Novy cannula into the tubal ostia, the inner sheathe (yellow in this picture) is then threaded through. (**c**) Laparoscopic chromopertubation is the gold standard for investigating tubal patency. After hysteroscopic tubal cannulation, chromopertubation using methylene blue is performed to confirm tubal patency

blockage may be affected by small sample size, patients with other contributing factors leading to infertility, and pregnancies achieved using ovulation induction regimens versus natural conception after surgical treatment of tubal blockage.

Decisions regarding tubal surgery versus in vitro fertilization (IVF) need to factor in safety, efficiency to achieving a successful pregnancy, cost-effectiveness, and patient's health history.

If proximal tubal occlusion is found with other existing infertility factors, such as advanced maternal age, presence of significant male factor, SIN, chronic salpingitis or obliterative fibrosis, IVF is the most appropriate therapeutic strategy [2]. Management of proximal tubal occlusion must account for other variables including integrity of distal tube, presence of pelvic disease, and other infertility diagnoses [35].

References

1. Wallach EE, Musich JR, Behrman SJ. Surgical management of tubal obstruction at the uterotubal junction. Fertil Steril. 1983;40(4):423–41.
2. Das S, Nardo LG, Seif MW. Proximal tubal disease: the place for tubal cannulation. Reprod Biomed Online. 2007;15(4):383–8.

3. Eddy CA. Tubal physiology and microsurgery. Aust N Z J Obstet Gynaecol. 1981;21(3):129–33.
4. Sweeney WJ. The interstitial portion of the uterine tube—its gross anatomy, course, and length. Obstet Gynecol. 1962;19(1):3–8.
5. Avner Hershlag MPD, DeCherney AH. Tubal physiology: an appraisal. J Gynecol Surg. 1989;5(1):3–25.
6. L V. The intramural part of the fallopian tube. Int J Fertil. 1959;4:309–14.
7. F.E. L. Upper genital tract infections in women. In: Nelson ALWJ, Wysocki S, editors. Sexually transmitted diseases current clinical practice. Totowa, NJ: Humana Press; 2006. p. 183–203.
8. Weström L. Effect of acute pelvic inflammatory disease on fertility. Am J Obstet Gynecol. 1975;121(5):707–13.
9. Jenkins CS, Williams SR, Schmidt GE. Salpingitis isthmica nodosa: a review of the literature, discussion of clinical significance, and consideration of patient management. Fertil Steril. 1993;60(4):599–607.
10. Sasson IE, Taylor HS. Stem cells and the pathogenesis of endometriosis. Ann N Y Acad Sci. 2008;1127:106–15.
11. Giudice LC, Kao LC. Endometriosis. Lancet. 2004;364(9447):1789–99.
12. Qi H, Zhang H, Zhang D, Li J, Huang Z, Zhao X, et al. Reassessment of prevalence of tubal endometriosis, and its associated clinicopathologic features and risk factors in premenopausal women received salpingectomy. Eur J Obstet Gynecol Reprod Biol X. 2019;4:100074.
13. Kerin JF, Surrey ES, Williams DB, Daykhovsky L, Grundfest WS. Falloposcopic observations of endotubal isthmic plugs as a cause of reversible obstruction and their histological characterization. J Laparoendosc Surg. 1991;1(2):103–10.
14. Dessole S, Meloni GB, Capobianco G, Manzoni MA, Ambrosini G, Canalis GC. A second hysterosalpingography reduces the use of selective technique for treatment of a proximal tubal obstruction. Fertil Steril. 2000;73(5):1037–9.
15. Simpson WL Jr, Beitia LG, Mester J. Hysterosalpingography: a reemerging study. Radiographics. 2006;26(2):419–31.
16. Papaioannou S. A hypothesis for the pathogenesis and natural history of proximal tubal blockage. Hum Reprod. 2004;19(3):481–5.
17. Swart P, Mol BW, van der Veen F, van Beurden M, Redekop WK, Bossuyt PM. The accuracy of hysterosalpingography in the diagnosis of tubal pathology: a meta-analysis. Fertil Steril. 1995;64(3):486–91.
18. Thurmond AS, Novy M, Rösch J. Terbutaline in diagnosis of interstitial fallopian tube obstruction. Investig Radiol. 1988;23(3):209–10.
19. Hurd WW, Wyckoff ET, Reynolds DB, Amesse LS, Gruber JS, Horowitz GM. Patient rotation and resolution of unilateral cornual obstruction during hysterosalpingography. Obstet Gynecol. 2003;101(6):1275–8.
20. Honoré GM, Holden AE, Schenken RS. Pathophysiology and management of proximal tubal blockage. Fertil Steril. 1999;71(5):785–95.
21. Holz K, Becker R, Schürmann R. Ultrasound in the investigation of tubal patency. A meta-analysis of three comparative studies of Echovist-200 including 1007 women. Zentralbl Gynakol. 1997;119(8):366–73.
22. Schlief R, Deichert U. Hysterosalpingo-contrast sonography of the uterus and fallopian tubes: results of a clinical trial of a new contrast medium in 120 patients. Radiology. 1991;178(1):213–5.
23. Bij de Vaate AJ, Brölmann HA, van der Slikke JW, Emanuel MH, Huirne JA. Gel instillation sonohysterography (GIS) and saline contrast sonohysterography (SCSH): comparison of two diagnostic techniques. Ultrasound Obstet Gynecol. 2010;35(4):486–9.
24. Jeanty P, Besnard S, Arnold A, Turner C, Crum P. Air-contrast sonohysterography as a first step assessment of tubal patency. J Ultrasound Med. 2000;19(8):519–27.
25. Grant A. Infertility surgery of the oviduct**presented at the eighteenth annual meeting of the Pacific Coast Fertility Society Phoenix, Arizona, 1970. Fertil Steril. 1971;22(8):496–503.
26. Fayez JA. Comparison between tubouterine implantation and tubouterine anastomosis for repair of cornual occlusion. Microsurgery. 1987;8(2):78–82.
27. Gomel V. Tubal reanastomosis by microsurgery. Fertil Steril. 1977;28(1):59–65.
28. Winston RM. Microsurgical tubocornual anastomosis for reversal of sterilisation. Lancet. 1977;1(8006):284–5.
29. Practice Committee of the American Society for Reproductive Medicine. Role of tubal surgery in the era of assisted reproductive technology: a committee opinion. Fertil Steril. 2021;115(5):1143–50.
30. Ellis H. The cause and prevention of postoperative intraperitoneal adhesions. Surg Gynecol Obstet. 1971;133(3):497–511.
31. Thurmond AS. Pregnancies after selective salpingography and tubal recanalization. Radiology. 1994;190(1):11–3.
32. Novy MJ, Thurmond AS, Patton P, Uchida BT, Rosch J. Diagnosis of cornual obstruction by transcervical fallopian tube cannulation. Fertil Steril. 1988;50(3):434–40.
33. Hou HY, Chen YQ, Li TC, Hu CX, Chen X, Yang ZH. Outcome of laparoscopy-guided hysteroscopic tubal catheterization for infertility due to proximal tubal obstruction. J Minim Invasive Gynecol. 2014;21(2):272–8.
34. De Silva PM, Chu JJ, Gallos ID, Vidyasagar AT, Robinson L, Coomarasamy A. Fallopian tube catheterization in the treatment of proximal tubal obstruction: a systematic review and meta-analysis. Hum Reprod. 2017;32(4):836–52.
35. Gomel V. The place of reconstructive tubal surgery in the era of assisted reproductive techniques. Reprod Biomed Online. 2015;31(6):722–31.

Diagnosis and Surgical Management of Adenomyosis

8

Audrey O. Chang and Linnea R. Goodman

Introduction

Adenomyosis, a benign gynecologic disease often observed in women within their reproductive age, is defined as the presence of endometrial glands and stroma within the myometrium. The German pathologist Carl von Rokitansky provided the first description of adenomyosis in 1860, followed by the influential book "Adenomyoma of the Uterus" published in 1908 by the Canadian gynecologist Thomas Stephen Cullen in which he described 100 cases [1]. Despite knowledge of the condition for over a century, the diagnosis, treatment, and impact of adenomyosis on reproductive outcomes remain enigmatic. Once believed to be a disease associated with multiparous women at the end of their reproductive age, there has been a shift to identifying adenomyosis earlier in women suffering from pain, abnormal uterine bleeding, and infertility.

Pathogenesis

The precise etiology and pathophysiology of adenomyosis is unclear and multiple theories exist, one of which involves the idea of endometrium invading predisposed myometrium during periods of regeneration and healing. This is supported by increased incidence of adenomyosis after repeated sharp curettage during interruption or removal of pregnancy as this can disrupt the endometrial-myometrial border and support implantation and survival of endometrium in the myometrium [2]. Another theory suggests that there may be changes that occur in the uterine junctional zone during pregnancy, such as angiogenesis, that can aggravate existing adenomyosis, supported by data that show sharp curettage in the non-pregnant uterus does not increase the risk of adenomyosis [2].

As adenomyosis has increasingly been observed in nulliparous women, investigation into additional theoretical etiologies has been undertaken over the past few decades. There is support based on animal studies that hormonal and genetic factors may play a role in the development of adenomyosis. One such finding is the association of adenomyosis with early tamoxifen exposure in mice, which raises the possibility that events in-utero can lead to adenomyosis from estrogenic effects [3]. Other hormones such as prolactin, FSH, and oxytocin may also have roles in the development of adenomyosis [4, 5].

There is thought to be an association between endometriosis and adenomyosis as they both involve ectopic endometrium with some MRI studies approximating up to one-third of patients diagnosed with adenomyosis having concurrent

A. O. Chang · L. R. Goodman (✉)
Department of Obstetrics and Gynecology, Division of Reproductive Endocrinology and Infertility, University of North Carolina Hospitals, Chapel Hill, NC, USA
e-mail: Audrey.Chang@unchealth.unc.edu

S. R. Lindheim, J. C. Petrozza (eds.), *Reproductive Surgery*,
https://doi.org/10.1007/978-3-031-05240-8_8

findings of endometriosis [6–8] and up to 80–90% concurrence of endometriosis in patients with adenomyosis [9, 10]. In addition, there are data to support that adenomyosis develops earlier in women with prior evidence of endometriosis [11]. In women with endometriosis, there have been documented hyperperistaltic contractions of the uterine musculature and an increased intrauterine pressure, which may help to sustain the infiltration of endometrium into the myometrium and support the development of adenomyosis [12, 13].

Presentation

The most common clinical presentations of adenomyosis include heavy menstrual bleeding and dysmenorrhea, which can occur in up to 60% and 30% of women, respectively [14]. Heavy menstrual bleeding is suspected to be due to the extra surface area of endometrial tissue in the enlarged uterus, while dysmenorrhea may be due to swelling of the endometrial tissue within the myometrium. Patients can also present with chronic pelvic pain, back pain, dyspareunia, and infertility, with approximately one-third lacking symptoms [14].

Diagnosis

There is no standardized histologic diagnosis of adenomyosis. Some pathologists use definitions of endometrial glands presenting deeper than one-fourth of the thickness of the myometrium or deeper than one-half of a lower-power field [2.5 mm] to define the disorder [15]. In gross appearance, the uterus is usually firm, enlarged, and somewhat globular with the cut surface of the myometrium occasionally containing hemorrhagic foci (Fig. 8.1). Under microscopy, the ectopic endometrium may form islands within the myometrium surrounded by myometrial hypertrophy (Fig. 8.2).

While the gold standard for the diagnosis of adenomyosis remains histological examination of a surgical specimen, improved resolution of imaging including MRI and 3D transvaginal ultrasound has led to promising non-invasive positive predictive values [16–18]. MRI has traditionally led the field for non-invasive imaging of adenomyosis with increased spatial and contrast resolution allowing for clearer focus on the uterine junctional zone, which is a transitional zone between the endometrium and myometrium. A review of 57 studies examining the utility of ultrasound and MRI for evaluation of

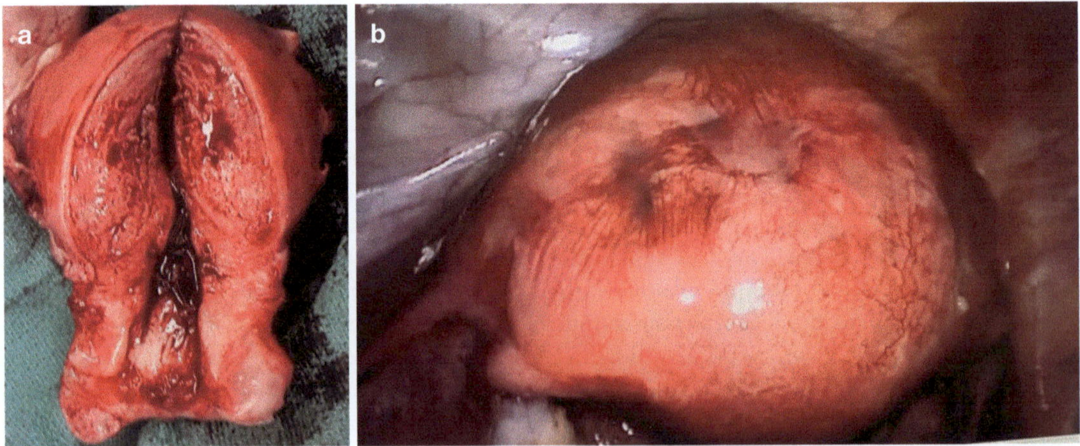

Fig. 8.1 (**a**) Cross-section of diffuse adenomyosis of the uterus at time of hysterectomy (**b**), Enlarged and boggy uterus at time of laparoscopy. (Courtesy of Rebecca Flyckt, MD, University Hospitals, Cleveland)

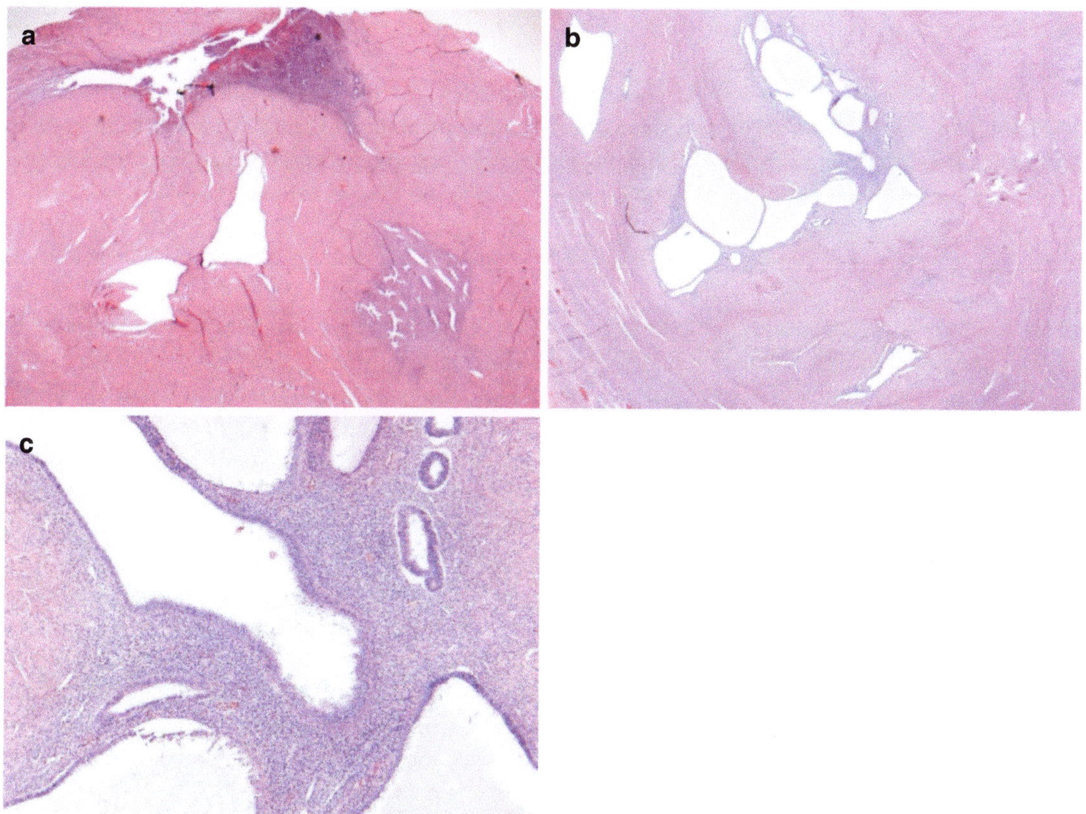

Fig. 8.2 Histologic appearance of adenomyosis at 1× (**a**), 2× (**b**) and 10× (**c**). (Courtesy of UNC pathology department)

adenomyosis characterized adenomyosis into three subtypes: internal adenomyosis, external adenomyosis, and adenomyomas and reported a pooled sensitivity of 77% and specificity of 89% for all subtypes [17]. Other quoted sensitivities and specificities of MRI range from 88–93% and 67–99%, respectively [16, 19, 20].

Defining features of adenomyosis on MRI include diffuse or focal thickening of the junctional zone, forming an ill-defined area of low signal intensity occasionally with embedded bright foci on T2-weighted images in which compartments with water appear bright and compartments with fat appear dark [21, 22]. On histology, the areas of low signal intensity correspond with smooth muscle hyperplasia, and bright foci on T2-weighted images correspond to islands of ectopic endometrial tissue which can vary depending on current treatments and current

phase of the menstrual cycle. Additional defining features of adenomyosis include the presence of adenomyoma, defined as localized, circumscribed forms of adenomyosis and may manifest as intramural or protrusions into the uterine cavity. On MRI, adenomyomas can have low signal intensity on T2-weighted images, similar to leiomyomas. However, small areas of high signal intensity, representing ectopic endometrial tissue, shift suspicion more toward adenomyoma. Another variant of adenomyoma includes polypoid adenomyoma, which presents as a hypointense polypoid mass with hyperintense foci on T2-weighted images on MRI [23]. Overall, adenomyomas have a high rate of misdiagnosis so clinical suspicion should remain vigilant (Fig. 8.3).

In comparison to MRI, ultrasound is a more cost-effective tool to evaluate intrauterine pathology. Transabdominal ultrasound has a high specificity [95–97.5%] but low sensitivity [30–63%] due to limited image resolution [23]. There is a wide range of reported sensitivity and specificity of transvaginal ultrasound [TVUS] for diagnosis of adenomyosis ranging from 53–89% and 50–99%, respectively [16, 17, 20, 24–29]. If there is an adenomyoma present, then sensitivity [33%] and specificity [78%] of TVUS drop, likely due to resemblances with myomas [19].

Sonographic findings of adenomyosis on TVUS include the following: globular uterine enlargement that is not explained by the presence of leiomyomata, cystic anechoic lakes in myometrium, uterine wall thickening [which can show anterior-posterior asymmetry], sub-endometrial echogenic linear striations [due to invasion of endometrial glands into sub-endometrial tissue leading to a hyperplastic reaction causing linear striations fanning out from the endometrium], heterogeneous uterine texture, obscuring of the endometrial/myometrial border, and thickening of the transition zone [≥12 mm] [30–34]. Sun et al. [2010] demonstrated that sub-endometrial echogenic linear striations, a heterogeneous

myometrial echotexture, and myometrial anterior-posterior asymmetry showed greater accuracy for diagnosing adenomyosis and sub-endometrial linear striations has the highest diagnostic accuracy with sensitivity of 91.8%, positive predictive value of 67.8%, and negative predictive value of 92.9%. A globular uterine shape was the most specific feature at 78.1%, but had poor sensitivity at 50.6% [33].

Color doppler ultrasound is a useful tool to evaluate the involvement of vascular structures. Three-dimensional ultrasound [3DUS] allows visualization of the uterus in a coronal view similar to MRI. Previously established criteria for the 3D US diagnosis of adenomyosis are the presence of one or more of the criteria depicted in Fig. 8.4 [33].

While a meta-analysis of eight studies revealed that there is no improved accuracy when utilizing 2D versus 3D TVUS [35], a recent study evaluating the accuracy of 3D TVUS diagnosing adenomyosis in 54 women without any pretreatment showed those with two diagnostic ultrasound features had an accuracy of 90% [sensitivity 92%, specificity 83%, PPV 99%, and NPV 71%] when

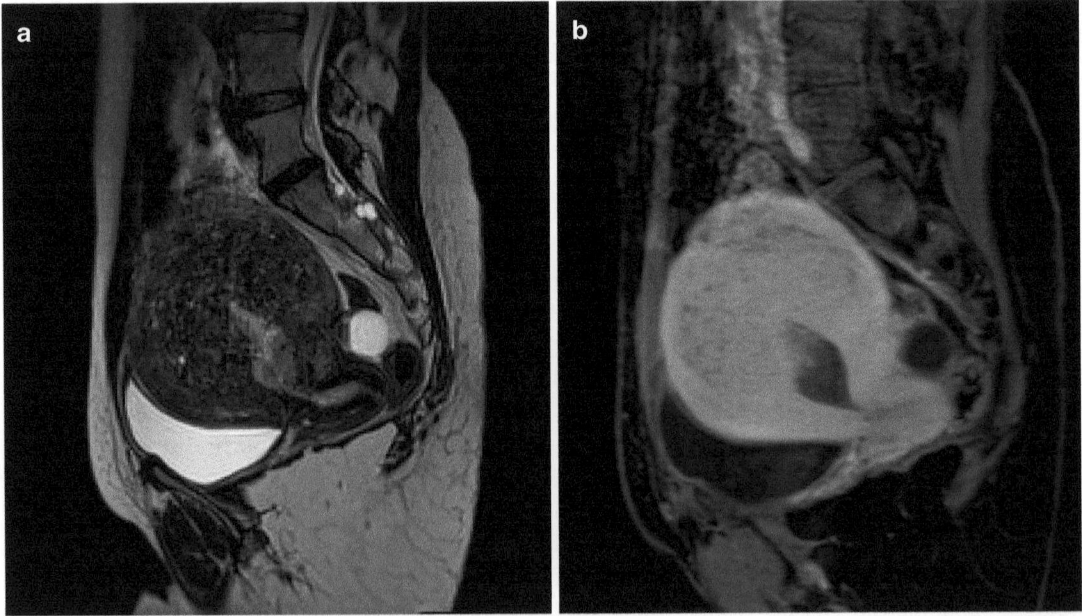

Fig. 8.3 (**a**) T2 MRI image of adenomyosis, (**b**) Post-contrast T1 MRI image of adenomyosis. (Courtesy of UNC radiology department)

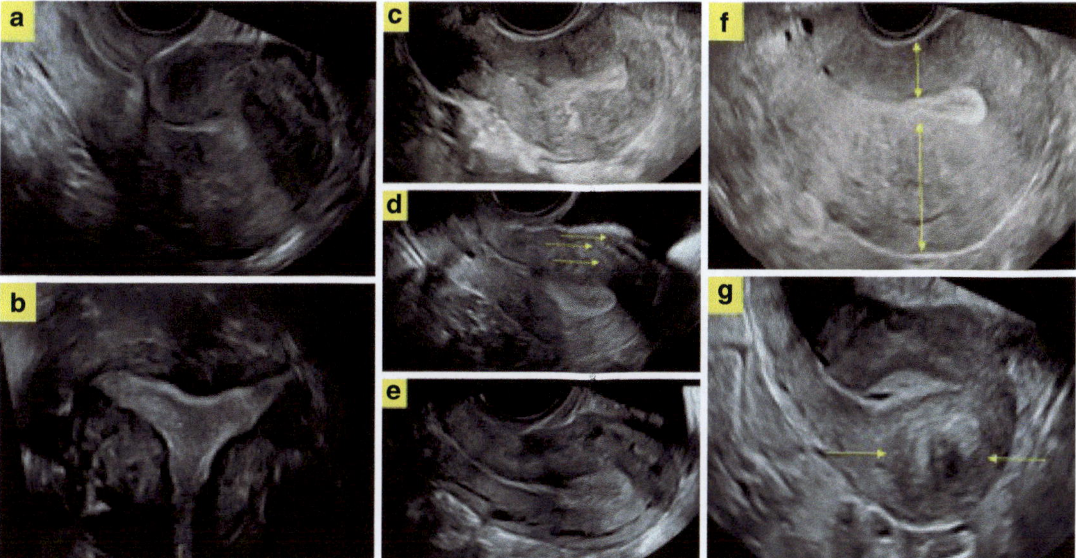

Fig. 8.4 (**a**) Globulous aspect of the uterus, defined as a global increase in uterine myometrial thickness not caused by fibroids or other pathologic uterine condition. (**b**) Irregular endometrium-myometrium interphase, or lack of a clearly visualized neat contour of the endometrial basal layer and the underlying myometrium, with no or incomplete visualization of the junction zone [JZ]. (**c**) Heterogeneous myometrial texture, or alternating hyperechogenic and hypoechogenic areas in terms of myometrial thickness without a precise margin, along with thin acoustic shadows with a radial pattern that are not induced by fibroids or intramyometrial hyperechogenic foci. (**d**) Linear striations from the endometrium to the myometrium, or hyperechogenic lines crossing the myometrial thickness, visible from the endometrial–myometrial interphase, and/or. (**e**) Presence of intramyometrial cysts, or areas with myometrial thickness of ≥ 1 mm and negative for color Doppler [power Doppler or high-definition Doppler]. (**f**) Uterine asymmetry, defined as thickening of the anterior uterine wall vs. the posterior, or vice versa. (**g**) Adenomyoma, defined as a heterogeneous nodular mass lacking well-defined margins and without internal calcifications

compared to histopathologic features of targeted biopsy specimens of the uterus [36].

Other forms of diagnosis include endometrial biopsy via utero-spirotome employed during hysteroscopy, which allows for direct visualization of the endometrial surface [37] (Fig. 8.5). Visualized endometrial findings such as hypervascularization, strawberry pattern, endometrial defects, and submucosal hemorrhagic cysts are suggestive of adenomyosis [37]. A Trophy hysteroscope allows for biopsy of these areas using the Spirotome, which has a distal corkscrew that can cut through layers of the endometrium, the inner myometrium, and the outer myometrium and biopsy tissue (Fig. 8.6). The Trophy hysteroscope can be loaded with the Spirotome or hysteroscopic 5 French instruments without removing the instrument. The spirotome contains a trocar with cutting cannula and receiving needle with helix. The helix can penetrate a distance up to 20 mm with a 1 cm corkscrew. It is inserted under ultrasound guidance to obtain a one centimeter cut of tissue and has a sensitivity of 54% and specificity of 78% [37]. The lower sensitivity may be attributable to false negatives in the cases of deep adenomyosis, but it does have the advantage of leaving the outer myometrium intact.

Adenomyosis and Fertility Outcomes

An association between adenomyosis and fertility has not been fully established; however, recent studies suggest that adenomyosis may have a negative impact on fertility. With more readily available uterine-sparing means of diagnosis, studies have aimed to determine the effect of adenomyosis on fertility with mixed results. Several publications have reported a negative impact on

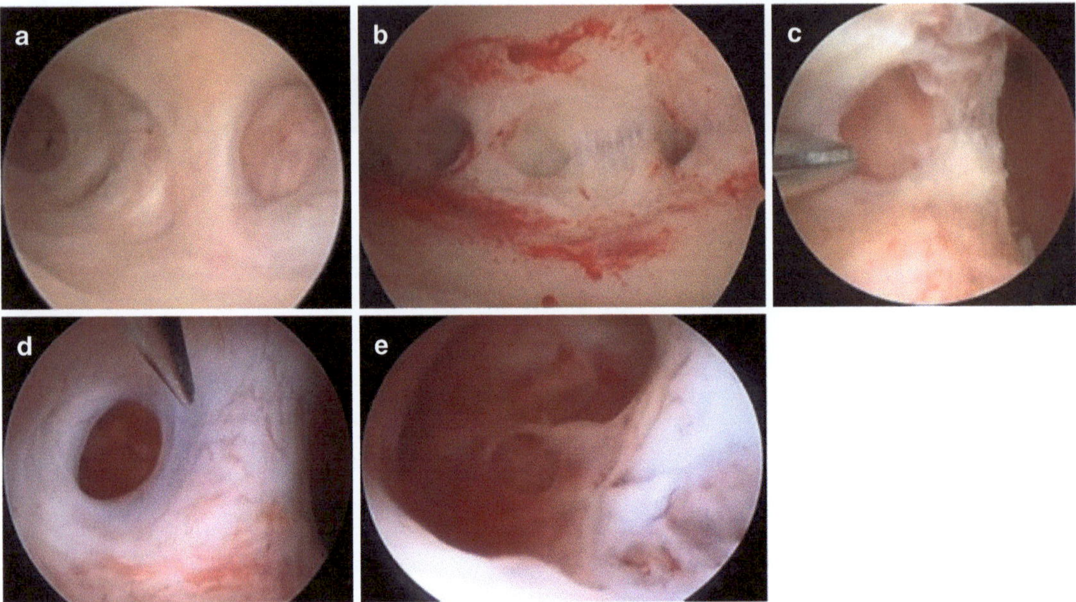

Fig. 8.5 Adenomyotic hysteroscopic images become pathognomic after sub-endometrial exploration: (**a**) visible endometrial defects on uterine septum; (**b**) after incision different cystic structures become visible; (**c**) incision of lateral wall of T-uterus reveals the presence of adeno-myotic cyst; (**d**) formation of cyst, still small opening is present; and (**e**) opening of this defect shows the inner sight of the cyst. (From Gordts and Campo et al. with permission)

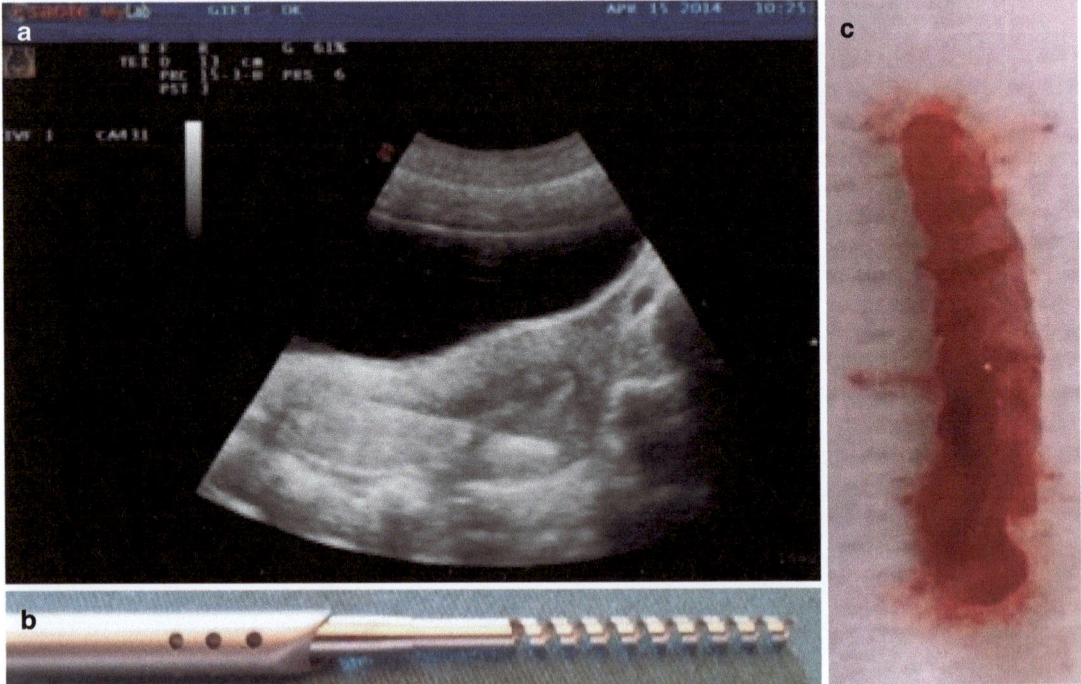

Fig. 8.6 Use of utero-spirotome under ultrasound guidance. (**a**) ultrasound-guided insertion of spirotome; (**b**) spirotome with 1 cm corkscrew; (**c**) biopsy obtained after use of spirotome. (From Gordts and Campo et al. with permission)

both spontaneous and assisted pregnancy outcomes in women with adenomyosis compared to age-matched controls [38, 39], while others have not [40, 41].

A meta-analysis including nine studies of in-vitro fertilization [IVF] outcomes in women with and without adenomyosis aimed to investigate an association [38]. In these studies, where adenomyosis was diagnosed via MRI or TVUS, there was a total of 1865 women, 665 of whom were enrolled in four prospective observational studies and 1200 in five retrospective studies. The clinical pregnancy rate was 123/304 [40.5%] in women with adenomyosis after IVF versus 628/1262 [49.8%] in women without adenomyosis. Pooling of the results yielded a risk ratio of 0.72 [95% CI 0.55–0.95], concluding that women with adenomyosis had a 28% reduction in the likelihood of a clinical pregnancy after IVF. Miscarriage rate, a secondary outcome studied, was observed in 77/241 women with adenomyosis [31.9%] verses 97/687 [14.1%] in women without with a pooled RR of 2.12 [95% CI 1.20–3.75].

Recently, a retrospective cohort study by Sharma et al. [2019] evaluated 973 women undergoing fertility treatment [39]. These women were divided into four groups: only endometriosis [n = 355], endometriosis and adenomyosis [n = 88], only adenomyosis [n = 64], and tubal factor infertility as controls [n = 466]. The clinical pregnancy rate in women with only endometriosis was 36.6%, women with endometriosis and adenomyosis 22.7%, women with only adenomyosis 23.4%, and control group 34.6%. The miscarriage rates and live birth rates were 14.6%, 35%, 40%, 13.0% and 26.5%, 11.4%, 12.5%, and 27.5% in those groups, respectively. The live birth rates between controls and women with only adenomyosis [p = 0.01] and women with both endometriosis and adenomyosis [p = 0.002] were statistically significant. The conclusion of this study was that the addition of adenomyosis contributed negatively to fertility outcomes.

Alternatively, Benaglia et al. [2014] evaluated implantation rates in 49 women with asymptomatic adenomyosis diagnosed by TVUS and 49 controls [40]. In the women with adenomyosis,

24 out of 76 embryos transferred implanted [32%] compared to 16 out of 76 [21%] in the controls, with an odds ratio of 1.73 [95% CI 0.83–3.77]. This study concluded that implantation rate was not affected by asymptomatic adenomyosis diagnosed by TVUS. Mijatovic et al. [2010] reached the same conclusion evaluating IVF outcomes in women with surgically proven endometriosis and adenomyosis diagnosed via TVUS [41]. This retrospective study encompassed 74 infertile patients with endometriosis, of which 90.4% of them were diagnosed with severe stage endometriosis and of these, 27% of these women had adenomyosis. There were no significant differences found in IVF outcomes compared to the women with and without adenomyosis.

A systematic review of the current literature on fertility-sparing treatment of adenomyosis was published in 2018 [42]. The review included 16 studies, with 533 patients included in six studies that looked at surgical management of adenomyosis and an additional 1052 patients in 10 studies evaluating outcomes of artificial reproductive technology in this population. The surgical methods for diffuse adenomyosis included adenomyomectomy with unilateral salpingectomy, microsurgical adenomyomectomy, adenomyomectomy with continuous horizontal mattress technique, and laparoscopic adenomyomectomy with laser. The spontaneous pregnancy rate with these various surgical techniques was low [18.2%]. A higher pregnancy rate was observed when surgery was followed by 24 weeks of GnRH-agonist (a) therapy [40.7% vs. 15.0%, p = 0.002]. In the pooled analysis of studies looking at exclusively artificial reproductive technology [ART] for the treatment of adenomyosis-associated infertility, there was an overall clinical pregnancy rate of 36.1%. When comparing the long and short stimulation protocol of ART in these patients, there were higher rates of clinical pregnancy [43.3% vs 31.8%, respectively; p = 0.0001], higher live birth/ ongoing pregnancy rate [43% vs 23.1%; p = 0.005], and lower frequency of miscarriage [18.5% vs 31.1%; p < 0.0001] with long GnRH-a downregulation protocols. Overall, the data are limited by heterogeneity of disease, a wide variety of treatment protocols and surgical methods, additional infertility diagnosis, and lack of long-term follow-up.

A recent study [43] evaluated 3D TVUS diagnosis and associated reproductive outcomes of adenomyosis by five independent reproductive endocrinology and infertility specialist reviewers of 648 patients undergoing a single thawed euploid blastocyst transfer. The 3D US was performed on the day prior to transfer, with only fair inter-rate agreement of US assessment of adenomyosis. In addition, there were no differences in clinical pregnancy, miscarriage, or live birth rates in patients with adenomyosis compared to those without adenomyosis, suggesting that routine screening for adenomyosis in patients undergoing frozen embryo transfer is not necessary.

Overall, the data regarding adenomyosis and fertility are mixed and a concrete association or causal mechanism of deleterious effect has yet to be elucidated.

Management

The definitive treatment for adenomyosis in women who have completed childbearing is hysterectomy. Other treatment modalities include hormonal management, uterine debulking surgery, adenomyomectomy, and uterine artery embolization [UAE]. Hormonal management includes levonorgestrel-releasing IUD, continuous use of oral contraceptive pills, high-dose progestins, and gonadotrophic receptor hormone agonists (Table 8.1).

The levonorgestrel-releasing IUD [LNG-IUD] works to treat adenomyosis-associated bleeding and pain by reducing the thickness of the myometrial junctional zone and total uterine volume [44–46]. It is thought to cause decidualization and an increase in apoptosis in the endometrial glands and stroma, as well as a local effect on adenomyosis by causing atrophy of adenomyotic lesions by downregulating estrogen receptors. This also prevents further stimulation by estrogens [47]. Sheng et al. looked at the overall satisfaction rate of LNG-IUD after three years in 94 women with moderate to severe dysmenorrhea associated with adenomyosis using a visual analog scale [VAS] to evaluate dysmenorrhea. The VAS dropped from a baseline score of 77.9 +/− 14.7 to 11.8 +/− 17.9 after 36 months of the LNG-IUD [$P < 0.001$]. After these 36 months, the overall satisfaction rate was 72.5% [48]. In another study that looked at uterine volume in 47 women with adenomyosis, they found that there was a significant decrease in mean uterine volume at 12 and 24 months after LNG-IUD insertion, but no significant differences after 36 months [49]. In a randomized controlled trial that evaluated 62 women with adenomyosis-related pain and bleeding, combined oral contraceptives [COCs] and LNG-IUD were both found to decrease pain and menstrual bleeding; however, the LNG-IUD was overall more effective [50]. One study looked at uterine volume as a predictor for LNG-IUD success and found that uterine volume >150 mL was associated with LNG-IUD treatment failure [51].

Table 8.1 Medical management options for adenomyosis

Class	Mechanism of action	Effects	Supporting evidence
LNG-IUD	Decidualization of endometrial tissue Downregulate estrogen receptors to cause atrophy of adenomyotic lesions	Reduces thickness of JZ Reduces total uterine volume	45–52
COCs	Decidualization of endometrial tissue	Amenorrhea	53
NETA	Inhibits estrogen-induced VEGF Decidualization of endometrial tissue	Reduces bleeding	54, 55
GnRH agonist	Antiproliferative effect Antiestrogen effect	Reduces bleeding Reduces uterine size	53

LNG-IUD levonorgestrel-releasing intrauterine device; *COCs* combined oral contraceptives; *NETA* norethindrone; *GnRH* gonadotropin-releasing hormone

Combined oral contraceptive pills [COCs] work to relieve the symptoms of adenomyosis via decidualization and subsequent atrophy of the endometrium. There are no well-conducted RCTs that support the pharmacological treatment of adenomyosis using COCs despite the common use of them off-label to treat adenomyosis-related symptoms [52]. Norethindrone acetate [NETA] is a studied progestin for treatment of adenomyosis symptoms, although there have been few studies that have compared NETA to other progestins or drugs. It works by inhibiting estrogen-induced VEGF in endometrial stroma, thus reducing bleeding and pain [53]. In a small retrospective chart review of 28 women taking NETA for adenomyosis-related symptoms, patients showed maximum response at three months of treatment with NETA, which was maintained throughout treatment. The study utilized "three weeks on, one week off" regimen to minimize the side effect of breakthrough bleeding. Both dysmenorrhea and bleeding were significantly improved while being treated with NETA [54].

GnRH-a has multiple mechanisms of action which can combine to alleviate symptomatic adenomyosis [52]. Mainly, it is thought to have an antiproliferative effect on the myometrium via the action of GnRH receptors that are expressed on the adenomyotic lesions. In addition, it has a systemic and local anti-estrogenic effect through central downregulation and suppression of gonadotropin section. This can result in uterine size reduction and an improvement in pelvic pain and bleeding. The side effects of GnRH-a include hypoestrogenic effects, such as vasomotor symptoms, decreased bone mineral density, and genital atrophy. Therefore, add-back therapy can be considered to mitigate these side effects in cases of prolonged use.

Potential treatment options necessitating more study include: selective progesterone receptor modulators (SPRMs), aromatase inhibitors (AI), and danazol. SPRMs demonstrate progesterone agonist and antagonist activities in the endometrium. They can reduce pain, bleeding, and inhibit development of adenomyosis but need more investigation. AIs block the conversion of testosterone to estrogen. Aromatase has been found in the endometrium of women with endometriosis, adenomyosis, and leiomyomas but not in healthy women [55, 56]. Again, additional studies are needed. Danazol has antigonadotropic properties, creating a low estrogen environment, and increases free testosterone levels.

While UAE is uterus sparing, it should be reserved for women who have also completed childbearing. Clinical studies have shown that UAE has been successful in improving heavy menstrual bleeding [57, 58]. In a systemic review of UAE on adenomyosis outcomes, improvement of symptoms occurred in 83.1% [872/1049] of patients [59]. Further prospective studies regarding UAE as a treatment option for adenomyosis are needed.

Surgical Management

For women who desire to become pregnant in the future, there are options for uterus-sparing resections of adenomyosis. An MRI prior to the surgery is often obtained to determine the extent and location of adenomyosis. Depending on size, location, diffusiveness of adenomyosis, and surgeon preference, minimally invasive and open techniques have been described including wedge resection of the uterine wall, transverse H-incision on the fundus with resection of the adenomyosis, Osada's triple-flap method, and asymmetric dissection [60].

In the classic wedge resection technique via laparotomy, parts of the serosa and adenomyoma are removed via wedge resection. The defect that is created by the resection is then sutured together with the remaining muscular layer and serosa. One retrospective study [61] found that the rate of relief of dysmenorrhea was 88.9% and of menorrhagia was 50.0% with a mean follow-up time of 27.6 months. The relapse rate by ultrasonography was 69.2% during this follow-up time.

Another partial reduction approach is the transverse H incision of the uterine wall [62]. Using this method, a transverse incision is made on the uterine fundus. The serosa is separated from the underlying myometrium, and then the adenomyoma tissue is removed after widely opening the bilateral uterine serosa. The defect is closed in one or two layers, using a tension-less suturing technique. The first layer is for hemostasis and to close the defect. In a study by Fujishita, this method was applied to six patients who desired to preserve fertility. Perforation occurred in one patient [17%], and one patient spontaneously conceived four months following the procedure. Fujishita also reported on another 41 patients who underwent the H-incision technique, of which 31 attempted to conceive. Of these, 12 [38.7%] achieved a clinical pregnancy, five [16.1%] miscarried, and seven [22.5%] reported a live birth [60]. Another study looked at 57 women who underwent adenomyomectomy via the H-incision technique in combination with intra-operative LND-IUD placement. Of the 53 patients that followed up, there was an 88.9% complete remission rate for dysmenorrhea at 36 months. Menstrual flow and uterine volume were also significantly decreased [63].

The triple flap method is effective for diffuse adenomyosis as well as nodular adenomyosis [64] (Fig. 8.7). The uterus is bisected in the sagit-tal plane through the adenomyosis until the uterine cavity is reached. Adenomyotic tissue is excised and the endometrial lining is first reapproximated with interrupted sutures. Then on one of the sides of the bisected uterus, the myometrium and serosa are reapproximated in the antero-posterior plane with interrupted sutures. The contralateral side of the uterine wall is brought over the reconstructed first side in order to cover the suture line. The myometrium of the underlying flaps is denuded of the overlying serosa. The uterine wall is reconstructed without overlapping suture lines via this triple flap method in order to prevent uterine rupture in subsequent pregnancies [60, 64, 65]. In a study of 104 women with severe adenomyosis who underwent this method of treatment, all patients had a return to normal menses and there was a significant improvement in dysmenorrhea. There were 26 women in this study who desired fertility; 16 became pregnant and 14 [53.8%] delivered a healthy baby at term. There were no cases of uterine rupture. Adenomyosis symptoms recurred in four patients out of the 104 [64].

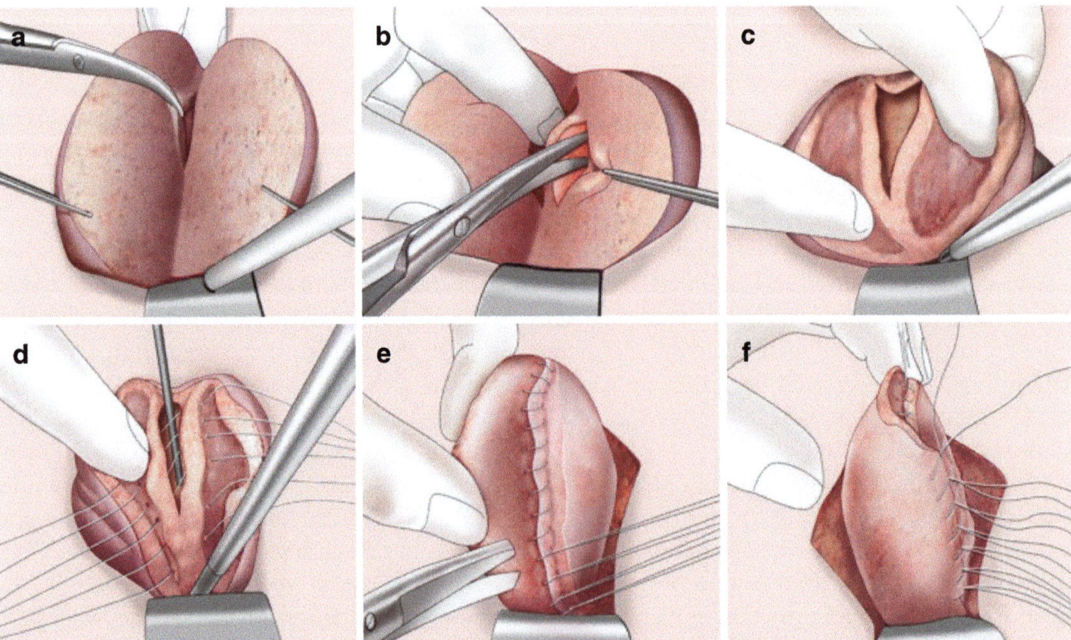

Fig. 8.7 Osada's triple-flap method. (**a**) The uterus is bivalved over the section of diffuse adenomyosis; (**b**) Cold scissors are used to undermine adenomyosis tissue which is excised; (**c**) Direct palpation to ensure adaquate tissue to repair; (**d**) The endometrial lining is reapproximated with interrupted surgures; (**e**) On one side of the bisected uterus, the myometrium and serosa are repproximated in the antero-posterior plane; (**f**) The myometrium of the underlying flaps is denuded of the overlying serosa and the uterine wall is reconstructed. (From Osada et al. with permission)

The asymmetric dissection method dissects the uterus longitudinally (Fig. 8.8). The uterine fundus is retracted upward and the uterine adenomyoma is then dissected into slices. From the incision, the myometrium is dissected diagonally, followed by a transverse incision to open the uterine cavity. The adenomyotic lesions are excised to >5 mm of the inner myometrium and this process is repeated on the outer side lesion. The uterine cavity is then closed and reconstructed. There have been five cases of uterine rupture out of 1349 cases of patients who underwent this surgical technique as of 2016 [60].

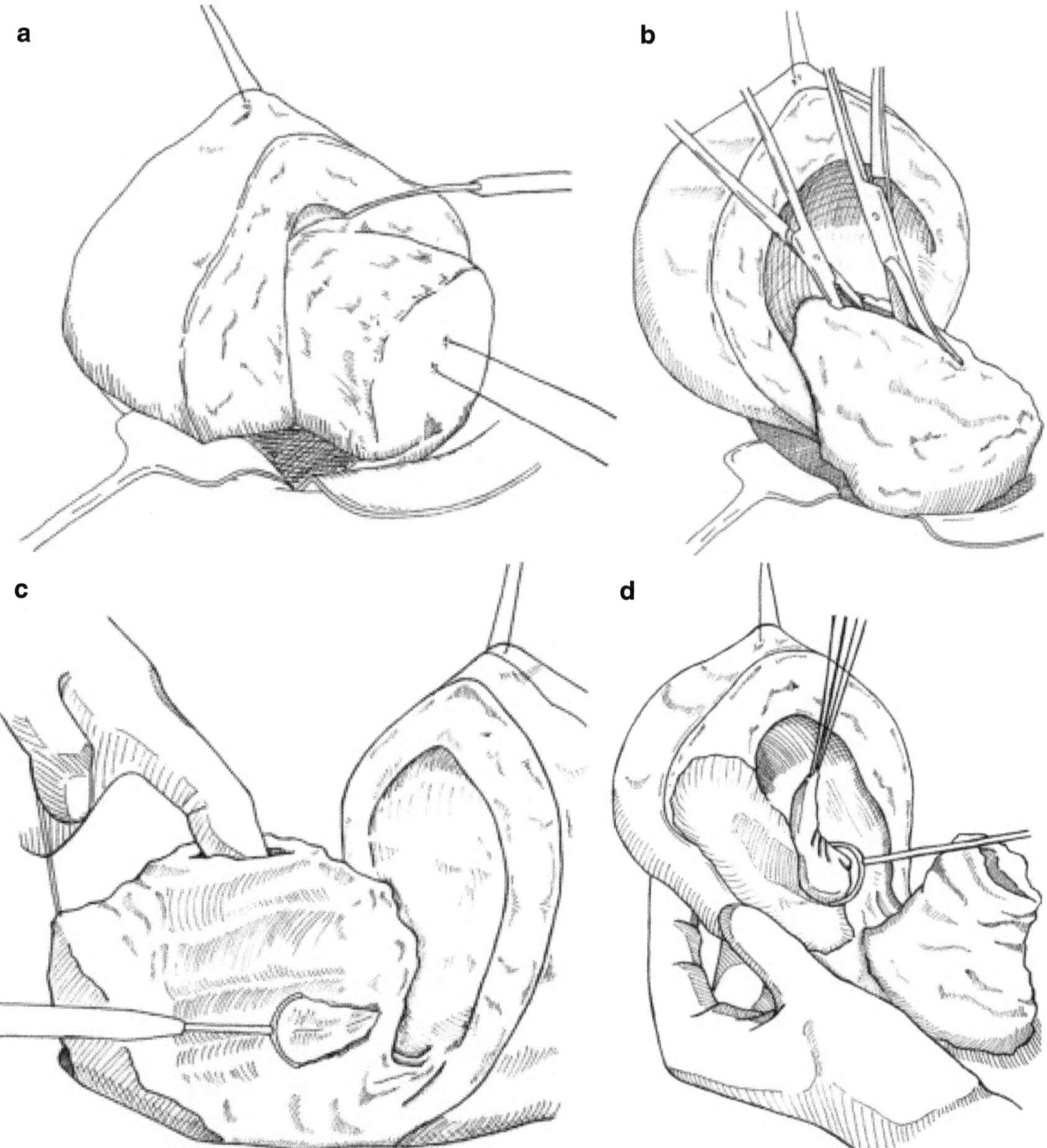

Fig. 8.8 Asymmetric dissection method. (**a**) Uterus is dissected; (**b**) Uterine cavity is opened; (**c**) Inner side lesion is excised; (**d**) Outer side lesion is excised; (**e**) Lesion is sutured; (**f**) Uterus is rejoined. (From Osada et al. with permission, adapted from Nishida et al. Conservative surgical management for diffuse uterine adenomyosis [63])

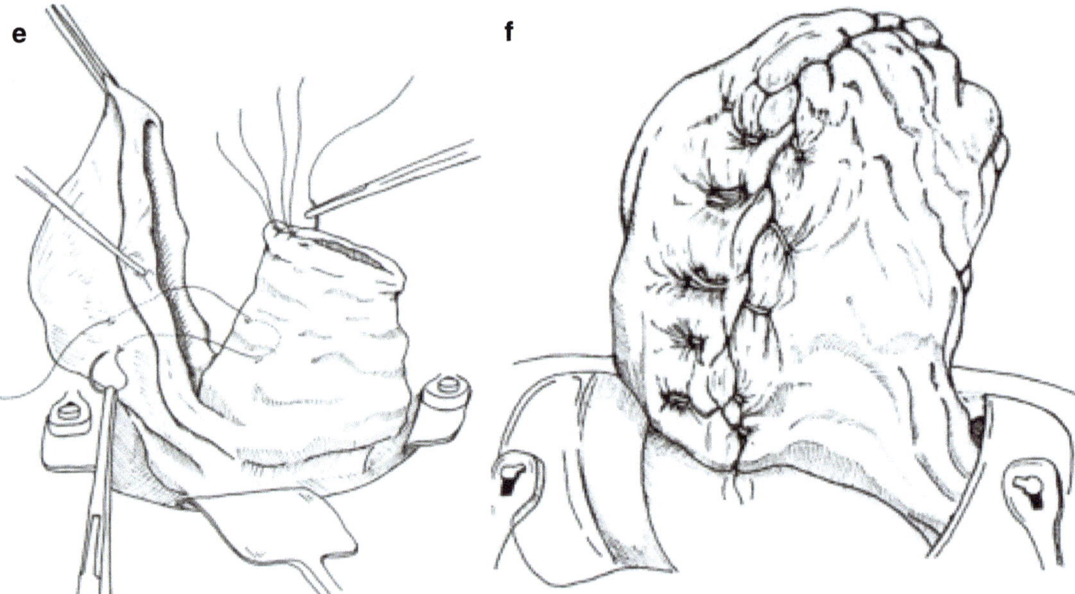

Fig. 8.8 (continued)

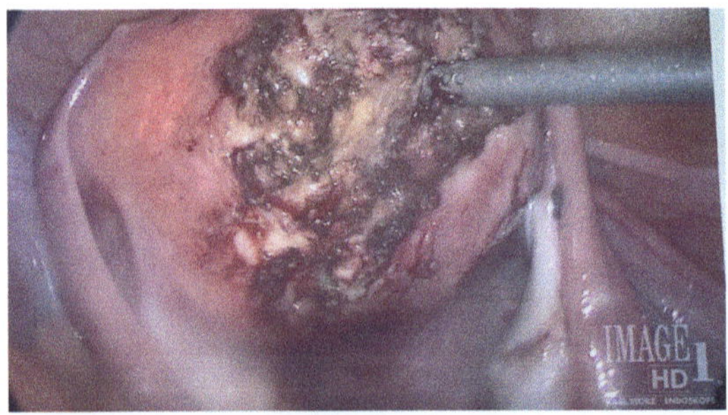

Fig. 8.9 Laparoscopic resection of adenomyosis demonstrating the ill-defined borders. (Courtesy of Rebecca Flyckt, MD, University Hospitals, Cleveland)

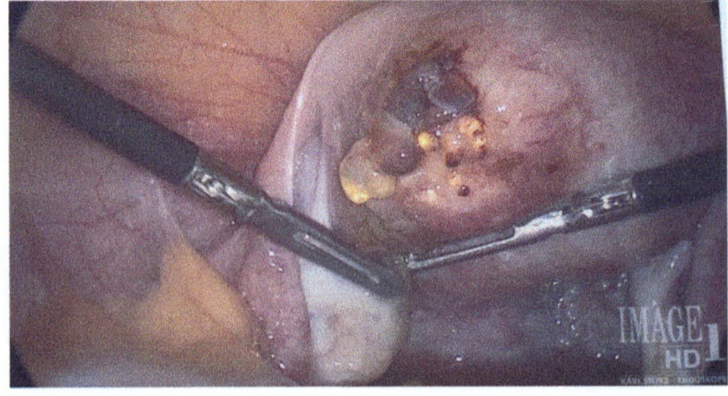

Fig. 8.10 Adenomyoma protruding from serosa viewed laparoscopically. (Courtesy of Rebecca Flyckt, MD, University Hospitals, Cleveland)

Laparoscopic methods of adenomyosis resection include a longitudinal or transverse incision of the uterine wall and then resection of the adenomyoma [66] (Figs. 8.9 and 8.10). Suturing of the uterine wall can occur in two or more layers using the double-flap method. An incision is made in the midline of the fundal serosal surface and carried in the sagittal plane until the uterine cavity is reached. The incision is also carried along the posterior and anterior uterine walls to reach the internal cervical os. The adenomyotic tissue is removed, and then the endometrial lining is reapproximated. The double-flap closure entails bringing the first flap in one side wall of the uterus into the second flap of the other side such that the myometrium and endometrium are covered. The serosal surface of the underlying flaps is stripped to ensure that only myometrial flaps are overlapping [67].

In a study [68] that looked at 141 women who underwent laparoscopic adenomyomectomy, of whom 102 desired fertility, there was a 31.4% [32/102] clinical pregnancy rate. When these women were divided into two age groups [≤39 and ≥40 years old], the clinical pregnancy rates were 41.3% and 3.7%, respectively. In the older group, 5/6 of the pregnancies resulted in miscarriages. The women who had successful clinical pregnancies were all delivered via elective cesarean section. IVF outcomes were also analyzed on women who had a history of IVF failures. In the younger age group, 60.8% had a postoperative clinical pregnancy versus 7.1% in the older group. There were no cases of uterine ruptures in this cohort, but there were 2 cases of placenta accreta that resulted in postpartum hysterectomies.

The risk of uterine rupture after adenomyomectomy is not insignificant. One literature review has suggested the rate to be as high as 6.0% [69]. Other reviews have reported rates anywhere from 1 to 3% [70]. Factors that appear to contribute to rate of uterine rupture after adenomyomectomy include the method of uterine reconstruction, interval length to pregnancy after adenomyomectomy, skill of the surgeon, and removal method [60].

Other experimental treatment options include MRI-guided focused ultrasound surgery [MRgFUS] and ultrasound-guided transvaginal radiofrequency ablation. MRgFUS is a non-invasive procedure that delivers a concentrated quantity of ultrasound energy to deep tissue areas, avoiding thermal effects to the surrounding tissues [71]. Several studies have demonstrated the safety and efficacy of this technique [72–77]. Ultrasound-guided transvaginal radiofrequency ablation is another promising minimally invasive technique that could be used to treat adenomyosis especially in patients who desire future fertility; however, more data are needed [78–80].

Conclusion

Despite long-term knowledge of the presence of endometrial glands and stroma within hypertrophic myometrium defining the condition of adenomyosis, the diagnosis, treatment, and impact of adenomyosis on reproductive outcomes remain somewhat mysterious. Once thought mainly a disease associated with multiparous women at the tail end of reproductive age, there has been a shift to identifying uterine shape and consistency deviations consistent with adenomyosis earlier in women suffering from pain, bleeding irregularities, and subfertility.

While the gold standard for the diagnosis of adenomyosis remains histological examination of a surgical specimen, improved resolution of imaging including MRI and 3D transvaginal ultrasound has led to promising non-invasive positive predictive values. With more readily available uterine-sparing means of diagnosis, studies have aimed to determine the effect of adenomyosis on fertility with mixed results.

With increased diagnosis and unclear delineation of the deleterious effects on reproductive outcomes, it is currently unknown which subset of asymptomatic patients would benefit from treatment. For patients with symptoms, treatment options such as hormonal manipulation and surgery can provide symptomatic relief. Overall, more prospective data are needed to combat the heterogeneity of disease, the wide variety of treatment protocols and surgical methods, and the lack of long-term follow-up to allow more insight into this enigmatic condition.

References

1. Benagiano G, Brosens I. History of adenomyosis. Best Pract Res Clin Obstet Gynaecol. 2006;20(4):449–63.
2. Benagiano G, Habiba M, Brosens I. The pathophysiology of uterine adenomyosis: an update. Fertil Steril. 2012;98(3):572–9.
3. Vannuccini S, Tosti C, Carmona F, Huang SJ, Chapron C, Guo SW, et al. Pathogenesis of adenomyosis: an update on molecular mechanisms. Reprod Biomed Online. 2017;35(5):592–601.
4. Mechsner S, Grum B, Gericke C, Loddenkemper C, Dudenhausen JW, Ebert AD. Possible roles of oxytocin receptor and vasopressin-1α receptor in the pathomechanism of dysperistalsis and dysmenorrhea in patients with adenomyosis uteri. Fertil Steril. 2010;94(7):2541–6.
5. Mori T, Singtripop T, Kawashima S. Animal model of uterine adenomyosis: is prolactin a potent inducer of adenomyosis in mice? Am J Obstet Gynecol. 1991;165(1):232–4.
6. Larsen SB, Lundorf E, Forman A, Dueholm M. Adenomyosis and junctional zone changes in patients with endometriosis. Eur J Obstet Gynecol Reprod Biol. 2011;157(2):206–11.

7. Puente JM, Fabris A, Patel J, Patel A, Cerrillo M, Requena A, et al. Adenomyosis in infertile women: prevalence and the role of 3D ultrasound as a marker of severity of the disease. Reprod Biol Endocrinol. 2016;14(1):60. Published 2016 Sep 20.

8. Zacharia TT, O'Neill MJ. Prevalence and distribution of adnexal findings suggesting endometriosis in patients with MR diagnosis of adenomyosis. Br J Radiol. 2006;79(940):303–7.

9. Kissler S, Zangos S, Wiegratz I, Kohl J, Rody A, Gaetje R, et al. Utero-tubal sperm transport and its impairment in endometriosis and adenomyosis. Ann N Y Acad Sci. 2007;1101:38–48.

10. Kunz G, Beil D, Huppert P, Noe M, Kissler S, Leyendecker G. Adenomyosis in endometriosis--prevalence and impact on fertility. Evidence from magnetic resonance imaging. Hum Reprod. 2005;20(8):2309–16.

11. Kunz G, Herbertz M, Beil D, Huppert P, Leyendecker G. Adenomyosis as a disorder of the early and late human reproductive period. Reprod Biomed Online. 2007;15(6):681–5.

12. Kunz G, Beil D, Huppert P, Leyendecker G. Structural abnormalities of the uterine wall in women with endometriosis and infertility visualized by vaginal sonography and magnetic resonance imaging. Hum Reprod. 2000;15(1):76–82.

13. Leyendecker G, Bilgicyildirim A, Inacker M, Stalf T, Huppert P, Mall G, et al. Adenomyosis and endometriosis. Re-visiting their association and further insights into the mechanisms of auto-traumatisation. An MRI study. Arch Gynecol Obstet. 2015;291(4):917–32.

14. Li JJ, Chung JPW, Wang S, Li TC, Duan H. The investigation and management of Adenomyosis in women who wish to improve or preserve fertility. Biomed Res Int. 2018;2018:6832685. Published 2018 Mar 15

15. Zoloudek C, Norris H. Mesenchymal tumors of the uterus. In: Kurman RJ, editor. Blaustein's pathology of the female genital tract. New York, NY: Springer-Verlag; 1994. p. 373–408.

16. Bazot M, Cortez A, Darai E, Rouger J, Chopier J, Antoine JM, et al. Ultrasonography compared with magnetic resonance imaging for the diagnosis of adenomyosis: correlation with histopathology. Hum Reprod. 2001;16(11):2427–33.

17. Bazot M, Daraï E. Role of transvaginal sonography and magnetic resonance imaging in the diagnosis of uterine adenomyosis. Fertil Steril. 2018;109(3):389–97.

18. Meredith SM, Sanchez-Ramos L, Kaunitz AM. Diagnostic accuracy of transvaginal sonography for the diagnosis of adenomyosis: systematic review and metaanalysis. Am J Obstet Gynecol. 2009;201(1):107.e1–107.e1076.

19. Dueholm M, Lundorf E. Transvaginal ultrasound or MRI for diagnosis of adenomyosis. Curr Opin Obstet Gynecol. 2007;19(6):505–12.

20. Ascher SM, Arnold LL, Patt RH, Schruefer JJ, Bagley AS, Semelka RC, et al. Adenomyosis: prospective comparison of MR imaging and transvaginal sonography. Radiology. 1994;190(3):803–6.

21. Takeuchi M, Matsuzaki K. Adenomyosis: usual and unusual imaging manifestations, pitfalls, and problem-solving MR imaging techniques. Radiographics. 2011;31(1):99–115.

22. Tamai K, Koyama T, Umeoka S, Saga T, Fujii S, Togashi K. Spectrum of MR features in adenomyosis. Best Pract Res Clin Obstet Gynaecol. 2006;20(4):583–602.

23. Tamai K, Togashi K, Ito T, Morisawa N, Fujiwara T, Koyama T. MR imaging findings of adenomyosis: correlation with histopathologic features and diagnostic pitfalls. Radiographics. 2005;25(1):21–40.

24. Dueholm M. Transvaginal ultrasound for diagnosis of adenomyosis: a review. Best Pract Res Clin Obstet Gynaecol. 2006;20(4):569–82.

25. Brosens JJ, de Souza NM, Barker FG, Paraschos T, Winston RM. Endovaginal ultrasonography in the diagnosis of adenomyosis uteri: identifying the predictive characteristics. Br J Obstet Gynaecol. 1995;102(6):471–4.

26. Fedele L, Bianchi S, Dorta M, Arcaini L, Zanotti F, Carinelli S. Transvaginal ultrasonography in the diagnosis of diffuse adenomyosis. Fertil Steril. 1992;58(1):94–7.

27. Reinhold C, McCarthy S, Bret PM, Mehio A, Atri M, Zakarian R, et al. Diffuse adenomyosis: comparison of endovaginal US and MR imaging with histopathologic correlation. Radiology. 1996;199(1):151–8.

28. Reinhold C, Atri M, Mehio A, Zakarian R, Aldis AE, Bret PM. Diffuse uterine adenomyosis: morphologic criteria and diagnostic accuracy of endovaginal sonography. Radiology. 1995;197(3):609–14.

29. Reinhold C, Tafazoli F, Mehio A, Wang L, Atri M, Siegelman ES, et al. Uterine adenomyosis: endovaginal US and MR imaging features with histopathologic correlation. Radiographics. 1999;19 Spec No:S147–60.

30. Atri M, Reinhold C, Mehio AR, Chapman WB, Bret PM. Adenomyosis: US features with histologic correlation in an in-vitro study. Radiology. 2000;215(3):783–90.

31. Cunningham RK, Horrow MM, Smith RJ, Springer J. Adenomyosis: a sonographic diagnosis. Radiographics. 2018;38(5):1576–89.

32. Sakhel K, Abuhamad A. Sonography of adenomyosis. J Ultrasound Med. 2012;31(5):805–8.

33. Sun YL, Wang CB, Lee CY, Wun TH, Lin P, Lin YH, et al. Transvaginal sonographic criteria for the diagnosis of adenomyosis based on histopathologic correlation. Taiwan J Obstet Gynecol. 2010;49(1):40–4.

34. Van den Bosch T, Dueholm M, Leone FP, Valentin L, Rasmussen CK, Votino A, et al. Terms, definitions and measurements to describe sonographic features of myometrium and uterine masses: a consensus opinion from the Morphological Uterus Sonographic Assessment [MUSA] group. Ultrasound Obstet Gynecol. 2015;46(3):284–98.

35. Andres MP, Borrelli GM, Ribeiro J, Baracat EC, Abrão MS, Kho RM. Transvaginal ultrasound for

the diagnosis of Adenomyosis: systematic review and meta-analysis. J Minim Invasive Gynecol. 2018;25(2):257–64.

36. Luciano DE, Exacoustos C, Albrecht L, LaMonica R, Proffer A, Zupi E, et al. Three-dimensional ultrasound in diagnosis of adenomyosis: histologic correlation with ultrasound targeted biopsies of the uterus. J Minim Invasive Gynecol. 2013;20(6):803–10.

37. Gordts S, Grimbizis G, Campo R. Symptoms and classification of uterine adenomyosis, including the place of hysteroscopy in diagnosis. Fertil Steril. 2018;109(3):380–388.e1.

38. Vercellini P, Consonni D, Dridi D, Bracco B, Frattaruolo MP, Somigliana E. Uterine adenomyosis and in vitro fertilization outcome: a systematic review and meta-analysis. Hum Reprod. 2014;29(5):964–77.

39. Sharma S, Bathwal S, Agarwal N, Chattopadhyay R, Saha I, Chakravarty B. Does presence of adenomyosis affect reproductive outcome in IVF cycles? A retrospective analysis of 973 patients. Reprod Biomed Online. 2019;38(1):13–21.

40. Benaglia L, Cardellicchio L, Leonardi M, Faulisi S, Vercellini P, Paffoni A, et al. Asymptomatic adenomyosis and embryo implantation in IVF cycles. Reprod Biomed Online. 2014;29(5):606–11.

41. Mijatovic V, Florijn E, Halim N, Schats R, Hompes P. Adenomyosis has no adverse effects on IVF/ICSI outcomes in women with endometriosis treated with long-term pituitary down-regulation before IVF/ICSI. Eur J Obstet Gynecol Reprod Biol. 2010;151(1):62–5.

42. Rocha TP, Andres MP, Borrelli GM, Abrão MS. Fertility-sparing treatment of Adenomyosis in patients with infertility: a systematic review of current options. Reprod Sci. 2018;25(4):480–6.

43. Neal S, Morin S, Werner M, Gueye NA, Pirtea P, Patounakis G, et al. Three-dimensional ultrasound diagnosis of adenomyosis is not associated with adverse pregnancy outcomes following single thawed euploid blastocyst transfer: a prospective cohort study [published online ahead of print, 2020 Apr 29]. Ultrasound Obstet Gynecol. 2020; https://doi.org/10.1002/uog.22065.

44. Fraser IS. Non-contraceptive health benefits of intrauterine hormonal systems. Contraception. 2010;82(5):396–403. https://doi.org/10.1016/j.contraception.2010.05.005.

45. Sabbioni L, Petraglia F, Luisi S. Non-contraceptive benefits of intrauterine levonorgestrel administration: why not? Gynecol Endocrinol. 2017;33(11):822–9.

46. Fedele L, Bianchi S, Raffaelli R, Portuese A, Dorta M. Treatment of adenomyosis-associated menorrhagia with a levonorgestrel-releasing intrauterine device. Fertil Steril. 1997;68(3):426–9.

47. Maruo T, Laoag-Fernandez JB, Pakarinen P, Murakoshi H, Spitz IM, Johansson E. Effects of the levonorgestrel-releasing intrauterine system on proliferation and apoptosis in the endometrium. Hum Reprod. 2001;16(10):2103–8.

48. Sheng J, Zhang WY, Zhang JP, Lu D. The LNG-IUS study on adenomyosis: a 3-year follow-up study on the efficacy and side effects of the use of levonorgestrel intrauterine system for the treatment of dysmenorrhea associated with adenomyosis. Contraception. 2009;79(3):189–93.

49. Cho S, Nam A, Kim H, Chay D, Park K, Cho DJ, et al. Clinical effects of the levonorgestrel-releasing intrauterine device in patients with adenomyosis. Am J Obstet Gynecol. 2008;198(4):373.e1–373.e3737.

50. Shaaban OM, Ali MK, Sabra AM, Abd El Aal DE. Levonorgestrel-releasing intrauterine system versus a low-dose combined oral contraceptive for treatment of adenomyotic uteri: a randomized clinical trial. Contraception. 2015;92(4):301–7.

51. Lee KH, Kim JK, Lee MA, Ko YB, Yang JB, Kang BH, et al. Relationship between uterine volume and discontinuation of treatment with levonorgestrel-releasing intrauterine devices in patients with adenomyosis. Arch Gynecol Obstet. 2016;294(3):561–6.

52. Vannuccini S, Luisi S, Tosti C, Sorbi F, Petraglia F. Role of medical therapy in the management of uterine adenomyosis. Fertil Steril. 2018;109(3):398–405.

53. Okada H, Okamoto R, Tsuzuki T, Tsuji S, Yasuda K, Kanzaki H. Progestins inhibit estradiol-induced vascular endothelial growth factor and stromal cell-derived factor 1 in human endometrial stromal cells. Fertil Steril. 2011;96(3):786–91.

54. Muneyyirci-Delale O, Chandrareddy A, Mankame S, Osei-Tutu N, von Gizycki H. Norethindrone acetate in the medical management of adenomyosis. Pharmaceuticals. 2012;5(10):1120–7.

55. Kitawaki J, Noguchi T, Amatsu T, Maeda K, Tsukamoto K, Yamamoto T, Fushiki S, Osawa Y, Honjo H. Expression of aromatase cytochrome P450 protein and messenger ribonucleic acid in human endometriotic and adenomyotic tissues but not in normal endometrium. Biol Reprod. 1997;57(3):514–9.

56. Yamamoto T, Noguchi T, Tamura T, Kitawaki J, Okada H. Evidence for estrogen synthesis in adenomyotic tissues. Am J Obstet Gynecol. 1993;169(3):734–8.

57. Liang E, Brown B, Kirsop R, Stewart P, Stuart A. Efficacy of uterine artery embolisation for treatment of symptomatic fibroids and adenomyosis - an interim report on an Australian experience. Aust N Z J Obstet Gynaecol. 2012;52(2):106–12.

58. Zhou J, He L, Liu P, Duan H, Zhang H, Li W, et al. Outcomes in Adenomyosis treated with uterine artery embolization are associated with lesion vascularity: a long-term follow-up study of 252 cases. PLoS One. 2016;11(11):e0165610. Published 2016 Nov 2.

59. de Bruijn AM, Smink M, Lohle PNM, Huirne JAF, Twisk JWR, Wong C, et al. Uterine artery embolization for the treatment of Adenomyosis: a systematic review and meta-analysis. J Vasc Interv Radiol. 2017;28(12):1629–1642.e1.

60. Osada H. Uterine adenomyosis and adenomyoma: the surgical approach. Fertil Steril. 2018;109(3):406–17.

61. Sun AJ, Luo M, Wang W, Chen R, Lang JH. Characteristics and efficacy of modified adenomyomectomy in the treatment of uterine adenomyoma. Chin Med J. 2011;124(9):1322–6.

62. Fujishita A, Masuzaki H, Khan KN, Kitajima M, Ishimaru T. Modified reduction surgery for adenomyosis. A preliminary report of the transverse H incision technique. Gynecol Obstet Investig. 2004;57(3):132–8.

63. Gao Y, Shan S, Zhao X, Jiang J, Li D, Shi B. Clinical efficacy of adenomyomectomy using "H" type incision combined with Mirena in the treatment of adenomyosis. Medicine (Baltimore). 2019;98(11):e14579.

64. Osada H, Silber S, Kakinuma T, Nagaishi M, Kato K, Kato O. Surgical procedure to conserve the uterus for future pregnancy in patients suffering from massive adenomyosis. Reprod Biomed Online. 2011;22(1):94–9.

65. Nishida M, Takano K, Arai Y, Ozone H, Ichikawa R. Conservative surgical management for diffuse uterine adenomyosis. Fertil Steril. 2010;94(2):715–9.

66. Takeuchi H, Kitade M, Kikuchi I, Shimanuki H, Kumakiri J, Kitano T, et al. Laparoscopic adenomyomectomy and hysteroplasty: a novel method. J Minim Invasive Gynecol. 2006;13(2):150–4.

67. Kim JK, Shin CS, Ko YB, Nam SY, Yim HS, Lee KH. Laparoscopic assisted adenomyomectomy using double flap method. Obstet Gynecol Sci. 2014;57(2):128–35.

68. Kishi Y, Yabuta M, Taniguchi F. Who will benefit from uterus-sparing surgery in adenomyosis-associated subfertility? Fertil Steril. 2014;102(3):802–807.e1.

69. Morimatsu Y, Matsubara S, Higashiyama N, Kuwata T, Ohkuchi A, Izumi A, et al. Uterine rupture during pregnancy soon after a laparoscopic adenomyomectomy. Reprod Med Biol. 2007;6(3):175–177. Published 2007 Aug 6.

70. Dubuisson JB, Fauconnier A, Deffarges JV, Norgaard C, Kreiker G, Chapron C. Pregnancy outcome and deliveries following laparoscopic myomectomy. Hum Reprod. 2000;15(4):869–73.

71. Al Hilli MM, Stewart EA. Magnetic resonance-guided focused ultrasound surgery. Semin Reprod Med. 2010;28(3):242–9.

72. Dev B, Gadddam S, Kumar M, Varadarajan S. MR-guided focused ultrasound surgery: a novel non-invasive technique in the treatment of adenomyosis −18 month's follow-up of 12 cases. Indian J Radiol Imag. 2019;29(3):284–8.

73. Jayaram R, Subbarayan K, Mithraprabhu S, Govindarajan M. Heavy menstrual bleeding and dysmenorrhea are improved by Magnetic Resonance Guided Focused Ultrasound Surgery [MRgFUS] of adenomyosis. Fertil Res Pract. 2016;2:8. Published 2016 May 16

74. Fan TY, Zhang L, Chen W, Liu Y, He M, Huang X, et al. Feasibility of MRI-guided high intensity focused ultrasound treatment for adenomyosis. Eur J Radiol. 2012;81(11):3624–30.

75. Fukunishi H, Funaki K, Sawada K, Yamaguchi K, Maeda T, Kaji Y. Early results of magnetic resonance-guided focused ultrasound surgery of adenomyosis: analysis of 20 cases. J Minim Invasive Gynecol. 2008;15(5):571–9.

76. Kim KA, Yoon SW, Lee C, Seong SJ, Yoon BS, Park H. Short-term results of magnetic resonance imaging-guided focused ultrasound surgery for patients with adenomyosis: symptomatic relief and pain reduction. Fertil Steril. 2011;95(3):1152–5.

77. Yoon SW, Kim KA, Cha SH, Kim YM, Lee C, Na YJ, et al. Successful use of magnetic resonance-guided focused ultrasound surgery to relieve symptoms in a patient with symptomatic focal adenomyosis. Fertil Steril. 2008;90(5):2018e.13.

78. Nam JH. Pregnancy and symptomatic relief following ultrasound-guided transvaginal radiofrequency ablation in patients with adenomyosis. J Obstet Gynaecol Res. 2020;46(1):124–32.

79. Hai N, Hou Q, Ding X, Dong X, Jin M. Ultrasound-guided transcervical radiofrequency ablation for symptomatic uterine adenomyosis. Br J Radiol. 2017;90(1069):20160119.

80. Zhou M, Chen JY, Tang LD, Chen WZ, Wang ZB. Ultrasound-guided high-intensity focused ultrasound ablation for adenomyosis: the clinical experience of a single center. Fertil Steril. 2011;95(3):900–5.

Jenna M. Rehmer, Natalia C. Llarena,
Christine Hur, and Jeffrey M. Goldberg

Introduction

Tubal factor infertility accounts for 25–35% of female factor infertility [1]. Proximal tubal blockage, resulting from obstruction, such as spasm or mucous plug, or occlusion, secondary to salpingitis isthmica nodosa or fibrosis, accounts for 10–25% of tubal disease. The majority of tubal disease is due to distal obstruction, with over 50% secondary to salpingitis, usually as a sequela of ascending sexually transmitted *Chlamydia trachomatis* and/or *Neisseria gonorrhoeae* infections. Other causes of pelvic inflammation such as perforated bowel, prior ectopic pregnancy, septic abortion, endometritis, surgery or trauma to fallopian tubes, and endometriosis may also lead to distal tubal occlusion.

At initial insult of salpingitis, the fallopian tube becomes inflamed leading to cell necrosis with loss of the ciliated tubal epithelium. The inflammation also causes the fimbriae to agglutinate resulting in distal obstruction of the fallo-

pian tube. Pelvic adhesions may develop as well. The physiological serous secretions of tubal epithelium then accumulate within the occluded tube resulting in a hydrosalpinx. The number and severity of salpingitis episodes adversely affects the potential for fertility. A prospective cohort study of 1309 women in Sweden showed a relative risk (RR) for infertility of 7.0 after 1 infection, 16.2 after 2, and 28.3 after 3 infections. In this same study, in women with only one pelvic inflammatory disease (PID) episode, the severity of infection was directly correlated with infertility with RRs of 1, 1.8, and 5.6 for mild, moderate, and severe infections, respectively [2].

Between 2015 and 2018, in the United States, the Centers for Disease Control and Prevention data show chlamydia and gonorrhea rates increased 11.9% and 37.2%, for a total of 692.7 and 145.8 cases per 100,000 females respectively. Up to 10% of untreated chlamydial infections progress to clinically diagnosed PID and the risk with untreated gonococcal infection is even higher [3–5]. A retrospective cohort study, with 38,193 women, examined the incidence of hospitalization for PID following chlamydia and/or gonorrhea diagnosis and found an incidence rate of 13.9 per 1000 person-years of follow-up (95% CI 12.6–15.1) for woman with a chlamydia diagnosis. The incidence rate for gonorrhea diagnosis was 50.8 per 1000 person-years of follow-up (95% CI 36.0–65.6) [6].

Supplementary Information The online version contains supplementary material available at [https://doi.org/10.1007/978-3-031-05240-8_9].

J. M. Rehmer · N. C. Llarena · C. Hur ·
J. M. Goldberg (✉)
The Cleveland Clinic, Women's Health Institute,
Cleveland, OH, USA
e-mail: rehmerj@ccf.org; llarenn@ccf.org;
hurc@ccf.org; goldbej@ccf.org

Risk factors for PID include sexual intercourse, multiple partners, history of PID, vaginal douching, menses, cigarette smoking, and substance abuse. Risk of PID is inversely related to age, with younger age being associated with greater risk. The use of barrier contraceptives reduce PID risk with condoms being the most effective [7]. Hydrosalpinges can be treated surgically to improve fertility. There are several surgical options for achieving patency in obstructed fallopian tubes, depending on the location and pathogenesis of the blockage. This chapter reviews these procedures and the factors that must be considered in distal tubal disease when deciding between surgical repair and salpingectomy followed by in vitro fertilization (IVF).

Diagnosis

Hydrosalpinx is most commonly asymptomatic, though it can present as chronic pelvic pain. Many women remain undiagnosed until presenting to a physician for infertility. The basic work up for infertility consists of an evaluation to exclude ovulatory disorders, semen abnormalities, and other major reproductive problems including uterine and tubal pathology. A history of sexually transmitted infections, PID, ectopic pregnancy, ruptured appendix, or prior pelvic surgery raises the index of suspicion for tubal factor infertility.

The standard first-line diagnostic test to evaluate tubal patency is hysterosalpingography (HSG) [8]. For this test, X-ray contrast medium is injected transcervically while observing the flow of contrast medium into the uterus and through the fallopian tubes under fluoroscopic visualization. It is important to eliminate air bubbles in contrast fluid prior to injecting and to inject with a slow, low pressure to prevent proximal tubal spasms. This technique is easily performed, relatively low cost, and has a minimal radiation exposure. Results are interpreted instantaneously by the performing physician and discussed with the patient. Contraindication, risks, benefits, and alternatives to HSG are outlined in Table 9.1.

Table 9.1 Risk, benefits, contraindications, and alternatives to HSG

Risks
Pain, normally limited and mild
Radiation exposure; low risk
Vasovagal reactions
Post-procedure PID; increased with hydrosalpinges
Granuloma formation with oil-based contrast
Oil embolism with oil-based contrast
Benefits
Non-invasive assessment of tubal patency with diagnostic information about tubal blockage location and tubal anatomy
Uterine cavity evaluation
Fertility enhancement
Contraindications
Bleeding/menstruation; relative contraindication
Active pelvic infection
Known or suspected endometrial carcinoma
Pregnancy
Alternatives
3D sono-hysterosalpingography or hysterosalpingo-contrast sonography (HyCoSy)
Hysteroscopy and laparoscopy with chromopertubation
Perryscope air infusion into saline during office hysteroscopy

In addition to its diagnostic potential, HSG provides a therapeutic effect. A 2020 Cochrane review concluded tubal flushing with oil-soluble contrast media (OSCM) and water-soluble contrast media (WSCM) are both superior to no treatment, with an ongoing pregnancy OR of 3.59 in the OSCM group and OR 1.14 in the WSCM group [9].

There has been much debate in the literature surrounding the fertility-enhancing effect of tubal flushing HSG with OSCM versus WSCM. A 2017 multicenter, randomized trial in the Netherlands with 1119 women showed higher rates of ongoing pregnancy and live births among women who underwent HSG with OSCM (39.7% and 38.8%) compared HSG with WSCM (29.1% and 28.1%) [10]. While this difference is significant, OSCM has a high viscosity, resulting in slower tubal filling and sometimes necessitates a late film 24 hours later, higher cost per case, and it is associated with rare, albeit significant, risks including granulomatous formation and pulmonary emboli. WSCM also provides superior detailed imaging of the internal architecture of the tubal mucosal folds and ampullary rugae as seen in Figs. 9.1 and 9.2 [9]. WSCM is also generally cheaper than OSCM.

The negative predictive value of HSG is high; when HSG results show tubal patency it is a highly accurate and reliable test [11]. However, when HSG suggests tubal occlusion, physicians should be aware this is less reliable, especially for proximal occlusion. A prospective study assessing 40 infertile women with proximal tubal obstruction found that 60% of women had bilateral tubal patency documented with a second

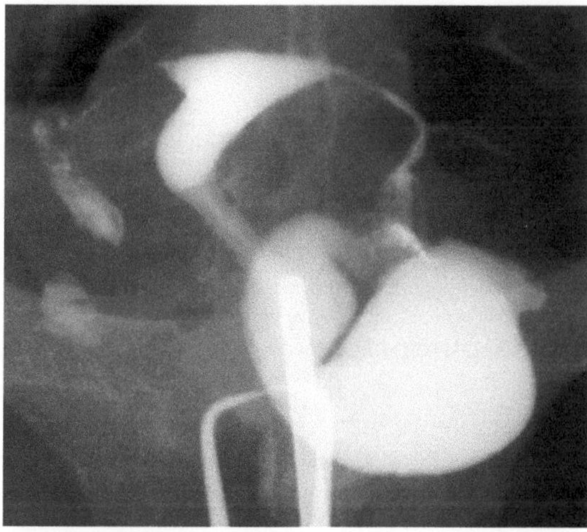

Fig. 9.1 Bilateral hydrosalpinx on hysterosalpingogram. Severely dilated distal left fallopian tube with complete loss of normal tubal mucosal folds and blunted ampullary segment. Neosalpingostomy on the left fallopian tube is unlikely to reveal normal tubal architecture. Salpingectomy should be considered first line for the left fallopian tube

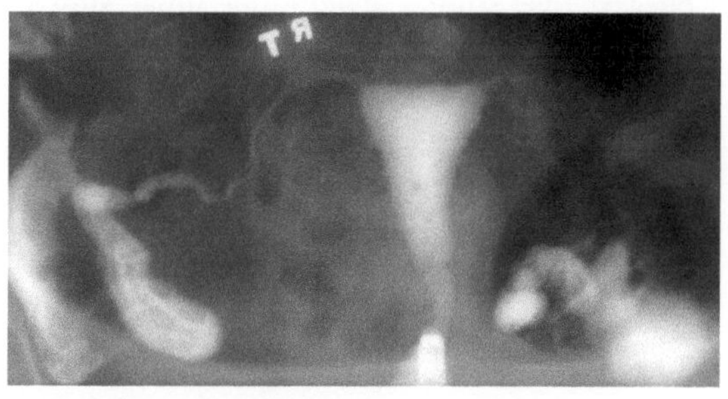

Fig. 9.2 Hysterosalpingogram with bilateral hydrosalpinx. Normal internal architecture of the tubal mucosal folds and ampullary rugae are still visible making this patient a candidate for neosalpingostomy

HSG one month later. Using laparoscopy as the gold-standard test to confirm tubal occlusion, a meta-analysis published in 2014 of nine studies allowed direct comparison of the accuracy of HSG. Pooled estimates of sensitivity and specificity for HSG were 0.94 (95% CI: 0.74–0.99) and 0.92 (95% CI: 0.87–0.95) respectively [12].

There are alternatives to HSG:

- *Sono-HSG*: The aforementioned meta-analysis also compared sono-HSG to laparoscopy and found pooled estimates of sensitivity and specify of sono-HSG to be 0.92 (95% CI: 0.82–0.96) and 0.95 (95% CI: 0.90–0.97), respectively [12]. This is comparable to HSG. This test is a valid alternative to HSG and can provide additional details on pelvic anatomy with simultaneous transvaginal ultrasonography. However, clinicians must remember that it does not reveal the tubal anatomy, hydrosalpinx diameter, presence of mucosal folds, SIN, or peri-tubal adhesions. Most commonly used contrast medium is saline with air bubbles introduced by agitation of saline prior to instillation. Other options available on the market include FemVue® Saline-Air device, which introduces a consistent mixture of saline and air contrast, ExEm© Foam, and SonoVue®.
- *Hysteroscopy and laparoscopy with chromopertubation*: The gold standard for uterine cavity assessment is hysteroscopy and for determining tubal patency, it is chromopertubation via laparoscopy. Even that, however, is not perfect with one study showing a 2% spontaneous pregnancy rate among women diagnosed with bilateral tubal occlusion by laparoscopy [13]. Laparoscopy also allows for the concurrent diagnosis and treatment of other pelvic pathology which may impair fertility such as pelvic adhesions and endometriosis.

Impact of Hydrosalpinx on IVF

It is clear that hydrosalpinges negatively impact pregnancy rates in women undergoing IVF. Two large meta-analyses including over 5000 patients each demonstrated that implantation, clinical pregnancy, and delivery rates per transfer decrease by 50% in the presence of a hydrosalpinx [14, 15]. Further, four randomized trials and a Cochrane review show that salpingectomy prior to IVF doubles clinical pregnancy rates (RR 2.02, 95% CI: 1.44 to 2.82) [16–19]. Proximal tubal occlusion surgically prior to IVF also increases clinical pregnancy rates (RR 3.21, 95% CI: 1.72 to 5.99) [17, 19], and current ASRM guidelines recommend salpingectomy or proximal tubal occlusion prior to IVF in women who are not candidates for reparative tubal surgery [1].

Interrupting the communication between the uterus and the hydrosalpinx, either by salpingectomy or proximal tubal occlusion, restores IVF outcomes; therefore, the negative effect of hydrosalpinx appears to be caused by the fluid itself (this is discussed in greater detail in the salpingectomy and proximal tubal occlusion sections). Several mechanisms have been proposed to account for the impact of hydrosalpinx on IVF outcomes, including direct embryotoxicity, impaired endometrial receptivity, and mechanical flushing [20–23].

The impact of hydrosalpinx fluid on embryo development has been tested by exposing both human and mouse embryos to human hydrosalpinx fluid in vitro. Mouse embryos cultured in the presence of human hydrosalpinx fluid aspirated at the time of laparoscopy showed higher rates of developmental arrest and degeneration compared to control embryos grown in conventional culture media [21]. Similarly, human embryos exposed to hydrosalpinx fluid showed a 50% reduction in blastulation rate compared to controls [24].

In addition to direct embryotoxicity, several lines of evidence suggest that hydrosalpinx fluid reduces endometrial receptivity by altering the profile of cytokines and growth factors necessary for implantation. Specifically, integrin $\alpha_v\beta_3$ is present both at the surface of the embryo and on the endometrial surface epithelium during the luteal phase of spontaneous cycles [22]. Integrin $\alpha_v\beta_3$ is thought to activate matrix metalloproteinases and plasminogen activators that allow for trophoblastic invasion and adherence of the embryo to the endometrial surface. Women with hydrosalpinges show decreased endometrial expression of integrin $\alpha_v\beta_3$, which may contribute to failed implantation after embryo transfer [25]. Additionally, HOXA10 is a transcription factor regulated by estrogen and progesterone that is expressed in the human endometrium and is critical for embryo implantation [26]. Whereas hydrosalpinx fluid decreases the expression of HOXA10 [21], a small prospective trial shows that salpingectomy restores HOXA10 expression in the endometrium [26]. The presence of hydrosalpinx has also been shown to reduce endometrial and subendometrial blood flow, as measured by Doppler ultrasound [27, 28]. Together, these data support the hypothesis that hydrosalpinges reduce pregnancy rates after IVF by impairing endometrial receptivity.

Finally, hydrosalpinx fluid may also prevent physical contact between the embryo and endometrial surface and act as a mechanical barrier to implantation [20].

Neosalpingostomy

The decision to proceed with neosalpingostomy to re-establish tubal patency versus IVF has many variables that must be considered when counseling patients. These include maternal age; coexisting fertility factors, especially male factor; number of desired children; the risks of surgery and IVF, as well as treatment costs and inconvenience [1]. Data comparing direct outcomes are limited due to the nature of reporting and lack of uniform registries for tubal surgery outcomes. Retrospective studies examining tubal surgery outcomes are heterogeneous, dated, and report success as percentage of patients conceiving within a given time interval, whereas pregnancy rates after IVF are reported per stimulation cycle initiated.

The benefits of IVF are high success rates, with the 2017 SART National Summary (SART. org) reporting a 42.7% live birth rate after first embryo transfer per retrieval in woman <35 years of age with tubal factor diagnosis, 28.4% for age 35–37, and 22.1% for age 38–40. However, IVF can be considerably more expensive, especially where insurance coverage is not mandated, and more than one cycle may be required to achieve the desired number of children. While the overall safety of IVF is well established, there have been reported fetal and neonatal risks including congenital malformations, preterm delivery, low birth weight, and increased maternal risk including multiple pregnancies and pre-eclampsia [29–31].

Successful neosalpingostomy allows for repeated attempts at spontaneous conception and multiple conceptions all without medical intervention following surgery. However, the risks of ectopic pregnancy and tubal re-occlusion should be discussed with the patient.

The extent of tubal disease is directly correlated with outcomes. Favorable prognosis patients have minimal adnexal adhesions, tubal dilation of <3 cm, pliable thin tubal walls, preservation of mucosal folds seen on HSG, and normal appearing fimbria and mucosal endosalpinx upon opening the tube [1]. The preservation of mucosal folds and endosalpinx are probably the most important parameter intraoperatively. Brosens and Puttemans described a tubal scoring system where stage 1 is normal, stage 2 has decreasing mucosal folds, in stage 3 there are intra-ampullary focal adhesions, and in stage 4 and 5 the folds are absent and ampulla contains increased adhesions. https://www.sciencedirect.com/science/article/pii/S2667164620300038#bib4 A 2014 study following 434 patient after laparoscopic neosalpingostomy reported a 5-year live birth rate of 53.1% for stage 1, 43.1% for stage 2, 24.0% for stage 3, and 23.1% for stage 4. No significant difference was found in ectopic pregnancy rate in relation to tubal stage: 5.6% in stage 1, 11.0% in stage 2, 11.4% in stage 3, and 6.2% in stage 4 [32].

When used indiscriminately, neosalpingostomy results in a 10–60% pregnancy rate and up to a 21% ectopic rate. This has led many to abandon the procedure [33]. However, when limited to appropriate good prognosis patients, those classified as having mild disease, the clinical pregnancy rate (CPR) ranges from 58 to 77% with ectopic pregnancy rates of 2–8% [34]. Table 9.2 summarizes five studies looking at CPR and ectopic rates based on patient prognosis.

Table 9.2 Summary of five studies evaluating clinical pregnancy rates and ectopic pregnancy rates following salpingostomy based upon patient prognosis

Prognosis	Number of patients	Clinical pregnancy rate	Ectopic pregnancy rate
Good	104	67%	3%
Intermediate	141	24%	28%
Poor	196	10%	31%

Rates are reported as average [35–39]

Young patients with no other significant factors and mild tubal disease possess the best potential for spontaneous intrauterine pregnancy following salpingostomy.

Patients should be consented preoperatively for both salpingostomy and salpingectomy, as the final decision is made upon direct visualization of the fallopian tube during laparoscopy. Neosalpingostomy is performed via laparoscopy using microsurgical technique. The principles of microsurgery are attention to gentle tissue handling, irrigation to prevent tissue desiccation, meticulous hemostasis with limited electrosurgical energy, avoidance of foreign body contamination, and use of a fine non-reactive suture placed without unnecessary tension to prevent tissue ischemia. There is no evidence to support any advantage of robotic surgery over conventional laparoscopy for this indication. Preoperative intravenous antibiotics should be administered given an increased history of prior infectious etiology and risk of stimulating chronic salpingitis infection.

Surgery begins in the same fashion as routine gynecological laparoscopy; to reduce risk of trocar-related injury a Foley catheter and orogastric tube are placed for decompression of the bladder and stomach. A uterine manipulator with chromopertubation capabilities is placed. This surgery can be completed through one 5 mm umbilical port and two additional 5 mm operative ports, one in each lower quadrant.

The first step in the surgery, as seen in Video 9.1, is a detailed survey of the anatomy and complete excision of all adhesions. Transcervical chromopertubation is performed to confirm proximal tubal patency and delineate distal tubal anatomy. It is recommended that the distal mesosalpinx is injected with dilute vasopressin (20 units in 100 mL of injectable saline). This provides vasoconstriction of nearby vessels, improving hemostasis and limiting the need for electrosurgical energy and potential thermal injury. The neosalpingostomy is performed at the most distal end of the hydrosalpinx by incising with a unipolar needle on 35 watts cutting current which provides a high-power density to limit thermal spread. The incision is widely opened to fully assess the endosalpinx and to mobilize the tubal ends for suturing. If normal tubal mucosa is present, the edges of the tube are fully everted and sutured to adjacent tubal serosa with 4-0 delayed absorbable suture using intracorporeal knot tying. In order to tie intracorporeally with only 2 contralateral operative ports, the surgeon and assistant work together to complete the knot. Alternatively, a 3rd accessory port can be placed to increase suturing agility and stabilization of the tube. A small half circle (SH) needle is used, and the suture end curvature is straightened using hemostats to form a ski needle. This facilitates passage of the needle through the 5 mm port. Alternatively, a half-curved (ski needle) suture could be used or the SH needle can be placed directly into the abdomen via the trocar incision. Tubal patency is confirmed by chromopertubation. To aid in the prevention of postoperative adhesions, an adhesive barrier such as Interceed (Ethicon, Somerville, NJ), a self-adhering absorbable sheet of oxidized regenerated cellulose, is placed over the tube. Alternative techniques to the aforementioned technique, include 1) opening the distal hydrosalpinges with cold scissors to avoid electrosurgical energy, and 2) fixating the opened tube by heating the serosal surfaces of the tube around the fimbrial ostium (flowering of Bruhat). Outcomes of these alternatives are compared in Table 9.3.

Postoperatively, patients are instructed to wait two cycles prior to attempting conception. Patients are also given ectopic pregnancy precautions which include early pregnancy assessment of HCG trends and ultrasound to identify pregnancy location. If the patient is not pregnant following six months of timed intercourse, tubal patency should be reassessed using HSG. If re-

Table 9.3 Clinical pregnancy outcomes following neosalpingostomy using varying surgical techniques; summarization of published data [38]

Surgical technique	PregnancyN, (%)	Intrauterine pregnancy N, (%)	Ectopic pregnancy N, (%)
Cold scissors, eversion with suture	9, (39%)	5, (19%)	4, (15%)
Unipolar needle, Bruhat eversion	13, (48%)	10, (37%)	3, (11%)
Unipolar needle, eversion with suture	15, (52%)	14, (48%)	1, (3%)

occlusion has occurred, salpingectomy prior to IVF would be recommended as repeat operations for distal occlusion have exceptionally low success rates [40].

While neosalpingostomy is more commonly considered in patients who desire natural conception, consideration can be given for it as an alternative approach to management of hydrosalpinx in the IVF patient. A non-randomized prospective study found no difference in clinical pregnancy rate in IVF patients with hydrosalpinges treated with salpingectomy versus salpingostomy. In this study group, the overall CPR was 50% after IVF in patients who underwent bilateral salpingectomy and 63.3% in patients with at least one function tube, with a spontaneous pregnancy rate of 30.4% [41]. This study shows a potential benefit of conservative surgical management in IVF patients with unilateral hydrosalpinges.

Salpingectomy

Patients with poor prognosis for spontaneous conception following neosalpingostomy include those with extensive adhesions, tubal dilation >3 cm, thick fibrotic walls, and no normal luminal mucosa upon opening the tube. For these patients, IVF success rates far exceed those of neosalpingostomy with attempted spontaneous conception. As previously noted, salpingectomy

Table 9.4 Summary of treatment options for hydrosalpinx

Salpingectomy	Tubal ligation	Salpingostomy
Proven efficacy in RCTs	Proven efficacy in RCTs	Limited data
Cannot conceive without IVF	Cannot conceive without IVF	Spontaneous conception possible
Risk(s): may decrease ovarian reserve	Risk(s): hydrosalpinx may enlarge	Risk(s): tubal re-occlusion and ectopic pregnancy
For mod-severe hydrosalpinges	For hydrosalpinges with extensive adhesions	For mild hydrosalpinges only

overcomes the adverse effect of hydrosalpinges on embryo implantation and restores IVF pregnancy rates back those of matched controls without hydrosalpinx (Table 9.4) [42].

Salpingectomy is performed endoscopically with a 5 mm port in each lower quadrant bilaterally and a 10 mm port in the umbilicus to extract the fallopian tube(s). The proximal tube is ligated and divided and the mesosalpinx is serially ligated and divided. This can be accomplished with any preferred modality such as reusable bipolar graspers and scissors, harmonic scalpel, or via vessel sealing device such as LigaSure (Covidien, Minneapolis). It is important to remain as close to the tube as possible to avoid compromising the vascular supply to the ovary which could result in diminished ovarian reserve. However, an RCT found no significant difference in ovarian reserve following prophylactic bilateral salpingectomy using conservative surgery versus wide excision of the mesosalpinx [43]. Following this minimally invasive surgery, patients may begin IVF with the next menstrual cycle.

Proximal Tubal Ligation

Salpingectomy is widely considered the gold standard in treating hydrosalpinx prior to IVF. However, proximal tubal ligation has been found to be an acceptable alternative, particularly for patients with extensive pelvic adhesions. Two randomized control trials (RCT) demonstrated proximal tubal ligation as an effective way of improving pregnancy rates in women with hydrosalpinx with clinical outcomes comparable to salpingectomy [17, 44]. A recent Cochran review concluded that proximal tubal ligation may provide an equally effective and safer alternative to salpingectomy (Table 9.4) [19].

There has been some debate as to whether the technique of proximal tubal ligation may affect clinical outcomes. A prospective RCT of 88 patients found a significant increase of day 3 FSH and a decrease in antral follicle count (AFC) and ovarian volumes in women who underwent tubal ligation by electrosurgery as compared to those who underwent tubal ligation by mechanical clips [45]. Other studies have reported decrease in ovarian response and increase in gonadotropin dosing following tubal ligation using electrosurgery [46, 47]. While additional studies are required to determine the best technique for tubal ligation in this clinical scenario, limited studies at this time suggest that ligation without electrosurgery may have less impact on subsequent ovarian function.

As noted above, there is a concern that salpingectomy may lead to diminished ovarian reserve. An RCT of 165 participants with hydrosalpinges randomized women to proximal tubal ligation or salpingectomy ($n = 83$ and $n = 82$, respectively). This study found there was a statistically significant decrease in postoperative serum anti-Mullerian hormone (AMH) (3.7 ng/ml v. 2.6 ng/mL; $p < 0.001$) and AFC (10.6 v 8.6; $p < 0.001$) in women who underwent salpingectomy, a trend not identified in women who underwent proximal tubal ligation. This same study found women undergoing salpingectomy required a greater dose of gonadotropins (3901 v. 3260; $p < 0.001$) over a longer period of stimulation (11.3 v. 10.2; $p < 0.001$). Otherwise, these authors could not find a significant difference in rate of implantation, clinical pregnancy, miscarriage, or live birth rate between these two groups [44]. Overall, the authors found proximal tubal ligation to be a superior treatment of hydrosalpinx when compared to salpingectomy. While some studies have indicated similar findings [48], others were unable to confirm that there was any difference between the two treatment options [49]. At this time, the evidence continues to support the use of proximal tubal ligation as a comparable alternative treatment of hydrosalpinx.

When performing a tubal ligation for treatment of a hydrosalpinx, there is a theoretical risk of continued expansion of hydrosalpinges [1]. Without the ability to drain through the uterine cavity, there is concern fluid will continue to build within the hydrosalpinx resulting in worsening distention and possibly secondary pain. To reduce this risk, the hydrosalpinx can be fenestrated to the fullest extent possible at the time of proximal tubal ligation.

Hysteroscopic Proximal Tubal Occlusion

In patients where laparoscopy is not feasible or carries a high risk for complications, hysteroscopic tubal occlusion primarily through the use of the Essure® device has been utilized to treat hydrosalpinges prior to IVF. While this has been successfully described in some small studies, there is concern that the trailing coils may carry an IUD-like contraceptive effect by limiting embryo implantation. One study found that only 17% of women had complete tissue encapsulation without identification of intrauterine coils by hysteroscopy at 1 year, and only 25% with complete tissue encapsulation by 13–43 months [50].

A 2017 meta-analysis comparing IVF outcomes following Essure® vs laparoscopic salpingectomy or proximal tubal ligation for hydrosalpinges concluded that the implantation rates and clinical pregnancy and live birth rates were significantly lower and the miscarriage rates significantly higher with Essure® [51]. The Essure® rates were essentially the same as untreated hydrosalpinges.

Of note, in December of 2018, Bayer distribution announced that the Essure® device would no longer be sold or distributed. This was due to recent post-market studies demonstrating that women had higher rates of chronic abdominal pain and abnormal bleeding following Essure® placement when compared to those who underwent other forms of tubal ligation. Currently, there is no device on the market that allows for hysteroscopic proximal tubal occlusion.

Alternatives to Salpingectomy: Aspiration and Sclerotherapy

Aspiration of hydrosalpinx fluid at the time of retrieval has been evaluated as a less invasive alternative to salpingectomy [52–54]; however, both retrospective studies and randomized trials have demonstrated mixed results (Table 9.5) [52, 55–57]. Among three randomized trials, two showed a statistically significant improvement in clinical pregnancy rates after aspiration of hydrosalpinx fluid and one showed a trend toward improvement that did not reach statistical significance [52, 54, 57]. When these randomized trials were pooled in a 2020 Cochrane review, they showed an overall increased clinical pregnancy rate after aspiration of hydrosalpinx fluid (OR: 1.67, 95% CI: 1.10, 2.55); however, the data were deemed to be of poor quality [19].

Sclerotherapy via instillation of ethanol or tetracycline into the hydrosalpinx following aspiration of the fluid was suggested as a method to limit fluid re-accumulation and increase the effectiveness of aspiration. A prospective trial of 339 women comparing sclerotherapy to no intervention showed improved rates of implantation and clinical pregnancy in the sclerotherapy group (26.4% vs 8.8% and 43.1% vs 16.0%, respectively, $p < 0.01$). Another prospective study of 482 women compared sclerotherapy to both salpingectomy and aspiration and showed that, although there was no difference in outcomes between the salpingectomy and sclerotherapy groups, women in the aspiration only group had significantly lower implantation and clinical pregnancy rates [58]. A meta-analysis including 10 studies confirmed these findings. Interestingly, this study demonstrated that rates of fluid re-accumulation after aspiration with and without sclerotherapy were comparable at 20–30% [59]. To date, there have been no ran-

Table 9.5 Summary of data from Cochrane review on treatment for hydrosalpinges prior to in vitro fertilization [17]

Intervention	CPR	OR for clinical pregnancy, (95% CI)	Number of included patients
Salpingectomy versus No tubal surgery	Salpingectomy: 100/256 (39.0%) No tubal surgery: 37/199 (18.6%)	2.02, (1.44–2.82)	Salpingectomy ($n = 256$) No tubal surgery ($n = 199$)
Tubal occlusion versus No tubal surgery	Tubal occlusion: 51/128 (39.8%) No tubal surgery: 10/81 (12.3%)	3.21, (1.72–5.99)	Tubal occlusion ($n = 128$) No tubal surgery ($n = 81$)
Aspiration of fluid versus No aspiration	Aspiration: 54/176 (30.7%) No aspiration 24/135 (17.8%)	1.67, (1.10–2.55)	Transvaginal aspiration ($n = 176$) No aspiration ($n = 135$)

domized trials of sclerotherapy prior to IVF. Although salpingectomy or proximal tubal ligation remains the gold standard for treatment of a poor-prognosis hydrosalpinx prior to IVF, aspiration appears to be superior to no intervention, and sclerotherapy may yield better results than aspiration [58, 59].

Conclusion

- Distal fallopian tube disease accounts for a significant portion of female factor infertility.
- HSG remains the standard first-line test for assessing tubal patency. It has a high negative predictive value, but positive predictive value remains low due to false-positive finding of proximal tubal occlusion. It is superior to other non-invasive imaging modalities for evaluating tubal architecture.
- There is a lack of adequate data comparing pregnancy outcomes with tubal surgery versus IVF.
- Laparoscopic neosalpingostomy for the treatment of good prognosis hydrosalpinges in young women with no other significant infertility factors should be recommended.
- For older, reproductive aged women with significant tubal disease IVF is the treatment of choice.
- Hydrosalpinges reduce IVF pregnancy rates by 50%. Laparoscopic salpingectomy or tubal occlusion should be performed in cases of irreparable hydrosalpinges to improve IVF

pregnancy rates. More data are needed on aspiration with sclerotherapy.

Bibliography

1. Practice Committee of the American Society for Reproductive Medicine. Role of tubal surgery in the era of assisted reproductive technology: a committee opinion. Fertil Steril. 2015;103(6):e37–43.
2. Westrom L. Effect of pelvic inflammatory disease on fertility. Venereology. 1995;8(4):219–22.
3. Haggerty CL, Gottlieb SL, Taylor BD, Low N, Xu F, Ness RB. Risk of sequelae after Chlamydia trachomatis genital infection in women. J Infect Dis. 2010;201 Suppl 2:S134–55.
4. Oakeshott P, Kerry S, Aghaizu A, Atherton H, Hay S, Taylor-Robinson D, et al. Randomised controlled trial of screening for Chlamydia trachomatis to prevent pelvic inflammatory disease: the POPI (prevention of pelvic infection) trial. BMJ. 2010;8(340):c1642.
5. Price MJ, Ades AE, De Angelis D, Welton NJ, Macleod J, Soldan K, et al. Risk of pelvic inflammatory disease following Chlamydia trachomatis infection: analysis of prospective studies with a multistate model. Am J Epidemiol. 2013;178(3):484–92.
6. Reekie J, Donovan B, Guy R, Hocking JS, Jorm L, Kaldor JM, et al. Hospitalisations for pelvic inflammatory disease temporally related to a diagnosis of Chlamydia or gonorrhoea: a retrospective cohort study. PLoS One. 2014;9(4):e94361.
7. Pelvic inflammatory disease: guidelines for prevention and management. MMWR Recomm Rep. 1991;40(RR-5):1–25.
8. Practice Committee of American Society for Reproductive Medicine. Diagnostic evaluation of the infertile female: a committee opinion. Fertil Steril. 2012;98(2):302–7.
9. Wang R, Watson A, Johnson N, Cheung K, Fitzgerald C, Mol BWJ, et al. Tubal flushing for subfertility. Cochrane Database Syst Rev. 2020;10:CD003718.

10. Dreyer K, van Rijswijk J, Mijatovic V, Goddijn M, Verhoeve HR, van Rooij IAJ, et al. Oil-based or water-based contrast for Hysterosalpingography in infertile women. N Engl J Med. 2017;376(21):2043–52.

11. Evers JLH, Land JA, Mol BW. Evidence-based medicine for diagnostic questions. Semin Reprod Med. 2003;21(1):9–15.

12. Maheux-Lacroix S, Boutin A, Moore L, Bergeron ME, Bujold E, Laberge P, et al. Hysterosalpingosonography for diagnosing tubal occlusion in subfertile women: a systematic review with meta-analysis. Hum Reprod. 2014;29(5):953–63.

13. Mol BW, Collins JA, Burrows EA, van der Veen F, Bossuyt PM. Comparison of hysterosalpingography and laparoscopy in predicting fertility outcome. Hum Reprod. 1999;14(5):1237–42.

14. Zeyneloglu HB, Arici A, Olive DL. Adverse effects of hydrosalpinx on pregnancy rates after in vitro fertilization-embryo transfer. Fertil Steril. 1998;70(3):492–9.

15. Camus E, Poncelet C, Goffinet F, Wainer B, Merlet F, Nisand I, et al. Pregnancy rates after in-vitro fertilization in cases of tubal infertility with and without hydrosalpinx: a meta-analysis of published comparative studies. Hum Reprod. 1999;14(5):1243–9.

16. Déchaud H, Daurès JP, Arnal F, Humeau C, Hédon B. Does previous salpingectomy improve implantation and pregnancy rates in patients with severe tubal factor infertility who are undergoing in vitro fertilization? A pilot prospective randomized study. Fertil Steril. 1998;69(6):1020–5.

17. Kontoravdis A, Makrakis E, Pantos K, Botsis D, Deligeoroglou E, Creatsas G. Proximal tubal occlusion and salpingectomy result in similar improvement in in vitro fertilization outcome in patients with hydrosalpinx. Fertil Steril. 2006;86(6):1642–9.

18. Strandell A, Lindhard A, Waldenström U, Thorburn J, Janson PO, Hamberger L. Hydrosalpinx and IVF outcome: a prospective, randomized multicentre trial in Scandinavia on salpingectomy prior to IVF. Hum Reprod. 1999;14(11):2762–9.

19. Melo P, Georgiou EX, Johnson N, van Voorst SF, Strandell A, Mol BWJ, et al. Surgical treatment for tubal disease in women due to undergo in vitro fertilisation. Cochrane Database Syst Rev. 2020;10:CD002125.

20. Savaris RF, Pedrini JL, Flores R, Fabris G, Zettler CG. Expression of alpha 1 and beta 3 integrins subunits in the endometrium of patients with tubal phimosis or hydrosalpinx. Fertil Steril. 2006;85(1):188–92.

21. Mukherjee T, Copperman AB, McCaffrey C, Cook CA, Bustillo M, Obasaju MF. Hydrosalpinx fluid has embryotoxic effects on murine embryogenesis: a case for prophylactic salpingectomy. Fertil Steril. 1996;66(5):851–3.

22. Strandell A, Lindhard A. Why does hydrosalpinx reduce fertility? The importance of hydrosalpinx fluid. Hum Reprod. 2002;17(5):1141–5.

23. Daftary GS, Taylor HS. Hydrosalpinx fluid diminishes endometrial cell HOXA10 expression. Fertil Steril. 2002;78(3):577–80.

24. Strandell A, Sjögren A, Bentin-Ley U, Thorburn J, Hamberger L, Brännström M. Hydrosalpinx fluid does not adversely affect the normal development of human embryos and implantation in vitro. Hum Reprod. 1998;13(1O):2921–5.

25. Meyer WR, Castelbaum AJ, Somkuti S, Sagoskin AW, Doyle M, Harris JE, et al. Hydrosalpinges adversely affect markers of endometrial receptivity. Hum Reprod. 1997;12(7):1393–8.

26. Daftary GS, Kayisli U, Seli E, Bukulmez O, Arici A, Taylor HS. Salpingectomy increases peri-implantation endometrial HOXA10 expression in women with hydrosalpinx. Fertil Steril. 2007;87(2):367–72.

27. Ng EHY, Chan CCW, Tang OS, Ho PC. Comparison of endometrial and subendometrial blood flows among patients with and without hydrosalpinx shown on scanning during in vitro fertilization treatment. Fertil Steril. 2006;85(2):333–8.

28. Cheng F, Li T, Wang Q-L, Zhou H-L, Duan L, Cai X. Effects of hydrosalpinx on ultrasonographic parameters for endometrial receptivity during the window of implantation measured by power color Doppler ultrasound. Int J Clin Exp Med. 2015;8(4):6103–8.

29. Hansen M, Kurinczuk JJ, Milne E, de Klerk N, Bower C. Assisted reproductive technology and birth defects: a systematic review and meta-analysis. Hum Reprod Update. 2013;19(4):330–53.

30. Kamath MS, Kirubakaran R, Mascarenhas M, Sunkara SK. Perinatal outcomes after stimulated versus natural cycle IVF: a systematic review and meta-analysis. Reprod Biomed Online. 2018;36(1):94–101.

31. Pandey S, Shetty A, Hamilton M, Bhattacharya S, Maheshwari A. Obstetric and perinatal outcomes in singleton pregnancies resulting from IVF/ICSI: a systematic review and meta-analysis. Hum Reprod Update. 2012;18(5):485–503.

32. Audebert A, Pouly JL, Bonifacie B, Yazbeck C. Laparoscopic surgery for distal tubal occlusions: lessons learned from a historical series of 434 cases. Fertil Steril. 2014;102(4):1203–8.

33. Taylor RC, Berkowitz J, McComb PF. Role of laparoscopic salpingostomy in the treatment of hydrosalpinx. Fertil Steril. 2001;75(3):594–600.

34. Daniilidis A, Balaouras D, Chitzios D, Theodoridis T, Assimakopoulos E. Hydrosalpinx: tubal surgery or in vitro fertilisation? An everlasting dilemma nowadays; a narrative review. J Obstet Gynaecol. 2017;37(5):550–6.

35. Boer-Meisel ME, te Velde ER, Habbema JD, Kardaun JW. Predicting the pregnancy outcome in patients treated for hydrosalpinx: a prospective study. Fertil Steril. 1986;45(1):23–9.

36. Donnez J, Nisolle M. 5 CO2 laser laparoscopic surgery. Baillieres Clin Obstet Gynaecol. 1989;3(3):525–43.

37. Schlaff WD, Hassiakos DK, Damewood MD, Rock JA. Neosalpingostomy for distal tubal obstruction: prognostic factors and impact of surgical technique. Fertil Steril. 1990;54(6):984–90.

38. Oh ST. Tubal patency and conception rates with three methods of laparoscopic terminal neosalpingostomy. J Am Assoc Gynecol Laparosc. 1996;3(4):519–23.

39. Rock JA, Katayama KP, Martin EJ, Woodruff JD, Jones HW. Factors influencing the success of salpingostomy techniques for distal fimbrial obstruction. Obstet Gynecol. 1978;52(5):591–6.

40. The American Fertility Society classifications of adnexal adhesions, distal tubal occlusion, tubal occlusion secondary to tubal ligation, tubal pregnancies, müllerian anomalies and intrauterine adhesions. Fertil Steril. 1988;49(6):944–55.

41. Chanelles O, Ducarme G, Sifer C, Hugues J-N, Touboul C, Poncelet C. Hydrosalpinx and infertility: what about conservative surgical management? Eur J Obstet Gynecol Reprod Biol. 2011;159(1):122–6.

42. Johnson N, van Voorst S, Sowter MC, Strandell A, Mol BWJ. Surgical treatment for tubal disease in women due to undergo in vitro fertilisation. Cochrane Database Syst Rev. 2010;(1):CD002125.

43. Venturella R, Morelli M, Lico D, Di Cello A, Rocca M, Sacchinelli A, et al. Wide excision of soft tissues adjacent to the ovary and fallopian tube does not impair the ovarian reserve in women undergoing prophylactic bilateral salpingectomy: results from a randomized, controlled trial. Fertil Steril. 2015;104(5):1332–9.

44. Stadtmauer LA, Riehl RM, Toma SK, Talbert LM. Cauterization of hydrosalpinges before in vitro fertilization is an effective surgical treatment associated with improved pregnancy rates. Am J Obstet Gynecol. 2000;183(2):367–71.

45. Goynumer G, Kayabasoglu F, Aydogdu S, Wetherilt L. The effect of tubal sterilization through electrocoagulation on the ovarian reserve. Contraception. 2009;80(1):90–4.

46. Carmona F, Cristóbal P, Casamitjana R, Balasch J. Effect of tubal sterilization on ovarian follicular reserve and function. Am J Obstet Gynecol. 2003;189(2):447–52.

47. Bulent Tiras M, Noyan V, Ozdemir H, Guner H, Yildiz A, Yildirim M. The changes in ovarian hormone levels and ovarian artery blood flow rate after laparoscopic tubal sterilization. Eur J Obstet Gynecol Reprod Biol. 2001;99(2):219–21.

48. Nakagawa K, Ohgi S, Nakashima A, Horikawa T, Irahara M, Saito H. Laparoscopic proximal tubal division can preserve ovarian reserve for infertility patients with hydrosalpinges. J Obstet Gynaecol Res. 2008;34(6):1037–42.

49. Ni L, Sadiq S, Mao Y, Cui Y, Wang W, Liu J. Influence of various tubal surgeries to serum antimullerian hormone level and outcome of the subsequent IVF-ET treatment. Gynecol Endocrinol. 2013;29(4):345–9.

50. Kerin JF, Munday D, Ritossa M, Rosen D. Tissue encapsulation of the proximal Essure micro-insert from the uterine cavity following hysteroscopic sterilization. J Minim Invasive Gynecol. 2007;14(2):202–4.

51. Xu B, Zhang Q, Zhao J, Wang Y, Xu D, Li Y. Pregnancy outcome of in vitro fertilization after Essure and laparoscopic management of hydrosalpinx: a systematic review and meta-analysis. Fertil Steril. 2017;108(1):84–95.e5.

52. An J, Ni Y, Liu X, Gao X, Wang Y. Effects of Tansvaginal aspiration of Hydrosalpinx combined auricular point sticking on IVF-ET outcomes. Zhongguo Zhong Xi Yi Jie He Za Zhi. 2015;35(6):682–5.

53. Fouda UM, Sayed AM. Effect of ultrasound-guided aspiration of hydrosalpingeal fluid during oocyte retrieval on the outcomes of in vitro fertilisation-embryo transfer: a randomised controlled trial (NCT01040351). Gynecol Endocrinol. 2011;27(8):562–7.

54. Hammadieh N, Coomarasamy A, Ola B, Papaioannou S, Afnan M, Sharif K. Ultrasound-guided hydrosalpinx aspiration during oocyte collection improves pregnancy outcome in IVF: a randomized controlled trial. Hum Reprod. 2008;23(5):1113–7.

55. Van Voorhis BJ, Sparks AE, Syrop CH, Stovall DW. Ultrasound-guided aspiration of hydrosalpinges is associated with improved pregnancy and implantation rates after in-vitro fertilization cycles. Hum Reprod. 1998;13(3):736–9.

56. Sowter MC, Akande VA, Williams JA, Hull MG. Is the outcome of in-vitro fertilization and embryo transfer treatment improved by spontaneous or surgical drainage of a hydrosalpinx? Hum Reprod. 1997;12(10):2147–50.

57. Fouda UM, Sayed AM, Abdelmoty HI, Elsetohy KA. Ultrasound guided aspiration of hydrosalpinx fluid versus salpingectomy in the management of patients with ultrasound visible hydrosalpinx undergoing IVF-ET: a randomized controlled trial. BMC Womens Health. 2015;27(15):21.

58. Song X-M, Jiang H, Zhang W-X, Zhou Y, Ni F, Wang X-M. Ultrasound sclerotherapy pretreatment could obtain a similar effect to surgical intervention on improving the outcomes of in vitro fertilization for patients with hydrosalpinx. J Obstet Gynaecol Res. 2017;43(1):122–7.

59. Cohen A, Almog B, Tulandi T. Hydrosalpinx Sclerotherapy before in vitro fertilization: systematic review and meta-analysis. J Minim Invasive Gynecol. 2018;25(4):600–7.

10

Matthew K. Wagar and Bala Bhagavath

Introduction

In 2018, 31.9% of all deliveries in the United States were cesarean deliveries [1]. As the absolute number of cesarean deliveries increases, the sequelae are also expected to increase. Cesarean scar defect (CSD), also referred to as uterine isthmocele or niche, is an iatrogenic defect within the myometrium at the site of a prior hysterotomy. CSDs are increasingly recognized contributors to abnormal uterine bleeding, pelvic pain, and infertility. Various diagnostic criteria and choice of imaging modality have been proposed in the evaluation of suspected CSD. Numerous surgical approaches to CSD repair have been described with improvements noted in fertility and symptomatology. This chapter will focus on the presentation, subsequent complications, and surgical management of CSDs.

Prevalence and Risk Factors

The exact prevalence of CSD is not fully elucidated in the literature. Differences in diagnostic criteria, imaging modalities and likely subclinical presentation of CSDs contribute to the variability in reported prevalence of this condition

[2]. Bij De Vaate et al. noted a prevalence of 24% to 70% and 56% to 84% when the presence of a CSD was assessed using transvaginal ultrasound (TVUS) and saline-infused sonohysterography (SIS), respectively [3]. As expected, less stringent definitions of uterine CSD have resulted in higher reported prevalence. In a random population of patients with a history of one or more cesarean deliveries, Vikhareva Osser et al. defined a CSD as "any indentation or other defect in the scar" reporting a high prevalence of 84% with SIS and 70% with TVUS [4]. Although lack of specific diagnostic criteria and population heterogeneity are likely to have contributed to a wide range of reported prevalence, the incidence is nonetheless likely very high.

Interestingly, several risk factors for the development of uterine CSD have been described, but because of their relatively recent identification as a pathologic correlate, the relative weight of each of these factors remains uncertain. The pathogenesis of uterine CSD is likely a combination of patient and surgical factors. A meta-analysis conducted by Tulandi et al. in 2016 determined that a history of multiple cesarean deliveries was the main risk factor for the development of CSD [5]. Multiple cesarean deliveries have also been noted to contribute to wider and larger CSDs than a history of one prior cesarean [2]. Other risk factors identified affecting the development of the CSD include cesarean delivery during active labor, lower fetal station at delivery, use of oxytocin

M. K. Wagar · B. Bhagavath (✉)
Department of OBGYN, University of Wisconsin-Madison, Madison, WI, USA
e-mail: mwagar@wisc.edu; bbhagavath@wisc.edu

S. R. Lindheim, J. C. Petrozza (eds.), *Reproductive Surgery*,
https://doi.org/10.1007/978-3-031-05240-8_10

augmentation, and duration of labor >5 hours [2]. Yazicioglu et al. conducted a randomized controlled trial comparing full-thickness (endometrial inclusion) with split-thickness (endometrium exclusion) closure of the myometrial defect at cesarean delivery and evaluated the development of CSD on postoperative day 40 to 42 using TVUS [6]. Defects were noted in 68.8% of patients with split-thickness closure compared to 44.7% of patients with full-thickness closure, reaching statistical significance. This evidence suggests the risk of CSD may be reduced with incorporation of the endometrium into hysterotomy repair. Other methods of uterine closure at time of cesarean have been evaluated as possible risk factors contributing to CSD including single-layer vs. double-layer closure; however evidence remains insufficient to classify either as contributory or protective against CSD development. Additionally, a retroverted uterus has been associated with CSD occurrence and confirmed in other studies [4, 7–8]. The proposed pathologic mechanism has been suggested that this might contribute to tensile issues and perhaps impaired perfusion on healing hysterotomies, increasing the likelihood of defect development.

Signs, Symptoms, and Complications of Cesarean Scar Defects

A significant portion of cesarean CSDs remain asymptomatic, confounding reported rates in the population. The most common presenting symptom is postmenstrual bleeding with up to 82% of patients with imaging diagnosed CSD experiencing postmenstrual bleeding or spotting [5]. Additionally, a correlation between the size of the defect and degree of spotting has been noted. The mechanism of abnormal uterine bleeding secondary to CSD is likely to be multifactorial. Postmenstrual bleeding is proposed to occur secondary to the accumulation of menstrual fluid within the defect itself with impaired passage secondary to myometrial deficiency at the site in

question. The development of fibrotic tissue below the CSD may further impede the flow of menstrual products, and the development of newly formed blood vessels adjacent to and within the CSD may further exacerbate the problem [9]. Other common presenting symptoms include dysmenorrhea, pelvic pain, and dyspareunia. Many of these symptoms are routine complaints in office-based gynecology and may exist in tandem with other etiologies for pelvic pain and abnormal uterine bleeding. Despite this, in the absence of other explanations and with a history of one or more cesarean deliveries, cesarean scar defect should be considered. Patients may also present with infertility, and an association with CSD has been noted [10, 11].

Infertility

A correlation between secondary infertility and the presence of a CSD has been well documented in the literature [9, 12, 13]. Two theories as to the mechanism of infertility in patients with CSD exist. First, the persistence of retained menstrual blood within the CSD secondary to myometrial contractile dysfunction is thought to affect cervical mucus, transport of sperm, and blastocyst implantation [12]. Second, persistence of menstrual blood is felt to contribute to a state of chronic inflammation within the CSD and surrounding endometrium in turn contributing to oxidative stress and further inhibiting implantation. In 2011, Gubbini et al. reported a prospective case series including 41 patients presenting with cesarean scar defects and secondary infertility who underwent hysteroscopic revision of their CSD with all patients achieving a pregnancy within 12 to 24 months following isthmoplasty (repair of the CSD) [13]. Given these findings, in the absence of other contributing factors, CSD can be considered a cause of secondary infertility warranting intervention. The revision of cesarean scar defects to restore future fertility can be considered with choice of surgical modalities discussed later in this chapter.

Ectopic Pregnancy

As the absolute number of women with a history of prior cesarean rises, so does the rate of cesarean scar ectopic pregnancy (CSP) [14]. While a still relatively rare occurrence, cesarean scar ectopic pregnancy remains difficult to diagnose, often confused with incomplete abortion, low implanted intrauterine pregnancies, and cervical ectopic pregnancies [2]. Common symptoms in the presentation of CSP include painless vaginal bleeding, abdominal pain, and in many cases no symptoms at all [15]. Diagnosis is established with TVUS. Two types of CSP have been described: Type 1, or endogenic CSP, where the gestational sac grows inward toward the cervicoisthmic space and Type 2, or exogenic CSP, where the gestational sac grows outward toward the bladder and anterior abdominal wall. Differentiation allows for adequate counseling and recommendations for management. Options for management include medical, surgical, and uterine artery embolization (UAE) and a combination of these approaches. In general, expectant management is not recommended given the high likelihood of morbidity. Medical management of CSP includes intragestational or intramuscular medications, with methotrexate being the most often utilized agent both systemically and locally. Candidates for medical management ideally should be less than 8 weeks of gestation, have absent fetal cardiac activity, and possess greater than 2-mm myometrium between the bladder and gestational sac [15]. Although uterine artery embolization (UAE) has also been utilized for the treatment of CSP, given its known detrimental impact on future fertility, it should not be utilized as first-line treatment for patients desiring future pregnancy. UAE is ideally reserved for patients with identified arteriovenous malformations or significant bleeding. Surgical management includes hysteroscopic resection and laparoscopic, transvaginal, or laparotomy excision of the sac with first-line methods favoring the least invasive techniques. Adequate treatment involves complete resection of the CSP and surrounding scar tissue in order to optimize future fertility.

Effects on Gynecologic Procedures

The presence of a CSD presents implications for gynecologic procedures. The presence of a CSD may alter the route of hysterectomy due to worrisome adhesions between the defect and anterior abdominal wall or bladder. Additionally, concerns regarding intrauterine instrumentation have been raised with reports in the literature of uterine perforation in the setting of CSD at the time of dilation and evacuation [16]. Similarly, placement of intrauterine devices may be altered or present an elevated risk of uterine perforation in the presence of a CSD [17]. Much attention has been given to the practice of endometrial ablation in the setting of prior cesarean delivery; however no specific studies have evaluated endometrial ablation in patients with diagnosed CSDs. Retrospective evidence reports no difference in procedural complication in patients with a history of cesarean delivery compared to controls undergoing endometrial ablation [18, 19]. Further evidence is needed to characterize the presence of a CSD and effect on gynecologic procedures.

Other Complications

The relationship between cesarean scar defects and placenta accreta has yet to be investigated. Notably, residual myometrial thickness is likely a factor in the development of uterine rupture; however further prospective evidence is needed to substantiate this claim [5]. Reports of endometriosis and adenomyosis in histologic specimens containing CSDs have been reported; however associations between these entities and cesarean section have not been supported in retrospective literature [7]. Case reports of abscess formation at the site of prior hysterotomies have been reported and theorized to be related to retained menstrual products within a CSD as a nidus for infection [20]. Further evidence is needed to determine CSD relationship to other pelvic pathologies.

Diagnosis

At present, there are no standardized criteria for the diagnosis of cesarean scar defects. A common descriptor is a triangular anechoic disruption of the myometrium at the site of a prior hysterotomy. Large defects have been defined variably including residual myometrial thickness <50% of wall thickness, with one study noting a cutoff of myometrial thickness <2.2 mm by TVUS and <2.5 mm by SIS – the latter allowance of 0.3 mm to account for distension artifact secondary to fluid used for distention [4].

Imaging Studies

Currently no consensus exists in regard to diagnosis of CSD. Common imaging modalities employed in aiding the diagnosis include TVUS, SIS, and hysteroscopy. Diagnosis via hysterosalpingogram (HSG) has also been reported but is less commonly utilized. In all cases, imaging serves several purposes. First, establishing the presence of a myometrial defect in the context of symptoms allows for inclusion of the CSD in the pathogenesis of a patient's complaints. Second, imaging evaluates for other anatomic etiologies such as polyps and fibroids that may be contributing to presenting symptoms. Third, evaluation of the defect dimensions and anatomy allows for effective counseling and preoperative planning if intervention is planned. Finally, imaging may alter proposed treatment based on findings.

Transvaginal Ultrasound

TVUS is the most common initial technique utilized for identification of CSD [2]. Findings on ultrasound can include a wedge defect with inward protrusion of the uterine scar, hematoma, or even retraction of the scar. The presence of hypoechoic fluid within this defect may be useful for diagnosis, but the absence of debris does not exclude the presence of a CSD. Ideally, if TVUS is to be used for aiding diagnosis, an attempt to obtain images during the early follicular phase should be made since the accumulation of menstrual blood within the defect enables its visualization without the need for fluid infusion [3]. Additionally, TVUS may be useful in scenarios where the use of intrauterine contrast or fluid is contraindicated such as pregnancy.

Saline Infusion Sonohyterogram

When available, SIS should be utilized and considered standard for the diagnosis of CSD. CSDs are more likely to be detected on SIS when compared with TVUS, and SIS increases the sensitivity and specificity for detection of CSDs due to enhancement of the defect from intrauterine fluid [21]. El-Mazny et al. reported in symptomatic women SIS demonstrated a sensitivity of 87% and specificity of 100% for the diagnosis of cesarean scar defect when compared to direct visualization with hysteroscopy [22]. Positive predictive value and negative predictive value were reported at 100% and 95%, respectively, with an overall accuracy of 96% [22]. However, defects on average have been noted to be 1 to 2 mm larger when visualized on SIS compared to TVUS secondary to distension pressure from infused saline [4]. Therefore, reliance on solely TVUS is not recommended given the superior ability of SIS to characterize CSDs requiring laparoscopic revision that would otherwise appear amenable to hysteroscopic resection. Notably common appearances of CSD on SIS reflected triangular anechoic defects in the myometrium, with semicircular shapes being second most common in appearance. SIS further aides the clinician in completing an infertility evaluation and assessing for structural pathology such as tubal blockage, leiomyomas, and endometrial polyps that may contribute to a multifactorial etiology of presenting symptoms.

Hysteroscopy

Diagnosis of CSD can also be made using hysteroscopy, where defects may appear as an outward bulge occurring along the anterior wall of the uterine isthmus [23]. Frequently this can be seen inside the cervical canal and inferior to the internal os. This pouch may contain blood or residual blood products and may be surrounded by fibrotic tissue or a fibrotic ring. If the diagnosis of CSD is suspected based on prior imaging, diagnostic hysteroscopy should then be utilized for further characterization. The benefit of this method allows for diagnosis and treatment simultaneously, as is discussed further in "Hysteroscopic Revision of Cesarean Scar Defects." However, evaluation for other etiologies for the presenting symptoms including infertility should be undertaken prior to therapeutic intervention where a complete and thorough evaluation will influence choice of therapy. Additionally, without information about the thickness of the myometrium overlying the defect, hysteroscopic management may result in injury to the urinary bladder.

Hysterosalpingogram and Magnetic Resonance Imaging

HSG has been reportedly used in the diagnosis of CSD with images acquired from an oblique view with patients in left lateral decubitus position. Notably, no current comparative studies exist assessing HSG to other imaging modalities for the purpose of diagnosing CSD. Similarly, pelvic magnetic resonance imaging (MRI) has also been reported to delineate CSD, specifically in the context of surgical planning in the presence of other pathologic conditions including adenomyosis or leiomyomas [2].

Management

Numerous techniques have been described for the treatment and repair of symptomatic cesarean scar defect. Medical and surgical methods have been evaluated for the management of patients with symptoms such as abnormal uterine bleeding (AUB), pelvic pain, and secondary infertility. Notably no evidence currently exists to support the routine revision of asymptomatic CSD, and this practice is currently not recommended. Similarly, no evidence supporting the revision of CSD to prevent obstetric complications such as uterine rupture and placenta accreta spectrum of disorders currently exists and therefore is also not recommended. No association has been reported between the revision of CSD and an increase in obstetric complications such as uterine rupture.

Medical Management

Non-surgical options for management of AUB associated with CSD include hormonal regulation using oral-combined contraceptives (OCPs). Zhang et al. prospectively compared three surgical routes to OCPs and the levonorgestrel containing IUD in the management of CSDs [24]. Shorter duration of menstrual bleeding for all OCP groups, though no benefit in bleeding outcomes, was demonstrated from the levonorgestrel containing IUD [24]. The benefit of OCPs is likely secondary to endothelial functional improvement and stabilization. When compared to hysteroscopy, Florio et al. reported a greater reduction in pain, duration of AUB, and a higher degree of satisfaction in patients undergoing hysteroscopic revision when compared with patients receiving OCPs [11]. As such, OCPs remain a viable option for patients who do not have pain and do not desire pregnancy or surgical intervention for their symptoms.

Hysteroscopic Revision of Cesarean Scar Defects

Hysteroscopic revision of CSD appears to be the treatment of choice when residual myometrial thickness exceeds 3 mm; however a cutoff of as low as 2 mm has been reported as well [25]. When compared to laparoscopic and vaginal approaches, hysteroscopic revision demonstrates similar resolution of AUB and pelvic pain with less operative complications: 0.3% for hysteroscopy compared to 1.5% and 1.8% for vaginal and laparoscopic treatment, respectively [26]. In a randomized controlled trial comparing hysteroscopic revision to expectant management, Vervoort et al. found a significant reduction in postmenstrual bleeding and pain following hysteroscopic revision of CSD (4 days vs. 7 days and median pain score 2/10 vs. 7/10) [25]. Additionally, two case series evaluating the utility of hysteroscopic revision of CSD for treatment of secondary infertility found that between 80 and 100% of patients undergoing hysteroscopic repair conceived within 24 months of treatment [13, 23]. Hysteroscopic revision is favored given shorter procedure times, minimal recovery time, and relative ease of the procedure itself. Given the risk of uterine perforation and bladder injury with this approach, a cutoff of 3-mm residual myometrial thickness is recommended [15, 25].

Consent

Complication rates for this procedure are low and similar to other types of hysteroscopic procedures including uterine perforation, damage to other pelvic viscera, volume overload, electrolyte disturbances, and rarely gas embolism.

Patient Preparation

Hysteroscopic revision of CSD is ideally performed during the early follicular phase in order to adequately identify the defect and potentially visualize retained menstrual products within the defect itself. Preoperative antibiotics or venous thromboprophylaxis is typically not required [27].

Instruments

A resectoscope with a 90-degree loop electrode is ideal for excision of the cephalad and caudad edges of the CSD [28]. A rollerball electrode device can be considered for fulguration and ablation of abnormal vascularity at the base of the CSD. If a hysteroscope with an angled lens is utilized, care should be used to visualize the cavity with a 180-degree rotation so as not to miss a potential defect. A sims or weighted speculum can be used to help mitigate capacitive coupling thermal injury to the perineum. When available, utilization of transabdominal ultrasound may further reduce the risk of bladder injury and uterine perforation although this has not been evaluated prospectively.

Surgical Steps

1. *Anesthesia and patient positioning.* Most cases of hysteroscopic revision are performed as outpatient procedures under general or regional anesthesia. As with all hysteroscopic procedures, careful management of hysteroscopic fluids is imperative. Following adequate anesthesia induction, the patient is placed in standard dorsal lithotomy position.

2. *Media selection.* Bipolar loop electrodes may be used in a physiologic saline solution. However, the use of a monopolar electrode loop or rollerball electrocautery device warrants utilization of a nonelectrolyte solution such as 5% mannitol. As with any hysteroscopic procedure, fluid volume deficits should be periodically recorded during surgery.

3. *Identify anatomy.* Following cervical dilation and insertion of the resectoscope, the uterine cavity and CSD are identified. Almost invariably, the defect is just caudad to the internal cervical os, that is, it is within the cervical canal. Care should be made to complete a 180-degree rotation of the resectoscope to adequately visualize the CSD, which can be overlooked on angled lenses. It is also imperative that an angled lens be used to perform this evaluation as it may be completely missed using a 0-degree lens. Extra attention should be paid to identification of the cephalad and caudad fibrotic edges of the CSD.

4. *Resect the cephalad edge.* The loop electrode is introduced, and the cephalad edge of fibrosis is resected starting medially, in order to smooth the contour of the uterine cavity/cervical canal and CSD. The resection begins in the midline and is continued laterally, only involving the anterior wall of the uterine isthmus.

5. *Resect the caudad edge.* The loop electrode is then activated to resect the caudad edge of fibrosis again beginning in the midline and extending laterally along the anterior wall of the cervical canal. This facilitates drainage of debris from within the CSD. Contour following resection should be smooth between CSD and endocervical canal.

6. *Ablation of the CSD (If needed).* The rollerball electrode is then introduced, and the endometrium within the CSD is ablated so as to disrupt abnormal vascularity commonly present within the defect.

7. *Case completion.* Following completion of the revision, all instruments are removed from the uterus and vagina while evaluating for hemostasis. Postoperative recovery is rapid and typically without complication, consistent with other hysteroscopic procedures.

Laparoscopic Repair of CSD

Laparoscopy is another commonly utilized method in the surgical revision of CSDs. Donnez et al. prospectively described 38 patients undergoing laparoscopic revision of CSD with myometrial thickness assessed via TVUS and MRI [29]. A noted benefit to laparoscopy described in this study was the significant increase in mean myometrial thickness postoperatively (1.43 ± 0.7 mm to 9.62 ± 1.8 mm) [27]. Proponents of a laparoscopic approach note a theoretical reduction in the risk of uterine rupture during pregnancy due to this observation [30]. Similarly, when compared to hysteroscopic and vaginal approaches, laparoscopy has demonstrated similar rates of symptom resolution with minimal operative complications. Both conventional laparoscopic and robot-assisted approaches have been described. Laparoscopy appears to be the preferred method of treatment of symptomatic CSD when residual myometrial thickness is <3 mm in order to reduce risks of uterine perforation and bladder injury [31]. Additionally, laparoscopy allows for the diagnosis of chronic pelvic inflammatory disease or endometriosis which may also contribute to infertility. Thus, its utility as a surgical approach also benefits when multiple pathologies are suspected. Limitations to this approach include its relative complexity and therefore the need for surgeons to be skilled in minimally invasive surgery.

Patient Evaluation

Prior to surgery, evaluation of myometrial thickness is imperative. This can be accomplished reliably with TVUS or SIS. MRI has been used for this practice with similar results in residual myometrial measurements when compared to TVUS [29]. As such, TVUS is preferred given its relative low cost and ease of completion.

Counseling

Complication rates for this procedure are low (1.5%) and similar to other types of laparoscopic procedures including visceral injury, vascular injury, thermal injury, bladder injury subcutaneous emphysema, and wound complications [25].

Patient Preparation

Antibiotic prophylaxis is not currently required for laparoscopic repair of CSD [27]. Bowel preparation is not required [32]. Venous Thromboembolism (VTE) prophylaxis is not typically recommended; however sequential compression devices should be utilized for mechanical prophylaxis if length of surgery requires it.

Instruments

Most instruments required for laparoscopic repair of CSD will be readily available in a standard laparoscopy tray. A probe such as a uterine sound or a Hegar dilator should be available to aid in identifying the defect and to maintain cervical continuity with the uterine cavity during defect closure. All types of energy including CO2 laser have been used to open the scar and excise fibrotic tissue. Additionally, a Foley catheter should be placed for bladder decompression [33]. Robot-assisted laparoscopy can be used to achieve the same results [34].

Surgical Steps

1. *Anesthesia and patient positioning.* The patient is positioned in low lithotomy position for laparoscopic surgery. A bimanual examination is performed to determine uterine size, position, and flexion. Uterine mobility and size will determine placement of accessory ports.

2. *Abdominal access and pelvic inspection.* Primary and secondary trocars are placed in standard fashion. Typically, two to three accessory ports are required. Upon entry, inspection of the pelvis and upper abdomen

for other abdominopelvic pathologies should be undertaken first.

3. *Development of the vesicovaginal space.* Except in the most severe cases, the vesicovaginal fold of peritoneum has to be incised, and the bladder dissected off the uterus/upper cervix to identify the defect. The incision is extended along the length of the defect laterally.

4. *Identification of the defect.* The CSD is identified along the anterior wall of the uterus or cervix. Depending on the thickness of the overlying myometrium, identification of the defect may be easy or challenging. In case of thick overlying myometrium, a couple of strategies can be utilized to identify the defect as described in the section titled "Combined Procedures." One strategy is to blindly insert a uterine sound or cervical dilator through the cervix vaginally and attempt to pass the instrument through the defect, though this is not recommended. Another approach is to perform hysteroscopy simultaneously, identify the defect, and position the lens into the defect. The light cast by the hysteroscope can be identified abdominally to locate the defect (transillumination). Alternatively, a hysteroscopic scissor can be inserted through the instrument channel and gently poked through the roof of the defect to identify the location of the scar laparoscopically. The size of defect should be documented for correlation with imaging.

5. *Excision of fibrosis.* Using an appropriate energy source, the scar is opened transversely, and the caudal and cephalad areas of fibrosis excised to expose healthy-appearing myometrium. Given the relative avascularity, uterine artery occlusion is not typically indicated.

6. *Defect closure.* Closure of the defect is accomplished with a suggested two-layer myometrial closure followed by an optional third layer approximating the peritoneum. Barbed suture or Vicryl is used as closure material depending on surgeon preference. A one-layer approach for closure has not been previously described as is not recommended given findings of worsening defect development following split-thickness closure in primary hysterotomy repair [4].

Vaginal Approach to CSD Repair

A vaginal approach to CSD repair has been described in settings without hysteroscopic capabilities or surgical expertise familiar with laparoscopic or hysteroscopic methods. Luo et al. described a case series of 42 patients undergoing vaginal repair of CSD with over 90% experiencing resolution of presenting AUB and pelvic pain [35]. Complication rates for the vaginal approach are reported highest of the three major modalities (1.8%–2%) [26, 36]. Retrospective analysis of a cohort of 241 patients undergoing vaginal repair of CSD revealed up to 40% of patients with identifiable CSD on TVUS at 6-month postoperatively [36]. Zhang et al. evaluated vaginal and laparoscopic revision of CSD retrospectively and found shorter operative times for the vaginal approach comparatively, though in general a vaginal approach carries longer lengths given the use of indwelling urinary catheter maintenance for bladder decompression and vaginal packing [24]. That being said, when available resources, residual myometrial thickness, or surgical expertise preclude the use of hysteroscopic or laparoscopic CSD revision, a vaginal approach may be considered.

Patient Evaluation

Preoperative evaluation is similar to laparoscopic and hysteroscopic CSD repair.

Consent

Complication rates for this procedure are low but higher than other modalities (1.8% for vaginal CSD repair compared to 0.3% and 1.5% for hysteroscopic and laparoscopic CSD repairs, respectively). Complications include pelvic organ injury including vascular, bladder, ureteral, or bowel injury. Wound infections, postoperative hematomas, and blood loss requiring transfusion have also been reported [35, 36].

Patient Preparation

Antibiotic prophylaxis is recommended and is continued for 48 hours postoperatively as reported in the literature [35]. Antibiotic prophylaxis is similar to hysterectomy and can be accomplished with a first- or second-generation cephalosporin [27]. Mechanical and chemoprophylaxis for VTE are recommended while patients are admitted during surgical stay [37].

Surgical Steps

1. *Anesthesia and patient positioning.* The patient is positioned in dorsal lithotomy position after administration of regional or general anesthesia. A Foley catheter may be placed preoperatively or at the conclusion of the case.
2. *Vaginal wall incision.* After adequate exposure of the cervix, the anterior lip of the cervix is grasped using forceps, and a dilute epinephrine solution (1:2000) is injected in the vesico-cervical space to dissect the underlying connective tissue with hydrodissection. A probe such as a Hegar dilator is inserted into the uterine cavity. The vaginal mucosa of the anterior vaginal wall is incised transversely from the 9 o'clock to 3 o'clock position.
3. *Anterior peritoneal entry.* The anterior vaginal wall is grasped with an Allis clamp and elevated in the midline near the transverse incision. Tension is then placed on the cervix, and tissue bands within the vesico-cervical space are dissected, typically sharply with Metzenbaum scissors. The vesico-uterine reflection is identified and incised sharply with Metzenbaum scissors. Entry into the peritoneal cavity is confirmed with palpation.
4. *Identification of the defect.* The CSD is identified along the anterior isthmus, and the probe may be visualized through the peritoneum and residual myometrium if the scar is sufficiently thin.
5. *Excision of fibrosis.* Using dissecting scissors, the defect is opened, and the fibrotic edges resected to reveal healthy-appearing myometrium. If hematocele is encountered, the fluid should be evacuated.
6. *Defect closure.* Closure of the defect is completed with a two-layer myometrial closure. A uterine sound remains in place or is placed at conclusion of hysterotomy closure to confirm patency of the cervical canal/uterine isthmus.
7. *Peritoneal closure.* The bladder peritoneum is grasped and reapproximated using suture of surgeon's preference. The vaginal vault is then approximated to the cervix using continuous suture.
8. *Case completion.* The vagina is then packed with surgical gauze, and a Foley catheter placed at conclusion of the case if not placed preoperatively. Vaginal packing is removed 24 hours postoperatively with antibiotics continued for 48 hours postoperatively as reported in one case series [35]. While cystoscopy has not been described in prior approaches to CSD repair, utilization should be performed at the surgeon's discretion particularly in vaginal approaches where bladder peritoneum may not be readily visualized.

Combined Procedures

In scenarios where concern for adhesive disease and difficult vesico-uterine dissection occurs, combined approaches involving hysteroscopic and laparoscopic or laparoscopic and vaginal modalities have been described [38, 39]. A hysteroscopic and laparoscopic combined approach has been described, initially by Nirgianakis et al. in 2016 [38]. Their procedure termed the "rendezvous technique" functions on the principal of laparoscopic CSD identification via transillumination from a hysteroscopic light source. Called the "halloween sign," light emitted via the hysteroscopic lens transilluminates the overlying CSD and peritoneum providing added visualization of the defect to be revised. CSD revision and closure are similar between the combined techniques and their solo counterparts. Benefits to a combined approach include immediate postoperative assessment of CSD revision upon completion in the hysteroscopic combined group and careful visualization of bladder and vesico-uterine space dissection in the vaginal combined group. However, neither of these approaches has been validated against other surgical modalities, and further research is needed to investigate their utility in mitigating surgical complications.

Considerations for Pregnancy

No current evidence exists in regard to preconception counseling following uterine CSD repair. Many authors recommend or prescribe a 3-month course of OCPs to promote epithelialization of the revised CSD and prevent pregnancy, while the isthmus heals from revision [33]. However, neither this interval nor the need for OCP has been evaluated prospectively, and optimal timing for pregnancy has not been delineated. Furthermore, the course of resolution of inflammation secondary to a CSD has not been described, and thus recommendations for increasing fecundity do not exist within the literature. Notably no evidence currently exists to support the routine revision of asymptomatic CSD, and this practice is currently not recommended. Similarly, no evidence supporting the revision of CSD to prevent obstetric complications such as uterine rupture and placenta accreta spectrum of disorders currently exists and therefore is also not recommended. No association has been reported between the revision of CSD and an increase in obstetric complications such as uterine rupture.

Additionally, expert recommendation advises delivery via repeat cesarean section between 38 and 39 weeks of gestation to reduce the theoretical risk of uterine rupture [40]. Indeed, many reported pregnancy outcomes following CSD repair include delivery via repeat cesarean section at term. Prospective evidence assessing pregnancy outcomes following CSD revision via various surgical modalities would inform this body of evidence further.

Conclusion

CSD are increasingly recognized as the cause of various symptoms including irregular vaginal bleeding, dysmenorrhea, and infertility. Saline sonogram appears to be the best diagnostic test preoperatively, though caution needs to be entertained regarding residual myometrium and type of approach for repair. Surgical repair is likely to provide symptom relief. The best approach to repair remains debated but likely depends on the extent of defect. If there is adequate (currently defined as 3 mm) overlying myometrium, hysteroscopic repair may be appropriate. If the myometrium overlying the defect is very thin, a laparoscopic approach appears to be the best option.

References

1. Martin JA, Hamilton BE, et al. National Vital Statistics Reports Births: final data for 2013. Statistics (Ber). 2015;64(1):1–104.
2. Tower AM, Frishman GN. Cesarean scar defects: an underrecognized cause of abnormal uterine bleeding and other gynecologic complications. J Minim Invasive Gynecol. 2013;20(5):562–72. https://doi.org/10.1016/j.jmig.2013.03.008.
3. Bij De Vaatea. JM, Van Der Voet LF, Naji O, et al. Prevalence, potential risk factors for development and symptoms related to the presence of uterine niches following Cesarean section: systematic review. Ultrasound Obstet Gynecol. 2014;43(4):372–82. https://doi.org/10.1002/uog.13199.
4. Vikhareva Osser O, Valentin L. Risk factors for incomplete healing of the uterine incision after caesarean section. BJOG. 2010;117(9):1119–26. https://doi.org/10.1111/j.1471-0528.2010.02631.x.
5. Tulandi T, Cohen A. Emerging manifestations of Cesarean scar defect in reproductive-aged women. J Minim Invasive Gynecol. 2016;23(6):893–902. https://doi.org/10.1016/j.jmig.2016.06.020.
6. Yazicioglu F, Gokdogan A, Kelekei S, et al. Incomplete healing of the uterine incision after caesarean section: is it preventable? Eur J Obstet Gynecol Reprod Biol. 2006;124:32–6.
7. Wang CB, Chiu WW, Lee CY, et al. Cesarean scar defect: correlation between Cesarean section number, defect size, clinical symptoms and uterine position. Ultrasound Obstet Gynecol. 2009;34:85–9.
8. Ofili-Yebovi D, Ben-Nagi J, Sawyer E, et al. Deficient lower-segment cesarean section scars: prevalence and risk factors. Ultrasound Obstet Gynecol. 2008;31:72–7.
9. Morris H. Surgical pathology of the lower uterine segment caesarean section scar: is the scar a source of clinical symptoms? Int J Gynecol Pathol. 1995;14(1):16–20.
10. Calzolari S, Sisti G, Pavone D, Ciocia E, Bianchini N, Cozzolino M. Prevalence of infertility among patients

with Isthmocele and fertility outcome after Isthmocele surgical treatment: a retrospective study. Ochsner J. 2019;19(3):204–9. https://doi.org/10.31486/toj.18.0048.

11. Florio P, Gubbini G, Marra E, et al. A retrospective case-control study comparing hysteroscopic resection versus hormonal modulation in treating menstrual disorder due to isthmocele. Gynecol Endocrinol. 2011;27:434–8.

12. Gubbini G, Casadio P, Marra E. Resectoscopic correction of the "Isthmocele" in women with postmenstrual abnormal uterine bleeding and secondary infertility. J Minim Invasive Gynecol. 2008;15(2):172–5. https://doi.org/10.1016/j.jmig.2007.10.004.

13. Gubbini G, Centini G, Nascetti D, et al. Surgical Hysteroscopic treatment of Cesarean-induced Isthmocele in restoring fertility: prospective study. J Minim Invasive Gynecol. 2011;18(2):234–7. https://doi.org/10.1016/j.jmig.2010.10.011.

14. Timor-Tritsch I, Monteagudo A. Unforeseen consequences of the increasing rate of cesarean deliveries: early placenta accrete and cesarean scar pregnancy. A review. Am J Obstet Gynecol. 2012;207:14–29.

15. Glenn TL, Bembry J, Findley AD, et al. Cesarean scar ectopic pregnancy: current management strategies. Obstet Gynecol Surv. 2018;73(5):293–302. https://doi.org/10.1097/OGX.0000000000000561.

16. Lichtenberg ES, Frederiksen MC. Cesarean scar dehiscence as a cause of hemorrhage after second-trimester abortion by dilation and evacuation. Contraception. 2004;70:61–4.

17. Chamsy DJ, Kho KA. Perforated intra-abdominal IUDs: a large case series. J Minim Invasive Gynecol. 2011;18:92.

18. Goorah B, Didomizio L, Thiel J. Safety of NovaSure ablation in women with previous cesarean section. J Minim Invasive Gynecol. 2011;18:83–4.

19. Adkins RT, Bressman PI, Bressman PB, Lucas TL. Evaluation of the NovaSure endometrial ablation system in women with a history of cesarean section. J Minim Invasive Gynecol. 2011;18:24–46.

20. Boukrid M, Dubuisson J. Conservative management of a scar abscess formed in a Cesarean induced Isthmocele. Front Surg. 2016;3(7) https://doi.org/10.7196/samj.5357.

21. Thurmond AS, Harvey WJ, Smith SA. Cesarean section scar as a cause of abnormal vaginal bleeding: diagnosis by sonohysterography. J Ultrasound Med. 1999;18:13–6.

22. El-Mazny A, Abou-Salem N, El-Khayat W, Farouk A. Diagnostic correlation between sonohysterography and hysteroscopy in the assessment of uterine cavity after cesarean section. Middle East Fertl Soc J. 2011;16:72–6.

23. Fabres C, Aviles G, De La Jara C, et al. The cesarean delivery scar pouch: clinical implications and diagnostic correlation between transvaginal sonography and hysteroscopy. J Ultrasound Med. 2003;22:695–700.

24. Zhang X, Yang M, Wang Q, Chen J, Ding J, Hua K. Prospective evaluation of five methods used to treat cesarean scar defects. Int J Gynecol Obstet. 2016;134(3):336–9. https://doi.org/10.1016/j.ijgo.2016.04.011.

25. Vervoort A, van der Voet LF, Hehenkamp W, Thurkow AL, van Kesteren P, Quartero H, et al. Hysteroscopic resection of a uterine caesarean scar defect (niche) in women with postmenstrual spotting: a randomized controlled trial. BJOG. 2018;125:326–34.

26. Vitale SG, Ludwin A, Vilos GA, et al. From hysteroscopy to laparoendoscopic surgery: what is the best surgical approach for symptomatic isthmocele? A systematic review and meta-analysis. Arch Gynecol Obstet. 2020;301(1):33–52. https://doi.org/10.1007/s00404-020-05438-0.

27. Prevention of infection after gynecologic procedures. ACOG Practice Bulletin No. 195. American College of Obstetricians and Gynecologists. Obstet Gynecol. 2018;131:e172–89.

28. Sanders AP, Murji A. Hysteroscopic repair of cesarean scar isthmocele. Fertil Steril. 2018;110(3):555–6. https://doi.org/10.1016/j.fertnstert.2018.05.032.

29. Donnez O, Donnez J, Orellana R, Dolmans MM. Gynecological and obstetrical outcomes after laparoscopic repair of a cesarean scar defect in a series of 38 women. Fertil Steril. 2017;107(1):289–296.e2. https://doi.org/10.1016/j.fertnstert.2016.09.033.

30. Sipahi S, Sasaki K, Miller CE. The minimally invasive approach to the symptomatic isthmocele - what does the literature say? A step-by-step primer on laparoscopic isthmocele - excision and repair. Curr Opin Obstet Gynecol. 2017;29(4):257–65. https://doi.org/10.1097/GCO.0000000000000380.

31. Marotta ML, Donnez J, Squifflet J, Jadoul P, Darii N, Donnez O. Laparoscopic repair of post-cesarean section uterine scar defects diagnosed in nonpregnant women. J Minim Invasive Gynecol. 2013;20(3):386–91. https://doi.org/10.1016/j.jmig.2012.12.006.

32. Arnold A, Aitchison LP, Abbott J. Preoperative mechanical bowel preparation for abdominal, laparoscopic, and vaginal surgery: a systematic review. J Minim Invasive Gynecol. 2015;22(5):737–52. https://doi.org/10.1016/j.jmig.2015.04.003.

33. Donnez O, Jadoul P, Squifflet J, Donnez J. Laparoscopic repair of wide and deep uterine scar dehiscence after cesarean section. Fertil Steril. 2008;89(4):974–80. https://doi.org/10.1016/j.fertnstert.2007.04.024.

34. Yalcinkaya TM, Akar ME, Kammire LD, Johnston-Macananny EB, Mertz HL. Robotic-assisted laparoscopic repair of symptomatic Cesarean scar defect a report of two cases. J Reprod Med. 2011;27103:265–70.

35. Luo L, Niu G, Wang Q, Xie HZ, Yao SZ. Vaginal repair of Cesarean section scar diverticula. J Minim Invasive Gynecol. 2012;19(4):454–8. https://doi.org/10.1016/j.jmig.2012.03.012.

36. Chen H, Wang H, Zhou J, Xiong Y, Wang X. Vaginal repair of Cesarean section scar diverticula diagnosed in non-pregnant women. J Minim Invasive Gynecol.

2019;26(3):526–34. https://doi.org/10.1016/j.jmig.2018.06.012.

37. Prevention of deep vein thrombosis and pulmonary embolism. ACOG Practice Bulletin No. 84. American College of Obstetricians and Gynecologists. Obstet Gynecol 2007;110:42940.

38. Nirgianakis K, Oehler R, Mueller M. The Rendezvous technique for treatment of caesarean scar defects: a novel combined endoscopic approach. Surg Endosc. 2016;30(2):770–1. https://doi.org/10.1007/s00464-015-4226-6.

39. Klemm P, Koehler C, Mangler M, Schneider U, Schneider A. Laparoscopic and vaginal repair of uterine scar dehiscence following cesarean section as detected by ultrasound. J Perinat Med. 2005;33(4):324–31. https://doi.org/10.1515/JPM.2005.058.

40. Laganà AS, Pacheco LA, Tinelli A, Haimovich S, Carugno J, Ghezzi F. Global Congress on Hysteroscopy Scientific Committee. Optimal timing and recommended route of delivery after hysteroscopic management of isthmocele? a consensus statement from the Global Congress on Hysteroscopy Scientific Committee. J Minim Invasive Gynecol. 2018;25(4):558. https://doi.org/10.1016/j.jmig.2018.01.018.

Fertility-Enhancing Ovarian Cystectomy

Megan Gornet, Susan Nasab, and Mindy S. Christianson

Introduction

Ovarian cysts are one of the most common gynecologic diagnoses for women of reproductive age. According to some reports, 5–10% of women will undergo surgery for an ovarian mass in their lifetime [1]. Performing ovarian cystectomy while optimizing reproductive potential is an essential skill for the reproductive surgeon. Since the ovary has a finite number of oocytes that decreases over time, it is critical that ovarian cystectomy be performed in a manner that minimizes ovarian trauma. Patients must also be counseled regarding the potential impact of the procedure on ovarian reserve and subsequent future fertility [2]. Therefore, the approach to the fertility-enhancing ovarian cystectomy has several important considerations, including the type of ovarian cyst and individual patient factors.

Overview of Cysts in Women of Reproductive Age

Approximately 7% of women will have an ovarian cyst diagnosed at some point in their lives. The most common cysts encountered in women of reproductive age include simple cysts, serous or mucinous cystadenomas, endometriomas, and mature cystic teratomas. In large population studies, functional cysts and endometriotic cysts represent 32.8% of adnexal masses, while teratomas represent about 29.8% [3]. Endometriomas affect 17–45% of women with endometriosis and comprise 35% of surgical cases for benign ovarian cysts [3].

Preoperative Approach and Evaluation

The first step in evaluating a woman with an adnexal mass is attempting to diagnose the type of ovarian cyst, which requires an organized and thoughtful approach. It is imperative to identify adnexal masses that are suspicious for malignancy and therefore necessitate referral to a gynecologic oncologist. Important aspects of a preoperative evaluation include a thorough medical history, physical examination, imaging studies, and laboratory evaluation.

This constellation of findings will aid in appropriate patient selection and surgical approach for proceeding with fertility-sparing ovarian cystectomy.

M. Gornet · S. Nasab · M. S. Christianson (✉)
Department of Gynecology and Obstetrics, Johns Hopkins University School of Medicine, Baltimore, MD, USA
e-mail: mgornet2@jhmi.edu; shossei4@jhmi.edu; mchris21@jhmi.edu

© The Author(s), under exclusive license to Springer Nature Switzerland AG 2022
S. R. Lindheim, J. C. Petrozza (eds.), *Reproductive Surgery*,
https://doi.org/10.1007/978-3-031-05240-8_11

Medical History

In reproductive-aged women, performing a complete medical history, including a comprehensive menstrual, sexual, and family history, is essential. As the pathogenesis of most benign ovarian cysts derives from normal ovarian reproductive function, an in-depth understanding of each patient's symptoms and medical history can provide clues toward diagnosis or general malignancy risk and, by extension, eligibility for a fertility-sparing approach. For example, women with an endometrioma often report cyclical abdominal pain that worsens with menses or report a history of infertility, whereas women with other benign cysts or even malignancy often have less specific symptoms. Therefore, a comprehensive review of systems should be performed in the medical history. Symptoms that may prompt evaluation for malignancy include weight loss, subjective sweats or chills, early satiety, or persistent abdominal bloating.

Imaging

The utility of imaging evaluation prior to surgical management cannot be overstated. First and foremost, imaging allows the surgeon to evaluate whether surgical intervention is warranted and, furthermore, aids in determining an etiology of a mass on a scale from benign to malignant. Moreover, serial imaging assessment over time is invaluable as a fertility-sparing approach, as most functional ovarian cysts resolve spontaneously and therefore do not warrant surgical intervention.

Pelvic ultrasound is largely considered the imaging modality of choice for evaluation of an ovarian cyst, due mainly to its cost-effectiveness and proven diagnostic capabilities [4]. Features of an ovarian cyst on ultrasound that are considered abnormal or suspicious for malignancy include (1) ovarian volume greater than 10 cubic cm, (2) cyst volume greater than 10 cubic cm, (3) any solid area or papillary projection extending into the cavity of a cystic ovarian tumor of any size, or (4) any mixed (solid/cystic) component

within a cystic ovarian tumor [5]. Likewise, ultrasound characteristics indicative of benign ovarian cysts include a simple appearance with thin, smooth walls and the absence of solid components, septations, or central or internal blood flow on Doppler imaging. Cysts with these characteristics are likely to be benign [6–10]. Cysts of 10 cm or larger in diameter are generally considered an indication for surgical intervention, regardless of simple appearance [11]. Many simple cysts, even large ones, will spontaneously regress when monitored by serial ultrasound [12]. Depending on the clinical scenario, general ultrasound surveillance often occurs at 3-, 6-, and 12-month intervals.

While definitive diagnosis cannot be made without histopathological evaluation, simple, hemorrhagic, endometriotic, and mature dermoid (teratoma) cysts all have stereotypical findings on ultrasound studies. These features provide important information to the reproductive surgeon about eligibility for and likelihood of success for a fertility-sparing approach. On ultrasound, endometriomas typically show ground-glass echogenicity and lack papillary structures [13]. Mature cystic teratomas often demonstrate echogenicity associated with fat-fluid levels, thin echogenic bands from hair, as well as shadowing echogenicity from calcifications [14]. Ultrasound has reported a sensitivity of 58% and specificity of 99% in the diagnosis of mature teratomas [15].

If ultrasound findings are indeterminate, equivocal, or suboptimal, magnetic resonance imaging (MRI) is the next imaging modality of choice. MRI may have a superior ability to identify malignant masses as well as adnexal masses that are not ovarian in origin, such as myomas [5]. In addition to improved delineation of cyst morphology, other parameters such as signal intensity, T1, T2, and perfusion or diffusion-weighted imaging can overall improve diagnostic evaluation. As an example, most functional ovarian cysts (i.e., containing simple fluid) have low signal intensity on T1-weighted images and very high signal intensity on T2. This is in contrast to hemorrhagic cysts, which have high signal intensity on both T1 and T2 images.

Table 11.1 Classic imaging characteristics of various ovarian cysts

	Ultrasound	MRI	CT
Simple or functional cyst	Anechoic with thin, smooth walls	T1 low or intermediate signal intensity T2 high signal intensity	Generally not considered useful
Hemorrhagic cyst	"Lace-like" reticular echoes or intracystic solid clot Often see free pelvic fluid in the setting of rupture	T1 high signal intensity T2 intermediate to high signal intensity	Generally not considered useful
Endometrioma	Diffuse, low-level echoes Multiple loculations or hyperechoic wall foci Often multiple or bilateral ovarian lesions, cul-de-sac lesions, thicker cyst walls, in conjunction with dilated fallopian tube	T1 high signal intensity T2 low signal intensity Thickened, low signal intensity wall Adhesions to surrounding organs	Generally not considered useful
Mature cystic teratoma	Shadowing echogenicity Hyperechoic lines and dots ("dot-dot-dash") Fat-fluid or fluid-fluid level Rokitansky nodule: Densely echogenic protuberance projecting into cystic lumen	Rokitansky nodule Intratumoral fat with T1 high signal intensity, but signal decreases on fat-suppressed, T1-weighted images	Presence of fat attenuation Often dense calcifications Rokitansky nodule
Tubo-ovarian abscess	Mass (solid, cystic, or complex) in the adnexal region or cul-de-sac with an adjacent fluid collection	Hyperintense content on diffusion-weighted imaging	Adnexal thick-walled complex cystic mass and intense enhancement Surrounding peritoneal thickening and stranding

Citations [17–19]

In general, computed tomography (CT) is not indicated unless there is concern for malignancy, as it best used to identify metastatic disease or enlarged lymph nodes [16].

Please see Table 11.1 for details regarding classic imaging findings by cyst type.

Laboratory Evaluation

Preoperative laboratory evaluation can be used to screen for malignancy and increasingly ovarian reserve which is an important aspect of preoperative care. Beyond the standard laboratory assessment for surgical safety (complete blood count, type and screen, etc.), there are several laboratory assessments that can be considered.

For reproductive-aged women, serum cancer antigen 125 (CA 125) evaluation is not recommended routinely; rather, it should be evaluated only when there is concern regarding the appearance of adnexal mass on imaging. It should be noted

Table 11.2 Characteristics concerning for malignancy

	Possible features of malignancy
Ultrasound	Thick, irregular walls and septa Papillary projections Absence of shadowing Mixed or high echogenicity Central vascularity/pattern of flow Low systolic-diastolic Doppler variation
MRI	Improved identification of true papillary projections versus ultrasound

that CA 125 is less useful in predicting malignancy in premenopausal women than in postmenopausal women. This is complicated by the fact that benign causes of ovarian cysts such as endometriomvas can cause elevated CA 125 levels [20]. Reproductive surgeons should consider the CA 125 in addition to the aforementioned factors when deciding whether consultation with a gynecologic oncologist is warranted (19). Table 11.2 highlights characteristics of malignant ovarian masses.

For any child or adolescent with adnexal mass, biomarkers associated with germ cell tumors should be evaluated, as germ cell tumor is a common pathology in this age group. Specifically, these markers include human chorionic gonadotropin (hCG), lactate dehydrogenase (LDH), and alpha fetoprotein (AFP). If these markers are abnormal, suspicion for germ cell or sex cord stromal neoplasms should be raised, and referral to a gynecologic oncologist should be made.

Lastly, anti-Mullerian hormone (AMH) has increasingly been demonstrated to be a reliable marker of ovarian reserve and has also been predictive of ovarian responsiveness with in vitro fertilization. Importantly, it can be assessed at any time in the menstrual cycle.

Patient Selection and Preoperative Counseling

Preoperative counseling is extremely important as surgical management can have nontrivial outcomes on fertility, even with fertility-sparing approach.

The reproductive surgeon must take into account several individualized factors, related to the patient and to the cyst, in consideration of proceeding with ovarian cystectomy. Observation without surgical intervention is generally recommended when the appearance of the cyst on ultrasound suggests benign disease and the patient is asymptomatic [21–23]. Benign cysts on ultrasound that can be managed expectantly include simple physiologic cysts, suspected endometriomas, and mature cystic teratomas [24]. Women who are poor surgical candidates, such as those with medical comorbidities, may benefit from expectant management with ultrasound monitoring [4].

Currently, laparoscopic ovarian cystectomy is recommended as treatment for symptomatic women with ovarian endometriomas. A 2008 Cochrane review compared various surgical interventions for endometriomas and found that ovarian cystectomy has better pain improvement, higher spontaneous pregnancy rates, and less ovarian cyst recurrence than drainage or ablation of endometriomas [25].

It is widely hypothesized that ovarian cystectomy can impair a woman's ovarian reserve [26]. Ovarian reserve is best defined as the egg supply of a woman at a given point in time, taking into account that females are born with a finite number of eggs and the number of eggs decreases over time [27–30]. Ovarian reserve can be measured by labs including anti-Mullerian hormone (AMH) and cycle day 2–3 follicle-stimulating hormone (FSH), as well as antral follicle count on ultrasound [31]. AMH is a commonly used measurement of ovarian reserve because it can be tested any time during the menstrual cycle and is a reliable marker of long-term egg supply [31].

There are various reasons that ovarian cystectomy can decrease ovarian reserve. Mechanisms include inadvertently excising normal ovarian cortex while excising the ovarian cyst, causing loss of primordial follicles. This occurs more often with endometriomas than other ovarian cysts, due to scarring, adhesions, and lack of obvious surgical planes [32, 33]. For patients pursuing IVF treatment who have endometriomas, the risk of diminished ovarian reserve due to ovarian cystectomy must be balanced with the risk of proceeding with an egg retrieval with an intact endometrioma. It is imperative to counsel patients with large endometriomas who decide to pursue IVF regarding this risks associated with the presence of the endometrioma which include inability to access ovarian follicles and risk of rupture of the endometrioma which can lead to infection.

For women with an endometrioma considering surgical management, it is of critical importance to discuss the potential impact on ovarian reserve and subsequently fertility. One prospective study by Goodman et al. compared AMH levels between women with endometriomas, pelvic endometriosis, and no endometriosis, preoperatively, 1 month and 6 months postoperatively. They found that women with endometriomas had significantly lower AMH levels: 45% lower than women without endometriosis and 36% lower than the pelvic endometriosis group [34].

Elements to Include in Surgical Consent

Informed consent prior to ovarian cystectomy should always include the risk of oophorectomy. Although this is never the primary intention of a planned ovarian cystectomy, patients must be informed that in the unpredictable scenario of malignancy, uncontrollable bleeding, or otherwise unforeseen complications, oophorectomy may be necessary. Additionally, as described previously in this chapter, patients must be consented for the risk of decreased ovarian reserve following ovarian cystectomy, as well as the risk of recurrence of ovarian cysts, with estimates as high as 50% [35], and need for subsequent surgery.

Operative Techniques and Surgical Approach

Minimally invasive ovarian cystectomy is an effective and safe surgical approach for management of ovarian cysts. For reproductive-aged women, laparoscopic technique has been advocated as a preferred approach in women with ovarian cyst(s). Advantages include the ability to perform ovarian-sparing surgery, faster recovery, and less postoperative pain [36]. Both conventional laparoscopy and robotic-assisted laparoscopy can be performed, although conventional laparoscopy is generally preferred due to shorter operative time and decreased costs [37].

When performing laparoscopic ovarian cystectomy, key operative goals include minimizing blood loss while preserving as much healthy ovarian cortex as possible, as it harbors the ovarian follicular pool. It is also imperative to avoid inadvertent rupture of the ovarian cyst to avoid the spread of undiagnosed malignancy as well as to avoid the risk of chemical peritonitis, which may promote inflammation within the pelvis and lead to adhesion formation. Even with meticulous dissection in the hands of the most experienced surgeon, it can be challenging to avoid cyst rupture, especially with endometriotic cysts. Should cyst rupture occur, copious irrigation of the abdominal cavity with normal saline is prudent to reduce the risk of chemical peritonitis.

Laparoscopic cystectomy mainly requires standard laparoscopic instruments available in the majority of contemporary operating rooms. A uterine manipulator, placed vaginally, can help in moving the uterus and adnexa for improved visu-alization without occupying a laparoscopic port for handling. This enables an appropriate and more ergonomical surgical angle. Insufflation may be performed with Veress needle or open Hasson technique depending on the surgeon's preference, as there is no high-level evidence to suggest superiority of one technique versus the other. Primary port is most often placed using a 5- to 10-mm trocar and is commonly placed through an everted umbilicus. There is no evidence to support superiority with infraumbilical versus supraumbilical placement. There are several options for laparoscopic accessory ports. Most often, two accessory 5-mm trocars are needed for an ovarian cystectomy, placed in the right and left lower quadrants. If an additional trocar is required, a left-sided assist port between the left lower quadrant and the umbilicus can be helpful. Some surgeons may prefer a suprapubic assist port. Overall, port sites may vary depending on cyst size, prior surgical history, and the surgeon's preference. After entry, an abdominal survey is recommended to inspect the pelvis, bilateral adnexal regions, as well as the upper abdomen. It is crucial to perform a systematic diagnostic approach inspecting for any signs of malignancy prior to cyst removal. If there is any concern for malignancy at this point, peritoneal washings should be collected, and gynecologic oncology should be consulted intraoperatively.

Steps to the basic approach to ovarian cystectomy are highlighted in Fig. 11.1. After initial inspection, the target ovary is elevated and stabilized with an atraumatic grasper. Our preferred technique is to then score the ovarian cyst using monopolar scissors or monopolar hook at the cut setting of 30–50 watts. Optimally, the incision is made on the thinnest part of the cyst in a location distance from the ovarian blood supply or fallopian tube. Care should be taken to avoid transection through the cyst wall (i.e., entering the cyst cavity). After scoring, an incision is made, and the plane between the ovarian capsule and cyst wall is developed utilizing a combination of blunt and sharp dissection. A Maryland or other graspers can be used to develop the plane between the ovarian cortex and cyst wall. As the plane develops, the cortical incision may be extended further to aid in cyst removal. Hydrodissection can help

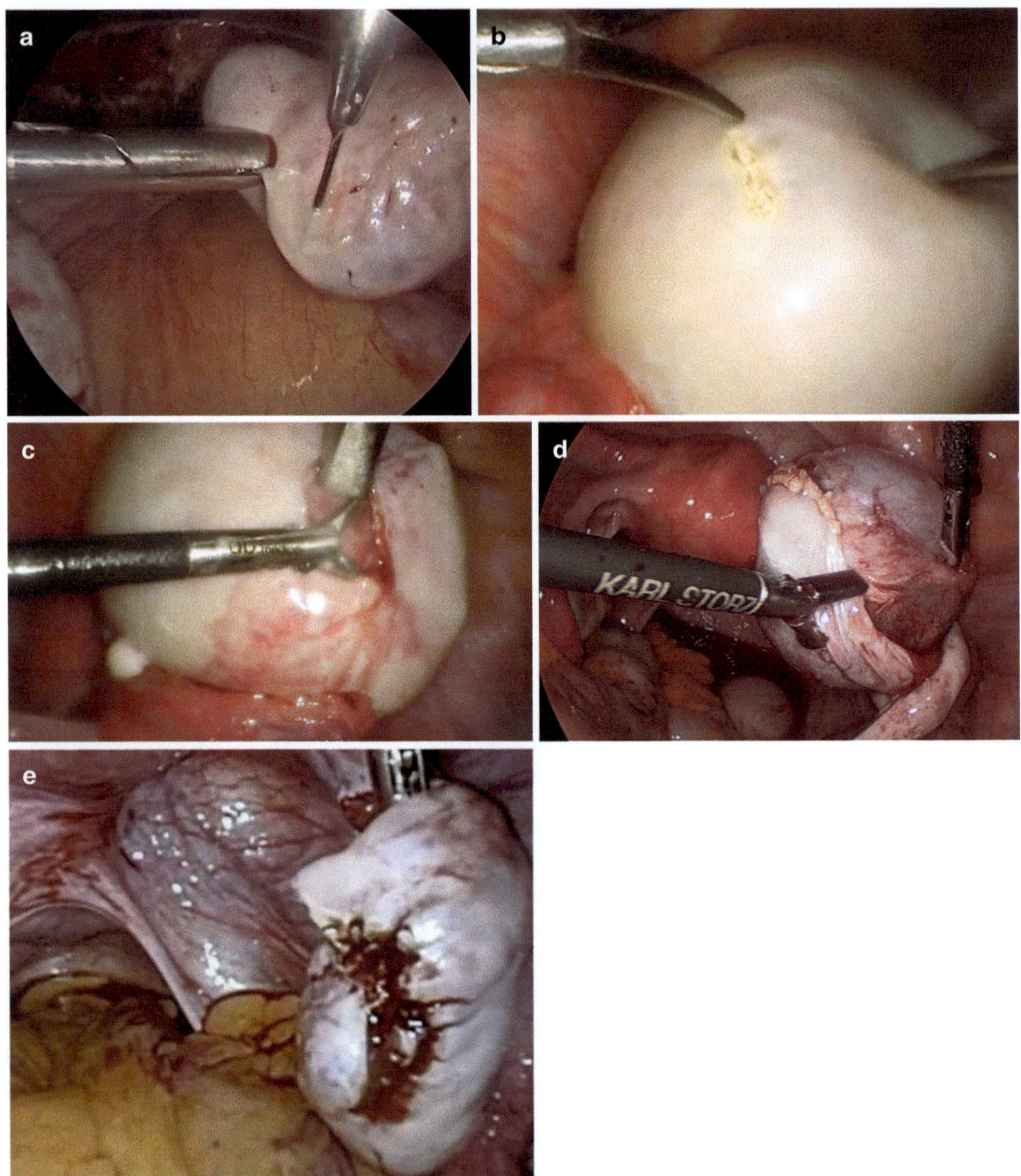

Fig. 11.1 Steps to perform laparoscopic ovarian cystectomy. (**a**) Some surgeons inject dilute vasopressin between the ovarian capsule and cyst wall prior to the incision to aid in plane development. (**b**) Monopolar scissors can be used to score the site of the incision. (**c**) After the initial incision, a Maryland or other graspers can be used to develop plane between the cortex and cyst wall. (**d**) Traction and countertraction combined with sharp and blunt dissection are used to gently separate the ovarian cortex and cyst wall. (**e**) Following excision of the ovarian cyst, the ovarian cortex can be allowed to heal primarily with loose anatomical reapproximation or surgical reapproximation with suture

develop planes and separate the cyst wall from the ovarian cortex in an atraumatic manner. Continued hydrodissection between the cortex and cyst wall can aid in cyst separation. Following excision of the ovarian cyst, it can be placed in an Endocatch bag or similar specimen removal device for ultimate removal from the abdominal cavity.

Following removal of an ovarian cyst, the ovarian cortex can be reapproximated or allowed to involute and heal on its own. The decision of ovarian repair versus primary healing depends on the surgeon's preference. Typically, the ovary is reapproximated in a running fashion with 3-0 or 4-0 monofilament suture. It's important to include the base of the ovary to ensure hemostasis and to collapse the cystic space. If the decision is made to allow the ovary to heal primarily, loose reapproximation in an anatomical fashion is recommended. While shown to reduce adhesion formation, at present, there is no conclusive evidence that the use of pharmacologic or fluid agents or anti-adhesive barriers improves ultimate pregnancy outcomes when used as an adjunct during pelvic surgery [PMID: **32683695**].

It is important to note that if there is any intraoperative concern for malignancy, there should be a low threshold to send a specimen for frozen section. Pelvic washings may also be collected at the start of the case and can be sent for cytology. While frozen section allows for a rapid albeit imperfect assessment for malignancy, it is accurate enough to aid in intraoperative decision-making and may reduce the extent of surgery in favor of a fertility-sparing approach in women ultimately diagnosed with a benign ovarian mass [38].

Approach to the Endometrioma

Laparoscopic ovarian cystectomy is the first-line surgical approach to remove endometriotic cysts. There are two common surgical methods for management of endometriomas: ablation and cystectomy. Ovarian cystectomy is described in detail as above. Unique considerations should be given to endometriotic cystectomy, in that often an endometrioma is formed by invagination of otherwise normal ovarian tissue rather than typical cystic changes.

Ablation technique is performed by cyst drainage followed by careful application of plasma energy in coagulation mode, at an average distance of 5 mm, with exposure time of 1–2 seconds. Complete cyst removal is not well achieved by an ablative technique and as a result is associated with a higher recurrence rate. A 2008 Cochrane review showed a reduced rate of recurrence of endometrioma (OR 0.41, 95% CI 0.18 to 0.93) as well as reduced requirement for further surgery (OR 0.21, 95% CI 0.05 to 0.79) compared to ablative surgery [**18425908**]. Multiple studies have demonstrated a lower incidence of recurrent symptoms such as pain, as well as a higher pregnancy rate when cyst is surgically managed with cystectomy rather than ablation [39]. It is worth noting that both cystectomy and ablation can cause a decline in AMH after endometrioma removal. Even though this decline is higher with cystectomy, specifically if the cyst is larger or bilateral, cystectomy results in higher pregnancy rate compared to ablation. Due to this advantage, ovarian cystectomy remains the gold standard surgical approach to treating an endometrioma [40].

Approach to the Mature Cystic Teratoma (Dermoid Cysts)

Similar to endometriomas, laparoscopic approach is the preferred mode of surgery to remove dermoid cysts. Several studies have demonstrated that AMH will inevitably decline postoperatively after ovarian cystectomy for dermoid cysts, irrespective of unilateral or bilateral location [41]. In contrast to endometriomas, cyst size has not been shown to impact ovarian reserve in the setting of surgical removal [42].

While it is a good surgical practice to avoid intraperitoneal rupture and spillage of cyst contents, it may be unavoidable. If cyst rupture does occur, copious irrigation is essential. This is especially true in the setting of ruptured teratomas, where cyst contents can be highly inflammatory and cause a chemical peritonitis. Following detachment of cyst, the specimen may be contained within a specimen bag and removed through the laparoscopic port. If cyst is too large to be delivered through the port itself, options include controlled cyst rupture within the specimen bag with drainage (via syringe or suction machine) or extension of an incision to accommodate the entirety of the intact cyst.

Special Considerations: Ovarian Cystectomy in the Pregnant Patient

Adnexal masses impact 0.05–3.2% of pregnant women [43–48]. The majority of ovarian cysts in pregnant women demonstrate a low risk of malignancy on imaging and can be managed expectantly. The vast majority of ovarian cysts resolve during pregnancy, with persistent cysts more likely to be those greater than 5 cm or with a complex appearance on ultrasound [43–45]. The most common types of ovarian cysts in pregnancy women include mature cystic teratomas and persistent corpus luteal cysts [48–50]. Of the pregnant women with persistent ovarian cysts, the prevalence of malignancy is roughly 1–3% [44, 47, 51, 52]. Non-contrast MRI is a valuable diagnostic imaging modality that can safely be used in pregnancy to identify malignant features if needed.

Overall, evaluation of the pregnant woman with an ovarian cyst is similar to nonpregnant premenopausal women, with the exception of avoiding CT for imaging assessment. If surgical intervention is indicated based on symptoms, laparoscopy or laparotomy can be considered. In the second and third trimester, trocar placement should be altered relative to the fundal height on exam. For initial entry, both Hassan and Veress needles have been effectively used, with careful attention to elevate abdominal wall during insertion. Intra-abdominal insufflation pressures of 12–15 mmHg have been used safely, without adverse outcomes [**28643072**].

Prior studies have demonstrated the safety and efficacy of laparoscopic ovarian cyst excision in the second trimester [53]. Persistent complex cysts or those larger than 5 cm can ideally be re-evaluated and removed in the postpartum period. In specific patient scenarios, cyst removal may be attempted during cesarean section in order to avoid an additional surgery in the future.

Special Considerations: Ovarian Cystectomy in Pediatric and Adolescent Patients

The approach to ovarian cysts in adolescents is similar to that in premenopausal women in that ovarian conservation should be prioritized. The majority of ovarian cysts in adolescents are benign and can be managed expectantly. For virginal or prepubertal adolescents, transvaginal ultrasound may not be able to be performed, in which case transabdominal ultrasound may provide limited visualization and characterization of the ovarian cyst [54]. Germ cell tumors are the most common malignancy in young patients [55, 56]. If a germ cell tumor is suspected, obtaining AFP, hCG, and LDH lab values are indicated [57]. Malignant ovarian masses are generally rare in the pediatric and adolescent population, with malignancy more common in pediatric patients [58].

Especially in the pediatric and adolescent population, who are at higher risk for later recurrence of pathology simply due to young age at diagnosis relative to expected life potential, consideration should be given to fertility preservation prior to any ovarian surgery. Techniques for fertility preservation may include oocyte or ovarian tissue cryopreservation. Furthermore, for these young patients who have already had ovarian surgery, such as oophorectomy or cystectomy, consultation with a reproductive endocrinologist postoperatively may be warranted to consider fertility preservation.

Postoperative Care

As it is known that there is a decrease in ovarian reserve following surgical removal for many types of cyst, effective and mindful postoperative care is essential. Especially given the serially increased consequence on ovarian reserve associated with reoperation for cyst recurrence, postoperative care geared toward prevention should be prioritized as much as primary surgical management. It has been estimated that recurrence rates for endometrioma may be as high as 50% [35]. Postoperative medical management to reduce recurrence is aimed at ovarian suppression and reduced menstrual flow. One meta-analysis investigating efficacy of various hormonal medication regimens for endometrioma recurrence following surgery found that GnRH agonists with Levonorgestrel intrauterine device was the most effective in lowering recurrence. This effectiveness was narrowly superior to continuous oral contraceptive pill use. However, notably, none of the hormonal regimens given as a short-term treatment (about 3–6 months) lowered endometrioma recurrence compared with expectant management [59]. This is an important consideration in women undergoing surgery for infertility, prior to proceeding with infertility treatment.

For those women who are pursuing assisted reproductive treatment in conjunction with surgery for ovarian cyst, there is often a debate about when it is safe to proceed with ovarian stimulation in the postoperative period. Consideration should be given to the patients such as specific approach, extent, and recovery course. Given the expected postoperative inflammation within the ovaries and pelvis, a postoperative recovery period of at least 4 weeks may be advised. There is a paucity of data on IVF outcomes relative to postoperative recovery period prior to ovarian stimulation.

References

1. National Institutes of Health Consensus Development Conference Statement. Ovarian cancer: screening, treatment, and follow-up. Gynecol Oncol. 1994;55(3 Pt 2):S4–14.
2. Legendre G, Catala L, Moriniere C, Lacoeuille C, Boussion F, Sentilhes L, et al. Relationship between ovarian cysts and infertility: what surgery and when? Fertil Steril. 2014;101(3):608–14.
3. Busacca M, Vignali M. Endometrioma excision and ovarian reserve: a dangerous relation. J Minim Invasive Gynecol. 2009;16(2):142–8.
4. American College of O, Gynecologists' Committee on Practice B-G. Practice Bulletin No. 174: Evaluation and Management of Adnexal Masses. Obstet Gynecol. 2016;128(5):e210–e26.
5. Farghaly SA. Current diagnosis and management of ovarian cysts. Clin Exp Obstet Gynecol. 2014;41(6):609–12.
6. Sokalska A, Timmerman D, Testa AC, Van Holsbeke C, Lissoni AA, Leone FP, et al. Diagnostic accuracy of transvaginal ultrasound examination for assigning a specific diagnosis to adnexal masses. Ultrasound Obstet Gynecol. 2009;34(4):462–70.
7. Castillo G, Alcazar JL, Jurado M. Natural history of sonographically detected simple unilocular adnexal cysts in asymptomatic postmenopausal women. Gynecol Oncol. 2004;92(3):965–9.
8. Ekerhovd E, Wienerroith H, Staudach A, Granberg S. Preoperative assessment of unilocular adnexal cysts by transvaginal ultrasonography: a comparison between ultrasonographic morphologic imaging and histopathologic diagnosis. Am J Obstet Gynecol. 2001;184(2):48–54.
9. Modesitt SC, Pavlik EJ, Ueland FR, DePriest PD, Kryscio RJ, van Nagell JR Jr. Risk of malignancy in unilocular ovarian cystic tumors less than 10 centimeters in diameter. Obstet Gynecol. 2003;102(3):594–9.
10. Guraslan H, Dogan K. Management of unilocular or multilocular cysts more than 5 centimeters in postmenopausal women. Eur J Obstet Gynecol Reprod Biol. 2016;203:40–3.
11. Brun JL, Fritel X, Aubard Y, Borghese B, Bourdel N, Chabbert-Buffet N, et al. Management of presumed benign ovarian tumors: updated French guidelines. Eur J Obstet Gynecol Reprod Biol. 2014;183:52–8.
12. Pavlik EJ, Ueland FR, Miller RW, Ubellacker JM, DeSimone CP, Elder J, et al. Frequency and disposition of ovarian abnormalities followed with serial transvaginal ultrasonography. Obstet Gynecol. 2013;122(2 Pt 1):210–7.
13. Van Holsbeke C, Van Calster B, Guerriero S, Savelli L, Paladini D, Lissoni AA, et al. Endometriomas: their ultrasound characteristics. Ultrasound Obstet Gynecol. 2010;35(6):730–40.
14. Patel MD, Feldstein VA, Lipson SD, Chen DC, Filly RA. Cystic teratomas of the ovary: diagnostic value of sonography. AJR Am J Roentgenol. 1998;171(4):1061–5.
15. Mais V, Guerriero S, Ajossa S, Angiolucci M, Paoletti AM, Melis GB. Transvaginal ultrasonography in the diagnosis of cystic teratoma. Obstet Gynecol. 1995;85(1):48–52.
16. Micco M, Sala E, Lakhman Y, Hricak H, Vargas HA. Role of imaging in the pretreatment evaluation

of common gynecological cancers. Womens Health (Lond). 2014;10(3):299–321.

17. Jeong YY, Outwater EK, Kang HK. Imaging evaluation of ovarian masses. Radiographics. 2000;20(5):1445–70.

18. Park SB, Lee JB. MRI features of ovarian cystic lesions. J Magn Reson Imaging. 2014;40(3):503–15.

19. Iraha Y, Okada M, Iraha R, Azama K, Yamashiro T, Tsubakimoto M, et al. CT and MR imaging of gynecologic emergencies. Radiographics. 2017;37(5):1569–86.

20. Kitawaki J, Ishihara H, Koshiba H, Kiyomizu M, Teramoto M, Kitaoka Y, et al. Usefulness and limits of CA-125 in diagnosis of endometriosis without associated ovarian endometriomas. Hum Reprod. 2005;20(7):1999–2003.

21. Suh-Burgmann E, Hung YY, Kinney W. Outcomes from ultrasound follow-up of small complex adnexal masses in women over 50. Am J Obstet Gynecol. 2014;211(6):623 e1–7.

22. Alcazar JL, Diaz L, Florez P, Guerriero S, Jurado M. Intensive training program for ultrasound diagnosis of adnexal masses: protocol and preliminary results. Ultrasound Obstet Gynecol. 2013;42(2):218–23.

23. Alcazar JL, Castillo G, Jurado M, Garcia GL. Is expectant management of sonographically benign adnexal cysts an option in selected asymptomatic premenopausal women? Hum Reprod. 2005;20(11):3231–4.

24. Kinkel K, Lu Y, Mehdizade A, Pelte MF, Hricak H. Indeterminate ovarian mass at US: incremental value of second imaging test for characterization—meta-analysis and Bayesian analysis. Radiology. 2005;236(1):85–94.

25. Hart RJ, Hickey M, Maouris P, Buckett W. Excisional surgery versus ablative surgery for ovarian endometriomata. Cochrane Database Syst Rev. 2008;2:CD004992.

26. Rustamov O, Krishnan M, Roberts SA, Fitzgerald CT. Effect of salpingectomy, ovarian cystectomy and unilateral salpingo-oopherectomy on ovarian reserve. Gynecol Surg. 2016;13:173–8.

27. Ding Y, Yuan Y, Ding J, Chen Y, Zhang X, Hua K. Comprehensive assessment of the impact of laparoscopic ovarian cystectomy on ovarian reserve. J Minim Invasive Gynecol. 2015;22(7):1252–9.

28. Ledger WL. Measurement of antimullerian hormone: not as straightforward as it seems. Fertil Steril. 2014;101(2):339.

29. Chang HJ, Han SH, Lee JR, Jee BC, Lee BI, Suh CS, et al. Impact of laparoscopic cystectomy on ovarian reserve: serial changes of serum anti-Mullerian hormone levels. Fertil Steril. 2010;94(1):343–9.

30. Raffi F, Metwally M, Amer S. The impact of excision of ovarian endometrioma on ovarian reserve: a systematic review and meta-analysis. J Clin Endocrinol Metab. 2012;97(9):3146–54.

31. Fleming R, Seifer DB, Frattarelli JL, Ruman J. Assessing ovarian response: antral follicle count versus anti-Mullerian hormone. Reprod Biomed Online. 2015;31(4):486–96.

32. Sugita A, Iwase A, Goto M, Nakahara T, Nakamura T, Kondo M, et al. One-year follow-up of serum antimullerian hormone levels in patients with cystectomy: are different sequential changes due to different mechanisms causing damage to the ovarian reserve? Fertil Steril. 2013;100(2):516–22. e3

33. Exacoustos C, Zupi E, Amadio A, Szabolcs B, De Vivo B, Marconi D, et al. Laparoscopic removal of endometriomas: sonographic evaluation of residual functioning ovarian tissue. Am J Obstet Gynecol. 2004;191(1):68–72.

34. Goodman LR, Goldberg JM, Flyckt RL, Gupta M, Harwalker J, Falcone T. Effect of surgery on ovarian reserve in women with endometriomas, endometriosis and controls. Am J Obstet Gynecol. 2016;215(5):589 e1–6.

35. Vercellini P, Somigliana E, Vigano P, De Matteis S, Barbara G, Fedele L. Post-operative endometriosis recurrence: a plea for prevention based on pathogenetic, epidemiological and clinical evidence. Reprod Biomed Online. 2010;21(2):259–65.

36. Alborzi S, Momtahan M, Parsanezhad ME, Dehbashi S, Zolghadri J, Alborzi S. A prospective, randomized study comparing laparoscopic ovarian cystectomy versus fenestration and coagulation in patients with endometriomas. Fertil Steril. 2004;82(6):1633–7.

37. El Khouly NI, Barr RL, Kim BB, Jeng CJ, Nagarsheth NP, Fishman DA, et al. Comparison of robotic-assisted and conventional laparoscopy in the management of adnexal masses. J Minim Invasive Gynecol. 2014;21(6):1071–4.

38. Morrison J, Lasserson T. Finding time to make the right decision: using frozen section to inform intraoperative management of suspicious ovarian masses. Cochrane Database Syst Rev. 2016;3:ED000109.

39. Beretta P, Franchi M, Ghezzi F, Busacca M, Zupi E, Bolis P. Randomized clinical trial of two laparoscopic treatments of endometriomas: cystectomy versus drainage and coagulation. Fertil Steril. 1998;70(6):1176–80.

40. Alammari R, Lightfoot M, Hur HC. Impact of cystectomy on ovarian reserve: review of the literature. J Minim Invasive Gynecol. 2017;24(2):247–57.

41. Salihoglu KN, Dilbaz B, Cirik DA, Ozelci R, Ozkaya E, Mollamahmutoglu L. Short-term impact of laparoscopic cystectomy on ovarian reserve tests in bilateral and unilateral endometriotic and non-endometriotic cysts. J Minim Invasive Gynecol. 2016;23(5):719–25.

42. Mohamed AA, Al-Hussaini TK, Fathalla MM, El Shamy TT, Abdelaal II, Amer SA. The impact of excision of benign nonendometriotic ovarian cysts on ovarian reserve: a systematic review. Am J Obstet Gynecol. 2016;215(2):169–76.

43. Bernhard LM, Klebba PK, Gray DL, Mutch DG. Predictors of persistence of adnexal masses in pregnancy. Obstet Gynecol. 1999;93(4):585–9.

44. Zanetta G, Mariani E, Lissoni A, Ceruti P, Trio D, Strobelt N, et al. A prospective study of the role of

ultrasound in the management of adnexal masses in pregnancy. BJOG. 2003;110(6):578–83.

45. Brady PC, Simpson LL, Lewin SN, Smok D, Lerner JP, D'Alton ME, et al. Safety of conservative management of ovarian masses during pregnancy. J Reprod Med. 2013;58(9–10):377–82.

46. Whitecar MP, Turner S, Higby MK. Adnexal masses in pregnancy: a review of 130 cases undergoing surgical management. Am J Obstet Gynecol. 1999;181(1):19–24.

47. Schmeler KM, Mayo-Smith WW, Peipert JF, Weitzen S, Manuel MD, Gordinier ME. Adnexal masses in pregnancy: surgery compared with observation. Obstet Gynecol. 2005;105(5 Pt 1):1098–103.

48. Platek DN, Henderson CE, Goldberg GL. The management of a persistent adnexal mass in pregnancy. Am J Obstet Gynecol. 1995;173(4):1236–40.

49. Bromley B, Benacerraf B. Adnexal masses during pregnancy: accuracy of sonographic diagnosis and outcome. J Ultrasound Med. 1997;16(7):447–52; quiz 53–4.

50. Sunoo CS, Terada KY, Kamemoto LE, Hale RW. Adnexal masses in pregnancy: occurrence by ethnic group. Obstet Gynecol. 1990;75(1):38–40.

51. Surampudi K, Nirmalan PK, Gundabattula SR, Chandran JB. Management of adnexal masses in pregnancy: our experience from a tertiary referral perinatal centre in South India. Arch Gynecol Obstet. 2015;291(1):53–8.

52. Balci O, Gezginc K, Karatayli R, Acar A, Celik C, Colakoglu MC. Management and outcomes of adnexal masses during pregnancy: a 6-year experience. J Obstet Gynaecol Res. 2008;34(4):524 8.

53. Balthazar U, Steiner AZ, Boggess JF, Gehrig PA. Management of a persistent adnexal mass in pregnancy: what is the ideal surgical approach? J Minim Invasive Gynecol. 2011;18(6):720–5.

54. Amies Oelschlager AM, Gow KW, Morse CB, Lara-Torre E. Management of large ovarian neoplasms in pediatric and adolescent females. J Pediatr Adolesc Gynecol. 2016;29(2):88–94.

55. Gupta B, Guleria K, Suneja A, Vaid NB, Rajaram S, Wadhwa N. Adolescent ovarian masses: a retrospective analysis. J Obstet Gynaecol. 2016;36(4):515–7.

56. Zhang M, Jiang W, Li G, Xu C. Ovarian masses in children and adolescents – an analysis of 521 clinical cases. J Pediatr Adolesc Gynecol. 2014;27(3):e73–7.

57. Papic JC, Finnell SM, Slaven JE, Billmire DF, Rescorla FJ, Leys CM. Predictors of ovarian malignancy in children: overcoming clinical barriers of ovarian preservation. J Pediatr Surg. 2014;49(1):144–7; discussion 7–8.

58. Hermans AJ, Kluivers KB, Wijnen MH, Bulten J, Massuger LF, Coppus SF. Diagnosis and treatment of adnexal masses in children and adolescents. Obstet Gynecol. 2015;125(3):611–5.

59. Wattanayingcharoenchai R, Rattanasiri S, Charakorn C, Attia J, Thakkinstian A. Postoperative hormonal treatment for prevention of endometrioma recurrence after ovarian cystectomy: a systematic review and network meta-analysis. BJOG. 2021;128(1):25–35.

Ovarian Transposition

12

Leigh A. Humphries, Anne E. Kim, and Divya K. Shah

Introduction

As cancer therapy and survival have improved greatly in recent decades, young women with cancer have increasingly prioritized long-term quality of life. Maintenance of future fertility after gonadotoxic chemotherapy or radiation treatment is often paramount. Radiation is of particular concern in this situation as it accelerates the decline in ovarian follicles, resulting in diminished ovarian reserve and rapid reproductive aging [1]. A radiation dose of 20 Gy or more can cause complete loss of ovarian function, even in young patients [2]. In many instances, the patient's abdomen and pelvis can be shielded with lead to minimize radiation-induced injury to the reproductive organs. However, in patients with certain malignancies, including cervical, vaginal, and anorectal cancers, as well as sarcomas and Hodgkin lymphoma, it is often necessary to irradiate the pelvis directly, leaving the ovaries susceptible to damage. This creates a significant burden for young women, who must confront the possibility of infertility and premature menopause as a side effect of cancer treatment.

Ovarian transposition is a surgical technique that addresses this problem by repositioning the ovaries away from the radiation field, most commonly to a peritoneal site above the pelvic brim. The ovarian blood supply is carefully dissected and preserved along its length to avoid ovarian infarction. The connection between the fallopian tube and ovary may be maintained to allow for unassisted conception in the future. Alternatively, oocyte retrieval either before or after ovarian transposition can facilitate the use of assisted reproductive technologies to achieve a future pregnancy.

This chapter describes the indications, techniques, and outcomes of ovarian transposition. The goal is to equip the reproductive surgeon to select appropriate candidates and achieve good surgical results.

L. A. Humphries · A. E. Kim
Department of Obstetrics and Gynecology, University of Pennsylvania, Philadelphia, PA, USA
e-mail: leigh.humphries@pennmedicine.upenn.edu; anne.kim@pennmedicine.upenn.edu

D. K. Shah (✉)
Division of Reproductive Endocrinology, Department of Obstetrics and Gynecology, University of Pennsylvania, Philadelphia, PA, USA
e-mail: Divya.Shah@pennmedicine.upenn.edu

Radiation Effects on the Ovary

The degree of radiation damage to the ovary depends on the patient's age, ovarian reserve, and radiation dose. Radiation therapy may target the total body, craniospinal, whole abdominal, or pelvic regions, all of which can impact the ovaries. Based on models that account for age-related decline in ovarian reserve, a dose of 2 Gy destroys roughly 50% of the ovarian follicles

© The Author(s), under exclusive license to Springer Nature Switzerland AG 2022
S. R. Lindheim, J. C. Petrozza (eds.), *Reproductive Surgery*,
https://doi.org/10.1007/978-3-031-05240-8_12

[3]. Ovarian reserve at the time of therapy is therefore important to determine the impact of a given dose. The estimated sterilizing dose at which complete ovarian failure occurs decreases with patient age: 20.3 Gy at birth, 18.4 Gy at 10 years old, 16.5 Gy at 20 years old, and 14.3 Gy at 30 years old [2]. Ovarian failure in this model was defined as lack of pubertal development or onset of premature menopause after radiation treatment. In another study of 94 patients who were followed for years after radiation treatment, no patients experienced premature menopause if the estimated ovarian dose was less than 1.5 Gy, while 14% experienced menopause at a dose of 1–10 Gy and 68% at a dose of over 12 Gy [4].

The doses to treat pelvic malignancies typically exceed the thresholds that cause ovarian failure. For example, most patients with Hodgkin lymphoma receive total doses of 20–30 Gy, while patients with cervical carcinoma may receive doses as high as 60 Gy. A single dose is more toxic than fractionated doses over time, yet premature ovarian failure is common even with fractionated dosing. By contrast, ovarian transposition can reduce the radiation dose to the ovary by 90–95%. The mean estimated dose sustained by transposed ovaries in most case series was less than 2–3 Gy [5, 6].

Candidate Selection

The ideal candidate for ovarian transposition is a patient less than 40 years old who requires pelvic radiation and no gonadotoxic chemotherapy and who also has a low risk of ovarian metastasis [7]. Some studies suggest using a lower threshold of 35 years old for women treated with external beam radiation to the pelvis, due to the higher gonadotoxicity of this modality [8]. Since younger women have higher ovarian reserve, they are less likely to suffer damage from low-level radiation scatter, which is inevitable even in transposed ovaries. Appropriate surgical candidates may have gynecologic cancers, such as cervical cancer, vaginal cancer, uterine cancer, and dysgerminomas, or nongynecologic cancers,

such as Hodgkin lymphoma, anorectal cancers, and sarcomas. Patients with cancers requiring craniospinal radiation, such as ependymomas or medulloblastomas, have also benefited from ovarian transposition.

The procedure is contraindicated in patients undergoing chemotherapy with a high risk of gonadotoxicity, such as alkylating agents, as these drugs will impair ovarian function regardless of their anatomic position. Ovarian transposition should also be avoided if there is moderate-to-high risk of ovarian metastasis, which can occur in stomach and colon cancers, advanced breast and cervical cancers, leukemia, neuroblastoma, and Burkitt lymphoma. In cases of cervical cancer, the risk of ovarian metastasis increases with the size of the tumor, such that ovarian transposition is only recommended in patients with small cervical masses less than 3 cm [7].

Surgical Approach: Laparotomy to Laparoscopy

Procedures to relocate and protect the ovaries from radiotherapy have been reported as early as the 1950s [9, 10]. Case reports at that time described exteriorizing the ovaries beneath the skin, suturing the ovaries to the psoas muscle or anterior abdominal wall, and even encasing the ovaries in lead shells prior to irradiation [9, 11, 12]. Such procedures were performed by laparotomy. By the 1980s, two dominant techniques had emerged: (1) medial transposition, in which the ovaries were sutured in the midline to the posterior uterus, and (2) lateral transposition, in which the ovaries were retracted cephalad and laterally and then sutured to the peritoneum [13–15]. These procedures successfully preserved menstruation (a proxy for ovarian function) after radiotherapy in most patients, yet the studies were small with limited follow-up; little or no pregnancy data; and notable complications, such as injury to the ovarian blood supply. Ovarian transposition by laparotomy also required extension of the incision and increased operative time, which limited its routine use [13].

In the 1990s, both the medial and lateral techniques were adapted for laparoscopy with good results in small case series [16–18]. Outpatient laparoscopic surgery allowed for quicker recovery, thus permitting immediate initiation of radiation therapy and decreasing the likelihood that the ovaries would migrate back into the pelvis. Despite these benefits, uptake of ovarian transposition was slow. As of 2003, only 46 cases of laparoscopic ovarian transposition had been reported in the literature [16]. Over the next decade, it became standard to perform ovarian transposition laparoscopically, with some surgeons utilizing robotic assistance [19, 20]. By 2019, observational studies had identified over 1150 patients with various malignancies who had undergone ovarian transposition by either laparoscopy or laparotomy [8, 21].

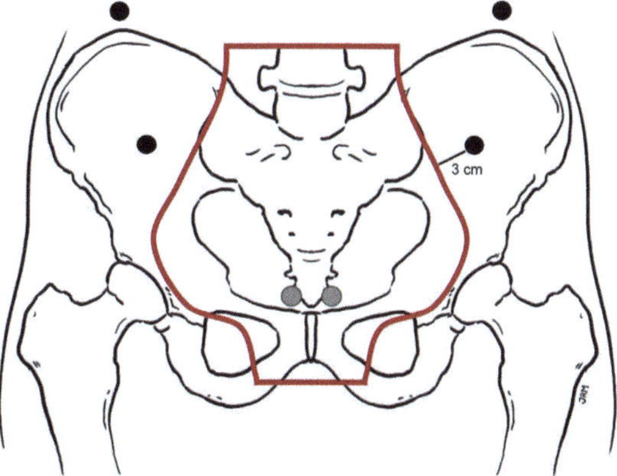

Fig. 12.1 Locations of ovarian transposition. In medial transposition (gray dots), the ovaries remain within the radiation field (outlined in red) and are attached behind the uterus, which acts as a shield. In lateral transposition, the ovaries are transposed laterally at least 3 cm outside of the radiation field, typically at positions above the pelvic brim or above the iliac crest (black dots)

Preoperative Considerations

Although ovarian transposition is typically performed laparoscopically, it can be performed during laparotomy if an abdominal incision is already planned for tumor removal. Robotic assistance may be helpful but is not typically necessary. Ovarian transposition should occur relatively close to the time of planned radiation therapy since there is a risk that the ovaries may migrate back into the radiation field.

Location of Transposition

The radiation oncologist should outline the radiation field preoperatively to indicate the ideal site for ovarian transposition. The success of the procedure is related to the distance between the transposed ovaries and the boundaries of the radiation field. To limit the ovarian dose to 4 Gy or less, the ovaries should be placed more than 3 cm from the target radiation border (Fig. 12.1) [6, 22]. Radio-opaque surgical clips should be applied at the inferior border of the ovaries to permit visualization by the radiation oncologist.

To achieve the adequate distance, the ovaries are typically elevated out of the pelvis and attached to the peritoneum laterally. Different lateral transposition sites have been reported, including the pelvic brim, paracolic gutters, and near the level of the lower kidney [16]. By contrast, medial transposition has been performed in patients with Hodgkin lymphoma requiring radiation in an inverted-Y field, which targets para-aortic, iliac, inguinal, and upper femoral lymph nodes [5]. With this technique, the ovaries are attached to the uterosacral ligaments and posterior uterus, and the uterus serves as a shield for the ovaries. Lateral transposition is the more commonly utilized technique as it is clinically appropriate for most cancer types and radiation fields and has also been associated with slightly lower radiation exposure to the ovaries (4.9 Gy after the medial technique vs. 3.25 Gy after the lateral technique) [23].

Management of Fallopian Tubes

There are three options for managing the fallopian tubes during ovarian transposition: (1) transposition with the ovary, (2) complete detachment from the ovary, and (3) removal via salpingectomy. In many cases, the fallopian tubes can be preserved and remain attached to

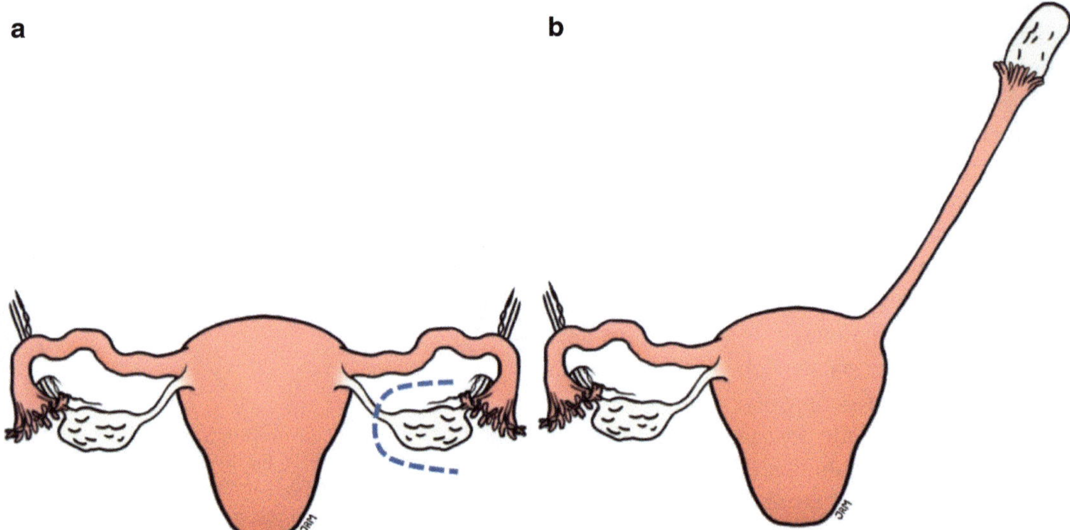

Fig. 12.2 Lateral ovarian transposition with preservation of the fallopian tube. (**a**) The utero-ovarian ligament is divided, followed by the mesovarium, which separates the ovary from the proximal tube in a c-shaped incision. Releasing the posterior peritoneum prevents tension and provides adequate mobility. (**b**) Once the vasculature has been dissected, the ovary is lifted superiorly and laterally to a new position above the pelvic brim, with the fallopian tube attached

the ovary (Fig. 12.2). The fimbriated end of the tube remains proximate to the ovary after transposition, thus permitting the possibility of unassisted conception. If the tube is fully detached from the ovary, there is greater mobilization of the ovary on the infundibulo-pelvic ligament, allowing for higher transposition above the pelvic brim or iliac crest. Bilateral salpingectomy has similar benefits in terms of increased mobilization and is common among patients for whom in vitro fertilization (IVF) is planned for future pregnancy. Salpingectomy also prevents future risks of developing paratubal cysts, hydrosalpinges, tubal torsion or infarction, and tubal metastasis; it is therefore preferable if spontaneous conception is not a priority.

Risks of the Procedure

In addition to standard risks of minor laparoscopy, such as bleeding, infection, injury to intraperitoneal structures, and port site hernia, there are risks specific to ovarian transposition. Injury or torsion of the ovarian vasculature can lead to ovarian ischemia and need for reoperation. Although very rare, ovarian metastasis within transposed ovaries has been reported [24, 25]. Also, since transposed ovaries are still functional, they may develop functional or hemorrhagic cysts, which can become symptomatic. Increased development of ovarian cysts was associated with ovarian transposition under the skin, but not with current techniques [21].

Surgical Technique: Lateral Ovarian Transposition

The general goals of ovarian transposition are to detach the ovaries from the uterus, mobilize the vascular pedicles, and suture the ovaries to new peritoneal locations. As medial transposition is less common and involves minimal surgical dissection before oophoropexy to the posterior-medial sites, this section focuses on the surgical technique for lateral ovarian transposition:

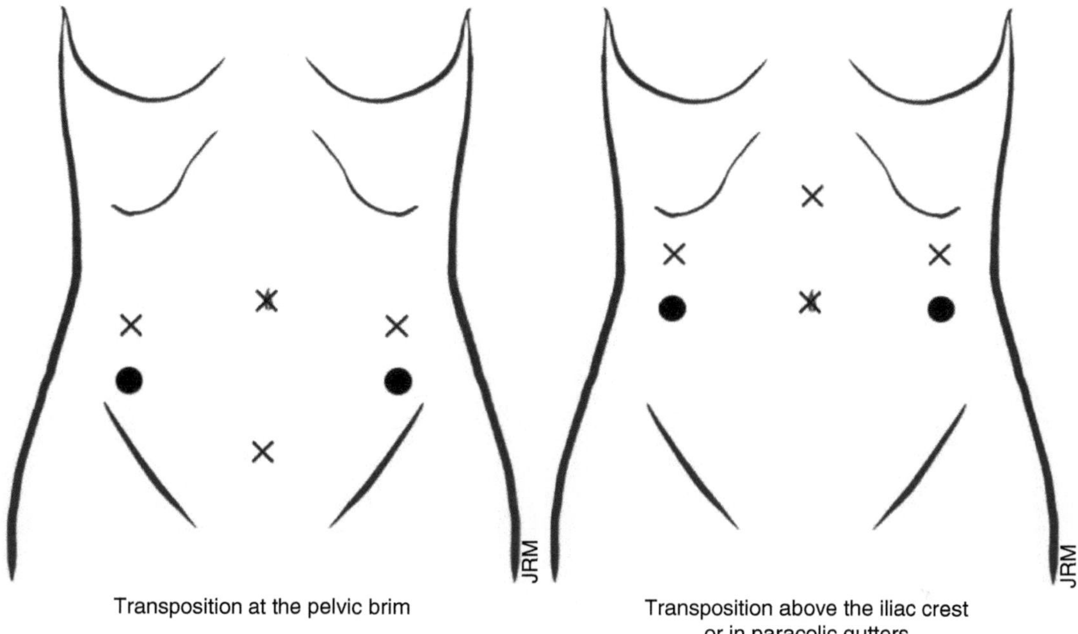

Transposition at the pelvic brim

Transposition above the iliac crest
or in paracolic gutters

Fig. 12.3 Laparoscopic port placement. Location of the laparoscopic ports (designated by X) depends on the intended location of the transposed ovaries (black dots). A more cephalad configuration could be adopted for performing transposition above the iliac crest or in the paracolic gutters

1. *Laparoscopic port placement*

   Specific port placement may differ based on the preferences of individual surgeons. One approach is to insert four laparoscopic ports in a diamond configuration: an umbilical port, two lateral ports, and a fourth midline port in either the suprapubic or supraumbilical region (Fig. 12.3). To allow for effective triangulation at the pelvic brim and to transpose the ovaries above the iliac crest, it may be important to position the ports more cephalad than is typical for pelvic surgery.

2. *Exposure at the pelvic brim*

   Perform an intraperitoneal survey to identify any evidence of metastatic disease or anatomic abnormalities. Identify the ureters through the peritoneum or following entry into the retroperitoneal space, where they can be found on the medial leaflet of the posterior broad ligament or at the pelvic brim crossing over the bifurcation of the common iliac vessels.

   Clear any adhesions or vital organs from the intended transposition sites for the ovaries. With the patient in Trendelenburg position, retract the bowel into the upper abdomen, and divide the physiologic adhesions between the sigmoid and the left pelvic sidewall. The sigmoid colon can then be retracted medially to expose the pelvic brim. Use external and intraperitoneal landmarks to confirm the intended locations for the ovaries sufficiently away from the planned radiation field. Mark the peritoneum at these sites (e.g., with monopolar cautery) in order to ensure the dissection proceeds to the appropriate level. The remaining steps of the ovarian transposition procedure are performed in the same way on each side (Fig. 12.4).

3. *Ovarian mobilization*

   If the fallopian tubes are being preserved, first coagulate and divide the utero-ovarian ligament with a vessel-sealing device. Extend the incision along the mesovarium to release the proximal tube from the ovary. An additional incision of the posterior peritoneum around the ovary may be needed to prevent tension on the ovary or vessels during trans-

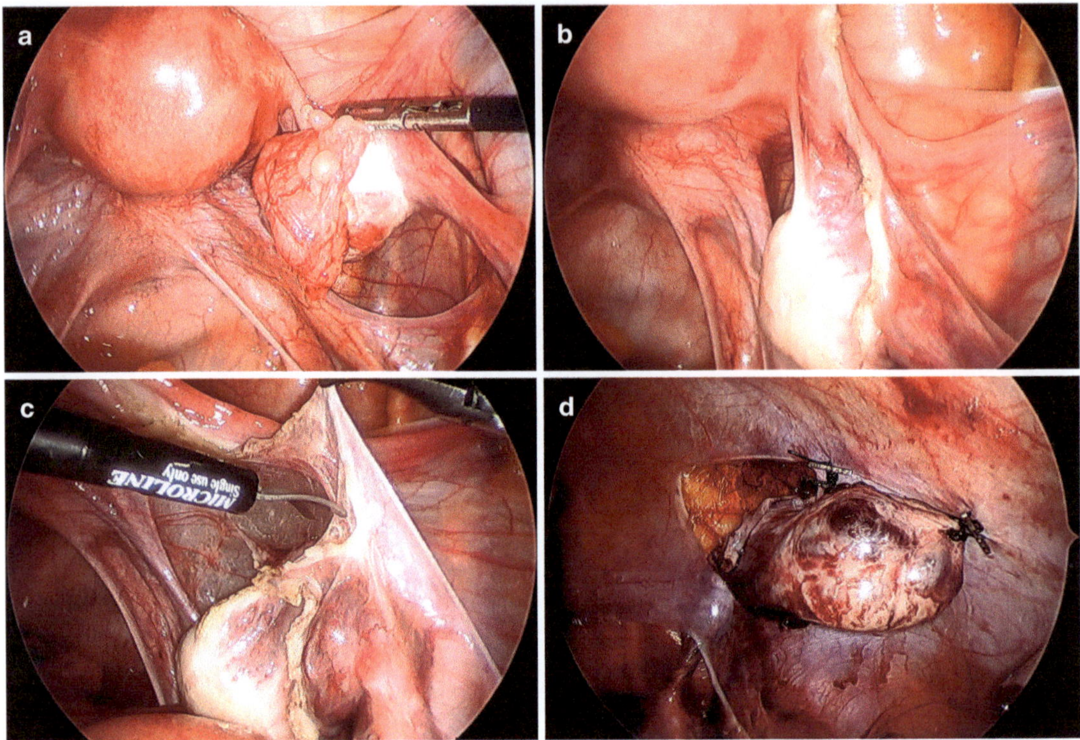

Fig. 12.4 Steps of ovarian transposition above the pelvic brim. (**a**) Identification of relevant anatomy, including the ovary, fallopian tube, utero-ovarian ligament, infundibulo-pelvic ligament, and ureter. (**b**) Removal of the fallopian tube. (**c**) Division of the utero-ovarian ligament and dissection of the peritoneum to mobilize the ovary and vessels. (**d**) Retroperitoneal tunneling of the ovary and attachment to the peritoneum with suture and metal clips

position. If the fallopian tubes are being preserved, grasp and rotate the ovary superiorly and laterally while still attached to its vascular supply and the distal fallopian tube. The laxity of the fallopian tube will ultimately permit it to be stretched to the pelvic brim. If the fallopian tubes are being removed, divide the mesosalpinx along its length to fully separate and remove the fallopian tube. Then coagulate and divide the utero-ovarian ligament, followed by mesovarium to mobilize the ovary on its vascular pedicle, as above.

4. *Development of the ovarian vascular pedicle*

   Grasp and elevate the ovary to expose its attachment to the infundibulo-pelvic ligament, which contains the ovarian vessels. Extend the incision in the posterior broad ligament cephalad along the infundibulo-pelvic ligament to free the vessels from their peritoneal attachments. Skeletonize the ovarian vessels with care to leave behind any surrounding fatty tissue that may contain lymph nodes. Gentle tissue handling is important to avoid injury to the blood supply and/or ovary. Develop the retroperitoneal space between the ureter and the ovarian vessels to the level of the bifurcation of the common iliac artery if the transposition site is near the pelvic brim or to the bifurcation of the aorta if the transposition site is the paracolic gutters.

5. *Tunneling through the retroperitoneum*

   Although this step is not universally performed, tunneling the ovary through the retroperitoneum is a useful way to secure the ovary at its new location (Fig. 12.5). Create a window in the peritoneum slightly caudal to the intended transposition site, and pass the ovary through this opening. The peritoneum functions as a "collar" to hold the ovary in place and may potentially prevent torsion or migra-

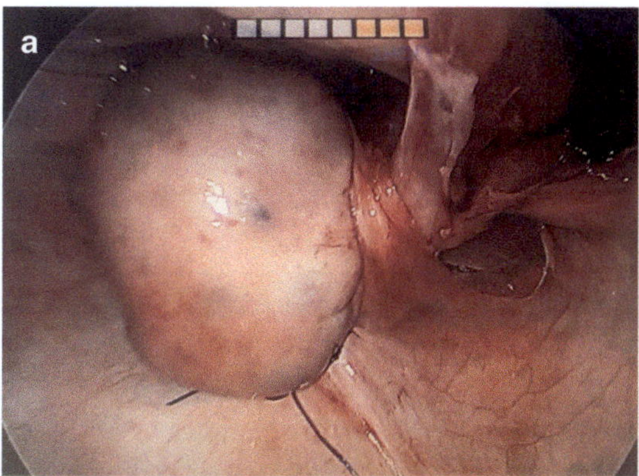

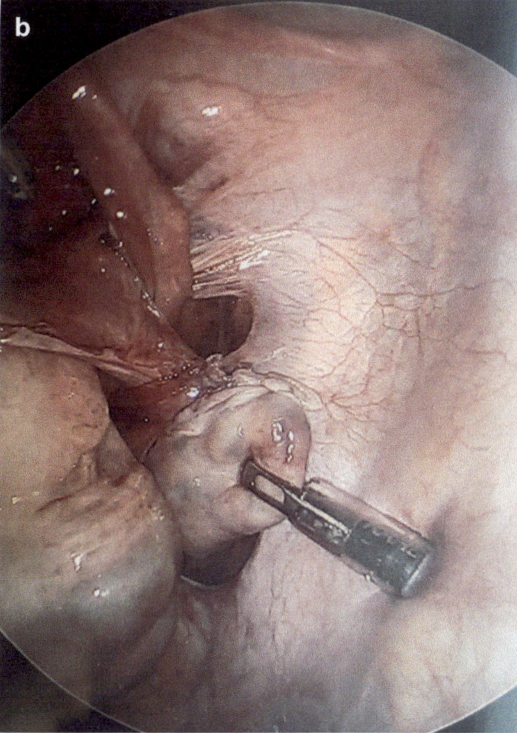

Fig. 12.5 Preservation of the fallopian tubes. The left ovary (**a**) and the right ovary (**b**) are tunneled through the window in the peritoneum above the pelvic brim, with the fallopian tubes left intact. (Photo courtesy of Rebecca Flyckt MD)

tion, though no evidence is available regarding these benefits. Good outcomes have been reported both with and without this step.

6. *Suturing the ovary*

Suture the ovary to the peritoneum with several interrupted stitches of nonabsorbable suture. Mark the lower limit of the ovaries with metal surgical clips to assist with radiologic detection at the time of radiation treatment.

Ovarian Function After Ovarian Transposition

Ovarian function after transposition is based on the absence of signs of ovarian failure, such as amenorrhea, menopausal symptoms, or rise in serum follicle-stimulating hormone (FSH) levels. However, there are no standardized definitions in the literature, with individual studies using different symptoms, laboratory cutoffs, and/or timing of hormone sample collection. There is also significant variability in patient characteristics, types of cancer and therapy, duration of follow-up, and surgical technique (e.g., laparotomy vs. laparoscopy, bilateral vs. unilateral transposition, medial vs. lateral transposition sites). No randomized controlled trials have been conducted to evaluate ovarian transposition, and most observational studies do not stratify by key confounders, such as age or duration of follow-up. Moreover, studies are limited by very small sample sizes, frequently less than ten patients. However, it is important to recognize that given the rarity of the procedure, it can take over a decade for a single institution to collect up to 30 cases [8].

Despite these limitations, systematic reviews have identified significant benefits and minimal risks of ovarian transposition [5, 21, 26]. Between 20% and 100% of women have successfully preserved ovarian function after transposition and radiation, with most studies reporting over 60% success rates. Patients who derived less benefit were older, had more extensive radiation therapy or surgery, or had ovaries that were transposed at shorter distances from the target radiation [5, 22]. Outcomes were most favorable for patients treated with vaginal brachytherapy as compared with external beam radiation therapy, pelvic radiation therapy, or radiation in combination with chemotherapy. A study of 95 patients with a median follow-up of 31 months after ovarian transposition found preserved ovarian function in

90% of those treated with brachytherapy as compared to 60% treated with external beam radiation therapy [7]. In that study, preserved ovarian function was defined as FSH less than 10 mIU/mL, E2 greater than 50 pg/mL, and visible ovarian follicles on pelvic ultrasound.

Ongoing ovarian function after transposition is impacted by patient age and may decline with time. A 2018 study showed that the overall ovarian survival rate had declined to 60% by 5 years after transposition among women with various pelvic malignancies [8]. The ovarian survival rate at 5 years was significantly impacted by patient age: 88% for age 25–30, 63% for age 31–35, and 43% for age 36–40. These rates were still notably higher than the 0% ovarian survival rate in similarly aged controls who had radiation without ovarian transposition. Another study from 2001 showed decreased ovarian function over time, with 65% preserved function at 1 year and 39% at 5 years [27]. The literature consistently demonstrates a greater loss of ovarian function after ovarian transposition in older women; the highest success rates are seen in women under the age of 35 [7, 8, 20]. It is worth noting that the ovarian transposition procedure itself does not appear to be the cause of ovarian damage or dysfunction. Follow-up of patients who underwent ovarian transposition but did not ultimately receive radiation therapy has demonstrated long-term preserved function in 87–100% [7, 8, 27].

The position of the transposed ovary is also critical to postoperative ovarian function. Multivariate analyses controlling for age, BMI, and radiation dose have demonstrated that the location of transposed ovary is the most significant determinant of intact ovarian function [28]. The goal of transposing the ovary as high and lateral as possible must be balanced with the need to avoid injury to the ovarian vessels. A minimum distance of 1.5 cm above the iliac crest was predictive of normal ovarian function after radiation in 31 patients followed for a median of 40 months. Another study of 21 patients found a significant correlation between post-treatment FSH level and the location of the transposed ovaries, with FSH levels less than 30 mIU/mL seen in patients with more superior locations of transposition

[29]. Most surgeons agree that the ovary should be placed at least 3 cm from the target radiation, based on the known impact of ovarian radiation dose, which at this distance is typically less than 4 Gy [22].

Pregnancy Outcomes After Ovarian Transposition

Few studies have reported pregnancy outcomes in cancer survivors after ovarian transposition. The largest report described a pregnancy rate of 32% (12/37 women), with 18 pregnancies occurring after ovarian transposition followed by external beam radiation therapy or brachytherapy [30]. In this case series, the ovaries were transposed laterally either during laparotomy or laparoscopy, and the fallopian tubes and uterus were left intact. Sixteen of the pregnancies were unassisted, and two were achieved using IVF. Five resulted in miscarriage. Of the unassisted pregnancies, 75% occurred with the ovaries still transposed out of the pelvis, showing that migration or repositioning of the ovaries was not necessary prior to spontaneous conception. Fourteen pregnancies were also reported after medial transposition in 11 women with Hodgkin lymphoma, which resulted in 12 live births (one twin birth) and 3 miscarriages [31]. Another study reported 3 pregnancies in 12 patients in whom the ovaries had been attached to the anterior abdominal wall and were later returned to the pelvis after radiation therapy [32]. These case series show that pregnancy and live birth are possible, but larger studies with long-term follow-up are needed to better quantify the impact of ovarian transposition on fertility preservation.

Concurrent Fertility Preservation Strategies

Ovarian transposition can be combined with other fertility preservation techniques, such as oocyte or embryo cryopreservation and ovarian tissue cryopreservation, to maximize reproductive potential in young cancer patients. Since limited data exist on live birth rates after oocyte and embryo cryopreservation specifically among cancer patients, success rates among women with infertility are frequently used for patient counseling [33]. It is clear that the likelihood of live birth relies on the number and quality of oocytes or embryos stored. Ovarian stimulation prior to ovarian transposition offers the benefit of being able to access the ovaries transvaginally at the time of oocyte retrieval. However, transabdominal oocyte retrieval is also possible after ovarian transposition [34–37]. In case reports, oocytes retrieved transabdominally from ovaries transposed as high as the paracolic gutters or the superior iliac spines have resulted in successful live births via gestational carriers [34–37]. Alternatively, relocation of the ovaries into the pelvis after completion of radiotherapy may facilitate transvaginal oocyte retrieval.

Ovarian tissue cryopreservation is an option for prepubertal patients and for patients who cannot or do not wish to delay cancer treatment in order to undergo ovarian stimulation and retrieval. This technique involves decortication of the ovary and dissection of tissue into strips that are then cryopreserved. Orthotopic transplantation of the thawed ovarian tissue is performed when fertility is desired. After transplantation, patients often resume menstruation and can have successful pregnancies, with live birth rates of about 25% in small case series. Ovarian tissue cryopreservation at the time of transposition of the contralateral ovary has been reported for fertility preservation in select candidates [38, 39].

Ovarian transposition does not prevent direct radiation exposure to the uterus, which may have its own detrimental effects, including the possibility of reduced uterine volume, myometrial fibrosis, and damage to the uterine vasculature or endometrium [1]. The degree to which uterine factors influence fertility outcomes after radiation is not known. Uterine transposition, or fixation of the uterus to the anterior abdominal wall, has been proposed in case reports as an adjunct to ovarian transposition, yet additional data on safety and efficacy are needed [40].

Conclusion

A multidisciplinary approach is essential to incorporate ovarian transposition into the care of patients with pelvic cancers. Women with cancer face unique barriers in access to fertility preservation and reproductive health, as they often lack adequate information and do not receive timely referrals to reproductive specialists [41]. This information is especially important for women undergoing pelvic radiation because they are at high risk of gonadal failure. Even for patients whose primary goal is not fertility, preserving ovarian function with ovarian transposition can help prevent symptoms and adverse health effects of premature menopause. Although there is still a risk of ovarian decline over time, especially for older women, ovarian transposition can significantly delay the onset of ovarian failure, which has important implications for quality of life. Therefore, the reproductive surgeon should offer and help prioritize ovarian transposition, in addition to other fertility preservation options, as part of the overall treatment plan in women requiring pelvic radiation.

References

1. Wo JY, Viswanathan AN. Impact of radiotherapy on fertility, pregnancy, and neonatal outcomes in female cancer patients. Int J Radiat Oncol Biol Phys. 2009;73(5):1304–12.
2. Wallace WH, Thomson AB, Saran F, Kelsey TW. Predicting age of ovarian failure after radiation to a field that includes the ovaries. Int J Radiat Oncol Biol Phys. 2005;62(3):738–44.
3. Wallace WH, Thomson AB, Kelsey TW. The radiosensitivity of the human oocyte. Hum Reprod. 2003;18(1):117–21.
4. Stillman RJ, Schinfeld JS, Schiff I, Gelber RD, Greenberger J, Larson M, et al. Ovarian failure in long-term survivors of childhood malignancy. Am J Obstet Gynecol. 1981;139(1):62–6.
5. Hoekman EJ, Broeders E, Louwe LA, Nout RA, Jansen FW, de Kroon CD. Ovarian function after ovarian transposition and additional pelvic radiotherapy: a systematic review. Eur J Surg Oncol. 2019;45(8):1328–40.
6. Mazonakis M, Damilakis J, Varveris H, Gourtsoyiannis N. Radiation dose to laterally transposed ovaries dur-

ing external beam radiotherapy for cervical cancer. Acta Oncol. 2006;45(6):702–7.

7. Morice P, Juncker L, Rey A, El-Hassan J, Haie-Meder C, Castaigne D. Ovarian transposition for patients with cervical carcinoma treated by radiosurgical combination. Fertil Steril. 2000;74(4):743–8.

8. Hoekman EJ, Knoester D, Peters AAW, Jansen FW, de Kroon CD, Hilders C. Ovarian survival after pelvic radiation: transposition until the age of 35 years. Arch Gynecol Obstet. 2018;298(5):1001–7.

9. Kovacev M. Exteriorization of ovaries under the skin of young women operated upon for cancer of the cervix. Am J Obstet Gynecol. 1968;101(6):756–9.

10. Ray GR, Trueblood HW, Enright LP, Kaplan HS, Nelsen TS. Oophoropexy: a means of preserving ovarian function following pelvic megavoltage radiotherapy for Hodgkin's disease. Radiology. 1970;96(1):175–80.

11. Batten R, Brown DE. Protection of ovaries from radiation. Lancet. 1956;270(6929):939–40.

12. Krebs, Blixenkrone-Moller N, Mosekilde V. Preservation of ovarian function in early cervical cancer after surgical lifting of the ovaries and radiation therapy. Acta Radiol Ther Phys Biol. 1963;1:176–82.

13. Gabriel DA, Bernard SA, Lambert J, Croom RD 3rd. Oophoropexy and the management of Hodgkin's disease. A reevaluation of the risks and benefits. Arch Surg. 1986;121(9):1083–5.

14. Husseinzadeh N, Nahhas WA, Velkley DE, Whitney CW, Mortel R. The preservation of ovarian function in young women undergoing pelvic radiation therapy. Gynecol Oncol. 1984;18(3):373–9.

15. Nahhas WA, Nisce LZ, D'Angio GJ, Lewis JL Jr. Lateral ovarian transposition. Ovarian relocation in patients with Hodgkin's disease. Obstet Gynecol. 1971;38(5):785–8.

16. Bisharah M, Tulandi T. Laparoscopic preservation of ovarian function: an underused procedure. Am J Obstet Gynecol. 2003;188(2):367–70.

17. Clough KB, Goffinet F, Labib A, Renolleau C, Campana F, de la Rochefordiere A, et al. Laparoscopic unilateral ovarian transposition prior to irradiation: prospective study of 20 cases. Cancer. 1996;77(12):2638–45.

18. Morice P, Castaigne D, Haie-Meder C, Pautier P, El Hassan J, Duvillard P, et al. Laparoscopic ovarian transposition for pelvic malignancies: indications and functional outcomes. Fertil Steril. 1998;70(5):956–60.

19. Iavazzo C, Darlas FM, Gkegkes ID. The role of robotics in ovarian transposition. Acta Inform Med. 2013;21(2):135–7.

20. Sioulas VD, Jorge S, Chern JY, Schiavone MB, Weiser MR, Kelvin JF, et al. Robotically assisted laparoscopic ovarian transposition in women with lower gastrointestinal cancer undergoing pelvic radiotherapy. Ann Surg Oncol. 2017;24(1):251–6.

21. Gubbala K, Laios A, Gallos I, Pathiraja P, Haldar K, Ind T. Outcomes of ovarian transposition in gynaecological cancers; a systematic review and meta-analysis. J Ovarian Res. 2014;7:69.

22. Lv XJ, Cheng XL, Tu YQ, Yan DD, Tang Q. Association between the location of transposed ovary and ovarian dose in patients with cervical cancer treated with postoperative pelvic radiotherapy. Radiat Oncol. 2019;14(1):230.

23. Grabenbauer GG, Girke P, Wildt L, Muller RG, Herbst M, Sauer R. Ovariopexy and the treatment of Hodgkin's disease. Strahlenther Onkol. 1991;167(5):273–6.

24. Morice P, Haie-Meder C, Pautier P, Lhomme C, Castaigne D. Ovarian metastasis on transposed ovary in patients treated for squamous cell carcinoma of the uterine cervix: report of two cases and surgical implications. Gynecol Oncol. 2001;83(3):605–7.

25. Sanjuan A, Martinez Roman S, Martinez-Zamora MA, Pahisa J. Bilateral ovarian metastasis on transposed ovaries from cervical carcinoma. Int J Gynaecol Obstet. 2007;99(1):64–5.

26. Mossa B, Schimberni M, Di Benedetto L, Mossa S. Ovarian transposition in young women and fertility sparing. Eur Rev Med Pharmacol Sci. 2015;19(18):3418–25.

27. Yamamoto R, Okamoto K, Yukiharu T, Kaneuchi M, Negishi H, Sakuragi N, et al. A study of risk factors for ovarian metastases in stage Ib–IIIb cervical carcinoma and analysis of ovarian function after a transposition. Gynecol Oncol. 2001;82(2):312–6.

28. Hwang JH, Yoo HJ, Park SH, Lim MC, Seo SS, Kang S, et al. Association between the location of transposed ovary and ovarian function in patients with uterine cervical cancer treated with (postoperative or primary) pelvic radiotherapy. Fertil Steril. 2012;97(6):1387–93.e1–2.

29. Yoon A, Lee YY, Park W, Huh SJ, Choi CH, Kim TJ, et al. Correlation between location of transposed ovary and function in cervical cancer patients who underwent radical hysterectomy. Int J Gynecol Cancer. 2015;25(4):688–93.

30. Morice P, Thiam-Ba R, Castaigne D, Haie-Meder C, Gerbaulet A, Pautier P, et al. Fertility results after ovarian transposition for pelvic malignancies treated by external irradiation or brachytherapy. Hum Reprod. 1998;13(3):660–3.

31. Terenziani M, Piva L, Meazza C, Gandola L, Cefalo G, Merola M. Oophoropexy: a relevant role in preservation of ovarian function after pelvic irradiation. Fertil Steril. 2009;91(3):935 e15–6.

32. Gareer W, Gad Z, Gareer H. Needle oophoropexy: a new simple technique for ovarian transposition prior to pelvic irradiation. Surg Endosc. 2011;25(7):2241–6.

33. Practice Committee of the American Society for Reproductive Medicine. Electronic address aao. Fertility preservation in patients undergoing gonadotoxic therapy or gonadectomy: a committee opinion. Fertil Steril. 2019;112(6):1022–33.

34. Agorastos T, Zafrakas M, Mastrominas M. Long-term follow-up after cervical cancer treatment and subsequent successful surrogate pregnancy. Reprod Biomed Online. 2009;19(2):250–1.

35. Giacalone PL, Laffargue F, Benos P, Dechaud H, Hedon B. Successful in vitro fertilization-surrogate pregnancy in a patient with ovarian transposition who had undergone chemotherapy and pelvic irradiation. Fertil Steril. 2001;76(2):388–9.
36. Steigrad S, Hacker NF, Kolb B. In vitro fertilization surrogate pregnancy in a patient who underwent radical hysterectomy followed by ovarian transposition, lower abdominal wall radiotherapy, and chemotherapy. Fertil Steril. 2005;83(5):1547–9.
37. Zinger M, Liu JH, Husseinzadeh N, Thomas MA. Successful surrogate pregnancy after ovarian transposition, pelvic irradiation and hysterectomy. J Reprod Med. 2004;49(7):573–4.
38. Martin JR, Kodaman P, Oktay K, Taylor HS. Ovarian cryopreservation with transposition of a contralateral ovary: a combined approach for fertility preservation in women receiving pelvic radiation. Fertil Steril. 2007;87(1):189 e5–7.
39. Arian SE, Goodman L, Flyckt RL, Falcone T. Ovarian transposition: a surgical option for fertility preservation. Fertil Steril. 2017;107(4):e15.
40. Ribeiro R, Rebolho JC, Tsumanuma FK, Brandalize GG, Trippia CH, Saab KA. Uterine transposition: technique and a case report. Fertil Steril. 2017;108(2):320–4 e1.
41. Jones G, Hughes J, Mahmoodi N, Smith E, Skull J, Ledger W. What factors hinder the decision-making process for women with cancer and contemplating fertility preservation treatment? Hum Reprod Update. 2017;23(4):433–57.

Imaging Modalities to Preoperatively Detect Fibroid Location

13

Thomas Winter

This short review addresses imaging modalities that may be employed to detect and properly characterize fibroids prior to uterine surgery.

Fibroids are common in women of reproductive age (Fig. 13.1), especially in black women [1]. Fibroids are multiple in as many as 84% of patients [2]. Hysteroscopic myomectomy is often the preferred therapy, but for this option to be appropriate accurate preoperative imaging is crucial.

Fibroids should be described with size measurements; where they are located in the standard three orthogonal planes (lower/isthmus, corpus, or fundus; left-right; and anterior-posterior), and site (e.g., submucosal, intramural, subserosal, and externally pedunculated). Various systems have been proposed to help with preoperative planning relative to the fibroid site. The easiest to understand is the simplified version of the European Society of Hysteroscopy classification schema, which reduces to: is the fibroid more than half in (Type 0 and Type I) or more than half out (Type II) of the endometrial cavity? The former will benefit from hysteroscopic resection, while the latter usually requires either an external myomectomy or a multistep hysteroscopic procedure. Other more detailed and elaborate classifi-

cation systems for reporting well-defined uterine masses are available, such as the FIGO classification illustrated in Fig. 13.2 [3]. Imaging is invaluable in preoperative planning and assigning fibroids to the appropriate site category.

Other entities besides fibroids may present as masses in the endometrium and myometrium. Besides a submucosal fibroid, the most common endometrial abnormality in a reproductive-endocrine-infertility (REI) population would be an endometrial polyp (assuming that one has ruled out transient filling defects such as blood clots or air bubbles), but one should always be alert for unusual and unexpected entities (Fig. 13.3). Similarly, well-defined focal myometrial abnormalities are almost always fibroids, but focal adenomyosis and uterine contractions may present as mimics. Adenomyosis can be challenging to accurately diagnose and image, even with magnetic resonance imaging (MRI). In general, Mullerian fusion and resorption abnormalities (septate uterus, bicornuate uterus, etc.) do not present as focal abnormalities [4], although a fundal intramural fibroid may occasionally mimic an arcuate uterus at ultrasound (US); an MRI can almost always distinguish between these two possibilities.

Furthermore, although many attempts have been made to do so, imaging generally cannot reliably distinguish between an ordinary leiomyoma and more malignant entities such as smooth muscle tumors of uncertain malignant potential

T. Winter (✉)
TCW, Abdominal Imaging Division, Department of Radiology and Imaging Science, University of Utah Health Sciences, Salt Lake City, UT, USA
e-mail: thomas.winter@hsc.utah.edu

© The Author(s), under exclusive license to Springer Nature Switzerland AG 2022
S. R. Lindheim, J. C. Petrozza (eds.), *Reproductive Surgery*,
https://doi.org/10.1007/978-3-031-05240-8_13

(STUMP) or leiomyosarcoma (LMS) [5–7]. The importance of this distinction has received much public visibility in recent years given the discus-sion over the pros and cons of fibroid morcella-tion [8]. Fortunately, although certainly an issue, LMS are less common in REI aged patients.

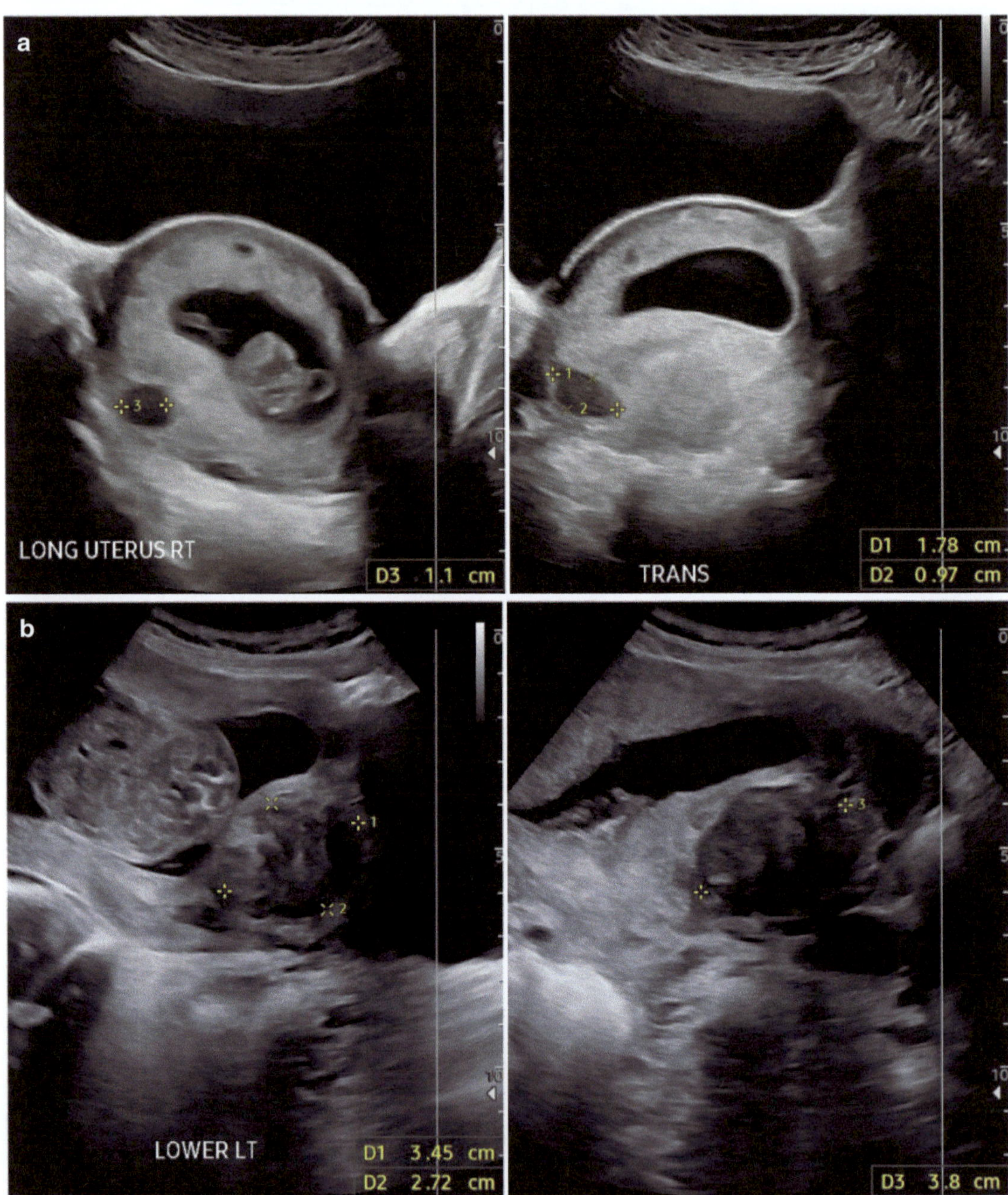

Fig. 13.1 Fibroids during pregnancy, 4 different patients. (**a**) Small incidental fibroid (yellow graticules) at the time of a routine first trimester dating scan. (**b**) Larger lower uterine segment fibroid (yellow graticules) at the time of a routine second trimester anatomy study. (**c**) 15-week pregnancy with a 7.2 × 7.0 × 6.9 cm large anterior lower uter-ine segment fibroid ("F") concerning for a risk of labor obstruction. (**d**) 34-week fetus with aqueductal stenosis ("V" denotes dilated lateral ventricle in this cephalic pre-sentation). Note how well this sagittal MRI shows the 9 cm degenerating anterior lower uterine segment fibroid ("F") ("B" is the urinary bladder)

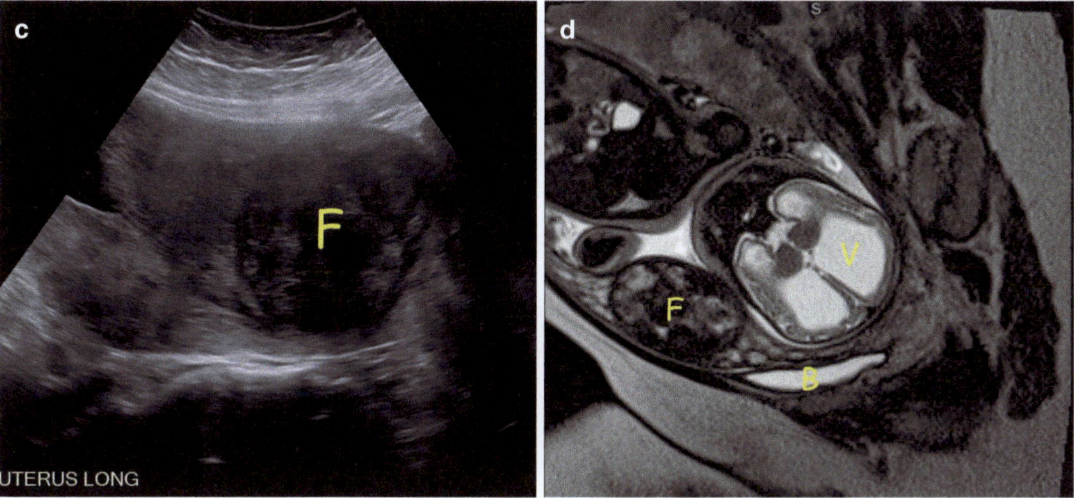

Fig. 13.1 (continued)

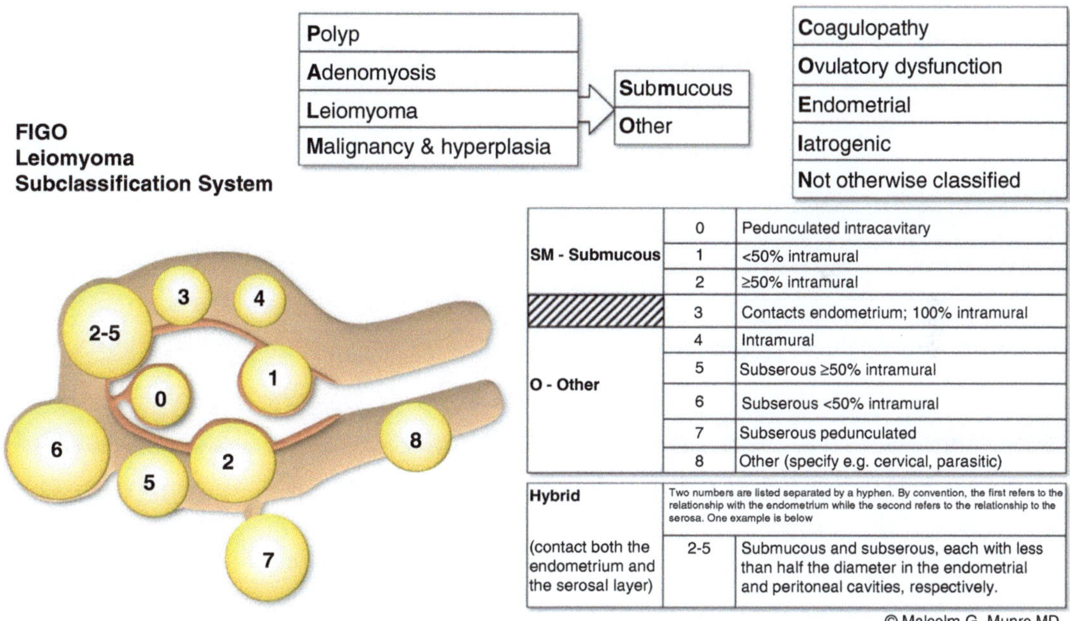

SM - Submucous	0	Pedunculated intracavitary
	1	<50% intramural
	2	≥50% intramural
	3	Contacts endometrium; 100% intramural
O - Other	4	Intramural
	5	Subserous ≥50% intramural
	6	Subserous <50% intramural
	7	Subserous pedunculated
	8	Other (specify e.g. cervical, parasitic)
Hybrid		Two numbers are listed separated by a hyphen. By convention, the first refers to the relationship with the endometrium while the second refers to the relationship to the serosa. One example is below
(contact both the endometrium and the serosal layer)	2-5	Submucous and subserous, each with less than half the diameter in the endometrial and peritoneal cavities, respectively.

© Malcolm G. Munro MD

Fig. 13.2 FIGO classification system for fibroids. (Reprinted with permission from Munro et al. [3])

While acknowledging that fibroids and uterine sarcomas have a similar appearance on imaging, and that it is unlikely that any given test will allow robust detection of sarcomas, Stewart [5] suggests the following imaging algorithm. If ultrasound depicts worrisome features (mixed echogenicity and hypoechoic regions; central necrosis; Doppler showing low resistance, high peak systolic velocity, and irregular distribution of vessels), move to contrast-enhanced MRI. Calcifications have been reported as being extremely rare in leiomyosarcomas, essentially ruling out the diagnosis [9]. A typical MRI appearance of a fibroid (homogeneously dark on T2-WI) has a high negative predictive value for LMS [10, 11]. Hemorrhage within a lesion is

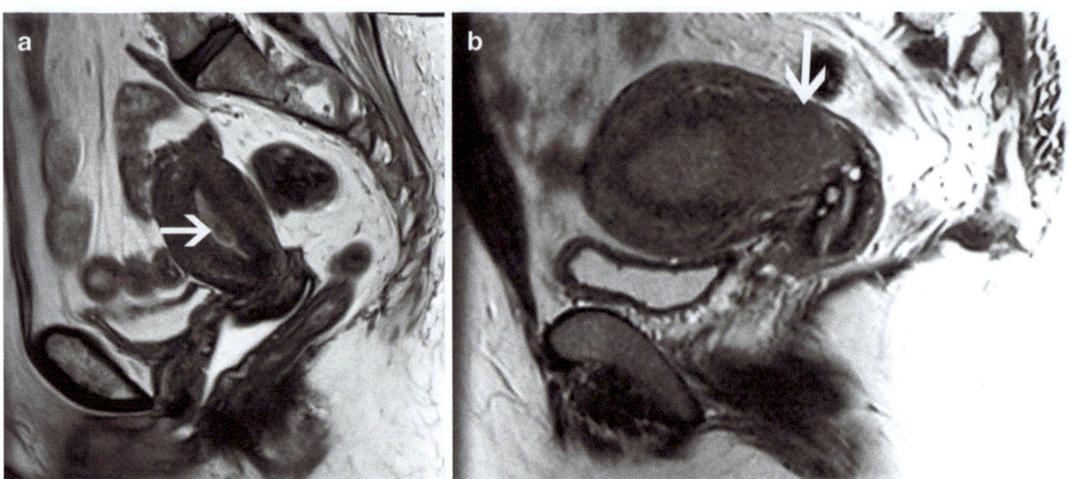

Fig. 13.3 Not a submucosal fibroid nor an endometrial polyp, but rather (**a**) a melanoma metastasis (arrow) (in a 29 yo) to the uterus and (**b**) advanced endometrial cancer (arrow) (in a 35 yo)

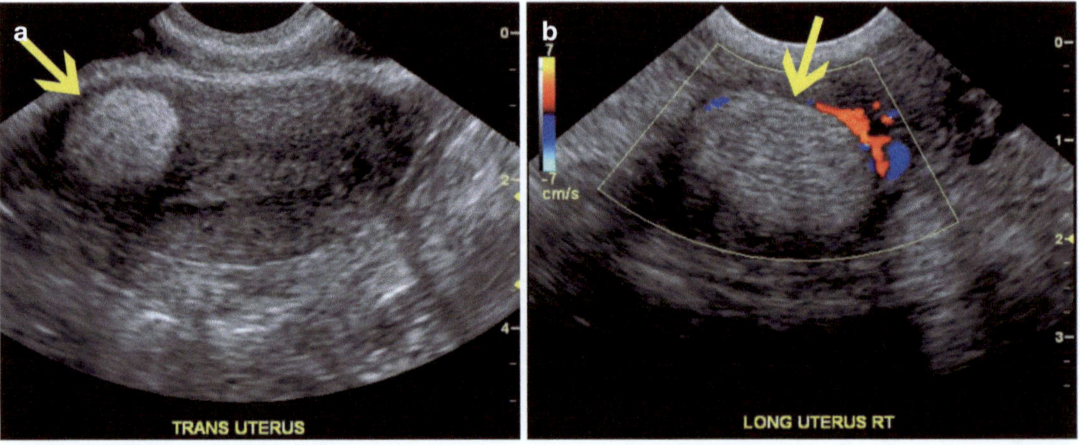

Fig. 13.4 Classic homogeneously echogenic avascular appearance of a lipoleiomyoma (arrow). TVUS transverse gray scale (**a**) and longitudinal CDU (**b**)

worrisome for LMS [10]. Diffusion weighted imaging (DWI) on MRI may help distinguish between typical and degenerating fibroids versus cellular leiomyomas and sarcomas [6, 10, 12–15]. The utility of PET to differentiate fibroid from LMS is mixed [6, 9, 16, 17]. It is important to remember that currently there are no pathognomonic features allowing reliable differentiation on any imaging technique [18].

There are various types of fibroids besides the common one, including cellular, mitotically active, atypical, and STUMP. Furthermore, myriad types of fibroid degeneration have been described, including cystic, hemorrhagic (carneous), lipoleiomyoma, hyaline, hydropic, myxoid, and coagulate necrosis. Imaging characterization of some of these entities is occasionally possible [19] (such as the characteristic US and MRI appearance of a lipoleiomyoma, Fig. 13.4). However, Arleo et al. concluded, "Nonetheless, the bottom line is that, at the present time, the diagnosis of a leiomyoma variant cannot be made with certainty until a pathologist, guided by recently updated 2014 World Health Organization criteria [20], thoroughly examines the specimen" [19].

The utility of various imaging techniques is reviewed below. Ultrasound and MRI are the mainstays in fibroid imaging.

Plain Films There is no role for plain films in the evaluation of potential uterine fibroids. However, fibroids may be suggested when pelvic calcifications are noted.

Computed Tomography (CT) Similarly, there is generally no utility for CT in the evaluation of potential uterine fibroids for preoperative planning (although calcified uterine fibroids are often seen incidentally during CT of the pelvis). CT is inferior to US and MRI for evaluation of the endometrium, myometrium, and adnexa. However, CT should be considered for other indications when global evaluation of the abdomen and pelvis is considered, for example, when looking for a drainable abscess or when worried about metastatic disease.

Hysterosalpingogram (HSG) Once the primary method to evaluate the endometrial cavity and uterus, HSG has long been surpassed in these arenas by US and MRI. HSG is essentially obsolete now for diagnostic uterine and endometrial evaluation, with the possible exception of assessing for tubal patency; however, even tubal patency is now starting to be performed with radiation-free ultrasound-based techniques using various tubal contrast agents [21–23]. HSG evaluation of the endometrial cavity has both false negative and false positive errors diagnostically, with a study by Wadhwa et al. [24] yielding a sensitivity and specificity of HSG in evaluating uterine cavity abnormalities of 45% and 87%, respectively, while corresponding values from the investigation by Acholonu et al. [25] were 58% and 26%. For example, hysteroscopy (considered the gold standard) may reveal synechiae, polyps, or myomas in substantial percentages of patients with normal HSGs, and conversely many women diagnosed as having an intrauterine filling defect by HSG will have a normal cavity by hysteroscopy. Even if a polypoid filling defect is seen at HSG, characterization (for example, between endometrial polyp and submucosal fibroid) is extremely difficult. Figure 13.5 shows two ~30-year-old REI patients with polypoid filling defects on tubal patency HSGs. The first (Fig. 13.5a) had an endometrial polyp, and the second (Fig. 13.5b) had endometrial cancer. Ultrasound, saline infusion sonohysterography (SIS), and MRI are much better than HSG at distinguishing between polyps, fibroids, cancer, air bubbles, etc.

Ultrasound Ultrasound alone (noting that transvaginal ultrasound should be performed routinely in all but very special cases) is good at detecting fibroids (Figs. 13.6 and 13.7), and has the advantages of being relatively inexpensive, well-tolerated, and without any ionizing radiation.

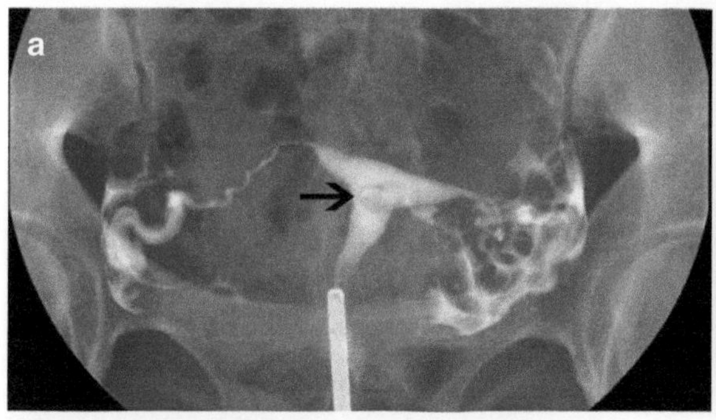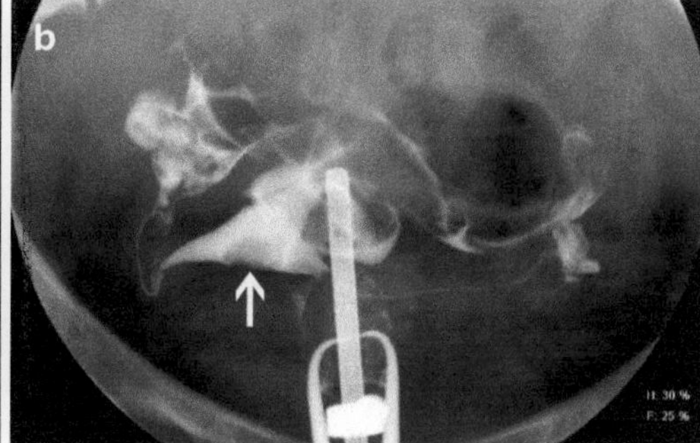

Fig. 13.5 The nonspecific nature of filling defects within the endometrial cavity as seen during HSG, illustrated in two patients undergoing HSG to assess tubal patency. The first (**a**) is a 32 yo; the filling defect (arrow) noted on the HSG turned out to be a benign endometrial polyp. The second (**b**) is a 35 yo; her filling defect represented endometrial cancer

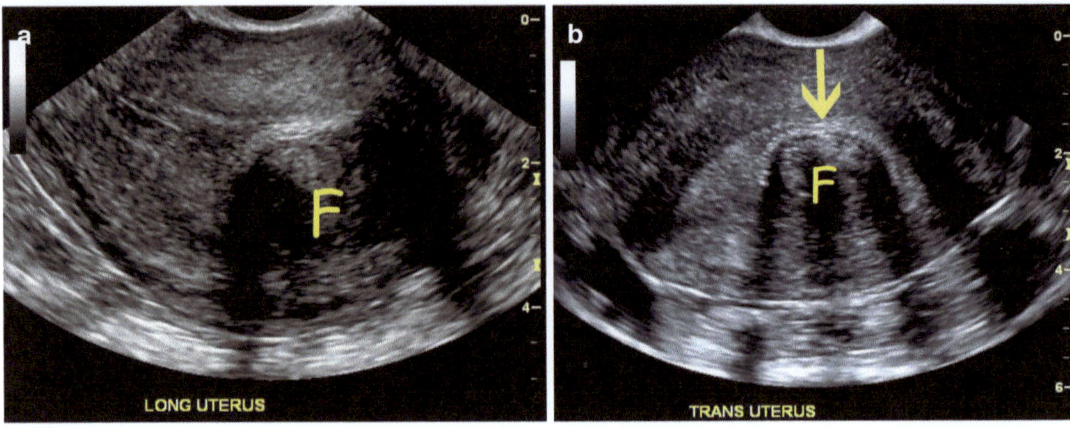

Fig. 13.6 Classic transvaginal US appearance ((**a**) longitudinal and (**b**) transverse) of a large submucosal fibroid ("F"). Note the displacement of the endometrium (arrow in **b**), and the fact that FIGO site classification may be difficult without SIS or MRI

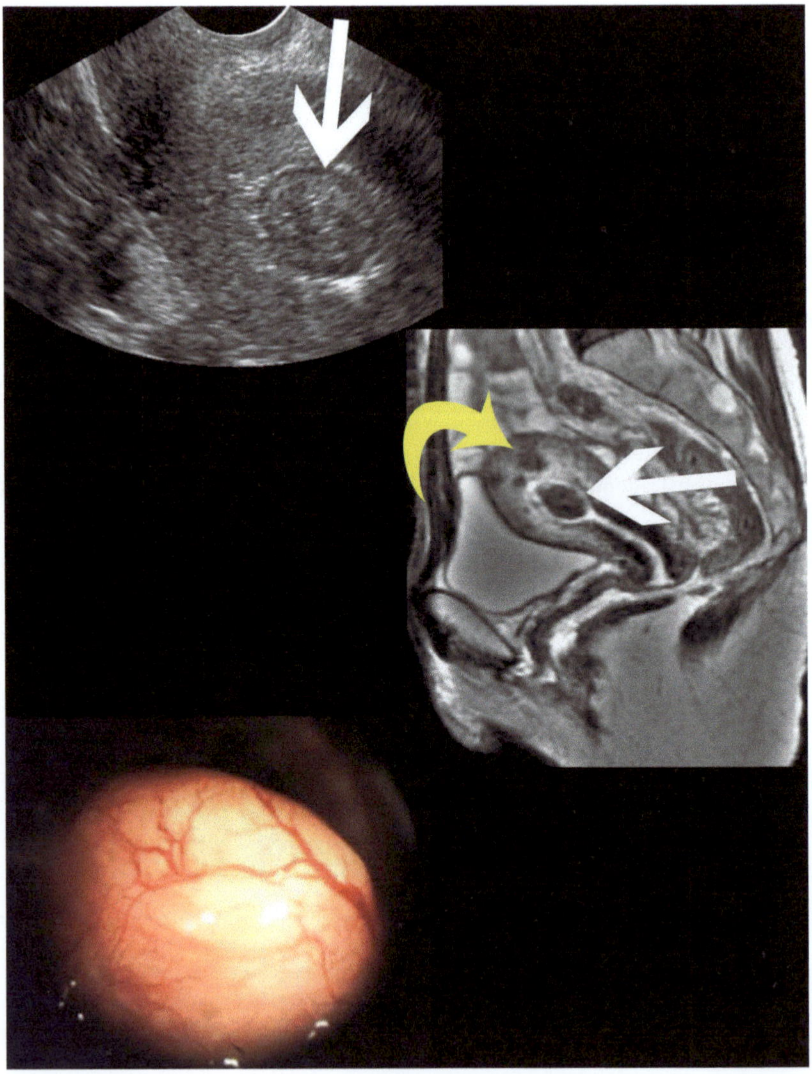

Fig. 13.7 Intracavitary fibroid at TVUS, MRI, and hysteroscopy. Note that the MR image shows three additional small intramural fibroids in the fundus that were not well seen at ultrasound (a curved yellow arrow denotes the largest of these three). (Reprinted with permission from Cooperberg [43])

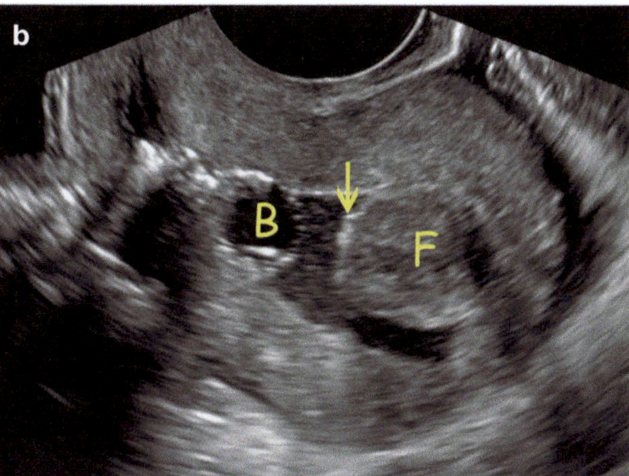

Fig. 13.8 Large type I intracavitary fibroid ("F") demonstrated on 3D ultrasound (**a**). However, please note how the true intracavitary relationship is better delineated on SIS (**b**) ("B" = SIS balloon, "F" = fibroid, and arrow denotes the thin cap of echogenic endometrium covering the more hypoechoic myometrium of the fibroid)

Fibroids usually present as comparatively well-defined, solid masses with a whorled appearance, relatively isoechoic to the rest of the myometrium, and typically with posterior acoustic shadowing [2]. 3D-ultrasound often provides an even more graphic display of fibroid site and position (Fig. 13.8). However, TVUS may be limited in large BMI individuals, in uteri that are in suboptimal position for US evaluation, and in uteri that are poorly seen due to obscuration by multiple, shadowing fibroids, adenomyosis, etc. Despite the widely acknowledged role of ultrasound in evaluating the endometrium, transvaginal ultrasound alone may not be adequate to fully evaluate endometrial abnormalities like submucosal fibroids and endometrial polyps [26–29].

Saline Infusion Sonohysterography First described by Nannini in 1981 [30], SIS provides a near optimum balance of cost, accessibility, and accuracy in the evaluation of women with submucosal fibroids: "The introduction of intracervical fluid (saline-infusion sonography) during transvaginal ultrasound is one of the most significant advances in ultrasonography of the past decade" [31].

The procedure has been referred to by a variety of names over time, including sonohysterography, hysterosonography, transvaginal sonography with fluid contrast augmentation, and saline infused sonography, but the underlying technique is straightforward [32]. If a balloon catheter is employed, which it often is not, the balloon may be inflated either in the endometrial cavity or within the cervix (with various pros and cons to each approach) [33, 34]. SIS performs well even in nonexpert hands [35, 36] and is considered as good as diagnostic hysteroscopy at detecting focal lesions in the uterine cavity, better tolerated, and has undeniable advantages in terms of time, cost, availability, convenience, risk of anesthesia and perforation, and the additional information provided regarding myometrium which is critical for surgical planning and adnexa over hysteroscopy [37]. An overall success rate of ~95% may be expected, although obviously this depends upon operator experience and patient factors [31]. Theoretical risks of potentially seeding malignancy [38] and causing endometriosis have not been borne out in widespread use, and the volume of fluid and pressure of instilled fluid in SIS are less than those needed in hysteroscopy. A 2015 consensus opinion attempted to standardize and define uterine fibroid imaging with ultrasound, aiming to help with both clinical practice and research [39]. These descriptive principles are equally relevant to MRI. SIS permits more accurate assessment of the extent of fibroid protrusion into the endometrial cavity than does US alone. Several examples of fibroids seen at SIS are given in Figs. 13.9, 13.10, 13.11, and 13.12.

Distinction between submucosal fibroids and other common endometrial pathologies such as polyps is usually possible, but may require direct visualization and biopsy in some cases. Fibroids are generally broad based, hypoechoic, with a thin hyperechoic cap/rim of overlying endometrium, more heterogeneous than fibroids, and often have multiple feeding vessels on color Doppler ultrasound (CDU). Endometrial polyps usually have a narrower base of attachment, are hyperechoic (matching the lining of the endometrial cavity in echogenicity), are more homogeneous, and often have only one feeding vessel at CDU. One must be aware of unusual entities that may present in the endometrium and inner myometrium as polypoid masses, including metastatic disease, especially from breast cancer. Also, note that fibroids can coexist with (and potentially obscure) endometrial cancer, even in REI age patients (Fig. 13.13).

Magnetic Resonance Imaging Pelvic MRI is the definitive "go-to" if one wishes to best define size, number, location, and site of uterine fibroids, particularly in the large BMI individual, or in a uterus with multiple fibroids, adenomyosis, IUD, suboptimal uterine position, etc., or anything that may potentially obscure ultrasound visualization [40]. For example, compare similarly sized large anterior lower uterine segment fibroids via US (Fig. 13.1c) vs. MRI (Fig. 13.1d); note how the anatomy is much better delineated with MRI. In certain scenarios, when US is not adequate, the more definitive assessment of size, number, location, and site of uterine fibroids provided by MRI may add clinical value. However, ultrasound (including SIS) may often be "good enough," more convenient, and readily available, and better use societal resources. Charges at our institution for a pelvic US (with TVUS) are $1700

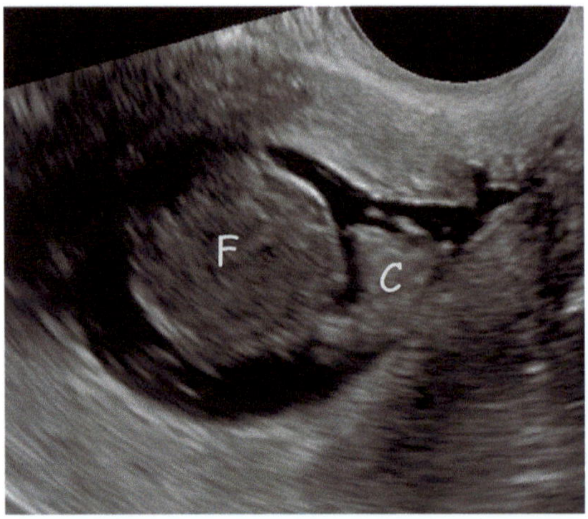

Fig. 13.9 Large intracavitary pedunculated fibroid ("F") with adjacent clot ("C"). The latter was mobile during the course of the SIS

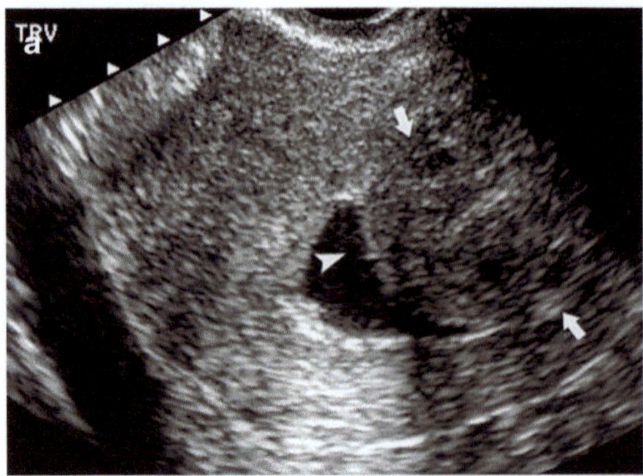
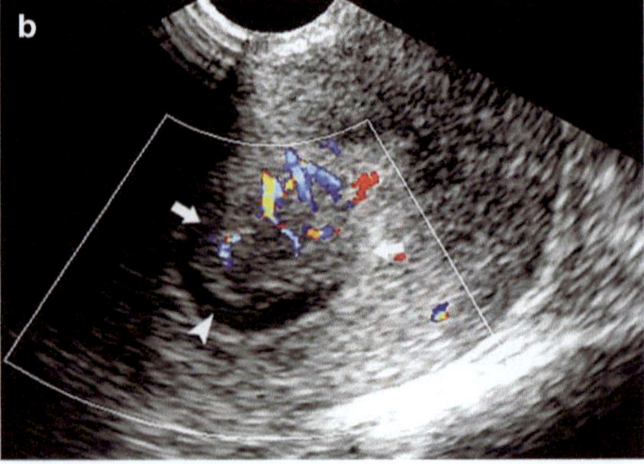

Fig. 13.10 Submucosal fibroid. Saline infusion sonohysterography shows a hypoechoic mass (arrows) with echogenic endometrium (arrowhead) draped over it. This is the typical appearance of a submucosal fibroid. (**a**), Gray scale image; (**b**), color Doppler image. (Reprinted with permission from Berridge and Winter [44])

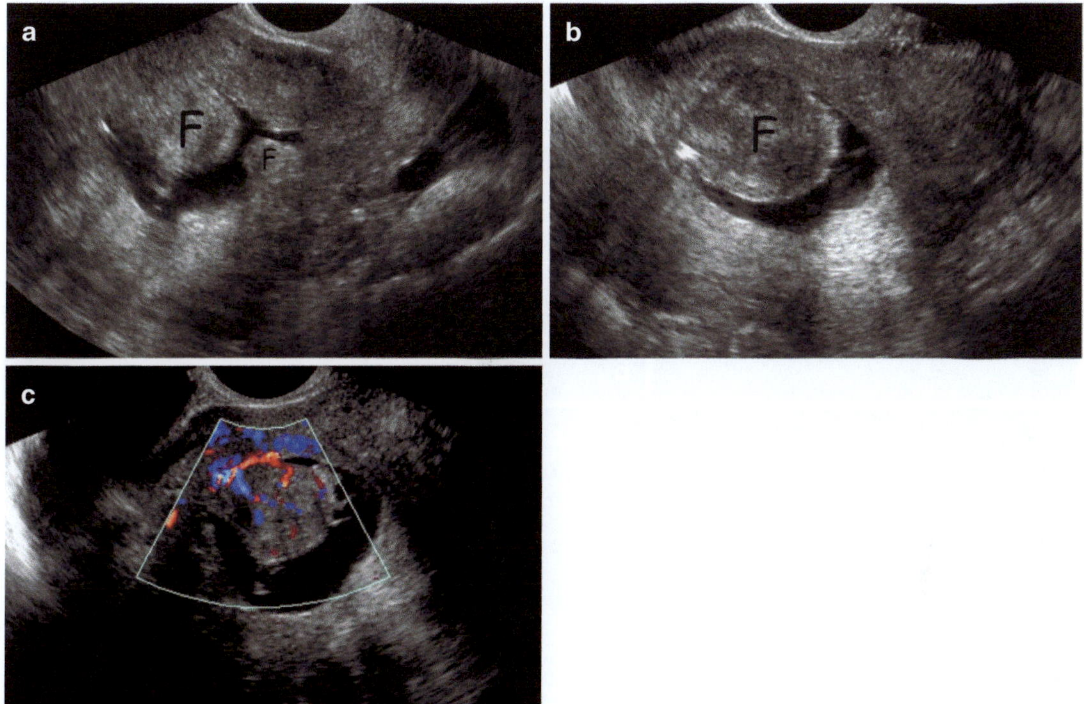

Fig. 13.11 Three SIS images from a 38 yo patient show multiple (**a**, **b**) fibroids ("F") projecting into the endometrial cavity. If more than 50% of the fibroid's surface projects into the endometrial cavity, it can be resected hysteroscopically. Note the multiple feeding vessels on the CDU (**c**) typical for fibroids, different than the single vessel commonly seen with an endometrial polyp. (Reprinted with permission from Berridge and Winter [44])

(hospital + professional, rounded to the nearest $100, and with the understanding that charges are a very imperfect metric for true costs); for an SIS $2700; and for a pelvic MRI $3000. Intravenous contrast (using one of a variety of gadolinium-based agents in the magnet) helps assess fibroid viability/necrosis, and is particularly useful if UAE is being contemplated or has been performed [41]. Start to finish, a pelvic MRI takes about 45–60 min. Attempts to combine the best features of SIS and MRI have been made, distending the uterine cavity with fluid via an indwelling catheter during the MRI and looking at tubal patency [42], but these have not entered widespread use due to a combination of technical difficulty, cost, and inconvenience. And, as always, one needs to be alert during pelvic MRI to the presence of unexpected findings that may change surgical management, e.g., worrisome adnexal masses that are not pedunculated fibroids,

non-fibroid pathology of the uterus as previously discussed, etc.

Normal uterine morphology at MRI on T2 weighted images (T2-WI) consists of high signal intensity endometrium, a thin surrounding dark band representing the junctional zone, with the remainder of the myometrium being intermediate in signal intensity. Fibroids as small as 5 mm [2] typically stand out extremely well as sharply demarcated dark (low signal intensity) masses against the intermediate normal myometrium. Cystic and myxoid degeneration often presents with areas of high T2 signal intensity (SI) within the fibroid. T1 weighted images are less useful in detecting fibroids (since fibroids tend to have similar signal intensity to normal myometrium on T1-WI), but have utility in characterizing degeneration and necrosis, particularly if intravenous gadolinium is administered. Carneous, red, and hemorrhagic degeneration often has high

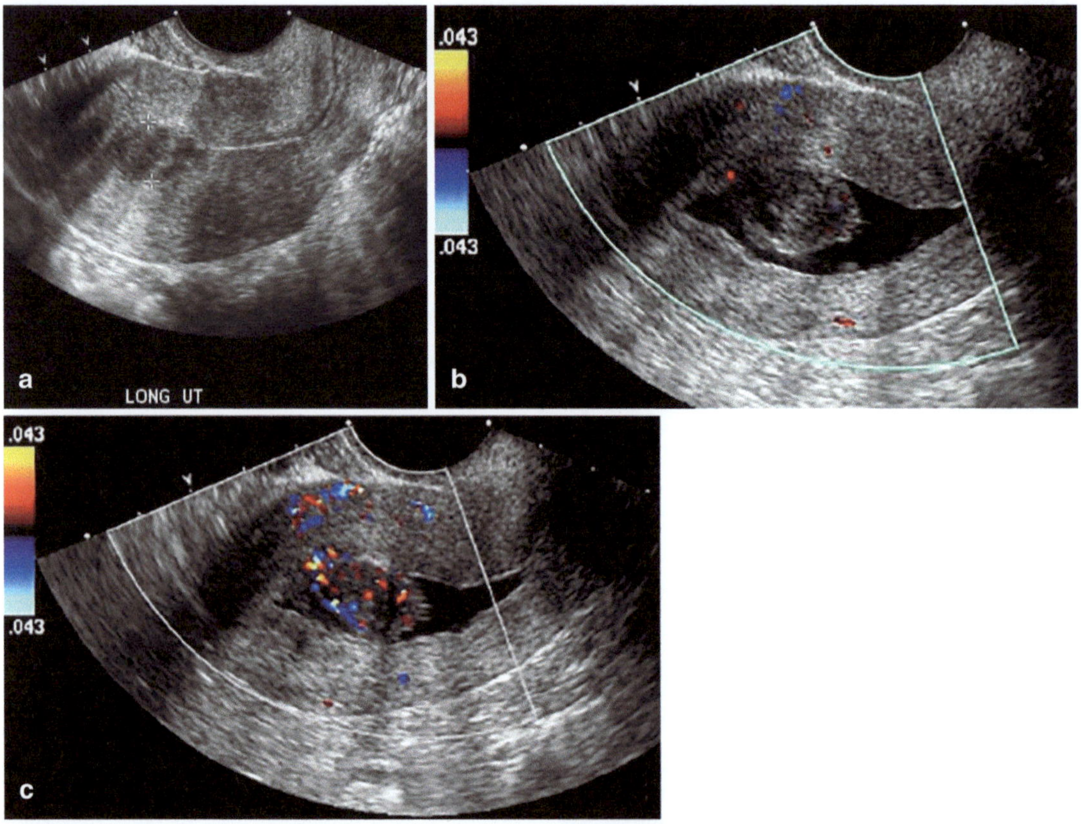

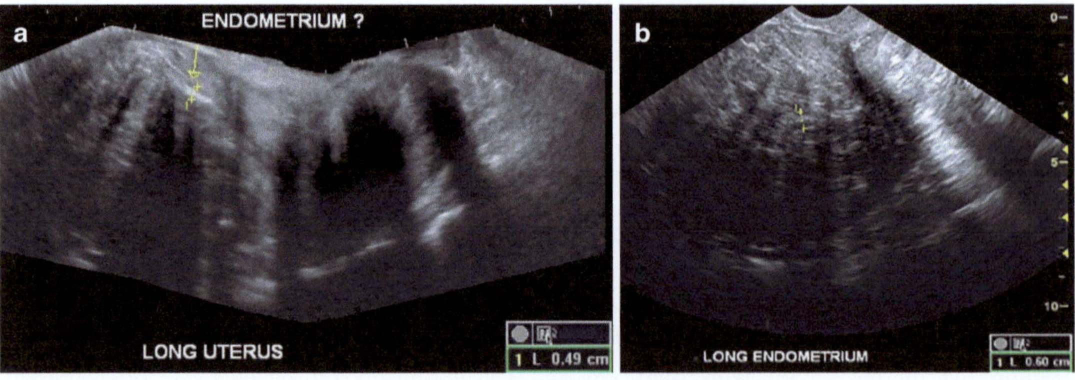

Fig. 13.12 Intracavitary fibroid on TVUS (**a**), followed by CDU images (**b**, **c**) obtained during SIS. Note how the fibroid's base of attachment and the extent of intracavitary protrusion are much better seen at SIS

Fig. 13.13 Fibroids obscuring a stage IIb endometrial cancer during TVUS. Extended field of view (**a**) and oblique longitudinal image (**b**). Note that the endometrial thickness was "measured," but obviously adequate evaluation of the endometrium and endometrial cavity cannot be obtained in a case like this

(bright) SI on T1 WI (but SI varies depending upon the age of the blood products). Multiplanar T2-WI is crucial in optimally determining fibroid location and site. Examples of uterine fibroids at pelvic MRI are seen in Figs. 13.14, 13.15, 13.16, and 13.17.

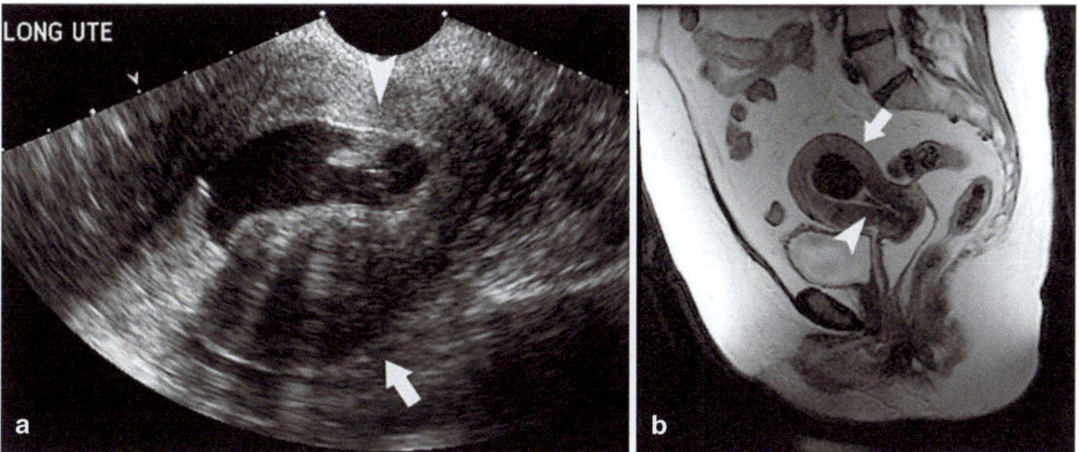

Fig. 13.14 Saline infusion sonohysterography and MRI of the pelvis show both a submucosal fibroid (arrow) and an endometrial polyp (arrowhead). (**a**), Gray scale SIS image; (**b**), MRI. Note how the MRI better depicts the predominantly intracavitary nature of the fibroid. (Reprinted with permission from Berridge and Winter [44])

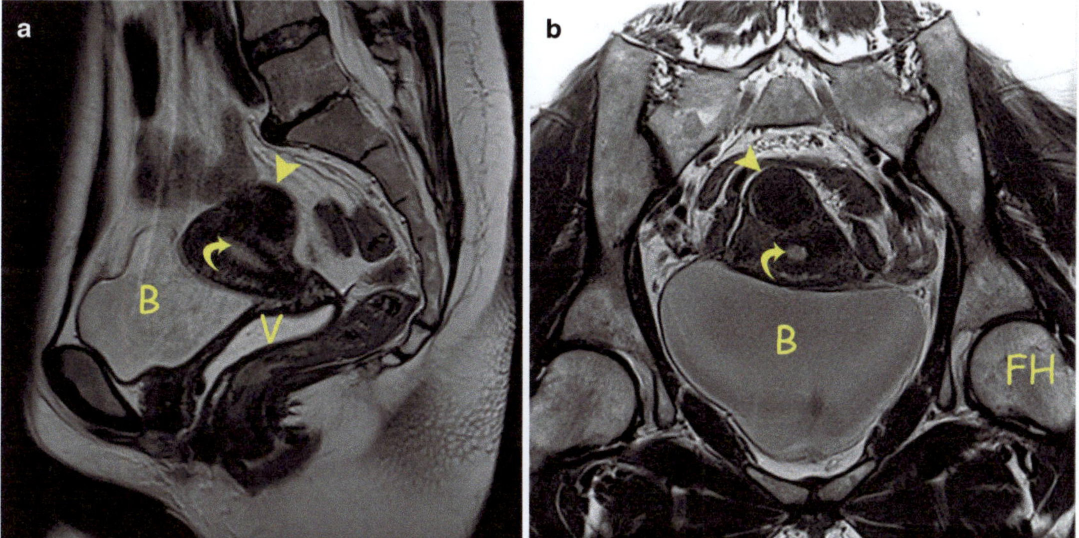

Fig. 13.15 The multiplanar capability of MRI is of great utility in fibroid assessment. (**a**) Sagittal T2-WI. Subserosal fibroid (yellow arrowhead) posterior to the bright endometrial cavity (curved yellow arrow) anteriorly. Also note the thin rim of dark junctional zone (not labeled) surrounding the endometrial cavity. "B" = urinary bladder, and "V" = high signal intensity gel placed immediately prior to the exam per vagina. (**b**) Oblique coronal ("short-axis") T2 WI. Custom prescribed imaging plane between the coronal and axial planes of the pelvis, this plane is true axial to the uterus and fibroid (yellow arrowhead). Curved yellow arrow again shows the high signal intensity normal endometrium. Note urinary bladder ("B") in midline, and femoral heads ("FH" denotes the left femoral head)

MRI can both predict and also assess the response of fibroids to uterine artery embolization (UAE), especially when intravenous gadolinium contrast is administered (Fig. 13.18). Pre-procedural fibroid high SI on T1-WI is a predictor of a poor response to UAE, while pre-

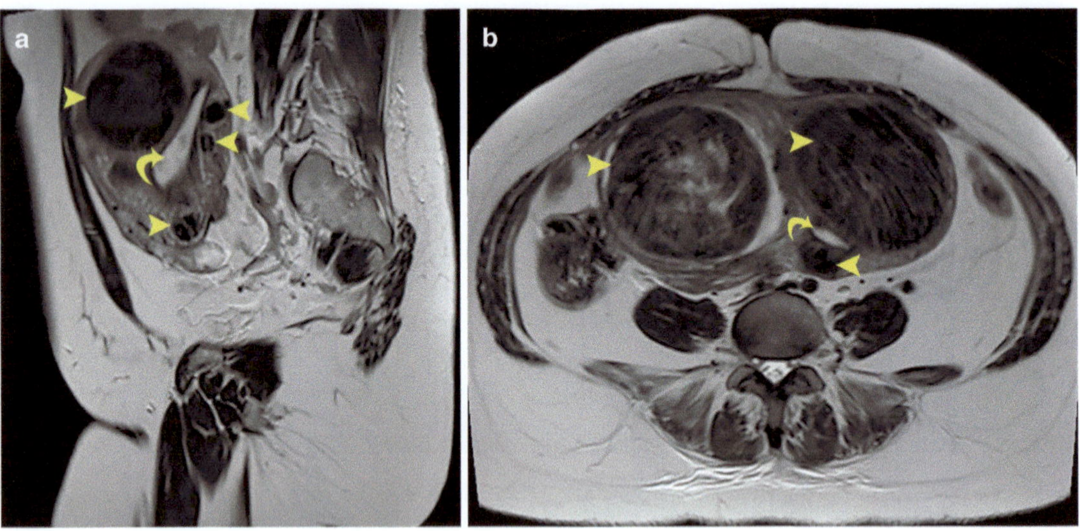

Fig. 13.16 Fibroids are multiple in as many as 84% of patients [2]. MRI can provide definitive fibroid number, size, location, and site. (**a**) Parasagittal T2-WI. One large and 3 additional smaller fibroids (yellow arrowheads) sur-round the bright endometrial cavity (curved yellow arrow). (**b**) Axial T2 WI. Two large and 1 additional smaller fibroid (yellow arrowheads) surround and dis-place the bright endometrial cavity (curved yellow arrow)

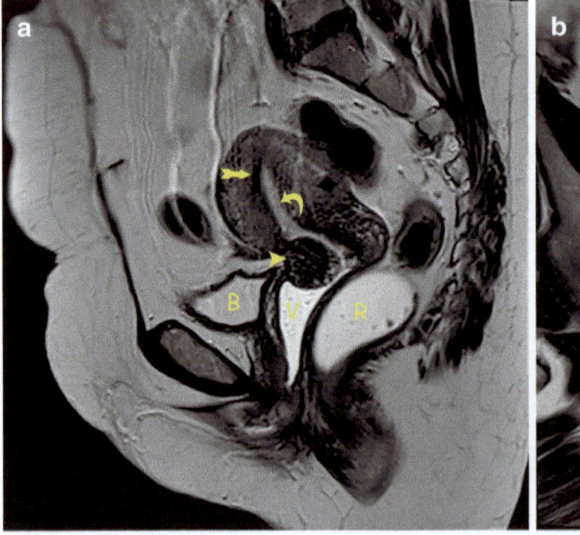
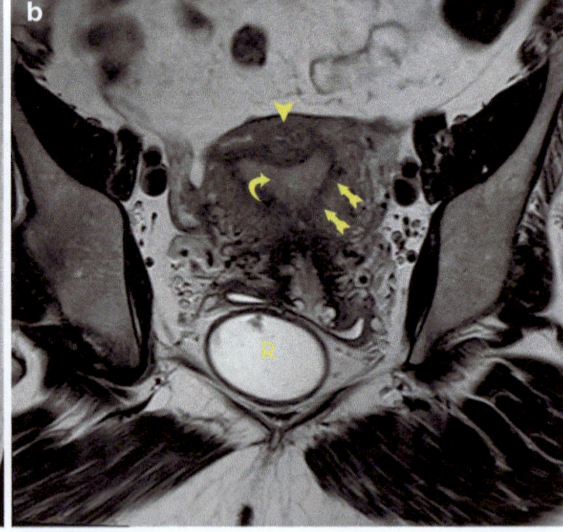

Fig. 13.17 Another example of multiple fibroids delin-eated at multiplanar imaging. One of the fibroids mimics an arcuate uterus. (**a**) Sagittal T2-WI. Low signal intensity anterior cervical fibroid (yellow arrowhead) nicely con-trasts with the bright endometrial cavity (curved yellow arrow). "B" = urinary bladder, "V" = high signal intensity gel placed immediately prior to the exam per vagina, and "R" = high signal intensity gel placed immediately prior to the exam per rectum (the latter is not routinely used for simple fibroid imaging). (**b**) Coronal T2 WI. Lower signal intensity fundal intramural fibroid (yellow arrowhead) might mimic an arcuate uterus at HSG or even ultrasound. The fibroid contrasts with the bright endometrial cavity (curved yellow arrow). Note the thin rim of dark junc-tional zone (yellow arrows) surrounding the endometrial cavity. "R" = high signal intensity gel placed immediately prior to the exam per rectum. (**c**) Axial T2 WI. Three low signal intensity intramural and subserosal fibroids (yellow arrowheads) contrast with the bright endometrial cavity (curved yellow arrow). Again note the thin rim of dark junctional zone (yellow arrows) surrounding the endome-trial cavity

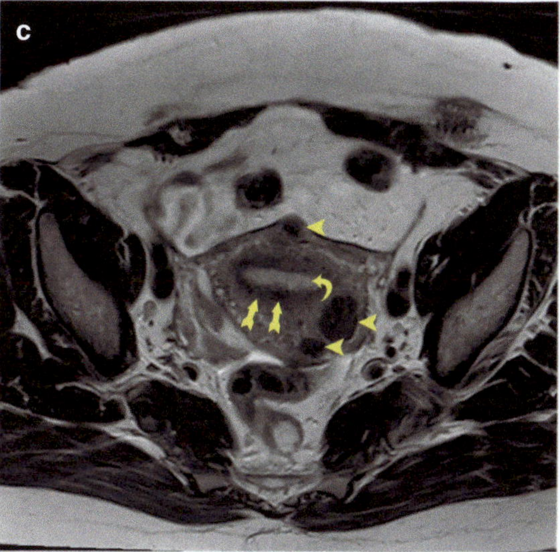

Fig. 13.17 (continued)

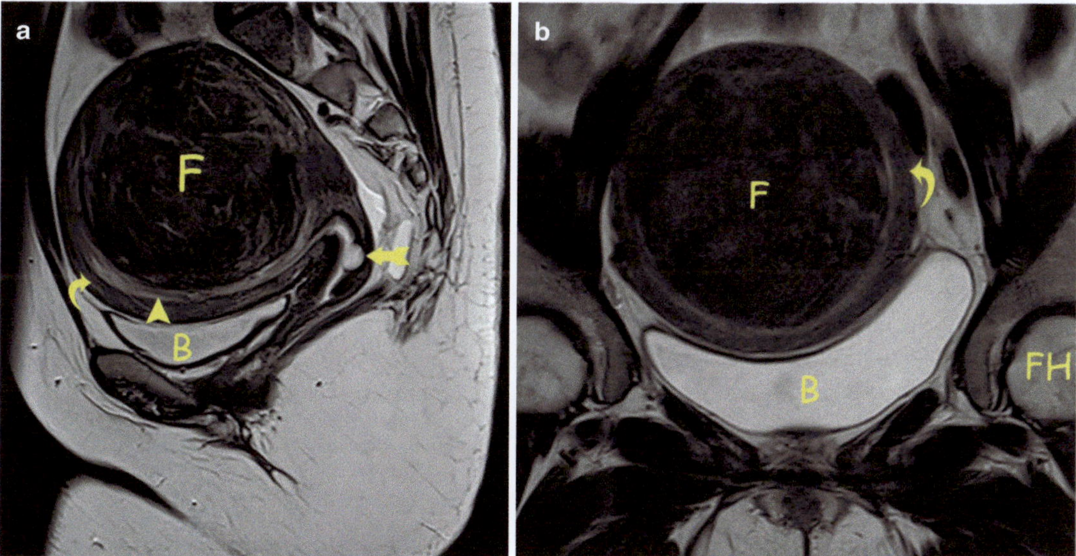

Fig. 13.18 Single large fibroid on MRI showing gadolinium contrast enhancement. (**a**) Sagittal T2-WI. Posterior intramural fibroid ("F") displaces the bright endometrial cavity (yellow arrowhead) anteriorly. Note how the fibroid, although heterogeneous, is darker (lower signal intensity) than the thin rim of normal myometrium (curved yellow arrow). "B" = urinary bladder. Yellow arrow denotes Nabothian cyst in the cervix, just posterior to the vertically oriented cervical canal. (**b**) Coronal T2 WI. Although coronal to the pelvis, this plane is axial to the uterine corpus, fundus, and dark fibroid ("F"). Curved yellow arrow again shows the slightly higher signal intensity normal myometrium. Note urinary bladder ("B") in midline, and femoral heads ("FH" denotes the left femoral head). (**c**) Sagittal T1 WI after the administration of intravenous gadolinium contrast. Posterior intramural fibroid ("F") displaces the dark endometrial cavity (yellow arrowhead) anteriorly. Note how the fibroid enhances less (lower signal intensity) and is more heterogeneous than the thin rim of normal myometrium (curved yellow arrow). Routine use of gadolinium may not help with fibroid detection, but is useful in the setting of UAE [2]

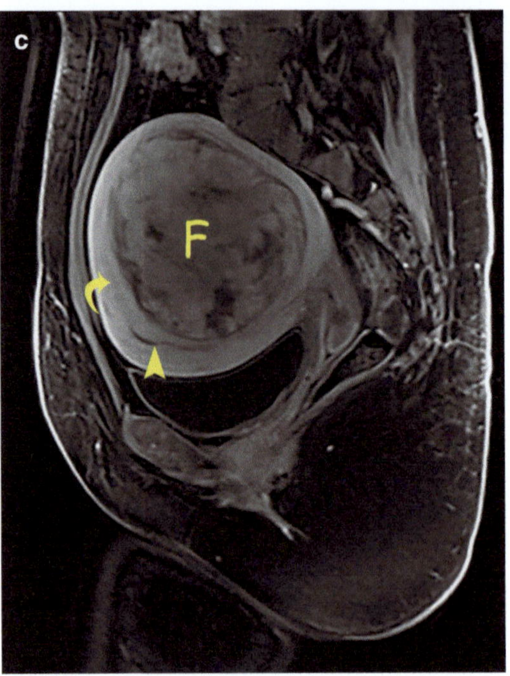

Fig. 13.18 (continued)

procedural fibroid high SI on T2-WI is a predictor of a good response to UAE [2]. Good contrast enhancement on T1-WI following intravenous gadolinium contrast administration prior to embolization is generally a predictor of a good response to UAE. MRI is also the guidance modality for the newer technique of noninvasive MRI-guided focused ultrasound ablation (AKA high-intensity focused ultrasound, HIFU), which directs very high energy ultrasound waves onto a fibroid, resulting in localized heating and cell death.

Hysteroscopy (HS) Obviously direct visualization with various and continually improving hysteroscopic fiberoptic technologies can play a role, but we focus on imaging evaluation in this chapter. Furthermore, ultrasound and MRI allow one to estimate depth of invasion into the myometrium (vide supra), something that is generally not robust with hysteroscopic techniques. To quote Bradley [31], "Compared with hysteroscopy, SIS more reliably predicts uterine fibroids' size and the depth of myometrial involvement."

Summary

The goal of preoperative fibroid imaging is to accurately assess fibroid size, number, position, and site to be able to offer optimal surgical management, and to ensure that no unexpected findings are present that will change the planned approach. Pelvic ultrasound (including TVUS) may be sufficient in very simple, uncomplicated cases. SIS provides much more definitive information. Pelvic MRI is the definitive "go-to" and may be used as a problem-solving tool in complex cases: multiple fibroids; when anatomy, particularly the relationship to the endometrium, is difficult to assess at ultrasound due to obscuration by shadowing fibroids, maternal habitus, or other factors; and when information about fibroid viability/necrosis (such as before and after UAE) is desired.

References

1. Stewart EA. Uterine fibroids. N Engl J Med. 2015;372(17):1646–55.
2. Wilde S, Scott-Barrett S. Radiological appearances of uterine fibroids. Indian J Radiol Imaging. 2009;19(3):222–31.
3. Munro MG, Critchley HOD, Fraser IS, Committee FMD. The two FIGO systems for normal and abnormal uterine bleeding symptoms and classification of causes of abnormal uterine bleeding in the reproductive years: 2018 revisions. Int J Gynaecol Obstet. 2018;143(3):393–408.
4. Bhagavath B, Ellie G, Griffiths KM, Winter T, Alur-Gupta S, Richardson C, et al. Uterine malformations: an update of diagnosis, management, and outcomes. Obstet Gynecol Surv. 2017;72(6):377–92.
5. Stewart E. Uterine fibroids (leiomyomas): differentiating fibroids from uterine sarcomas. In: Post T, editor. UpToDate. Waltham, MA: UpToDate; 2021.
6. DeMulder D, Ascher SM. Uterine leiomyosarcoma: can MRI differentiate leiomyosarcoma from benign leiomyoma before treatment? AJR Am J Roentgenol. 2018;211(6):1405–15.
7. Oh J, Park SB, Park HJ, Lee ES. Ultrasound features of uterine sarcomas. Ultrasound Q. 2019;35(4):376–84.
8. Rosenbaum L. N-of-1 policymaking — tragedy, trade-offs, and the demise of morcellation. N Engl J Med. 2016;374(10):986–90.
9. Van den Bosch T, Coosemans A, Morina M, Timmerman D, Amant F. Screening for uterine tumours. Best Pract Res Clin Obstet Gynaecol. 2012;26(2):257–66.

10. Thomassin-Naggara I, Dechoux S, Bonneau C, Morel A, Rouzier R, Carette MF, et al. How to differentiate benign from malignant myometrial tumours using MR imaging. Eur Radiol. 2013;23(8):2306–14.

11. Smith J, Zawaideh JP, Sahin H, Freeman S, Bolton H, Addley HC. Differentiating uterine sarcoma from leiomyoma: BET(1)T(2)ER check! Br J Radiol. 2021;94:20201332.

12. Tamai K, Koyama T, Saga T, Morisawa N, Fujimoto K, Mikami Y, et al. The utility of diffusion-weighted MR imaging for differentiating uterine sarcomas from benign leiomyomas. Eur Radiol. 2008;18(4):723–30.

13. Sun S, Bonaffini PA, Nougaret S, Fournier L, Dohan A, Chong J, et al. How to differentiate uterine leiomyosarcoma from leiomyoma with imaging. Diagn Interv Imaging. 2019;100(10):619–34.

14. Mendez RJ. MRI to differentiate atypical leiomyoma from uterine sarcoma. Radiology. 2020;297(2):372–3.

15. Abdel Wahab C, Jannot AS, Bonaffini PA, Bourillon C, Cornou C, Lefrere-Belda MA, et al. Diagnostic algorithm to differentiate benign atypical leiomyomas from malignant uterine sarcomas with diffusion-weighted MRI. Radiology. 2020;297(3):E347.

16. Kitajima K, Murakami K, Kaji Y, Sugimura K. Spectrum of FDG PET/CT findings of uterine tumors. AJR Am J Roentgenol. 2010;195(3):737–43.

17. Lakhman Y, Reinhold C. Malignant diseases of the uterus. In: Hodler J, Kubik-Huch RA, von Schulthess GK, editors. Diseases of the abdomen and pelvis 2018–2021: diagnostic imaging. Cham (CH): IDKD Book; 2018. p. 197–206.

18. Serno J, Meinhold-Heerlein I, Schrading S, Papathemelis T. Does any imaging method allow distinguishing between myoma and sarcoma? Curr Obstet Gynecol Rep. 2015;4(3):149–51.

19. Arleo EK, Schwartz PE, Hui P, McCarthy S. Review of leiomyoma variants. Am J Roentgenol. 2015;205(4):912–21.

20. Kurman R, Carcangiu M, Herrington C, Young R. WHO classification of tumours of female reproductive organs. 4th ed. Lyon, France: International Agency for Research on Cancer; 2014.

21. Luong E, Ludwin A, Winter T, Yaklic J, Maxwell RA, Bhagavath B, et al. Saline-air hysterosalpingo-contrast sonography is equivalent to the modified hysterosalpingogram following hysteroscopic sterilization. Ultrasound Q. 2020;36(2):138–45.

22. Robertshaw IM, Sroga JM, Batcheller AE, Martinez AM, Winter TC 3rd, Sinning K, et al. Hysterosalpingo-contrast sonography with a saline-air device is equivalent to hysterosalpingography only in the presence of tubal patency. J Ultrasound Med. 2016;35(6):1215–22.

23. van Rijswijk J, van Welie N, Dreyer K, van Hooff MHA, de Bruin JP, Verhoeve HR, et al. The FOAM study: is Hysterosalpingo foam sonography (HyFoSy) a cost-effective alternative for hysterosalpingography (HSG) in assessing tubal patency in subfertile women? Study protocol for a randomized controlled trial. BMC Womens Health. 2018;18(1):64.

24. Wadhwa L, Rani P, Bhatia P. Comparative prospective study of hysterosalpingography and hysteroscopy in infertile women. J Hum Reprod Sci. 2017;10(2):73–8.

25. Acholonu UC, Silberzweig J, Stein DE, Keltz M. Hysterosalpingography versus sonohysterography for intrauterine abnormalities. JSLS. 2011;15(4):471–4.

26. Laifer-Narin S, Ragavendra N, Parmenter EK, Grant EG. False-normal appearance of the endometrium on conventional transvaginal sonography: comparison with saline hysterosonography. AJR Am J Roentgenol. 2002;178(1):129–33.

27. Maheux-Lacroix S, Li F, Laberge PY, Abbott J. Imaging for polyps and leiomyomas in women with abnormal uterine bleeding. Obstet Gynecol. 2016;128(6):1425–36.

28. Neele SJ, Marchien van Baal W, van der Mooren MJ, Kessel H, Netelenbos JC, Kenemans P. Ultrasound assessment of the endometrium in healthy, asymptomatic early post-menopausal women: saline infusion sonohysterography versus transvaginal ultrasound. Ultrasound Obstet Gynecol. 2000;16(3):254–9.

29. Ragni G, Diaferia D, Vegetti W, Colombo M, Arnoldi M, Crosignani PG. Effectiveness of sonohysterography in infertile patient work-up: a comparison with transvaginal ultrasonography and hysteroscopy. Gynecol Obstet Investig. 2005;59(4):184–8.

30. Nannini R, Chelo E, Branconi F, Tantini C, Scarselli GF. Dynamic echohysteroscopy: a new diagnostic technique in the study of female infertility. Acta Eur Fertil. 1981;12(2):165–71.

31. Bradley L. Assessment of abnormal uterine bleeding: 3 office-based tools. OBG Manag. 2003;15:51–66.

32. Lindheim SR, Sprague C, Winter TC 3rd. Hysterosalpingography and sonohysterography: lessons in technique. AJR Am J Roentgenol. 2006;186(1):24–9.

33. Ahmadi F, Jahangiri N, Zafarani F, Vosough A. Pain perception and side effects during saline infusion sonohysterography with a balloon catheter: a randomized comparative study of cervical versus intrauterine catheter placement. J Ultrasound Med. 2020;39(9):1829–37.

34. Spieldoch RL, Winter TC, Schouweiler C, Ansay S, Evans MD, Lindheim SR. Optimal catheter placement during sonohysterography: a randomized controlled trial comparing cervical to uterine placement. Obstet Gynecol. 2008;111(1):15–21.

35. Dueholm M, Forman A, Jensen ML, Laursen H, Kracht P. Transvaginal sonography combined with saline contrast sonohysterography in evaluating the uterine cavity in premenopausal patients with abnormal uterine bleeding. Ultrasound Obstet Gynecol. 2001;18(1):54–61.

36. Parker JD, Alvero RJ, Luterzo J, Segars JH, Armstrong AY. Assessment of resident competency in the performance of sonohysterography: does the level of training impact the accuracy? Am J Obstet Gynecol. 2004;191(2):582–6.

37. Epstein E, Ramirez A, Skoog L, Valentin L. Transvaginal sonography, saline contrast sonohysterography and hysteroscopy for the investigation of women with postmenopausal bleeding and endometrium > 5 mm. Ultrasound Obstet Gynecol. 2001;18(2):157–62.
38. Berry E, Lindheim SR, Connor JP, Hartenbach EM, Schink JC, Harter J, et al. Sonohysterography and endometrial cancer: incidence and functional viability of disseminated malignant cells. Am J Obstet Gynecol. 2008;199(3):240.e1–.e8.
39. Van den Bosch T, Dueholm M, Leone FP, Valentin L, Rasmussen CK, Votino A, et al. Terms, definitions and measurements to describe sonographic features of myometrium and uterine masses: a consensus opinion from the Morphological Uterus Sonographic Assessment (MUSA) group. Ultrasound Obstet Gynecol. 2015;46(3):284–98.
40. Dueholm M, Lundorf E, Hansen ES, Ledertoug S, Olesen F. Evaluation of the uterine cavity with magnetic resonance imaging, transvaginal sonography, hysterosonographic examination, and diagnostic hysteroscopy. Fertil Steril. 2001;76(2):350–7.
41. Jha RC, Ascher SM, Imaoka I, Spies JB. Symptomatic fibroleiomyomata: MR imaging of the uterus before and after uterine arterial embolization. Radiology. 2000;217(1):228–35.
42. Sadowski EA, Ochsner JE, Riherd JM, Korosec FR, Agrawal G, Pritts EA, et al. MR hysterosalpingography with an angiographic time-resolved 3D pulse sequence: assessment of tubal patency. AJR Am J Roentgenol. 2008;191(5):1381–5.
43. Cooperberg P. The endometrium looks thick: what does that mean? In: Cooperberg P, Charboneau J, Winter T, editors. 2002 syllabus: categorical course in diagnostic radiology: findings at US –what do they mean? Oak Brook, IL: RSNA; 2002. p. 39–46.
44. Berridge DL, Winter TC. Saline infusion sonohysterography: technique, indications, and imaging findings. J Ultrasound Med. 2004;23(1):97–112; quiz 4–5.

Image-Based Surgery: Treating Fibroids You Can't See

14

Victoria S. Jiang and John C. Petrozza

Introduction

Over the last 100 years, gynecologic surgery has experienced an exponential growth of new procedures and surgical techniques thanks to developing technologies. Ultrasound technology has become a mainstay and gold standard for pelvic organ evaluation. With a gynecologic surgeon performing the first successful appendectomy (source), the integration of laparoscopy to general practice has been met with continual innovation, as new techniques, visualization methods, and imaging have led to improved patient outcomes and decreased patient morbidity and mortality. Laparoscopy has transformed surgical recovery from multiple days to same-day discharge and reduced blood loss for the same procedures historically done through large incisions. Paired with advancements in imaging, surgical visualization, preoperative planning, and intraoperative decision making has been revolutionized. We discuss the origins of ultrasound, and how new innovations in image processing and visualization in gynecologic surgery allow surgeons to have the vision to make decisions that improve patient care and outcomes.

V. S. Jiang · J. C. Petrozza (✉)
Department of Obstetrics and Gynecology, Division of Reproductive Endocrinology and Infertility, Massachusetts General Hospital, Harvard Medical School, Boston, MA, USA
e-mail: jpetrozza@mgh.harvard.edu

History of Ultrasound Imaging

The journey to our modern-day ultrasound technology began initially in the early nineteenth century with the characterization of sound. The speed of sound was first described in 1826 by Jean-Daniel Colladon, a Swiss physicist, at the Academie Royale de Science of Paris [1, 2]. Through a series of experiments involving an underwater bell and underwater ballistics in Lake Geneva, Colladon was credited with the birth of modern underwater acoustic science [1, 2]. These fundamental experiments were expanded upon by John William Strutt, who published *The Theory of Sound* in 1877, which became the foundation of ultrasound science. Shortly thereafter, in 1880, Jacques and Pierre Curie observed that an electric charge was generated proportional to the pressure that was applied to crystals of quartz or Rochelle salt, termed "piezoelectricity" [2, 3]. They also demonstrated that the crystal would vibrate if a rapidly changing electric potential was applied [2]. This principle serves as the basis for the use of piezoelectric crystals within modern ultrasound transducers that interconvert electric and mechanical energy [2].

These advances in underwater acoustics lead to interests in ocean floor mapping with echosounding. The sinking of the Titanic on April 15, 1912, paired with public outcry of the event lead to English meteorologist L. F. Richardson's research in airborne and ultrasonic underwater detection systems, and Canadian inventor Reginald Fessenden's electromagnetic moving-coil arrangement for iceberg detection [1, 2]. With growing international tensions, World War I lead to an international race in expanding underwater detection and mapping to advance naval efforts in identifying submarines and German U-boats [2]. Russian expatriate Constantin Chilowsky collaborated with French physicist Paul Langevin to pioneer the hydrophone [4] and the pulse-echo principle of Sound Navigating and Ranging (SONAR), which involved generating and receiving ultrasound waves [2]. SONAR became increasingly useful and popular for not only naval superiority but also industrial applications, with simultaneous research being conducted in many countries internationally. While most of the funding was exhausted with the end of World War I, Donald Sproule revolutionized the field with the first echo-sounder for the Royal Navy, which not only mapped the sea floor but also inadvertently detected the schools of fish along the way [5]. World War II revived interests in the development of ultrasound acoustics and transducers [2]. With the growing need for metal shipping hulls, ultrasound technology was optimized by industrial manufacturers for metal flaw detection, culminating in Tom Brown and Ian Donald developing the first handheld contact ultrasound device in the post-war era [2].

The advent of SONAR inspired the extension of ultrasonography to medical applications in the late 1930s. Karl Theodore Dussik, a neurologist and psychiatrist, alongside his brother Friederich Dussik initially used a 1.5 MHz transmitter to attempt to characterize the human brain and describe brain tumors. Unfortunately, the brothers were ultimately unsuccessful, as the variations in these "hyperphonograms" were likely due to bone thickness, setting back medical ultrasound development and funding for the next decade [5–7]. Medical research was also slowed from the fear of ultrasound to be destructive in nature. Supersonic sound experiments caused pain to the observer's hand and harmed schools of fish. In 1944, TJ Putnam and JG Lynn attempted and ultimately abandoned the of use

ultrasound as a neurosurgical tool alongside craniotomy for the destruction of brain tissue in Parkinson's disease [5].

Pursuit of medical applications continued with George D. Ludwig at the Naval Medical Research Institute. In collaboration with Francis Struthers and Horace Trent at the Naval Research Laboratory, and Ivan Greenwood at General Precision Laboratories, Ludwig used beef models and canine gallbladders to measure the impedance of ultrasound on soft tissue and was able to conduct in vivo experiments that examined implanted gall stones in muscle and canine gall bladder tissue [2, 8, 9]. This work, initially published in 1950 served as the basis for John Julian Wild and Douglass Howry, leaders in the field of early ultrasound.

During World War II, Wild was a notable surgeon who treated many soldiers that suffered spinal cord blast injuries that developed paralytic ileus. He used A-mode ultrasound imaging with a 15 MHz transducer to examine the layers of the small intestine to distinguish ileus from small bowel obstruction [2]. By examining changes in echogenicity between benign and malignant tissue [10, 11], Wild used ultrasound imaging to aid diagnosis of gastric cancer [10], a thigh tumor, and breast cancer [12]. While his published 1952 findings were hard to replicate due to the operator-dependent nature of ultrasound, he persevered in finding clinical applications within the field. He was credited with developing a scanning device to screen patients for breast cancer, the transrectal and transvaginal transducers, and contributing significantly to the development of two-dimensional ultrasonography [2].

Simultaneously, Howry applied ultrasound theory to develop ultrasound machines and related equipment within the field of radiology. Working through the Denver University Hospital with W. Roderic Bliss, Howry created the first B-mode scanner in 1949, a cumbersome machine that required a large water tank coupling system with a mounted transducer, a first of its kind to consistently provide accurate, reproducible results [2]. After several years of prototypes, attempts to remove shadowing, and collaborations, he was able to decouple the ultrasound machine from the water system in the late 1950s [2]. In 1961, he partnered with W. Wright and E Meyers to form Physionics Engineering which produced the first handheld contact scanner in the United States [13].

In 1955, Ian Donald, an obstetrician/gynecologist at the University of Glasgow who was familiar with SONAR and radar equipment from his Royal Air Force experience in World War II (42), applied A-mode ultrasound to differentiate between different types of tissues such as excised fibroids and ovarian cysts [2]. After developing the first contact compound scanner with gynecologist John McVicar, Donald published a landmark article in June 1958, "Investigation of Abdominal Masses by Pulsed Ultrasound," describing the use of ultrasound in diagnosis of a patient with a large mucinous ovarian cyst [14]. During his experiments, he found that a full urinary bladder provided an ideal natural acoustic window to improve transabdominal ultrasound evaluation of pelvic structures [14]. While at the University of Glasgow, Donald's contributions to the field were invaluable to the medical integration of ultrasound as a diagnostic tool in obstetrics and gynecology, visualizing small pelvic tumors, ectopic pregnancies, placentation locations, and being the first to measure fetal biparietal diameter for fetal growth.

Integrating Ultrasound into Gynecology

With the creation of handheld ultrasound probes, smaller ultrasound machines, and commercially available technology, ultrasound has made an invaluable impact on the field of the gynecology. Ultrasound has become the gold standard in evaluation of pelvic anatomy due to its ease of access, accuracy in characterizing pelvic organs, lack of radiation, and cost-effectiveness. With many clinics performing in-office ultrasounds, the use of ultrasound has become universal in both medical training and practice. As growing comfort in using this technology has expanded over the last 40 years, the use of ultrasound in gynecologic procedures and surgery is a natural extension of

the diagnostic in-office use. Continual development of different types of ultrasound probes has contributed to expanding its value as an adjunct in surgery. Two main avenues that have seamlessly integrated ultrasound include fertility treatment and fibroid care.

Outside of diagnostics, ultrasound was first described for use in fertility treatments such as assisted reproductive technology (ART) in 1987 [15]. Prior to ultrasound-guided oocyte aspiration, in vitro fertilization (IVF) was conventionally performed in the hospital with laparoscopic retrieval of oocytes under general anesthesia, which was cost-prohibitive to many patients especially in the context of need for repetitive cycles before successful live birth. Schulman et al. described performing oocyte retrieval under local anesthesia with transvaginal ultrasound-guided needle aspiration under local anesthesia, which revolutionized practice and cost efficiency. In this cohort of women, while not all women went to retrieval, the pregnancy rates were 26% per transfer, 16% per retrieval, and 13% per cycle started, with 9% continuing pregnancy and 10% infants per cycle initiated [15]. These rates were comparable to the time, with 10–20% live birth rate reported by the top, most successful institutions at that time [15]. This approach was subsequently universally accepted, and opened the door to outpatient oocyte aspiration, the gold standard method of retrieval today.

Alongside oocyte retrieval, ultrasound-guided embryo transfer served as another major landmark in the use of ultrasound imaging in ART. Stickler et al. [16] first described using transabdominal ultrasound to assist with embryo transfer in 1985. In 1997, Woolcott and Stanger [17] described that by using transabdominal ultrasound during embryo transfer, they were able to better visualize the path of the transfer catheter during embryo transfers. They found that the outer guiding cannula indented the endometrium in 17.4% of transfers, the transfer catheter abutted the fundal endometrium in 24.8% of transfers, the transfer catheter embedded in the endometrium in 33.1% of transfers, and accidental tubal transfer occurred in 7.4% of embryo transfers [17]. A hallmark study by Tang et al. in

2001 reported a prospective randomized controlled trial of 800 embryo transfers that compared clinical touch to transabdominal ultrasound-guided approach. While there was no significant difference in pregnancy rates between clinical touch and transabdominal ultrasound-guided embryo transfers, a slight improvement was seen of the pregnancy rate in the ultrasound group comparatively. Implantation rate, however, was significantly higher, improving from 12% in the clinical touch group to 15.3% in the ultrasound-guided group, with no difference in overall ectopic rates [18]. The authors posited that pregnancy rates are likely more affected by the specific catheter and techniques of individual clinicians, whereas ultrasound guidance can help with verification of the catheter placement and subsequent transfer.

Outside of ART, ultrasound has been serving as a used adjunctive surgical tool in seeking and treating myomas during laparoscopic myomectomy. Intraoperative ultrasound use during laparoscopic myomectomy was first described by Lin et al. in 2004. Use in gynecologic surgery with a laparoscopic ultrasound transducer was a natural extension of use in other surgical areas such as partial nephrectomy, particle liver resection, gallbladder surgery, and breast surgery. Lin et al. [19] initially described a case report involving a 44-year-old female with unexplained secondary infertility and a 2 cm intramural myoma noted with distortion of the endometrial cavity. At the time of laparoscopy, the fibroid was not able to be visualized due to normal-appearing uterine contour from size and location. Given limited tactile feedback from laparoscopic approach, the laparoscopic ultrasound transducer, which fits through a 12-mm port, was used to visualize the myoma and led to accurate subsequent resection [19]. Since this first case report, intraoperative ultrasound was evaluated by Angioli et al. [20], who evaluated its utility in 64 consecutive laparoscopic myomectomy cases. In this population, they showed that for patients with more than 6 fibroids, preoperative ultrasound efficiency was significantly

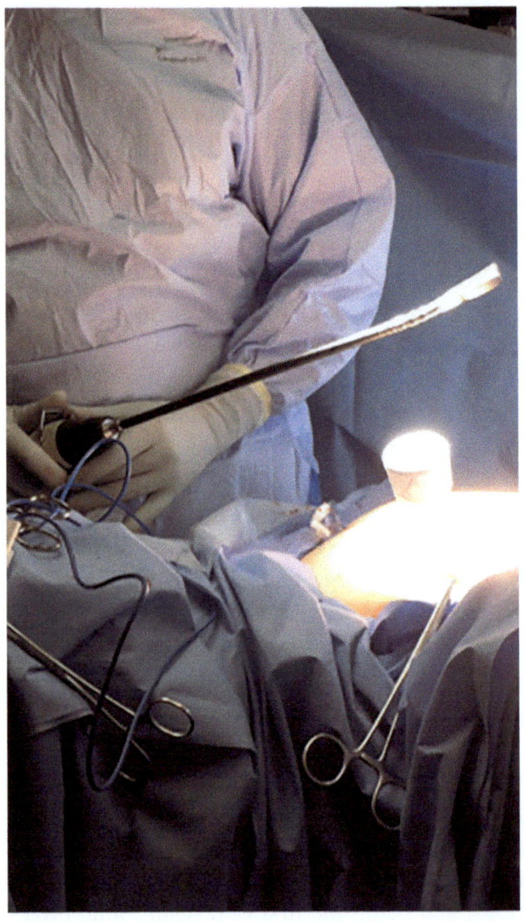

Fig. 14.1 Laparoscopic ultrasound transducer

decreased [20]. Additionally, after initial myomas were resected, residual fibroids were palpated, then subsequently underwent laparoscopic ultrasound. The mean number of residual fibroids noted with intraoperative ultrasound compared to intraoperative palpation was higher [20]. This study confirmed the usefulness of applying intraoperative laparoscopic ultrasound during laparoscopic myomectomy (Figs. 14.1 and 14.2).

Ultrasound technology has also been developed to try to integrate intraoperative ultrasound into abdominal procedures. Finger-grip 7.5 MHz ultrasounds with sterile sleeves have been developed for transabdominal procedures to maintain sterility during transabdominal procedures, with use reported in case series [21]. The use of this

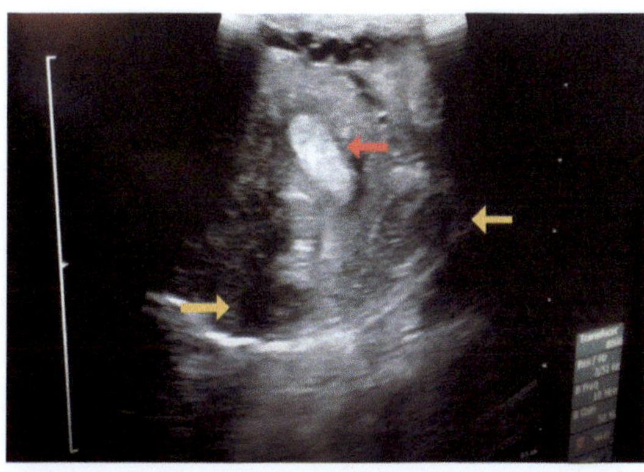

Fig. 14.2 Laparoscopic ultrasound image; red arrow—endometrium; white arrows—residual fibroids

finger-grip ultrasound can be useful in guiding dissection and tracking instruments in complex gynecologic surgery for both myomectomy and obstructive Mullerian abnormalities [21]. It can serve to assist with myometrial dissection and help avoid endometrial cavity invasion, and use may be extended to intraoperative anatomic identification, such as the ureter or uterine artery [21]. With continual innovation, ultrasound will continue to serve as a useful, inexpensive adjunct to gynecologic surgery for many decades to come.

Fluorescent Imaging: How Indocyanine Green Is the New Black

While white light imaging during laparoscopy and with overhead lights in the operating room has been the standard for several decades, new light sources paired with intraoperative fluorescence imaging has been helpful in discerning underlying pathology that may not be obvious to the naked eye or novice observer. Intraoperative fluorescence imaging with near-infrared indocyanine green has been a growing interest among many gynecologic surgeons for use in surgical treatment of gynecologic cancers and endometriosis.

Indocyanine green (ICG) is a fluorescent water-soluble, anionic, relatively hydrophobic, tricarbocyanine molecule that is commonly used as a medical dye in a wide variety of applications [22]. It was originally developed by the Kodak

research laboratories for near infra-red photography in 1955 and gained FDA approval for clinical use in 1959 [23]. Since the 1950s [24–26], ICG has been used to measure cardiac output [27, 28], to study retinal vessel anatomy [24], and measure liver functional reserve [29]. The standard clinical dose is 0.1–0.5 mg/mL/kg [23] and the dye becomes visible with either laser beam [30, 31] or near infra-red (NIR) light at around 820 nm and longer wave lengths [32]. After intravenous administration, ICG binds tightly to plasma proteins, allowing for visualization of the peritoneal and pelvic vascular system (24) several millimeters into blood of soft tissue.

In the treatment of endometriosis, ICG has been predominantly used as an adjunct to skilled surgical acumen in treatment of deep infiltrating endometriosis (DIE). DIE is commonly not adequately treated with medical management, and surgery is needed for symptom management [33]. While surgery is a safe option, it requires a high level of surgical skill and experience to adequately treat, as DIE can be difficult to visualize and adequately resect. In a study of 7 women with endometriosis conducted by Jayakumaran et al. [34], visualization and identification of endometriosis was 3.2 times greater with robotic NIR fluorescence imaging compared to traditional laparoscopic white light, and 2 times higher than robotic white light [34]. The ICG in this case allowed surgeons to better visualize endometriosis lesions due to ICG exposing vascular lesions and endometriotic angiogenesis underlying the peritoneum that may be otherwise missed. All patients in the small cohort had improvement in their pain postoperatively, and reduction of their symptoms to no or very mild symptoms at the 2–4 weeks postoperative visit [34]. Additionally, ICG has been useful in identifying peritoneal and visceral organ endometriosis lesions, allowing fluorescence for rectal and bowel lesions for resection and rectal shave procedures [35] (Fig. 14.3).

ICG is also used in the context of gynecologic surgery for sentinel lymph node mapping. Sentinel lymph node (SLN) mapping is already readily used in vulvar cancer [36]; endometrial and cervical cancers have limited studies show-

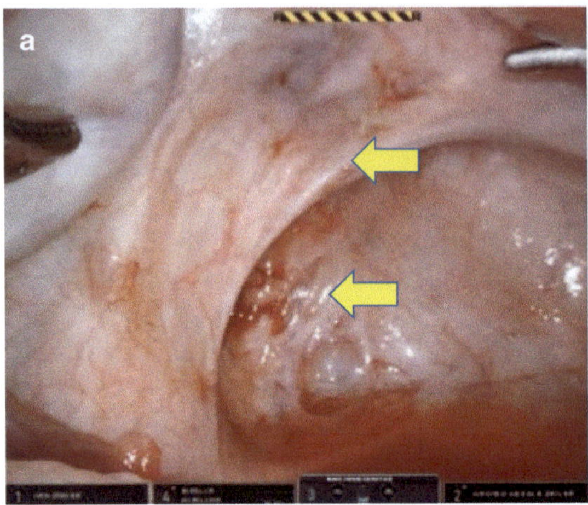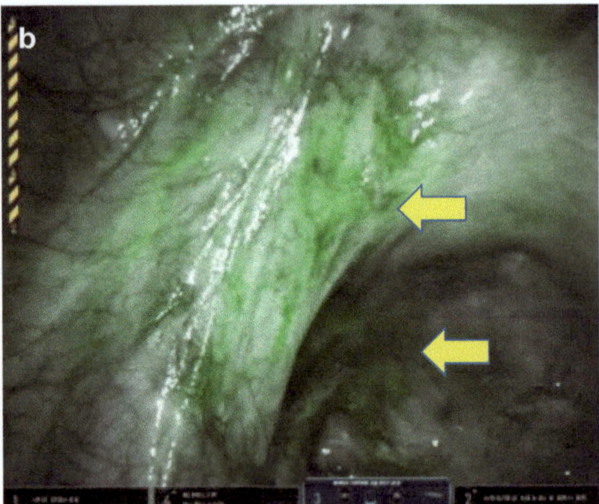

Fig. 14.3 (**a**) Pelvic endometriosis lesions using white light. (**b**) Pelvic endometriosis using near-infrared fluorescence with indocyanine green. Yellow arrows represent endometriosis. (Ref. [34]; [Reprinted by permission from Springer Nature: Springer [Robotic single-site endometriosis resection using near-infrared fluorescence imaging with indocyanine green: a prospective case series and review of literature] by Jayapriya Jayakumaran et al. [COPYRIGHT] (2019)])

ing the efficacy of sentinel lymph node mapping. ICG in NIR fluorescence has been studied as a more feasible and efficient tracer in comparison to the more expensive and complex combination of technetium 99 m radiocolloid and blue dye [37]. Several groups have examined its efficacy in SLN [38–40], and recently, Buda et al. [37] examined intracervical ICG injection feasibility for SLN mapping of endometrial and cervical cancer. A cohort of 49 patients with either early stage endometrial (Stage I) or cervical cancer (Stage 1A2 – 1B1) underwent minimally invasive surgery with pelvic and paraaortic lymph node dissection with intracervical ICG injection [37]. In this cohort, SLN detection with ICG alone demonstrated 100% detection rate and 86% rate of bilateral mapping. In average, 2 SLNs were mapped using ICG, ranging from 1 to 6. Advantages of the ICG mapping compared to the traditional blue dye technique include better intraoperative visualization of lymphatic channels, better penetration of the underlying structures, and nonstaining nature within the operative field [37]. ICG mapping serves as a useful tool, particularly in the obese population that may have obstructing overlying adiposity that may make lymphadenectomy difficult to complete.

Continuing studies into ICG with NIR fluorescence will show the potential in its utilization within the field of gynecology. Promising findings have shown its value in endometriosis surgery and SLN mapping in early-stage gynecologic cancer. As a versatile, nonradioactive, affordable, nonstaining fluorescent marker, ICG will become more widely available and used throughout laparoscopy as the camera and image processing continues to improve and expand to include NIR imaging.

3D Models and Augmented Reality: Seeing Is Believing

Prior to myomectomy, medical imaging with ultrasound and MRI has been essential in surgical planning and intraoperative decision-making. A key principle in myomectomy includes uterine incision site optimization, which includes determining the location, orientation, and length of the incision to minimize incisions and maximize access to underlying fibroids. Uterine incision optimization can be challenging particularly during laparoscopy, due to the size, number, location, and lack of tactile feedback, especially if the fibroid does not distort the surface of the uterus. In conjunction with ultrasound and MRI, the integration of 3D models and augmented reality has been a novel addition to enhance and complement both preoperative and intraoperative surgical planning.

Modern 3D printing has become more accessible to both laypeople and medical researchers, allowing for applications to be ever-expanding. In the medical field, 3D printed models can be a key component to surgical planning that can serve as an aid for both the surgeon and the patient to help visualize anatomy. Aluwee et al. [41] created five 3D printed uterine models for patients undergoing surgery for endometrioid adenocarcinoma. All five patients underwent 3-T MR imaging with 3D volume isotropic turbo spin-echo acquisition (VISTA) sequence with imaged obtained in the sagittal plane [41]. Contrast-enhanced MR angiography was also obtained using the bolus tracking technique [41]. 3D printed uterine models were created using fused deposition printers with polyol with isocyanate as printing material, and model validation was performed by obtaining CT images of the 3D physical models and comparing to previously obtained MR images for accuracy [41]. Through these models, they were able to reproduce low-cost, recyclable 3D uterine models that accurately displayed the underlying anatomy and lesions present, with minimal error [41]. Furthermore, they assessed the reliability and usefulness of their uterine models through patients and surgeon evaluations. The five patients, while a small sample size, described greater satisfaction with the 3D model with understanding their disease, the surgical procedures, and risk of complications [41]. Surgeons also described a favorable evaluation of the 3D model for preoperative counseling and visualizing positional relationships between the uterus and the underlying tumor [41]. Overall, 3D printing and modeling can serve as a useful additional to preoperative counseling and surgical planning as 3D printers become more widely available and used (Fig. 14.4).

While a physical three-dimensional model can be valuable for surgical planning prior to surgery,

integration of 3D models into real-time augmented reality is changing the practice of traditional laparoscopy throughout many fields. Augmented reality (AR) describes an interactive interface where computer-generated images are incorporated into real-life objects or the surrounding environment to enhance perceptual information. AR has been used in laparoscopy by integrating computer-generated images into endoscopic video monitors to allow surgeons to view subsurface structures [43–45]. AR systems have been developed for adrenalectomy [44], prostatectomy [46], liver resection [45, 47], endoscopic sinus surgery, and neurosurgery [48]; however, previously described systems have been limited to nonmobile organs visualized during surgery. Bourdel et al. based at the Centre Hospitalier de l'Université Estaing Clermont-Ferrand in France have described an AR system that can be used for a very mobile organ, such as the uterus, to enhance intraoperative myoma visualization for uterine incision optimization [49, 50].

The first AR system used for gynecologic surgery was aimed at improving laparoscopic myomectomy and addressed the challenge of uterine mobility with active manipulation. Bourdel et al. describe an intraoperative myoma visualization system that divided information into two main phases: the segmentation phase and the fusion phase [49, 51]. Initially, a radiologist takes the MRI imaging and separates the myomas from the uterine surface, from which a 3D mesh model is constructed [49, 51]. The fusion phase then involves fusing the 3D mesh model and overlaying it on real-time laparoscopic imaging, creating a semitransparent uterus where the surgeon can visualize the myomas underlying the serosal surface [49, 51] (Fig. 14.5).

The AR system was initially tested by testing 10 users with a 3D printed synthetic uterus with 6 embedded 2 cm myomas [49]. Synthetic MRI images were created of each myoma location, and the 10 users were asked to identify the closest distance using a laparoscopic pointer to the underlying myomas through a laparoscopic trainer using either the AR system or the synthetic MRI slices (which is considered gold stan-

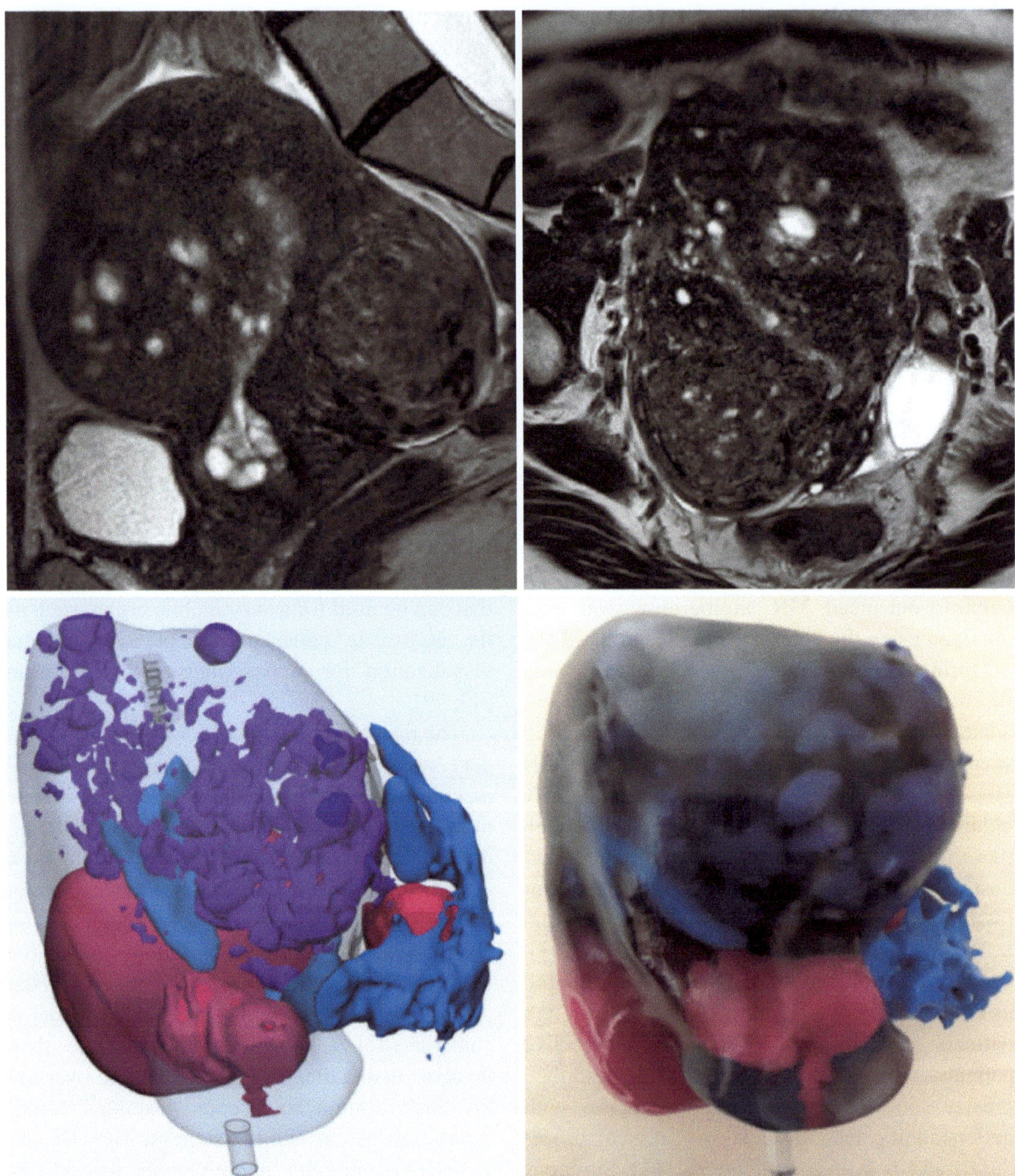

Fig. 14.4 MRI images on top row. Bottom row is 3D printed fibroid uterus with adenomyosis. Red areas represent fibroids and proximity to uterine cavity (blue area); purple area represents adenomyosis. (Ref. [42]; used with permission from Springer)

dard) [51]. While there was no significant difference in time to completion of the task, the mean accuracy of localization was improved by a factor of 20 [49].

The same system was then utilized in a surgical case and represents the first in vivo use of an AR system within gynecology [50]. First, T2-weighted MRI imaging was obtained, and the segmentation phase was performed with interactive segmentation software through radiology [49]. During standard laparoscopy with a 0^0 laparoscope, the uterus was visualized in several

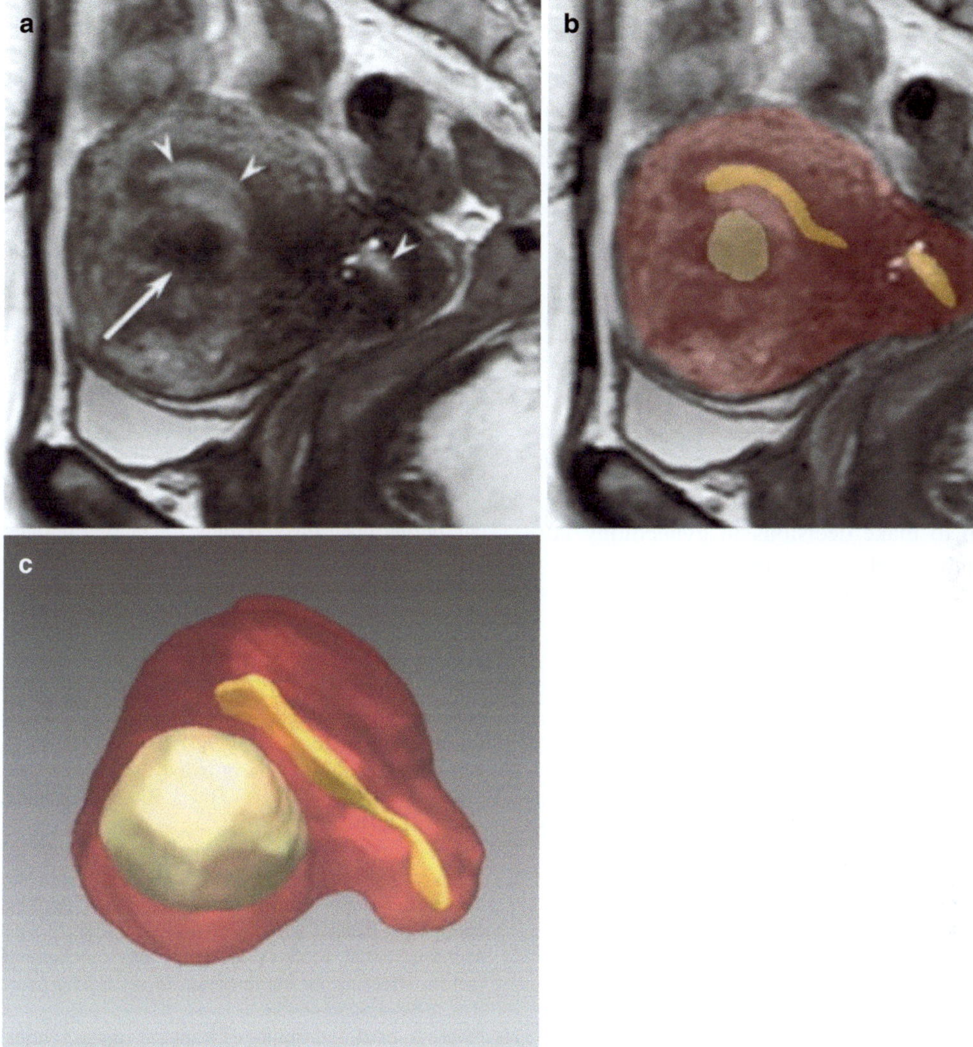

Fig. 14.5 3D surface-rendered MRI images. (**a**) small arrows represent endometrium and large arrow shows fibroid; (**b**) Soft yellow areas represent fibroids in relation to dark yellow endometrium; (**c**) 3D rendered image allows better resolution between soft yellow fibroid and dark yellow endometrium

different angles, and the AR software creates a 3D intraoperative mesh model of the uterus using "dense structure-from-motion" technology [50]. The AR myoma visualization was then overlaid on top of the laparoscopic images, providing real-time image feedback and allowing for the fusion stage. The system was tested on three patients initially, one with a dominant fundal 6 cm fibroid, and two patients with multiple, smaller myomas [49]. The system was a novel application of AR in gynecology which overcame many challenges of AR. The AR system did not require any additional laparoscopic hardware or artificial landmarks, and withstood motion artifact, blur, and laparoscope removal and reinsertion [50].

The use of augmented reality has been focused on improving efficiency of movement, minimizing error, and improving operator accuracy. It is focused on reducing natural limitations, enhancing spatial awareness, and identifying concealed vital structures [52]. AR integration has been shown to decrease operative time and improve surgical accuracy [53–55] in other fields. With this further integration to gynecology, AR serves as an opportunity to seamlessly complement the surgeon's skill, allowing for faster and safer surgeries for future generations.

Conclusions

Over the course of the last century, gynecologic surgery has changed immensely with the integration of technological advances. The integration of ultrasound into gynecology and subsequently into surgical practice has created safer and more precise procedures, opening the space for further advancements in image-based surgery. With new developments in the AR space, the ability to utilize vision to make decisions in gynecology is ever-expanding and will change not only the way we practice and operate, but also the safety and efficacy of the procedures we provide.

References

1. Hackmann WD. Underwater acoustics before the first world war. In: Seek and strike. London: Unipub; 1984. p. 1–10.
2. Newman PG, Rozycki GS. The history of ultrasound. Surg Clin North Am. 1998;78(2):179–95.
3. Hackmann WD. Introduction. In: Seek and strike. London: Unipub; 1984. p. xxiv–xv.
4. Hackmann WD. Underwater acoustics before the first world war. In: Seek and strike. London: Unipub; 1984. p. 73–95.
5. White DN. Neurosonology pioneers. Ultrasound Med Biol. 1988;14(7):541–61.
6. Meire HB, Farrant P. An historical review. In: Basic ultrasound. Wiley-Blackwell; 1995. p. 1–7.
7. Wells P. Developments in medical ultrasonics. World Med Electron. 1966;4:2721.
8. Ludwig GD, Struthers FW. Detecting gallstones with ultrasound. Electronics. 1950;23:172–8.
9. Ludwig GD, Struthers FW. The velocity of sound through tissues and the acoustic impedance of tissues. J Acoust Soc Am. 1950;22:862–6.
10. Wild JJ. The use of ultrasonic pulses for the measurement of biologic tissues and the detection of tissue density changes. Surgery. 1950;27(2):183–8.
11. Wild JJ, Reid JM. Diagnostic use of ultrasound. Br J Phys Med. 1956;19(11):248–57; passim.
12. Wild JJ, Reid JM. Further pilot echographic studies on the histologic structure of tumors of the living intact human breast. Am J Pathol. 1952;28(5):839–61.
13. Goldberg BB, Gramiak R, Freimanis AK. Early history of diagnostic ultrasound: the role of American radiologists. AJR Am J Roentgenol. 1993;160(1):189–94.
14. Donald I. Sonar–the story of an experiment. Ultrasound Med Biol. 1974;1(2):109–17.
15. Schulman JD, et al. Outpatient in vitro fertilization using transvaginal ultrasound-guided oocyte retrieval. Obstet Gynecol. 1987;69(4):665–8.
16. Strickler RC, et al. Ultrasound guidance for human embryo transfer. Fertil Steril. 1985;43(1):54–61.
17. Woolcott R, Stanger J. Potentially important variables identified by transvaginal ultrasound-guided embryo transfer. Hum Reprod. 1997;12(5):963–6.
18. Tang OS, et al. Ultrasound-guided embryo transfer: a prospective randomized controlled trial. Hum Reprod. 2001;16(11):2310–5.
19. Lin PC, Thyer A, Soules MR. Intraoperative ultrasound during a laparoscopic myomectomy. Fertil Steril. 2004;81(6):1671–4.
20. Angioli R, et al. Intraoperative contact ultrasonography during open myomectomy for uterine fibroids. Fertil Steril. 2010;94(4):1487–90.
21. Letterie GS, Catherino WH. A 7.5-MHz finger-grip ultrasound probe for real-time intraoperative guidance during complex reproductive surgical procedures. Am J Obstet Gynecol. 2002;187(6):1588–90.
22. Boni L, et al. Clinical applications of indocyanine green (ICG) enhanced fluorescence in laparoscopic surgery. Surg Endosc. 2015;29(7):2046–55.
23. Alander JT, et al. A review of indocyanine green fluorescent imaging in surgery. Int J Biomed Imaging. 2012;2012:940585.
24. Baillif S, et al. Retinal fluorescein and indocyanine green angiography and spectral-domain optical coherence tomography findings in acute retinal pigment epitheliitis. Retina. 2011;31(6):1156–63.
25. Mordon S, et al. Indocyanine green: physicochemical factors affecting its fluorescence in vivo. Microvasc Res. 1998;55(2):146–52.
26. Noura S, et al. Feasibility of a lateral region sentinel node biopsy of lower rectal cancer guided by indocyanine green using a near-infrared camera system. Ann Surg Oncol. 2010;17(1):144–51.
27. Desai ND, et al. A randomized comparison of intraoperative indocyanine green angiography and transit-time flow measurement to detect technical errors in coronary bypass grafts. J Thorac Cardiovasc Surg. 2006;132(3):585–94.
28. Reuthebuch O, et al. Novadaq SPY: intraoperative quality assessment in off-pump coronary artery bypass grafting. Chest. 2004;125(2):418–24.
29. Lim C, et al. Indocyanine green fluorescence imaging in the surgical management of liver cancers: current facts and future implications. J Visc Surg. 2014;151(2):117–24.
30. Spinoglio G, et al. Real-time near-infrared (NIR) fluorescent cholangiography in single-site robotic cholecystectomy (SSRC): a single-institutional prospective study. Surg Endosc. 2013;27(6):2156–62.

31. Daskalaki D, et al. Indocyanine green (ICG) fluorescent cholangiography during robotic cholecystectomy: results of 184 consecutive cases in a single institution. Surg Innov. 2014;21(6):615–21.

32. Luo S, et al. A review of NIR dyes in cancer targeting and imaging. Biomaterials. 2011;32(29):7127–38.

33. Practice Committee of the American Society for Reproductive, M. Treatment of pelvic pain associated with endometriosis: a committee opinion. Fertil Steril. 2014;101(4):927–35.

34. Jayakumaran J, et al. Robotic single-site endometriosis resection using near-infrared fluorescence imaging with indocyanine green: a prospective case series and review of literature. J Robot Surg. 2020;14(1):145–54.

35. Bourdel N, et al. Indocyanine green in deep infiltrating endometriosis: a preliminary feasibility study to examine vascularization after rectal shaving. Fertil Steril. 2020;114(2):367–73.

36. Van der Zee AG, et al. Sentinel node dissection is safe in the treatment of early-stage vulvar cancer. J Clin Oncol. 2008;26(6):884–9.

37. Buda A, et al. Sentinel lymph node mapping with near-infrared fluorescent imaging using indocyanine green: a new tool for laparoscopic platform in patients with endometrial and cervical cancer. J Minim Invasive Gynecol. 2016;23(2):265–9.

38. Jewell EL, et al. Detection of sentinel lymph nodes in minimally invasive surgery using indocyanine green and near-infrared fluorescence imaging for uterine and cervical malignancies. Gynecol Oncol. 2014;133(2):274–7.

39. Plante M, et al. Sentinel node mapping with indocyanine green and endoscopic near-infrared fluorescence imaging in endometrial cancer. A pilot study and review of the literature. Gynecol Oncol. 2015;137(3):443–7.

40. How J, et al. Comparing indocyanine green, technetium, and blue dye for sentinel lymph node mapping in endometrial cancer. Gynecol Oncol. 2015;137(3):436–42.

41. Sayed Aluwee S, et al. Evaluation of pre-surgical models for uterine surgery by use of three-dimensional printing and mold casting. Radiol Phys Technol. 2017;10(3):279–85.

42. Flaxman T, Cooke C, Miguel O, Sheikh A. A review and guide of to creating patient specific 3D printed anatomical models from MRI for benigh gynecologic surgery. 3D Print Med. 2021;7(1):17.

43. Pessaux P, et al. Robotic duodenopancreatectomy assisted with augmented reality and real-time fluorescence guidance. Surg Endosc. 2014;28(8):2493–8.

44. Marescaux J, et al. Augmented-reality-assisted laparoscopic adrenalectomy. JAMA. 2004;292(18):2214–5.

45. Pessaux P, et al. Towards cybernetic surgery: robotic and augmented reality-assisted liver segmentectomy. Langenbeck's Arch Surg. 2015;400(3):381–5.

46. Simpfendorfer T, et al. Augmented reality visualization during laparoscopic radical prostatectomy. J Endourol. 2011;25(12):1841–5.

47. Soler L, et al. Real-time 3D image reconstruction guidance in liver resection surgery. Hepatobiliary Surg Nutr. 2014;3(2):73–81.

48. Grimson WL, et al. An automatic registration method for frameless stereotaxy, image guided surgery, and enhanced reality visualization. IEEE Trans Med Imaging. 1996;15(2):129–40.

49. Bourdel N, et al. Augmented reality in gynecologic surgery: evaluation of potential benefits for myomectomy in an experimental uterine model. Surg Endosc. 2017;31(1):456–61.

50. Bourdel N, et al. Use of augmented reality in laparoscopic gynecology to visualize myomas. Fertil Steril. 2017;107(3):737–9.

51. Collins T, et al. Realtime wide-baseline registration of the uterus in laparoscopic videos using multiple texture maps. Berlin, Heidelberg: Springer Berlin Heidelberg; 2013.

52. Aluwee SA, Kato H, Zhou X, Hara T. Magnetic resonance imaging of uterine fibroids: a preliminary investigation into the usefulness of 3D-rendered images for surgical planning. Springerplus. 2015;4:384.

53. Moawad G, Tyan P, Louie M. Artificial intelligence and augmented reality in gynecology. Curr Opin Obstet Gynecol. 2019;31(5):345–8.

54. Murugesan YP, et al. A novel rotational matrix and translation vector algorithm: geometric accuracy for augmented reality in oral and maxillofacial surgeries. Int J Med Robot. 2018;14(3):e1889.

55. Vavra P, et al. Recent development of augmented reality in surgery: a review. J Healthc Eng. 2017;2017:457–72.

Cervical Fibroids

15

Joseph Findley and Callum Potts

Introduction

Uterine fibroids (also known as leiomyomas) are benign, monoclonal tumors arising from the myometrium. They are the most common benign gynecologic tumors, with a cumulative incidence approaching 70–80% for women by the age of 50 [1]. The inciting event for fibroid development remains speculative, though their proliferation has been found to be responsive to the ovarian steroids estrogen and progesterone [2]. Though fibroids can be asymptomatic, those that cause symptoms (including heavy and/or irregular menstrual bleeding, pelvic pain, pelvic pressure, and infertility) have the potential to significantly impact to quality of life. As such, fibroids are the leading indication for hysterectomy worldwide [3].

The vast majority of fibroids are found in the uterine corpus (95%), with approximately 5% occurring in the cervix [4]. Per the 2011 FIGO classification system, cervical fibroids are

J. Findley (✉)
Division of Reproductive Endocrinology and Infertility, University Hospitals Cleveland Medical Center, Cleveland, OH, USA
e-mail: Joseph.Findley@UHHospitals.org

C. Potts
Division of Reproductive Endocrinology and Infertility, University of Vermont Medical Center, Burlington, VT, USA
e-mail: Callum.Potts@UVMHealth.org

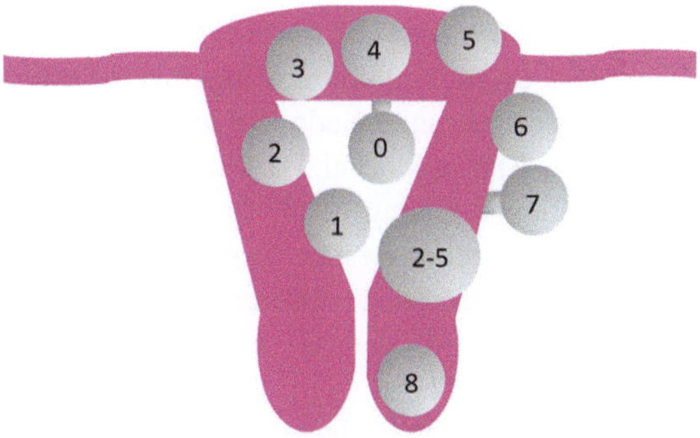

Fig. 15.1 Simplified diagram of the International Federation of Gynecology and Obstetrics (FIGO) uterine leiomyoma classification. Leiomyoma types: (0) Pedunculated intracavitary, (1) Submucosal and <50% intramural, (2) Submucosal and >50% intramural, (3) Intramural and contacts the endometrium, (4) Intramural, (5) Subserosal and >50% intramural, (6) Subserosal and <50% intramural, (7) Subserosal pedunculated, (8) Cervical or ectopic. For hybrid leiomyomas, two numbers are listed separated by a hyphen. The first number describes the leiomyoma's relation to the endometrium, and the second describes its relationship to the serosa

described in the ectopic type 8 category (Fig. 15.1) [5]. They may be further subclassified as extracervical (subserosal) or intracervical (intramural with or without submucosal components) [6]. A variety of interventional radiology and surgical techniques have been proposed for the management of uterine corpus fibroids, though their applicability to the management of cervical fibroids is less clear. By virtue of their location, cervical fibroids present additional challenges due to their proximity to the bladder, ureters, rectum, and the major vascular supply for the uterus [7].

Descriptions of surgical approaches for the management of cervical fibroids vary significantly in the available literature. With the relative infrequency of cervical fibroids compared with their uterine corpus counterparts, evidence for different techniques is present largely in the form of case reports or limited case series. Particular attention has been given to laparoscopic techniques due to their apparent non-inferiority to an abdominal approach with a similar risk for postoperative recurrence [8]. Takeuchi et al. report a series of 5 patients for a laparoscopic enucleation technique of intracervical fibroids that minimizes blood loss through clipping of the uterine artery [9], a surgical technique adopted in a series of 16 patients by Matsuoka et al. [10]. In a larger series of 28 patients, Chang et al. further delineated laparoscopic techniques by the location of the fibroid in the cervix, differentiating between anterior, posterior, central, lateral, and deep-rooted fibroids [11].

Other approaches have been considered. Vaginal and hysteroscopic myomectomies have been described [12, 13], particularly in situations where the fibroid is prolapsing through the cervical canal [14–16]. The abdominal approach, though less commonly reported, appears more favored for cervical fibroids that are either very large or pose particular surgical risks due to distortion of the anatomy or involvement of adjacent vasculature [17]. When the cervix is almost completely obliterated by the fibroid, radical abdominal trachelectomy has also been described [18, 19]. Hysterectomy remains an option where fertility is not desired or when uterine preservation is not possible [20].

Diagnosis

Similar to uterine fibroids, cervical fibroids may be asymptomatic or can present with symptoms such as abnormal bleeding or bulk symptoms related to physical pressure exerted on surrounding tissues. When present, this pressure is manifested by a sensation of pelvic or vaginal pressure, urinary frequency or urgency, and/or bowel dysfunction. Ureteral compression may present as unilateral or bilateral hydronephrosis. Significant distortion of the cervical canal can result in subfertility. A cervical fibroid may also prolapse into the vagina, presenting with acute and unrelenting pain and bleeding. A necrotic or degenerating fibroid may cause acute pain, fever, and abnormal discharge.

Evaluation for cervical fibroids should start with a thorough history and physical examination. Bowel and bladder symptoms should prompt consideration of alternative etiologies prior to surgical management. Rapid progression of symptoms thought to be related to rapid growth of the cervical mass raises concern for leiomyosarcoma, though malignancy is rare particularly amongst pre-menopausal women. Bi-manual pelvic examination is likely to demonstrate an enlarged, irregular uterus. Assessment of location and involvement with surrounding structures may be limited by discomfort and can often be more thoroughly evaluated under anesthesia.

Imaging

Medical imaging is an invaluable tool to aid in the assessment of uterine fibroids. As with fibroids arising from other areas in the uterus, cervical fibroids are best imaged using ultrasound and magnetic resonance imaging (MRI). Ultrasound is an excellent initial imaging modality as it is readily available and cost-effective. Ultrasound can provide valuable information about uterine fibroids based on variation in echotexture (Fig. 15.2a), use of color doppler imaging can provide information regarding internal vascularity and blood supply (Fig. 15.3), and saline infusion sonography can help to further delineate a fibroid's location relative to the uterine cavity or cervical canal. On the other hand, ultrasound is operator dependent, and imaging can be limited due to artifact, uterine positioning, and patient body habitus.

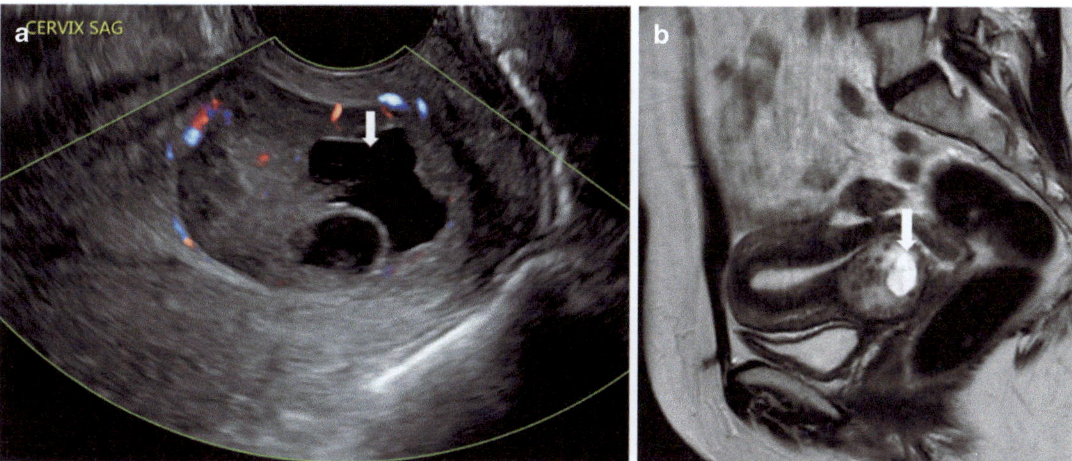

Fig. 15.2 Cervical fibroid showing cystic degeneration. (**a**) On ultrasound, cystic degeneration of the fibroid appears anechoic (arrow) compared to the surrounding fibroid tissue and cervical stroma. Use of color doppler can also help to differentiate degeneration from vasculature. (**b**) On T2-weighted MRI, cystic degeneration of this same fibroid demonstrates a hyperintense signal (arrow)

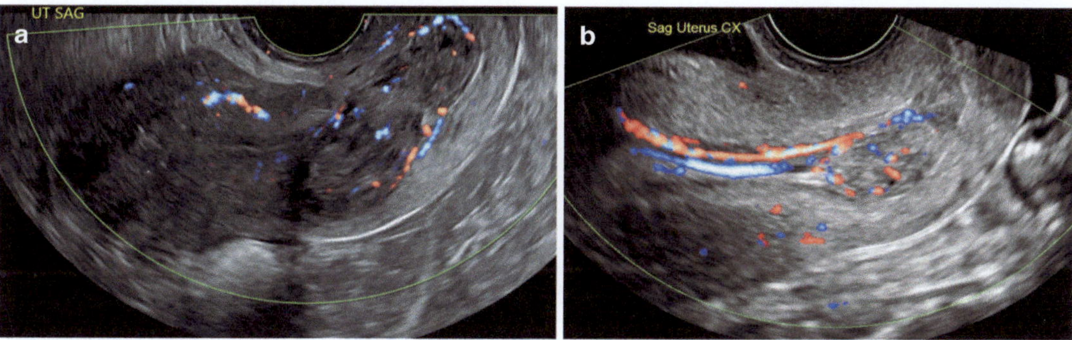

Fig. 15.3 Use of color doppler imaging can provide valuable information regarding the blood supply of fibroids, and can help differentiate between fibroids that arise from the cervical stroma (**a**) from fibroids that origi-nate in the uterine cavity and have prolapsed into the cervix (**b**). When fibroid prolapse occurs, a vascular stalk can often be identified, as seen in image B

Though MRI is less cost-effective, it can provide valuable information for pretreatment planning, especially when sonographic evaluation is limited. As MRI is less subject to the limitations of ultrasound, it can accurately define the size, borders, location, and number of fibroids that are present. MRI can also depict variation in fibroid composition by showing differences in signal intensity (Fig. 15.2b), as well as map the location and borders of adjacent pelvic structures such as the ureters, vasculature, bladder, and bowel (Fig. 15.4).

Surgical Approach

Presurgical Considerations

Comprehensive preoperative planning is critical for risk reduction and to allow for adequately informed counselling and consent. After a thorough history and physical examination, imaging with transvaginal pelvic ultrasound offers insight into the fibroid location, size, and association with surrounding structures. Pelvic MRI should be considered when there is particular concern

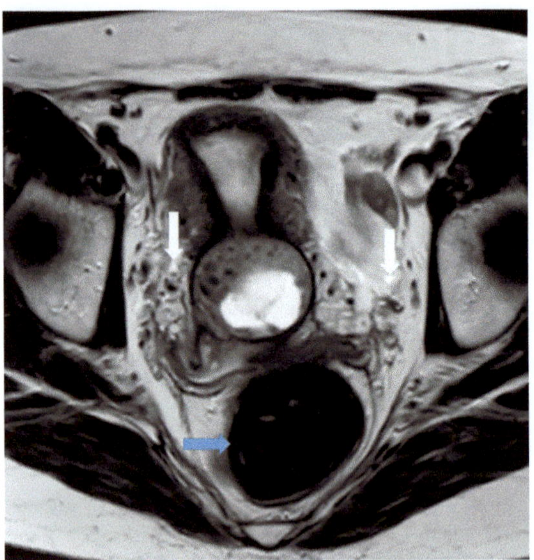

Fig. 15.4 Axial T2-weighted MRI showing a cervical uterine fibroid demonstrating the location of the ureters (white arrows) and rectum (blue arrow)

for fibroid size or impingement on other vital structures. If there is concern for anemia, laboratory assessment and correction with supplemental iron or blood transfusion is warranted. With significant risk for bleeding, blood products should be considered and available at the time of surgery. Patients should be counselled about the risk for hysterectomy and the impact surgery may have on future fertility.

Particularly large cervical fibroids, or cervical fibroids in locations more likely to obscure the identification of key pelvic structures like the ureters and uterine vessels, may be pretreated for 3–4 months with GnRH agonists or antagonists to reduce their volume. This technique should be applied judiciously, as there is some concern that GnRH agonist pretreatment may soften the fibroid and make the enucleation plane more difficult to define, thus increasing operative time [21]. The selective progesterone receptor modulator ulipristal acetate has been studied for fibroid volume reduction prior to surgery, though it is not currently recommended by the Food and Drug Administration (FDA) or European Medicines Agency (EMA) due to concerns regarding liver toxicity potentially requiring liver transplantation [22].

Abdominal

Myomectomy has traditionally been managed by laparotomy, and though newer minimally invasive techniques have increased in popularity and prevalence, abdominal myomectomy remains a central procedure for the reproductive surgeon. Though route preference is less well-defined for cervical fibroids, hospital and regional studies suggest uterine fibroids are approached abdominally in the majority of cases [23, 24]. Factors favoring an abdominal approach include surgeon skill and training, fibroid size (particularly fibroids greater than 10 cm in maximal diameter), extensive attachment to the cervix or uterus, concern for preexisting pelvic adhesive disease, and fibroids that lie predominantly above the level of the cervical-vaginal junction (Fig. 15.5) [17, 23].

Choice of abdominal incision varies by fibroid size, location, and other surgical risk factors, though the approach should optimize visualization of the expected surgical field. Pfannenstiel and Cherney incisions should provide adequate exposure for anterior cervical fibroids. Posterior fibroids and cases where safely accessing vital structures is expected to be difficult should prompt consideration of a vertical midline incision [17].

In our practices, we approach cervical fibroids from the midline to minimize risk of injury to lateral vital structures like ureters and uterine vessels when possible. Opening the retroperitoneal spaces allows for identification of the ureters, and ureterolysis may be required to mobilize them away from the operative site [17]. We prefer to use a serosal injection with dilute vasopressin (20 units in 100–200 mL of normal saline) at the beginning of the case to reduce blood loss. A longitudinal incision with a monopolar needle electrode is made through the serosa and carried down to the depth of the fibroid. The fibroid may then be grasped and, using traction and countertraction, enucleated from the surrounding stroma. Fibroid adhesions should be dissected sharply (for example, with a monopolar electrode or Metzenbaum scissors), as blunt or overly aggressive tissue manipulation may cause unnecessary entry into the endocervical canal or endometrial

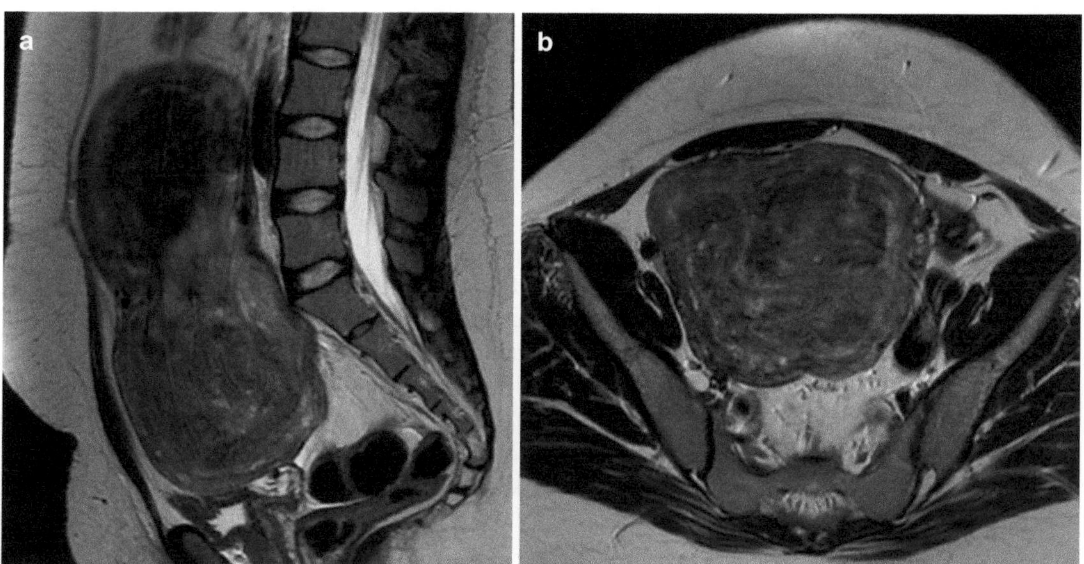

Fig. 15.5 Sagittal (**a**) and axial (**b**) T2-weighted MRI of myomatous uterus with a large fibroid encompassing a significant amount of the cervical stroma

cavity. Large feeding vessels may be suture ligated at their base to minimize blood loss. Meticulous attention to hemostasis during the fibroid enucleation helps to keep the operative field clear and reduce the risk of postoperative adhesion formation. Where possible, the fibroid should be removed intact to avoid iatrogenic spread of an undiagnosed malignancy.

Following removal of the fibroid, its cavity should be re-approximated with a multilayer closure to minimize dead-space (which promotes hematoma formation) and maximize tissue strength. The cervical stroma should be closed with an absorbable suture like 0-Vicryl (polyglactin 910). The overlying serosa is then closed with a finer suture, typically a 3-0 or 4-0 delayed-absorbable suture, employing a "baseball" stitch technique to reduce exposure of the suture material [17, 25]. Prior to abdominal closure, an adhesion barrier such as *Interceed®* (oxidized cellulose) is placed over the uterine incision line.

In rare cases, where the fibroid is so extensive as to obliterate the cervix, radical trachelectomy (either planned or as a rescue procedure) has been described as a means of preserving fertility [18, 19]. In their technique, Del Priore et al. dissect the ureters through the cardinal ligaments before ligating the uterine vessels. The lower uterine segment, cervix, and a portion of the upper vagina are then resected, and a running layer of absorbable suture is used to reestablish continuity between the vaginal margin and seromuscular margin of the remaining uterine corpus [19]. Where possible, the ectocervical portion of the vaginal apex should be preserved, and a Foley catheter may be utilized to assist in more accurately re-approximating the uterus to the upper vagina [18, 19]. Pregnancy outcomes after radical trachelectomy have been studied more extensively in the cervical cancer literature, and these highlight the importance of placing a cervical cerclage at the time of the trachelectomy for reducing the risk of cervical insufficiency, preterm premature rupture of membranes (PPROM), and preterm birth [26].

Laparoscopy

Laparoscopic myomectomy for uterine fibroids was first reported in 1979. This approach has the potential advantages of decreased blood loss and shorter hospital course compared with the abdominal approach, however laparoscopy is also associated with increased operative time [27]. Complication rates and postoperative fertility and obstetric outcomes are similar to abdominal myomectomy [23]. Despite its potential advantages, widespread adoption of the laparoscopic approach has been limited, likely due to surgeon experience and the technical skill required to perform laparoscopic myomectomies. As such, regional studies suggest utilization of laparoscopy in less than 50% of myomectomy cases [23, 24]. Patient selection tends to favor smaller fibroids, with several large series finding a mean or median maximal fibroid diameter of 5–7 cm [9, 10, 23]. For cases where laparoscopy is considered, pretreatment with GnRH analogues for 3–6 months may reduce the fibroid's volume to a degree that facilitates enucleation and subsequent morcellation. This approach should be taken with caution, as GnRH analogue therapy can distort the pseudocapsule and make laparoscopic dissection more challenging.

In our practices, laparoscopic cervical myomectomy is performed per the technique initially described by Takeuchi et al. [9], and modified by Matsuoka et al. [10]. A 5 or 10 mm trocar is placed at the umbilicus for the laparoscope, and additional 5 mm trocars are obtained in the bilateral lower quadrants. We then use an 11 mm trocar at Palmer's point in the left upper quadrant. An assistant sequentially dilates the cervix to 10 mm with Hegar cervical dilators, and utilizes either the Hegar dilator or a RUMI uterine manipulator (CooperSurgical Inc., Trumbull, CT) for manipulation during the procedure. Similar to the abdominal approach, dilute vasopressin is injected subserosally to reduce blood loss. If the cervical fibroid is particularly large and impacts the surrounding vital structures, the broad ligament may be opened for identification and dissection of the ureters away from the operative site. If there is concern for increased intraoperative blood loss, a temporary vessel clip may be applied to the uterine artery at this time.

Due to the excellent visualization of and access to the posterior field of the uterus with sharp uterine anteversion, a vertical incision made with a monopolar needle electrode in the posterior cervix can reach almost all posterior cervical fibroids. The incision is made to the depth of the fibroid, and lengthened until the entire fibroid is visualized [9]. The overlying tissue is pushed away from the capsule, and the fibroid is penetrated with a laparoscopic myoma screw or laparoscopic tenaculum to allow for traction and countertraction while its attachments are separated with the monopolar electrode [11]. The stalk of the fibroid should be identified, grasped, and suture ligated with 2-0 Vicryl for adequate hemostasis and to maintain clear visualization of the surgical field. The fibroid cavity may then be re-approximated in two layers with 2-0 Vicryl or a similar caliber absorbable barbed suture on a circular tapered needle, with the first layer involving the cervical endothelium and a small amount of stroma in an interrupted fashion, and the second layer involving the remaining stroma and overlying serosa in a running fashion. If vessel clips were applied, these are now removed, and the broad ligament closed with a 3-0 Vicryl in a running fashion [9, 10]. A specimen retrieval bag is then utilized to retrieve the fibroid using the left upper quadrant port, and it is brought to the anterior abdominal wall to allow for morcellation in the bag to minimize iatrogenic spread of an undiagnosed malignancy and facilitate removal [28].

Though most cervical fibroids removed laparoscopically are amenable to the posterior approach, this technique should be adapted depending on each patient's characteristics. Chang et al. describe different techniques for cervical fibroids in one of five specific locations (Table 15.1). They endorse an anterior approach for anterior cervical fibroids, with care taken to dissect the bladder away from the operative field. Additionally, they describe slight modifications to approach posterior, central, lateral, and deep-rooted cervical fibroids [11].

Robotic-Assisted Laparoscopy

The use of robotics is a recent innovation in the field of surgery, and may be considered an advancement along the spectrum of laparoscopic technologies. The *da Vinci®* Surgical System

Table 15.1 Surgical techniques for cervical fibroids depending on their location relative to the cervix [11]

Anterior	Separate bladder Anterior incision
Posterior	Separate ureters, uterine arteries, rectum Posterior incision
Central	(Separate surrounding structures depending on incision) Anterior or posterior incision
Lateral	Separate ureters, uterine arteries, rectum Incise over capsule laterally Bipolar coagulation of pedicular vessels
Deep-rooted	Transverse incision May require fibroid to be pushed into abdominal cavity from the vagina

(Intuitive Surgical, Inc., Sunnyvale, CA) was the first robot approved by the US Food and Drug Administration (FDA) for gynecologic applications in April of 2005. Since that time, this technology has been utilized for numerous different applications, as surgeons have sought to extend what can be done with a minimally invasive approach. In this vein, myomectomy is no different, and the use of robotics has been shown to be feasible and safe for the management of both small and large (>10 cm in diameter) fibroids alike [29]. Though previous literature cites cervical location of fibroids as an exclusion criterion for minimally invasive approach [30], robotic approach for management of cervical fibroids has recently been described [31]. Only experienced surgeons should use the robotic approach to manage cervical fibroids, and patients should be adequately counseled regarding the risks of bleeding, surgical complications, and conversion to laparotomy. In general, gynecologic procedures performed robotically have been associated with a 0–5% risk of conversion to laparotomy [32, 33], and laparoscopy for the removal of fibroids arising from the uterine corpus is estimated to have an 11.3% risk of conversion [34]. Though a minimally invasive approach with either conventional laparoscopy or robotic assisted laparoscopy can be attempted for the management of cervical fibroids, the rate of conversion to laparotomy in such cases would be expected to be higher given their technical challenges and proximity to vital structures.

The robotic approach is thought to have several advantages. A more delicate dissection is possible with the increased dexterity afforded by the robotic approach compared to conventional laparoscopy. With concerns expressed regarding the risk of uterine rupture following laparoscopic myometrial closure [35], the improved dexterity associated with the robotic approach may aid in ease of myometrial repair. Studies have found that blood loss, complications, and hospital stay following surgery are similar with robotic myomectomy compared to laparoscopic myomectomy [36, 37], and are lower compared to abdominal myomectomy [27]. Two major criticisms of the robotic approach are increased cost and potential increased operative time compared to laparotomy [38]. Data is conflicting regarding length of surgery when comparing robotic versus laparoscopic myomectomy, with some studies showing increased length of surgery with robotic approach [37], and others showing comparable operating times [36].

Our practices approach robotic myomectomy for cervical fibroids using the same principles we would for myomectomy via laparotomy. Preoperative anemia can be managed with the use of gonadotropin-releasing hormone agonists [27], and surgical planning can be supplemented with ultrasound and magnetic resonance imaging. Our institutions utilize the *da Vinci®* Surgical System (Intuitive Surgical, Inc., Sunnyvale, CA) for robotic procedures. Intraoperatively, we place our camera port at or above the umbilicus, with the camera port optimally being placed at a distance of 10–20 cm from the superior margin of the target anatomy. Additional robotic ports are placed 8–10 cm lateral to the camera port. An assistant port is typically placed in the suprapubic area to facilitate introduction and removal of sutures into the operative field under direct visualization (Fig. 15.6). Interventions to minimize intraoperative blood loss are employed as previously described. Attempts are made to minimize the size and number of incisions made on the uterus, and fibroids are enucleated using gentle traction/countertraction and meticulously dissecting healthy tissue away from pathology.

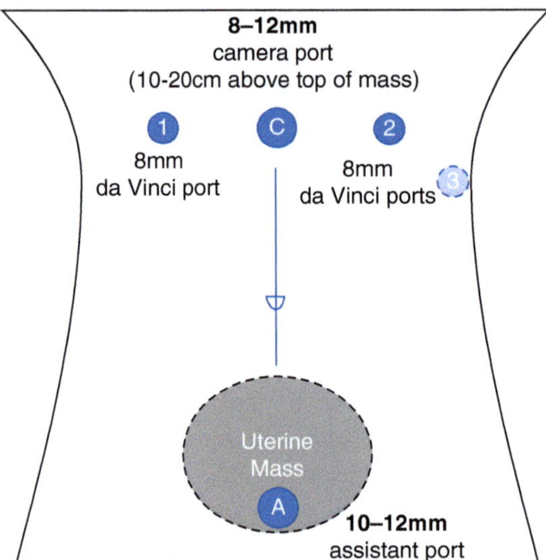

Fig. 15.6 Robotic port site placements. The camera port (C) (8–12 mm port) is placed approximately 10–20 cm above the target anatomy based on preoperative imaging and exam under anesthesia. Two 8 mm da Vinci ports are placed at the level of the camera port, each 8 cm lateral to the camera port as shown in the figure. A third 8 mm da Vinci port may be added 8 cm lateral (and inferior if space is limited) to the left abdominal da Vinci port for extra intraabdominal manipulation. A 10–12 mm assistant port (A) is placed in the operative field where introduction and removal of suture material can be performed under visualization with the camera

During dissection, care is taken to avoid avulsing myomas as this may result in excess damage to surrounding tissue. Additional attention is paid towards preservation of the endometrial cavity to avoid compromising future fertility. Breaches in the cavity are repaired using monofilament suture to minimize inflammation, and hysteroscopy is performed at the end of the procedure to ensure that portions of the cavity were not obliterated during the uterine repair. Incisions on the uterus are then closed in a multilayer fashion, with either 0-Vicryl or a similar gauge self-retaining suture such as *V-Loc®* (Covidien) or *Quill®* SRS (Angiotech) being utilized for myometrial repair. We typically close the serosal layer using a 2-0 or 3-0 monofilament suture in a baseball stitch fashion as previously described [17, 25]. Myomas are then removed from the abdomen through a small incision in the suprapubic area (following removal of the suprapubic port from the abdo-

men, this incision is extended as needed to facilitate leiomyoma removal). Attempts are made to minimize morcellation of myomas; however, if necessary, we morcellate in a bag. Prior to abdominal closure, an adhesion barrier such as *Interceed®* (oxidized cellulose) is placed over the uterine incision line.

Hysteroscopy

Commonly reserved for the treatment of submucosal leiomyomas, there is a paucity of literature describing treatment of cervical myomas by the hysteroscopic approach. Due to the nature and physical location of cervical fibroids, access via hysteroscopy may not be adequate or feasible in many cases. Maintaining a visual field with cervical fibroids is difficult as the tip of the hysteroscope is often either within the cervix, preventing fluid circulation, or its position within the cervix is difficult to maintain to safely allow for resection. In certain situations, however, a hysteroscopic approach may be reasonable. These would include cervical fibroids that are both smaller in size (<4–5 cm in diameter), fibroids that are located primarily within the cervical canal, and those that arise from the cervix but protrude into the endometrial cavity. Fibroids that prohibit hysteroscopic access due to complete obstruction of the cervical canal, those that are larger in size (>5 cm), or fibroids that do not protrude into the cervical canal are likely better approached by a different surgical route. Because the hysteroscopic approach does not afford surgeons the ability to repair the uterus after enucleation of a fibroid, fibroids that breach greater than 50% of the depth of the cervical stroma may also be more effectively managed with an alternative approach.

In the few instances where the hysteroscopic approach is thought to be preferable, patients should be adequately counseled regarding the risks associated with the hysteroscopic approach. Thorough preoperative evaluation including physical examination and imaging with US and/or MRI can provide in-depth information regarding fibroid burden, size, and location in relation to surrounding vital structures. Patient should also be informed of the relative limitations inherent to the hysteroscopic approach such as limited access in situations where fibroids completely obstruct the cervical canal, inability to visualize structures outside of the uterus, and the possible need to terminate the procedure prior to complete myoma resection due to excess fluid deficit. Complete fibroid resection may not be possible in a single procedure, and as such, more than one procedure may be required to obtain the desired result.

Preoperatively, treatment with GnRH agonists can be of some benefit in select patients. Though routine use of these medications is not recommended, treatment with GnRH-agonists for 3–4 months prior to surgery can help to optimize hemoglobin levels in patients who are found to be anemic, as well as reduce intraoperative blood loss [39]. These benefits must be weighed with the risk of adverse effects associated with these medications. Intraoperatively, use of vasoconstricting agents such as epinephrine of vasopressin can reduce procedural blood loss and fluid absorption. When added to local anesthetic, these agents can reduce the systemic absorption and toxicity of the anesthetic [40]. Additionally, injection of intracervical dilute vasopressin has been associated with a reduction in the force required for mechanical cervical dilation [41]. As described above, we utilize subepithelial injections of dilute vasopressin (20 units in 100–200 mL of normal saline) at the beginning of the case.

Our practice has been to utilize a resectoscope with a bipolar cutting loop and isotonic solution to minimize the risks associated with excess fluid deficit. Though the maximum permissible fluid deficit with isotonic solution is based solely upon expert opinion, most would agree that this maximum should be set at 2500 mL [42]. If the fluid deficit reaches 2000 mL with isotonic solution in a young, healthy patient, the surgeon should strongly consider stopping infusion of distension media and terminating the procedure. Termination of the procedure should be considered with lower fluid deficits in older patients or patients with impaired cardiac function to reduce the risk of fluid overload. If a bipolar resectoscope is not available, then hysteroscopy with a monopolar cutting loop and hypotonic solution can be considered. The maximum permissible fluid deficit with hypotonic distension media is reported to be 1000 ml, with a 750 ml fluid deficit being the point at which the surgeon should consider terminating the procedure [42].

During myoma resection, great care is taken to keep the operative filament of the cutting loop within the field of vision, and once activated, passes of the cutting loop are only made towards the operator. Activating the cutting loop while it is moving away from the operator places the patient at increased risk of uterine perforation and injury to adjacent vital structures such as the bladder, bowel, uterine vasculature, and ureters. Intraoperative bleeding can be further mitigated with electrocautery, suture ligation, or the application of ferric subsulfate solution (Monsel's paste) if the area of hemorrhage is able to be accessed [43]. In less accessible areas, a Foley catheter balloon or Cook® Cervical Ripening Balloon (Cook Medical, Bloomington, IN) can be used for tamponade.

Vaginal

Due to their low position in the uterus, and the relative inflexibility of the cervix, a vaginal approach may be considered for a cervical fibroid unable to be accessed with a hysteroscopic approach. Thomas and Magos describe a classification system for vaginal myomectomy procedures, of which surgery to correct prolapsing and intracervical fibroids represent Type 1 and Type 2 [13]. The vaginal route carries significant advantages over the more invasive abdominal approaches, including significantly lower risk for postoperative fever, shorter hospital stay, and shorter recovery time, though are limited in patients with significant vaginal or cervical abnormality [13].

Type 1 procedures are for pedunculated, prolapsed cervical fibroids, which are approached vaginally preferentially to other techniques [13]. These typically occur with relatively acute onset and often quite heavy vaginal bleeding, abnormal and malodorous vaginal discharge, vaginal pressure or pain, dyspareunia, and may present with concomitant ascending infection due to the forced dilation of the endocervical canal by the protruding fibroid stalk [13, 15, 16]. If the stalk is accessible, simply twisting the fibroid off its pedicle may be attempted, though this should be attempted cautiously with risk for avulsion injury to the underlying cervical tissue, and, when separated, bleeding feeding vessels may retract into the cervical stroma and be difficult to ligate. When feasible, clamping and ligating the fibroid stalk allows for a more controlled removal [44]. In our practices, we will attempt to suture ligate the stalk with an ENDOLOOP® Ligature (Ethicon, Inc., Somerville, NJ) or Surgitie Loop (Medtronic, Minneapolis, MN), and amputate the fibroid with either a monopolar cautery device, bipolar loop electrode, Mayo scissors, or a scalpel. Injection of dilute vasopressin could be considered to reduce the risk of excessive bleeding.

Type 2 vaginal myomectomy procedures may be used to access non-prolapsed cervical fibroids, and begin by dilating the cervix to allow for adequate visualization [13]. When mechanical dilation is not sufficient, hygroscopic dilation may be achieved with *Laminaria japonica* tents. Goldrath documents two case series with this method, whereby *Laminaria* tents are placed, replaced after 6 hours, and left in place overnight. These are then removed, and cervical myomectomy is performed under procedural sedation and local anesthetic by paracervical block. The fibroid is grasped and avulsed for removal, and any bleeding is made hemostatic with tamponade by placement of an intrauterine Foley catheter [45, 46].

Postoperative Considerations

In general, postoperative care for each route follows institution-based guidelines for myomectomy for uterine fibroids. However, several site-specific considerations are made in postoperative counseling for cervical myomectomies. If incisions are made in the cervix, patients should be encouraged to avoid sexual intercourse or vaginal insertions for 4–6 weeks, or longer if there is concern for inadequate healing. If there is concern for postoperative adhesion formation within the cervix, intrauterine catheter placement could be considered following the procedure, and postoperative diagnostic hysteroscopy could allow for complete visualization of the healed operative site.

Adequate healing time should also be allowed prior to attempting conception. After vaginal myomectomy of a prolapsing cervical fibroid, or vaginal or hysteroscopic resection of an intracervical fibroid, patients should wait at least 4 weeks before attempting conception to allow for resolution of the profound cervical dilation associated with these states. For abdominal, laparoscopic, and robot-assisted excisions involving repair of cervical stroma, our practices tend to follow practice guidelines developed for myomectomies addressing uterine fibroids [2]. After excisions of cervical fibroids with minimal disruption of the cervical stroma, we recommend waiting at least 3 months before attempting conception. For more extensive excisions requiring incision of >50% depth into the cervical stroma or with extensive cervical reconstruction, we recommend waiting at least 6 months before attempting conception. This follows albeit indirect evidence from MRI assessment of myometrial injury resolution following cesarean section [47].

Obstetric risks for future pregnancies vary based on the degree of cervical involvement of the fibroid and the route of excision. Where a significant portion of the cervix is reconstructed or removed during the myomectomy, close follow-up with an appropriate obstetric provider should be encouraged to monitor for cervical insufficiency, and placement of a cervical cerclage should be considered. Cervical cerclage at the time of the myomectomy could also be considered, and is recommended when trachelectomy is performed [26]. Risk for uterine rupture during pregnancy should also be considered when counseling patients regarding route of delivery. In general, unless cervical myomectomy is performed by vaginal or hysteroscopic route and disruption of the cervical stroma is minimal, we recommend cesarean section for all future deliveries.

Conclusion

Cervical fibroids are an uncommon manifestation of uterine fibroids (FIGO Type 8) which present unique surgical challenges. When future reproductive potential is desired, surgical resection by myomectomy should be considered. Planned route of approach should take into consideration fibroid size, its location within the cervix, the breadth of its attachment to the cervix, and its relative position to surrounding vital structures including ureters, major blood vessels, bladder, and bowel. Surgical teams should consider appropriate preoperative imaging and potential medical pretreatment, have adequate experience and technical expertise to complete the planned procedure, and be aware of additional techniques should intraoperative challenges be encountered (including conversion to laparotomy or rescue radical trachelectomy). Though these challenges are not insignificant, careful operative preparation allows cervical myomectomy to be a useful treatment modality in reducing symptomatology of cervical fibroids while retaining reproductive potential.

References

1. Baird DD, Dunson DB, Hill MC, Cousins D, Schectman JM. High cumulative incidence of uterine leiomyoma in black and white women: ultrasound evidence. Am J Obstet Gynecol. 2003;188(1):100–7.
2. Vilos GA, Allaire C, Laberge P-Y, Leyland N, Vilos AG, Murji A, et al. The management of uterine leiomyomas. J Obstet Gynaecol Can. 2015;37(2):157–78.
3. Khan AT, Shehmar M, Gupta JK. Uterine fibroids: current perspectives. Int J Women's Health. 2014;6:95–114.
4. Stovall T. Myomectomy. In: Mann W, Stoval T, editors. Gynecologic surgery. New York, NY: Churchill Livingstone; 1996. p. 445–61.
5. Munro MG, Critchley HO, Broder MS, Fraser IS. FIGO classification system (PALM-COEIN) for causes of abnormal uterine bleeding in nongravid women of reproductive age. Int J Gynaecol Obstet. 2011;113(1):3–13.
6. Sinha R, Sundaram M, Lakhotia S, Hegde A. Cervical myomectomy with uterine artery ligation at its origin. J Minim Invasive Gynecol. 2009;16(5):604–8.
7. Patel P, Banker M, Munshi S, Bhalla A. Handling cervical myomas. J Gynecol Endosc Surg. 2011;2(1):30–2.
8. Rossetti A, Sizzi O, Soranna L, Cucinelli F, Mancuso S, Lanzone A. Long-term results of laparoscopic myomectomy: recurrence rate in comparison with abdominal myomectomy. Hum Reprod. 2001;16(4):770–4.
9. Takeuchi H, Kitade M, Kikuchi I, Shimanuki H, Kumakiri J, Kobayashi Y, et al. A new enucleation method for cervical myoma via laparoscopy. J Minim Invasive Gynecol. 2006;13(4):334–6.
10. Matsuoka S, Kikuchi I, Kitade M, Kumakiri J, Kuroda K, Tokita S, et al. Strategy for laparoscopic cervical myomectomy. J Minim Invasive Gynecol. 2010;17(3):301–5.
11. Chang WC, Chen SY, Huang SC, Chang DY, Chou LY, Sheu BC. Strategy of cervical myomectomy under laparoscopy. Fertil Steril. 2010;94(7):2710–5.
12. Sims JA, Brzyski R, Hansen K, Coddington CC 3rd. Use of a gonadotropin releasing hormone agonist before vaginal surgery for cervical leiomyomas. A report of two cases. J Reprod Med. 1994;39(8):660–2.
13. Thomas B, Magos A. Subtotal hysterectomy and myomectomy – vaginally. Best Pract Res Clin Obstet Gynaecol. 2011;25(2):133–52.
14. Pollard RR, Goldberg JM. Prolapsed cervical myoma after uterine artery embolization. A case report. J Reprod Med. 2001;46(5):499–500.
15. Al-Shukri M, Al-Ghafri W, Al-Dhuhli H, Gowri V. Vaginal myomectomy for prolapsed submucous fibroid: it is not only about size. Oman Med J. 2019;34(6):556–9.
16. Ikechebelu J, Eleje G, Okpala B, Onyiaorah I, Umeobika J, Onyegbule O, et al. Vaginal myomectomy of a prolapsed gangrenous cervical leiomyoma. Niger J Clin Pract. 2012;15(3):358–60.
17. Booher M, Edelson M, Jaspan D, Goldberg J. Myomectomy of a large cervical fibroid in a patient desiring future fertility. OBG Management. 2018;30(10):20–4.
18. Wong J, Tan GHC, Nadarajah R, Teo M. Novel management of a giant cervical myoma in a premenopausal patient. BMJ Case Rep. 2017;2017:bcr2017221408.
19. Del Priore G, Klapper AS, Gurshumov E, Vargas MM, Ungar L, Smith JR. Rescue radical trachelectomy for preservation of fertility in benign disease. Fertil Steril. 2010;94(5):1910 e5–7.
20. Tian J, Hu W. Cervical leiomyomas in pregnancy: report of 17 cases. Aust N Z J Obstet Gynaecol. 2012;52(3):258–61.
21. Campo S, Garcea N. Laparoscopic myomectomy in premenopausal women with and without preoperative treatment using gonadotrophin-releasing hormone analogues. Human Reprod (Oxford, England). 1999;14(1):44–8.
22. EMA/593162/2020 - Ulipristal acetate for uterine fibroids: EMA recommends restricting use. European Medicines Agency; November 2020.
23. Gobern JM, Rosemeyer CJ, Barter JF, Steren AJ. Comparison of robotic, laparoscopic, and abdominal myomectomy in a community hospital. JSLS. 2013;17(1):116–20.

24. Chen I, Lisonkova S, Joseph KS, Williams C, Yong P, Allaire C. Laparoscopic versus abdominal myomectomy: practice patterns and health care use in British Columbia. J Obstet Gynaecol Can. 2014;36(9):817–21.

25. Guarnaccia MM, Rein MS. Traditional surgical approaches to uterine fibroids: abdominal myomectomy and hysterectomy. Clin Obstet Gynecol. 2001;44(2):385–400.

26. Kim M, Ishioka S, Endo T, Baba T, Akashi Y, Morishita M, et al. Importance of uterine cervical cerclage to maintain a successful pregnancy for patients who undergo vaginal radical trachelectomy. Int J Clin Oncol. 2014;19(5):906–11.

27. Barakat EE, Bedaiwy MA, Zimberg S, Nutter B, Nosseir M, Falcone T. Robotic-assisted, laparoscopic, and abdominal myomectomy: a comparison of surgical outcomes. Obstet Gynecol. 2011;117(2 Pt 1):256–65.

28. Devassy R, Cezar C, Krentel H, Verhoeven HC, Devassy R, de Wilde MS, et al. Feasibility of myomatous tissue extraction in laparoscopic surgery by contained in – bag morcellation: a retrospective single arm study. Int J Surg (London, England). 2019;62:22–7.

29. Lee C-Y, Chen IH, Torng P-L. Robotic myomectomy for large uterine myomas. Taiwan J Obstet Gynecol. 2018;57(6):796–800.

30. Prentice A, Taylor A, Sharma MA, Magos A. Laparoscopic versus open myomectomy for uterine fibroids. Cochrane Database Syst Rev. 2004;1

31. Javadian P, Juusela A, Nezhat F. Robotic-assisted laparoscopic cervicovaginal myomectomy. J Minim Invasive Gynecol. 2019;26(1):31.

32. Unger CA, Lachiewicz MP, Ridgeway B. Risk factors for robotic gynecologic procedures requiring conversion to other surgical procedures. Int J Gynaecol Obstet. 2016;135(3):299–303.

33. Carbonnel M, Goetgheluck J, Frati A, Even M, Ayoubi JM. Robot-assisted laparoscopy for infertility treatment: current views. Fertil Steril. 2014;101(3):621–6.

34. Dubuisson JB, Fauconnier A, Fourchotte V, Babaki-Fard K, Coste J, Chapron C. Laparoscopic myomectomy: predicting the risk of conversion to an open procedure. Human Reprod (Oxford, England). 2001;16(8):1726–31.

35. Falcone T, Bedaiwy MA. Minimally invasive management of uterine fibroids. Curr Opin Obstet Gynecol. 2002;14(4):401–7.

36. Bedient CE, Magrina JF, Noble BN, Kho RM. Comparison of robotic and laparoscopic myomectomy. Am J Obstet Gynecol. 2009;201(6):566.e1–5.

37. Nezhat C, Lavie O, Hsu S, Watson J, Barnett O, Lemyre M. Robotic-assisted laparoscopic myomectomy compared with standard laparoscopic myomectomy–a retrospective matched control study. Fertil Steril. 2009;91(2):556–9.

38. Advincula AP, Xu X, Goudeau S, Ransom SB. Robot-assisted laparoscopic myomectomy versus abdominal myomectomy: a comparison of short-term surgical outcomes and immediate costs. J Minim Invasive Gynecol. 2007;14(6):698–705.

39. Kamath MS, Kalampokas EE, Kalampokas TE. Use of GnRH analogues pre-operatively for hysteroscopic resection of submucous fibroids: a systematic review and meta-analysis. Eur J Obstet Gynecol Reprod Biol. 2014;177:11–8.

40. Phillips DR, Nathanson HG, Milim SJ, Haselkorn JS, Khapra A, Ross PL. The effect of dilute vasopressin solution on blood loss during operative hysteroscopy: a randomized controlled trial. Obstet Gynecol. 1996;88(5):761–6.

41. Phillips DR, Nathanson HG, Milim SJ, Haselkorn JS. The effect of dilute vasopressin solution on the force needed for cervical dilatation: a randomized controlled trial. Obstet Gynecol. 1997;89(4):507–11.

42. Munro MG, Storz K, Abbott JA, Falcone T, Jacobs VR, Muzii L, et al. AAGL practice report: practice guidelines for the management of hysteroscopic distending media: (replaces hysteroscopic fluid monitoring guidelines. J Am Assoc Gynecol Laparosc. 2000;7:167–8.). J Minim Invasive Gynecol. 2013;20(2):137–48.

43. World HO. Comprehensive cervical cancer control: a guide to essential practice. 2nd ed. Geneva: World Health Organization; 2014.

44. Golan A, Zachalka N, Lurie S, Sagiv R, Glezerman M. Vaginal removal of prolapsed pedunculated submucous myoma: a short, simple, and definitive procedure with minimal morbidity. Arch Gynecol Obstet. 2005;271(1):11–3.

45. Goldrath MH. Vaginal removal of the pedunculated submucous myoma: the use of laminaria. Obstet Gynecol. 1987;70(4):670–2.

46. Goldrath MH. Vaginal removal of the pedunculated submucous myoma. Historical observations and development of a new procedure. J Reprod Med. 1990;35(10):921–4.

47. Dicle O, Küçükler C, Pirnar T, Erata Y, Posaci C. Magnetic resonance imaging evaluation of incision healing after cesarean sections. Eur Radiol. 1997;7(1):31–4.

Adenomyomectomy by the Triple-Flap Method

16

Hisao Osada

Introduction

Adenomyosis is a common gynecological disorder characterized by the presence of heterotopic endometrial glands and stroma infiltrating the myometrium, with adjacent smooth muscle hyperplasia. Typical symptoms include dysmenorrhea, menorrhagia, chronic pelvic pain, dyspareunia, spontaneous miscarriage, and infertility. Adenomyosis tissue lacks a definite surgical plane, making its removal extremely difficult. It can be present as either an adenomyoma or diffuse adenomyosis, and, because it deeply invades the myometrium and lacks a definitive tissue plane, complete resection is essentially impossible.

As the symptoms of adenomyosis, such as dysmenorrhea and menorrhagia, can be severely debilitating, the conventional treatment has been hysterectomy, and the definitive diagnosis has been established pathologically. However, as more patients delay childbirth, the need for conservative, effective, uterine-sparing treatments has become increasingly important. With diagnostic modalities, such as transvaginal ultrasonography and magnetic resonance imaging (MRI), the diagnosis no longer needs to be pathologically confirmed at surgery [1].

The desire to preserve fertility has led to the development of excisional surgeries, the first of which was described in 1952 by Hyams [2]. Since then, a variety of cytoreductive surgical methods have been developed in an attempt to completely eradicate the disease while easing symptoms and conserving fertility. Initially, adenomyosis was removed in a classical "V-Shaped" wedge resection, and this later evolved into procedures where more complete resections were attempted. In 2004, Fujishita proposed a transverse "H" incision by laparotomy to remove mainly anterior adenomyosis [3]. In 2010, Nishida introduced an asymmetric dissection method in which the uterine cavity was opened to further remove adenomyotic tissue [4]. With the advent of more minimally invasive surgeries, laparoscopic adenomyomectomy has also been performed, especially for focal adenomyomas. Its effectiveness for treating disease, however, may carry a much greater risk compared to laparotomy [5]. Although adenomyomectomy is effective in treating symptoms and preserving fertility, its postoperative risks include a thin uterine wall, which may lead to uterine rupture, abnormal placentation (placenta accreta/percreta), and increased spontaneous abortion.

More recently, Grimbizis et al. have shown that surgical removal could ease the symptoms of dysmenorrhea and menorrhagia in 81% and 50% of patients, respectively [6]. More importantly, for many women, pregnancy became possible.

H. Osada (✉)
Natural ART Clinic Nihonbashi,
Chuo-ku, Tokyo, Japan

Therefore, the diagnosis and conservative management of adenomyosis are becoming much more relevant, not only for the treatment of symptoms, but also for the management of infertility.

The following cytoreductive surgery for adenomyosis, termed the "triple-flap method" (also known as "the Osada Procedure"), is a completely new method that differs from other surgical methods. This method involves the resection of massive amounts of diseased tissue while maintaining a normal myometrial thickness, creating a disease-free uterus, dramatically decreasing the incidence of postoperative complications, and showing no cases of uterine rupture thus far.

Indications and Preoperative Examinations

The triple-flap method was carried out by the author in 113 patients between June 1998 and August 2017 at the Department of Obstetrics and Gynecology of the Nihon University Hospital, Okada Hospital in Tokyo, Japan, and St. Luke's Hospital in St. Louis, Missouri, U.S.A.

In our practices, the indications for the method included severe dysmenorrhea and hypermenorrhea that are difficult to control with medication, infertility, recurrent miscarriages, and a desire to preserve the fertility of the uterus. In these cases, adenomyosis involved more than 80% of the anterior and/or posterior wall of the uterus. MRI preoperative examinations were performed to accurately grasp the location and extent of uterine adenomyosis and the position of the uterine cavity to determine the site, direction, and depth of the incision to be made into the uterus. Hysterosalpingography (HSG) was also performed to examine the patency of the fallopian tube and the shape and size of the uterine cavity (Fig. 16.1).

The Triple-Flap Method

Although laparoscopic adenomyomectomy can be used to treat focal adenomyosis, it entails a risk of residual tissue after the procedure. In

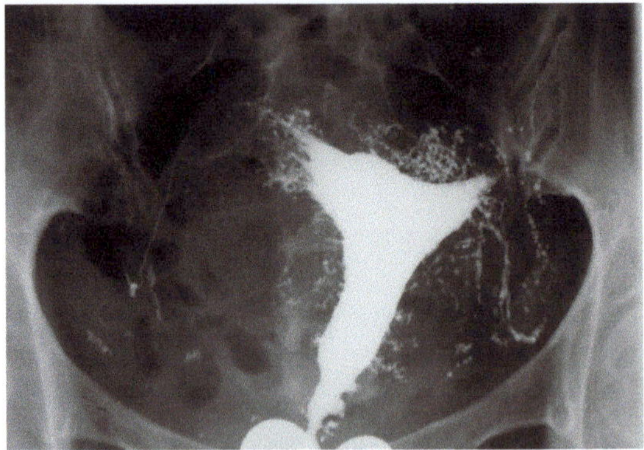

Fig. 16.1 Evaluation of uterine cavity size and shape of uterine adenomyosis by preoperative HSG

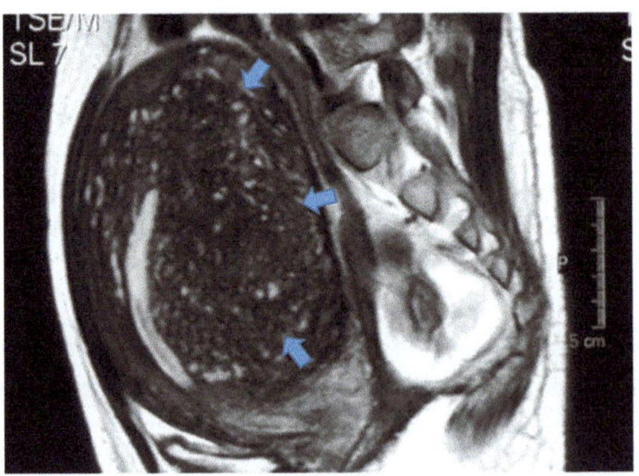

Fig. 16.2 MRI image of the posterior uterine wall with adenomyosis (The arrows indicate the location of the uterine wall)

diffuse adenomyosis, the border of the diseased tissue and the normal tissue can only be grasped by palpation. Reconstruction of the uterine wall using the triple-flap method is a delicate procedure because the flaps are sutured in layers. Therefore, to accurately remove diffuse adenomyosis tissue and perform triple-flap uterine wall reconstruction, laparotomy or laparoscopic-assisted laparotomy is necessary. Reconstruction of the uterus using this method can be accomplished for all forms of adenomyosis, including adenomyomas, anterior/posterior disease (Figs. 16.2 and 16.3), and global diffuse adenomyosis (Figs. 16.4 and 16.5) [7–13].

The main objectives of this procedure are as follows: (1) Removal of all adenomyoma tissues by visualization and palpation using a cold knife

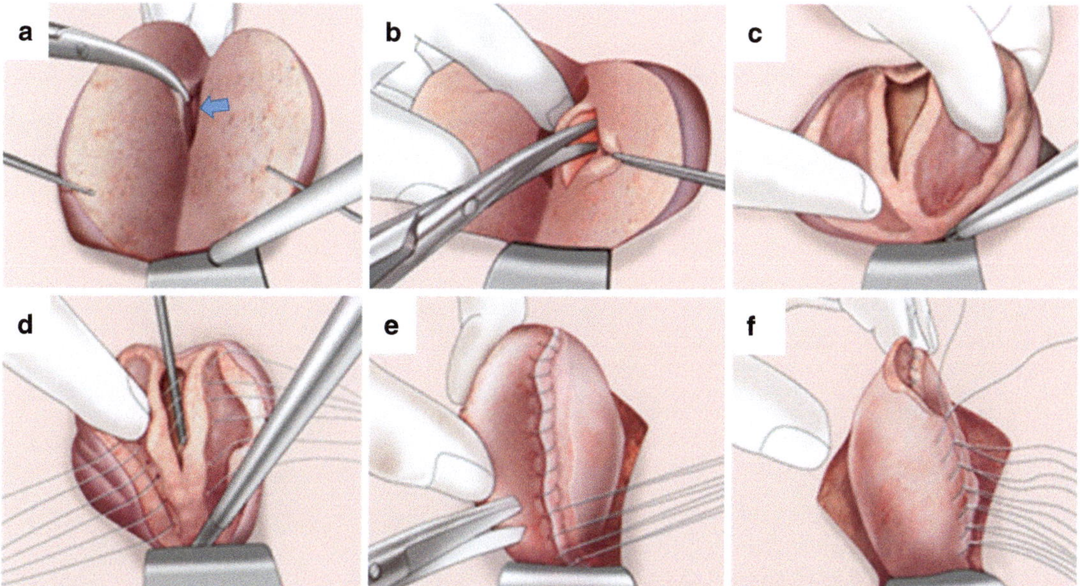

Fig. 16.3 (**a–f**) Schematic diagram of the triple-flap method applied to the posterior adenomyosis (The arrow indicates the location of the uterine cavity.) (**a**) Bisection of the uterus/adenomyosis, (**b**) Excision of adenomyotic tissue, (**c**) Copious irrigation, (**d**) Reconstruction of the uterine cavity (suturing the first layer), (**e**) Reconstruction of the uterine wall (suturing the second layer), (**f**) Reconstruction of the uterine wall (suturing the third layer)

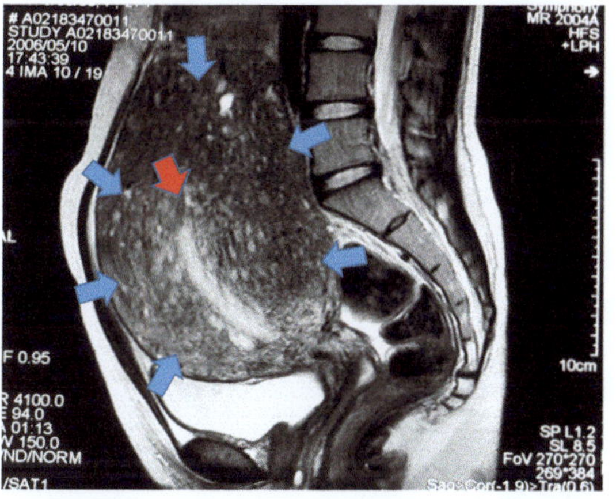

Fig. 16.4 MRI image of the anterior and posterior uterine wall with adenomyosis (The blue and red arrows indicate the location of uterine wall and cavity, respectively)

to avoid poor wound healing and possible suture failure; (2) Reconstruction of the functional uterine cavity through initiating metroplasty by opening the uterine cavity to preserve the thickness of the endometrial tissue flap and its functionality; (3) Reconstruction of the uterine wall in a non-overlapping manner to disperse the load (tension) in such a way as to prevent uterine rupture due to possible pregnancy.

The procedure for performing adenomyomectomy by the triple-flap method is divided into six steps.

Step 1: Diagnostic Laparoscopy

Laparoscopy allows observation of the inside of the pelvis to confirm the mobility of the uterus. If adhesions are found, laparoscopic adhesiolysis can be performed to free the uterus. This allows adenomyomectomy by the triple-flap method to be performed with a smaller laparotomy wound.

Key Point
1. Preoperative vaginal lavage is a necessary and effective procedure to prevent ascending vaginal infections during and after surgery. We use 0.025% benzalkonium chloride disinfectant solution for the lavage.

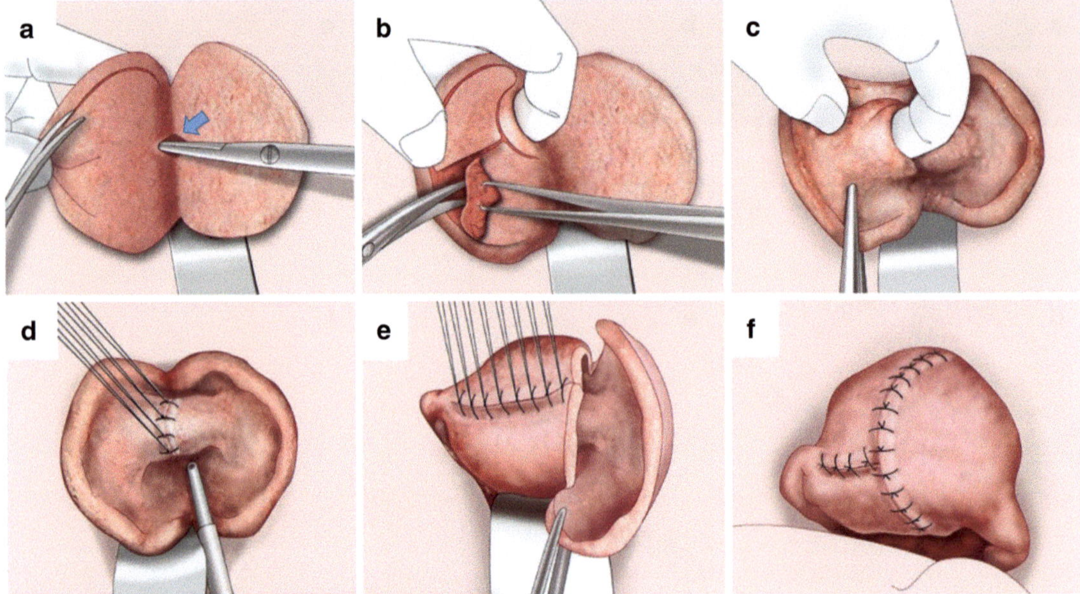

Fig. 16.5 (**a–f**) Schematic diagram of the triple-flap method applied to the anterior and posterior adenomyosis (The arrow indicates the location of the uterine cavity). (**a**) Bisection of the uterus/adenomyosis, (**b**) Excision of adenomyotic tissue, (**c**) Copious irrigation, (**d**) Reconstruction of the uterine cavity (suturing the first layer), (**e**) Reconstruction of the uterine wall (suturing the second layer), (**f**) Reconstruction of the uterine wall (suturing of the third layer)

Step 2: Exteriorization of the Uterus and Placement of a Tourniquet Around the Proximal Cervix

A transverse suprapubic incision (Pfannenstiel incision) is made to extraperitonealize the uterus. The typical length of the incision is approximately 10–15 cm, depending on the size of the uterus. From the incision, a rubber tube (pediatric tourniquet) is placed around the proximal cervix through the broad ligament, avoiding the infundibulopelvic ligament, to occlude the ascending uterine arteries to achieve better hemostasis (Fig. 16.6). (The infundibulopelvic ligament can be clamped with a Bulldog clamp when bleeding is severe, but it should be used only temporarily for a short period of time.) Next, two Martin forceps are used to grasp the uterine fundus (which contains the adenomyosis), and the uterus is pulled out of the abdominal wall through the Pfannenstiel incision.

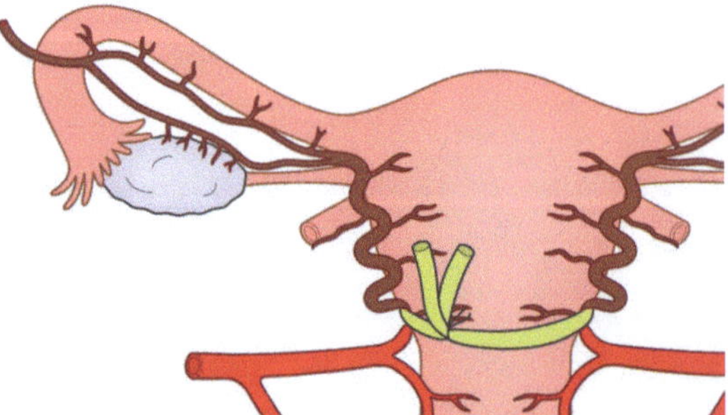

Fig. 16.6 A rubber tube is placed around the proximal cervix, thus encompassing the ascending uterine arteries and acting as a tourniquet. (With permission from Nakayama Shoten [13])

Key Points

1. Surgery on the uterus outside the abdominal cavity is made much easier with a small Pfannenstiel incision than a large open wound.
2. When a tourniquet is applied to the infundibulopelvic ligament, blood flow in the ovarian artery is completely blocked. Although it min-

imizes the bleeding, it may make microvascular bleeding challenging to see and could result in an increase in postoperative bleeding. Prolonged occlusion may have an adverse effect on the ovaries' function due to the ischemia.

3. As long-term tourniqueting leads to blood coagulation disorders, it is preferable to loosen the tourniquet every 2–3 h and resume blood flow for a brief period of time.

Step 3: Bisection of the Uterus/ Adenomyosis

The left and right sides of the apex of the enlarged uterus are grasped using Martin forceps. With a cold knife, the enlarged uterus is bisected in the sagittal midline incision of the fundus from the serosal surface through the adenomyotic tissue until the uterine cavity is accessed while pulling the Martin forceps to the left and right (Figs. 16.3a, 16.5a, 16.7, and 16.8). The use of a cold knife is preferable to using an electric knife, as the latter causes severe tissue damage due to burns which delay wound healing. The poorly defined boundaries of the adenomyosis are now visualized (Fig. 16.8). Then, Kelly forceps are inserted into the uterine cavity, which is now separated into left and right, and the size and shape of the uterine cavity are checked (Figs. 16.3a,

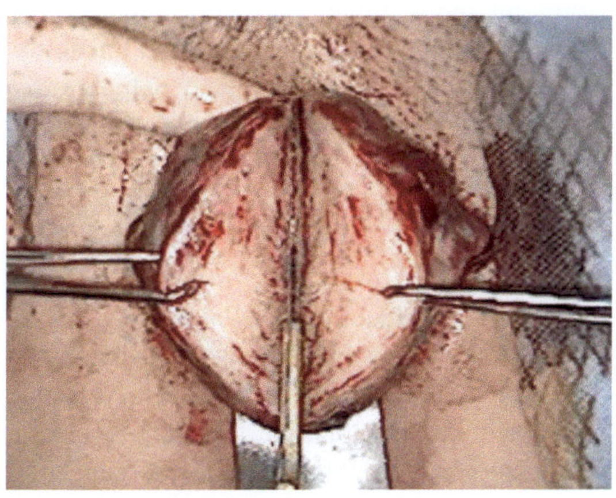

Fig. 16.7 Bisection of the uterus/adenomyosis

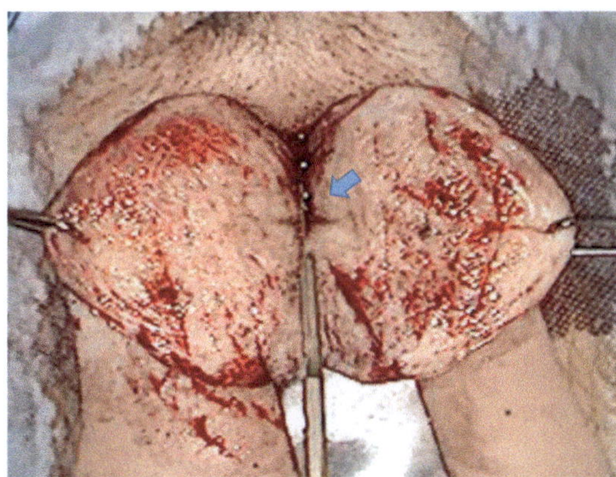

Fig. 16.8 Section to the uterine cavity (The arrow indicates uterine cavity)

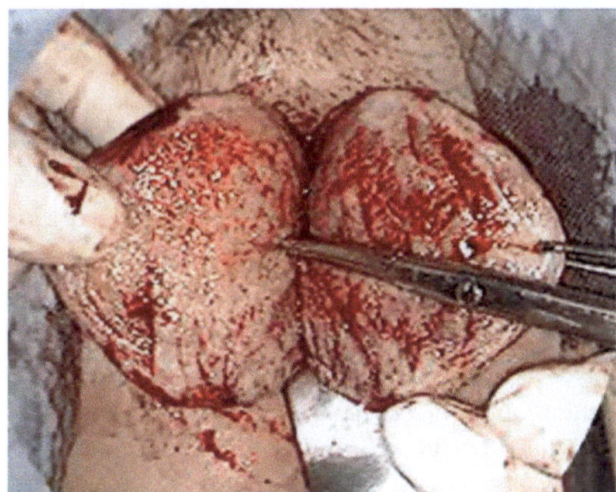

Fig. 16.9 Checking the uterine cavity

16.5a, and 16.9). In order to protect the interstitial part of the fallopian tubes, the fallopian tubes are located through the uterine cavity and a thin, soft catheter is inserted from the uterine ostium into each of the fallopian tubes.

Key Points

1. If the scalpel goes in the wrong direction, it will not reach the uterine cavity and performing the triple-flap method will become extremely difficult. Therefore, prior to creating the incision, it is necessary to confirm the position of the uterine cavity using MRI and HSG, and to determine correctly the scalpel incision.

2. Other methods of locating the uterine cavity to help determine the direction of the incision include a uterine manipulator, blue dye, and/or ultrasonography which is applied directly to the uterine wall.
3. Pulsating vascular bleeding is stopped by pinpoint coagulation.

Step 4: Excision of Adenomyotic Tissue

The adenomyotic lesion is removed by palpation under direct vision to create the inner endometrial flap (endometrial uterine muscle) for uterine cavity reconstruction and the serosal layer (serosal uterine muscle flap) for uterine wall reconstruction. The uterine cavity is sufficiently opened, allowing the insertion/placement of the index finger or the Kelly forceps to ensure an appropriate inner endometrial flap thickness and protect the cornual region (Figs. 16.3b, 16.5b, 16.10, and 16.11). The adenomyotic tissue is now demarcated by making an incision 1 cm from the surface of the serosal layer (Fig. 16.10) and 1 cm proximal to the endometrium (Fig. 16.11).

The adenomyotic tissues are grasped with Martin forceps, and all diseased tissue that lie between these 1 cm flaps is now removed with Metzenbaum scissors or a scalpel while ensuring the integrity of the serosal flap thickness by

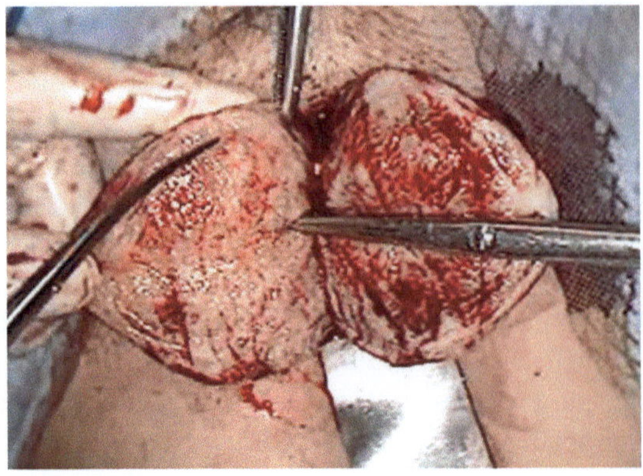

Fig. 16.10 Removing adenomyotic tissue using palm palpation

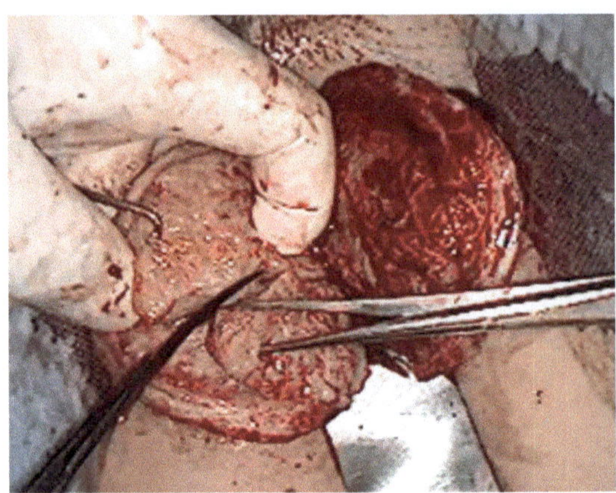

Fig. 16.11 Removing adenomyotic tissue using index finger palpation

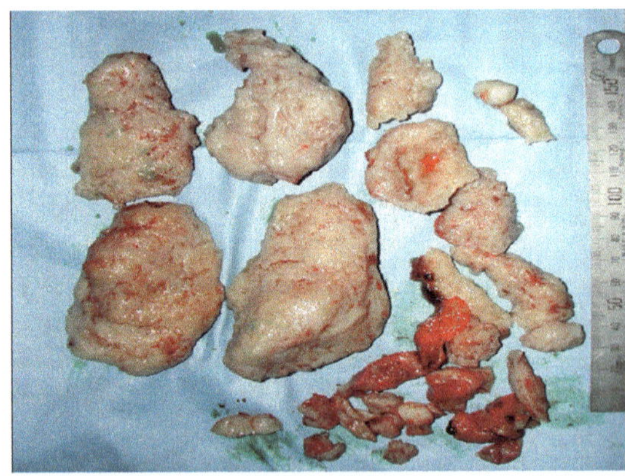

Fig. 16.12 Excised uterine adenomyotic tissue

palm palpation (Fig. 16.10) and the endometrium by index finger palpation (Fig. 16.11). Meticulous excision of any residual adenomyotic tissue is performed until all palpable diseased tissue is removed, and the surfaces of both flaps are smooth and free of disease (Fig. 16.12).

Key Points

1. Preserve oviductal patency as much as possible to allow postoperative spontaneous pregnancy by injecting methylene blue dye and/or inserting a stent into the fallopian tubes during surgery through the uterine ostium of the fallopian tube, taking care not to damage the tube.

2. Adenomyotic tissue is removed by separating it from the normal uterine muscle by pushing the scissors into the coarse tissue between the hard adenomyotic tissue and the normal myometrium.

Step 5: Reconstruction of the Uterine Wall by the Triple-Flap Method

The reconstruction of the uterine wall by the triple-flap method consists of the reconstruction of the uterine cavity (suturing the first layer of the uterine muscle) and reconstruction of the uterine wall (suturing the second and third layers of the uterine muscle).

As this surgery involves opening and manipulating the uterine cavity, there is a high probability of ascending infection from the vagina. Therefore, to prevent postoperative infection, it is necessary to copiously irrigate the surgical field throughout the entire process. In particular, when suturing the first layer of the uterine muscle, which closes the endometrium, it is necessary to thoroughly irrigate the uterine cavity, including the cervical canal, and remove tissue fragments and blood clots in the uterus (Figs. 16.3c, 16.5c, and 16.13). We use 3% D-Solbitol (UromaticS®) for irrigation, and also administer intravenous antibiotics (Cephalosporin). In addition, as the uterine wall is reconstructed by stacking three thin uterine muscle flaps, it is important to perform surgery with single interrupted sutures that cause less local blood flow obstruction.

Reconstruction of the Uterine Cavity (Suturing the First Layer of the Uterine Muscle)

The opened uterine cavity is closed with the endometrial flap (first flap suture) using 3–0 Vicryl (absorbable suture) and a taper-point needle (Ethicon, SH-1; 22 mm, 1/2 circle). Sutures are performed at 5–7 mm intervals by single interrupted sutures in a manner in which the sutures are not exposed to the uterine cavity (Figs. 16.3d, 16.5d, 16.14, and 16.15). If the uterine cavity has been enlarged, it should be reduced in size by partially trimming the intimal side of

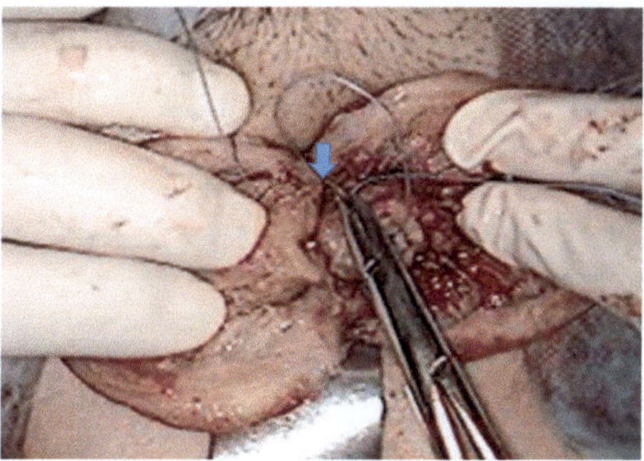

Fig. 16.14 Single interrupted sutures (The arrow indicates the two edges to be sutured)

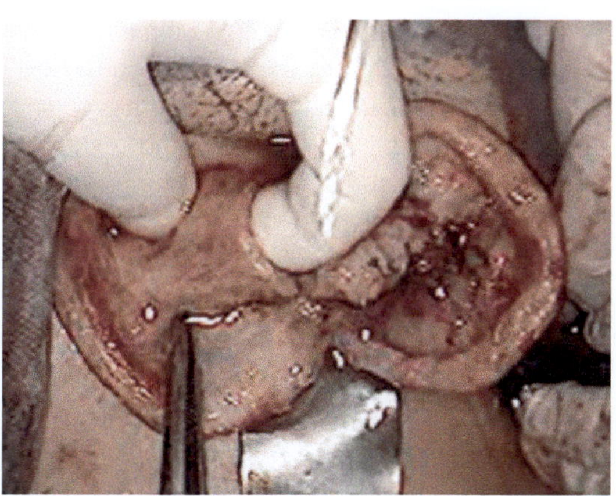

Fig. 16.13 Copious irrigation

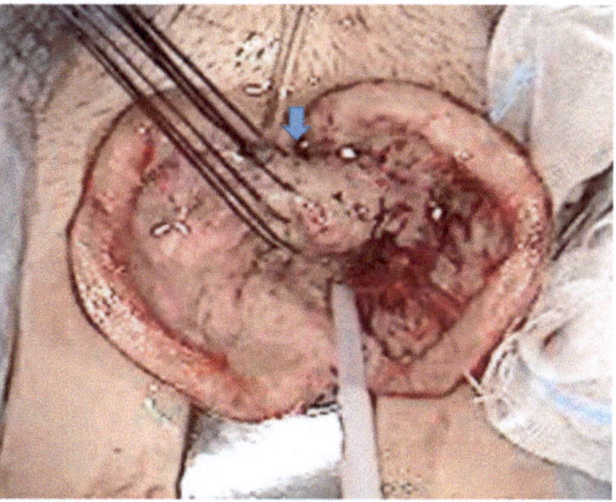

Fig. 16.15 Suturing the first layer of the uterine muscle (The arrow indicates the finished suturing)

the uterine muscle flap with reference to the preoperative HSG and MRI. At this time, suturing requires utmost care because too strong a suture may cause rupture of the uterine muscle, and too weak sutures may cause suture failure.

Key Points
1. To clean the opened uterine cavity, temporarily loosen the tourniquet on the cervix and irrigate deep into the cervix.
2. Insufficient irrigation of the uterine cavity may result in endometritis and uterine wall wound inflammation due to transvaginal infection after surgery and is likely to cause suture failure and surgical wound dehiscence.
3. During hysteroplasty, exposure of sutures to the uterine cavity can cause infection and induce complications, such as placenta accreta and suture failure (Fig. 16.14).
4. Failure of suturing in the first uterine muscle layer may induce recurrence of adenomyosis due to invasion of the endometrium into the muscular layer and placenta accreta due to postoperative pregnancy.

Reconstruction of the Uterine Wall (Suturing of the Second Uterine Muscle Layer)

The serosal flaps are now irrigated after the closure of the endometrium and are closed in a fashion that ensures that no two suture lines directly overlap each other. This is accomplished by first suturing one of the remaining myometrial/serosal flaps to the repaired endometrial flap in the anteroposterior plane with a single interrupted suture at 10–12 mm intervals using 2–0 Vicryl suture. Thus, the second flap is pulled toward the contralateral side (Figs. 16.3e, 16.5e, and 16.16).

Key Points
1. If the uterine muscle flap to be covered is too large, a dead space would be created between the uterine muscle flaps, causing hematoma and suture failure, which affects healing. Therefore, the serosal uterine muscle flap should be trimmed according to the size of the first layer of the uterine muscle and then sutured carefully.

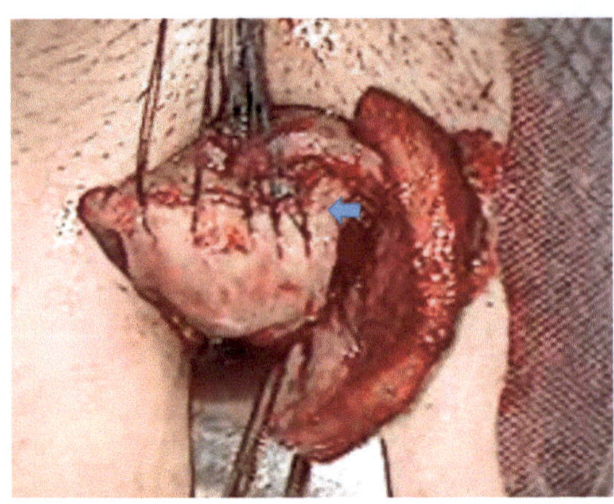

Fig. 16.16 Suturing the second uterine muscle layer (The arrow indicates where two edges have been brought together and sutured)

2. It is necessary to suture with utmost care so that the sutures are not exposed to the uterine cavity and placenta accreta is prevented.

Reconstruction of the Uterine Wall (Suturing of the Third Uterine Muscle Layer)

At this stage, the serosal uterine muscle flap on the other side is layered on the already sutured second uterine muscle layer to form the uterine wall of the third uterine muscle layer. Prior to the placement of this third and final flap, the serosal surface of the second flap must be removed to ensure proper wound healing of the myometrium (Fig. 16.17). This is accomplished by first marking the area to be denuded and then, with a scalpel, stripping the serosa off from the underlying myometrium. The third flap is now pulled over and secured to the second flap, assuring no overlapping suture lines, with interrupted suturing using 2–0 Vicryl, until the entire defect is closed and the serosa is reapproximated (Figs. 16.3f, 16.5f, and 16.18). After the reconstruction of the uterine wall is completed, the tourniquet is removed, the hole in the broad ligament is closed, and the Pfannenstiel transverse incision is closed.

Key Points
1. If sutures are exposed to the uterine cavity, a risk of inducing placenta accreta arises.

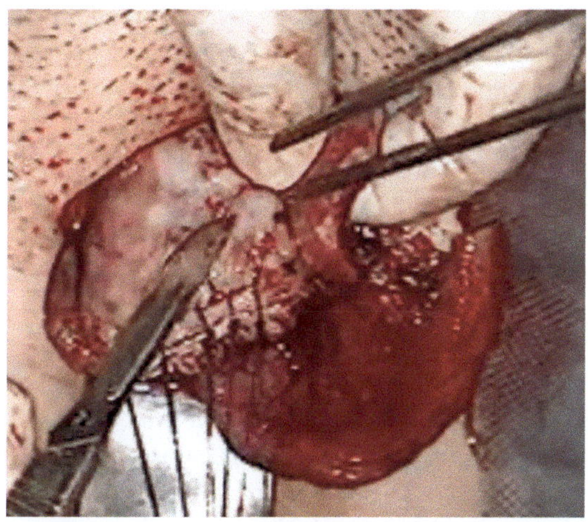

Fig. 16.17 Peeling the uterine serosal surface

remove tissue fragments and blood clots that cause adhesions by suction, and thoroughly irrigate the surgical field in the abdominal cavity (Fig. 16.19). The triple-flap method creates a large wound on the surface of the uterus, and vascular bleeding and oozing are often observed from the sutured parts and surfaces created by adhesiolysis. Pinpoint vascular bleeding is stemmed by coagulation. However, as oozing is difficult to stop, TachoComb®, an absorbable fibrin-collagen patch sheet, is applied for hemostasis (Fig. 16.20). After the operation, the position of the patient is frequently changed (alternately placed in the left and right lateral decubitus positions) to prevent adhesions, start-

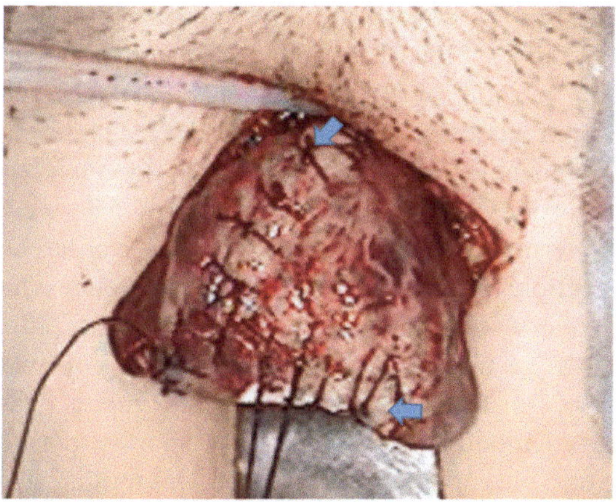

Fig. 16.18 Suturing the third uterine muscle layer (Arrows indicate where the serosal edge has been brought onto the denuded second layer and sutured)

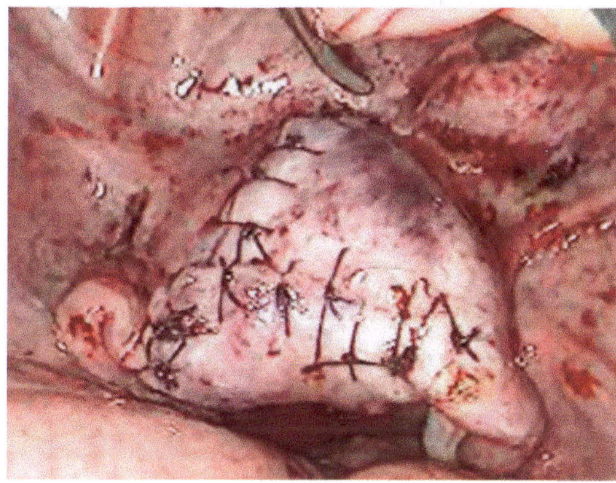

Fig. 16.19 Irrigating the surgical field in the abdominal cavity

2. To avoid inducing hematoma that causes suture failure of the wound, suturing must be performed with the utmost care so that there is no dead space between the uterine muscle flaps.
3. Insufficient suturing of the second and third uterine muscle layers poses a risk of uterine rupture.

Step 6: Final Laparoscopy and Adhesion Prevention

A final laparoscopic examination is performed again to observe the entire abdominal cavity,

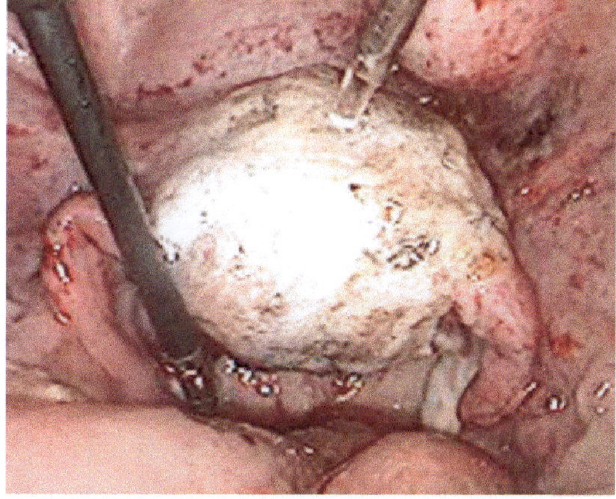

Fig. 16.20 TachoComb® was pasted on the uterine surface

ing immediately after being returned to the recovery room [7–13].

Figure 16.21 shows the condition of the wound on the uterine wall of a patient who conceived spontaneously after adenomyomectomy by the triple-flap method and delivered by cesarean section. This photograph was taken at the time of the cesarean section. No thinning of the uterine wall and no depression caused by scar tissue formation were observed.

Key Points

1. Care should be taken when using TachoComb®, as resting overnight without changing the position will cause strong adhesions.

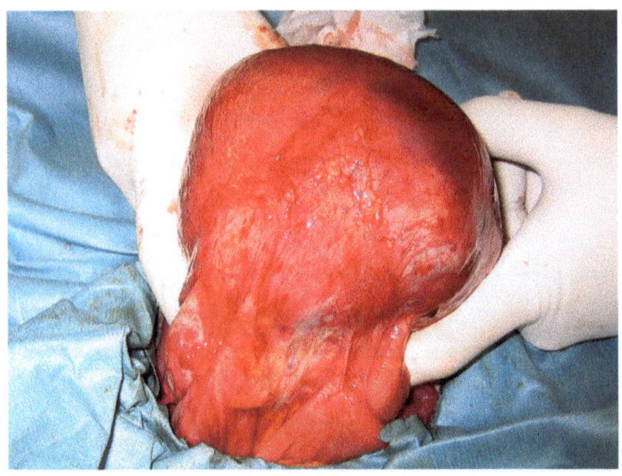

Fig. 16.21 The condition of the uterine wall observed during the cesarean section

2. When TachoComb® is used, preventing its adhesion effect is enhanced by alternating the resting position of the patient between left and right every 60 min for several hours immediately after she is returned to the room and then every 2–3 h for the next 2 days [7–13].

Results of the Triple-Flap Method

The effectiveness of the surgery on symptoms of dysmenorrhea and menorrhagia was evaluated postoperatively using a visual analog scale (VAS) (Fig. 16.22). The symptoms of both dysmenorrhea and menorrhagia had significantly improved.

The procedure also had a positive effect on infertility. Sixty-two out of the 113 patients wished to conceive following the triple-flap method. Of the 62 women, 32 became pregnant for a total of 46 pregnancies (7 conceived spontaneously and 39 by IVF/ET). Of the 46 pregnancies, 14 experienced a spontaneous abortion (14/46; 30.4%), and 32 (69.5%) went to term and were delivered by elective cesarean section (Table 16.1). Of the 32 patients who became pregnant and delivered babies, the average time from surgery to conception was 20.5 ± 21.4 months, and the range was 5–81 months. Incidentally, the shortest period from surgery to pregnancy was 5 months. The pregnancy was an unplanned, spontaneous

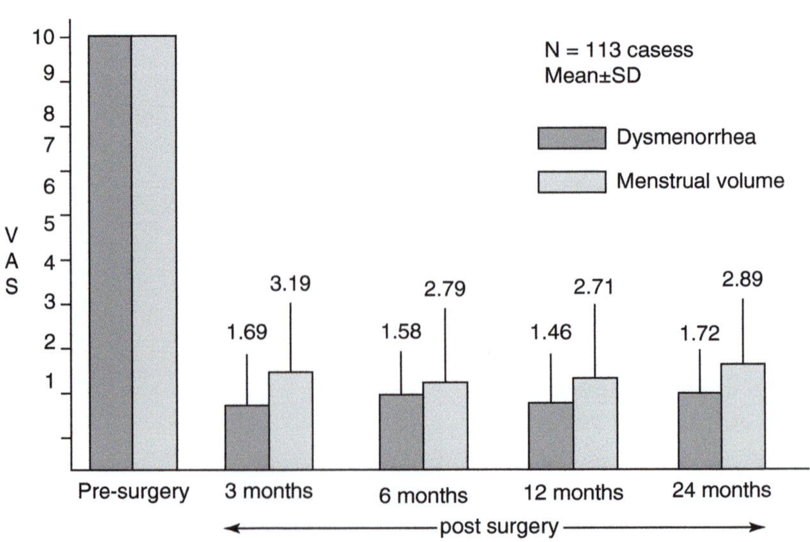

Fig. 16.22 VAS demonstrating the clinical postoperative efficacy of the triple-flap method for dysmenorrhea and hypermenorrhea

Table 16.1 Outcome of surgical treatment for severe cases of adenomyosis using the triple-flap method

	N	%
No. of patients	113	
Age of patients	38.2 ± 7.2	
No. of patients who wished to conceive	62/113	54.8
No. of patients who became pregnant	32/62	51.6
Total no. of pregnancies	46/62	74.1
Spontaneous pregnancies	7/46	15.2
IVF-ET	39/46	84.7
Birth and pregnancy outcome:		
Miscarriages[a]	14/46	30.4
Births by elective cesarean section	32/46	69.5
Spontaneous pregnancies	6/32	18.7
IVF-ET	26/32	81.2

[a]5 weeks × 8; 6 weeks × 2; 7 weeks × 1; 8 weeks × 2; 16 weeks × 1

pregnancy (twin pregnancy). Most importantly, there were no cases of uterine rupture during any of the pregnancies [12, 13].

Surgery-to-Pregnancy Interval

Whether the period of contraception after adenomyomectomy correlates with the occurrence of uterine rupture remains unclear. The risk of uterine rupture after uterine surgery and a trial of labor has been well established, with reported rates of uterine rupture at 0.27% after cesarean delivery [14]. In a study by Bujold et al., 1527 cesarean section deliveries with a subsequent trial of labor correlated the incidence of uterine rupture when the pregnancy occurred less than 24 months after the surgery to have a two to three fold increased risk of uterine rupture [15]. Following adenomyomectomy, the literature suggests that the contraceptive period varies by institution. Although there have been uneventful pregnancies when conception has occurred at a 3-month interval, most institutions recommend a period of 6–12 months. Interestingly, our literature review suggested that uterine rupture after adenomyomectomy included three cases of uterine rupture when pregnancy occurred within 3 months of surgery. Additionally, three uterine ruptures occurred between 3 and 6 months, two between 6 and 12 months, and eight over 1 year [5].

There is no agreed-upon recommendation in the literature for a compulsory waiting time before attempting conception. Our approach, using contrast-enhanced MRI and ultrasound Doppler imaging postoperatively, shows the evolution of resolving avascular areas in the uterus. Of the 113 patients who underwent adenomyomectomy using the triple-flap method, resolution of the avascular area occurred in 92 patients (81.4%) within 6 months and in 111 patients (98.2%) within 1 year. Interestingly, the resolution of vascularity in two patients required up to 2 years (Fig. 16.23a–h). These cases indicated that the return of vascularity might take up to 2 years, especially when there is massive resection of the uterine wall. Therefore, permission to attempt pregnancy is given when there is confirmation of the loss of the avascular area, ensuring the resumption of uterine blood flow [12].

Laparotomy Versus Laparoscopy

The published literature has not elucidated which type of procedure increases the risk of uterine rupture. There are many advantages and disadvantages of laparotomy, laparoscopy, or a combination of both methods. Nezhat et al. showed the efficacy of laparoscopy-assisted myomectomy as a safe alternative to myomectomy by laparotomy [16]. This approach is technically not as difficult to perform, may require less operative time, reduce blood loss and postoperative recovery time, and reduce adhesion formation. However, laparotomy, with or without laparoscopic assistance, allows for better closure of the uterine defect with multiple layers and more touch-sensitive monitoring of adequate remaining uterine tissue [10–13]. Laparoscopic adenomyomectomy may result in incompletely repaired muscle defects compared to laparotomy. Thus, the risk of uterine rupture is believed to increase during subsequent pregnancies following a laparoscopic approach [17–22]. Laparoscopic procedures also utilize powered instruments such as monopolar cautery, high frequency cutting instruments, and laser knives. In a review of the literature, there have been 24 cases reported of uterine rupture after adenomyosis surgery. Of these, 18 cases used powered instruments

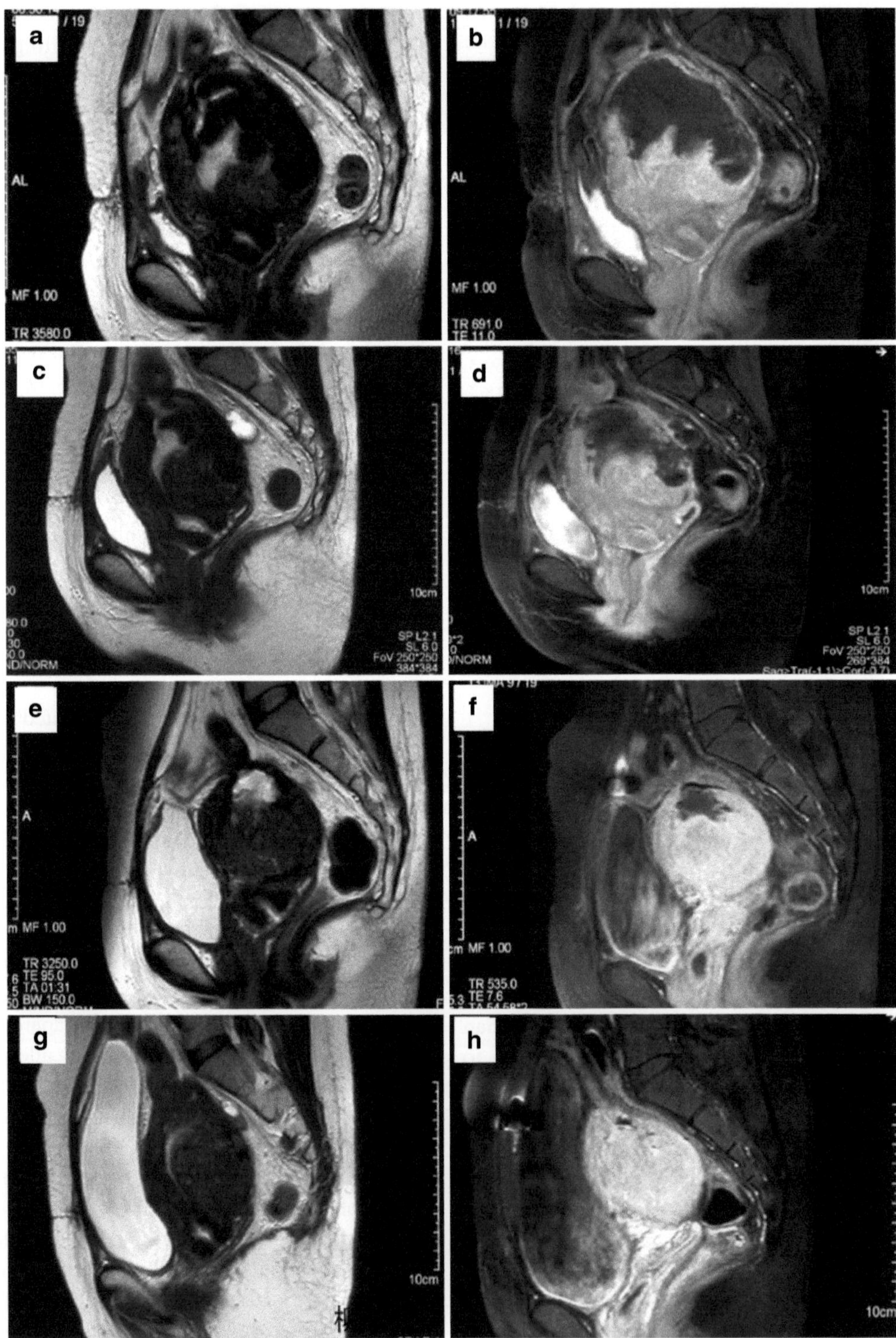

Fig. 16.23 (a–h) MRI image showing the circumferential vascular pattern of a myometrial lesion. (a–h) Contrast-enhanced MRI showing resumption of blood flow (loss of avascular area) after the surgery ((a, b) 2 months after surgery; (c, d) 6 months after surgery; (e, f) 12 months after surgery; (g, h) 2 years after surgery)

(eight monopolar/four laser knife/six high frequency), and six cases had no equipment described [5]. Therefore, the use of powered instruments in laparoscopy may also be associated with uterine rupture during pregnancy.

Wound Healing Disturbance Due to Excessive Electrocoagulation

Wound healing is generally a complex process involving inflammation, angiogenesis, new tissue formation, and tissue remodeling [23]. This process requires balanced collagen deposition and growth factor release from the injured site. Pathologic scarring (hypertrophic scarring) interferes with growth factor expression [24]. Uterine ruptures involving the scarred area after uterine fibroid surgery or cesarean section typically demonstrate abnormally high concentrations of collagen and fewer smooth muscle cells in the tissue near the rupture sites. As a result, there is a high possibility that the strength of the uterine muscle layer is diminished [23].

A detailed histologic investigation into the influence of electrocautery on wound healing has indicated that it may greatly interfere with wound healing and cause secondary uterine damage [25]. Other studies have reported a histological delay in wound healing associated with electrocautery compared with the use of a surgical blade. Power instruments such as the ultrasonically activated scalpel used in laparoscopy cause blood vessel sealing due to the presence of clots of heat-denatured proteins. These clots form highly cohesive agglomerates due to tissue protein degeneration that affects wound healing [26]. Therefore, use of an instrument that causes healing disorders may result in suture failure due to tissue necrosis, scarring, and excessive collagen deposition [27, 28].

Although removal of adenomyosis can be accomplished by laparotomy or laparoscopy, the latter exclusively uses powered instruments. To understand the need to decrease the use of electrocauterization, vasopressin injection has been used in conjunction with laparoscopic procedures to reduce the amount of hemorrhage [29, 30]. In our review of 24 uterine ruptures, all reported operative methods involved the use of powered instruments during laparotomy or laparoscopy [5]. Therefore, if the use of electrosurgical instruments affects wound healing, it seems logical to avoid them when possible.

Postoperative Recurrence and Pathological Examination of the Removed Uterus

Recurrence of adenomyosis was observed in four patients (3.8%) within 5 years postoperatively, and dysmenorrhea was controlled by drug therapy. By 15 years post-operation, three patients had a recurrence and underwent a hysterectomy. Of them, one had a recurrence 13 years postoperatively with ascites that was difficult to control and underwent hysterectomy (Fig. 16.24: center).

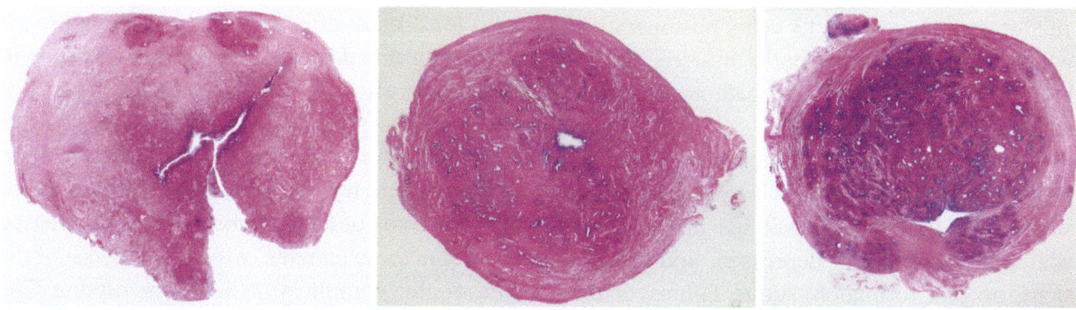

Fig. 16.24 Pathological findings of the uterine specimen removed by total hysterectomy due to recurrence after adenomyomectomy by the triple-flap method. *Left*: 10 years after surgery; *center*: 13 years after surgery; *right*: 9 years after surgery

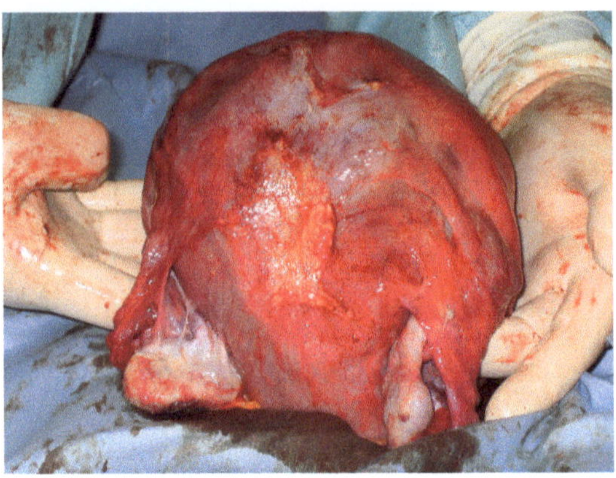

Fig. 16.25 The condition of the uterine wall of a patient who spontaneously conceived 5 months after the operation and gave birth by cesarean section 13 months after the operation

The remaining two patients had a recurrence at 10 years and 9 years postoperatively and underwent a hysterectomy due to suspected malignancy (Fig. 16.24: left and right, respectively).

Figure 16.25 shows the uterine wall wound of a patient who underwent adenomyomectomy by the triple-flap method at the age of 31 and spontaneously conceived twins at 5 months postoperatively (no thinning of the uterine wall was observed during the pregnancy). She had a premature rupture of the membranes at 34 weeks, 3 days of gestation, and underwent cesarean section on the same day. Figure 16.25 was photographed at the time of the cesarean section. In the wound of the uterine wall, a sheet-like hemostatic material (TachoComb®) applied to the sutured part was found, but no adhesion with the surrounding tissues was observed, and the uterine wall was flat with no depression. This patient had an aforesaid recurrence 13 years postoperatively with ascites and underwent a hysterectomy. In Fig. 16.24, the center is the pathological specimen of her removed uterus.

Laparotomic findings of the uterus of the three patients who underwent hysterectomy demonstrated that the surgical wounds of the uterine wall were flat and not depressed, and no adhesions, no scar formation, suture failure, or thinning of the uterine wall suture were observed in the pathological specimen of the removed uterus.

Pathological examination of the resected specimen revealed slight scarring at the microscopic level at the serosal suture on the surface of the uterus. No scar formation or suture failure was observed at the site where the uterine muscle flaps were presumed to have overlapped, and the uterine muscle flaps were integrated into the surrounding muscle layer. Although some disturbance in the running of smooth muscle fibers was observed at the same site, smooth muscles were evenly distributed and no decrease in uterine muscle fibers was observed.

No abnormality in the distribution of collagen fibers and elastic fibers was demonstrated by special staining, and the effect of the surgery was considered extremely minor. The endometrial wound was slightly depressed when viewed from the uterine cavity surface, but no rupture or scar formation of the endometrium was observed. In addition, no abnormality was observed in the muscular layer (junctional zone) just below the endometrium. Regarding the recurrence of adenomyosis, uterine adenomyotic tissue was scattered in the muscle layer in two patients, but it is unknown whether it was a recurrence or a remnant around the surgical site. One patient had a clear recurrence of adenomyosis.

Conclusion

Adenomyosis is a disabling disease in women that until recently had been treated with hysterectomy. However, an increasing number of patients are now wishing to preserve their uterus for childbearing or cultural reasons, necessitating the need for a more effective conservative approach in treating this disease. Such treatment needs to be not only effective but also decrease the risk of postoperative pregnancy complications such as uterine rupture. Thus far, the triple-flap method described here has not only significantly reduced the symptoms of adenomyosis but also increased fertility in these patients, with no incidence of the catastrophic complication of uterine rupture. The principles of laparotomy, avoidance of power instruments, complete resection of adenomyotic tissue, avoidance of overlapping suture lines, and adequate surgery-to-pregnancy interval assuring complete resolution of blood flow to the uterus are essential to a successful outcome.

Acknowledgements I would like to thank Drs. S. J. Silber, M. DeRosa, T. Kakinuma, M. Nagaishi, K. Kato, and S. Teramoto for their help in developing this new procedure. I would also like to thank K. Nakazato and A. Pinnington for their help in the preparation of the manuscript.

References

1. Novellas S, Chassang M, Delotte J, Toullalan O, Chevallier A, Bouaziz J, et al. MRI characteristics of the uterine junctional zone: from normal to the diagnosis of adenomyosis. Am J Roentgenol. 2011;196:1206–13.
2. Hyams LL. Adenomyosis: its conservative surgical treatment (hysteroplasty) in young women. N Y State J Med. 1952;52:2778–83.
3. Fujishita A, Masuzaki H, Khan KN, Kitajima M, Ishimaru T. Modified reduction surgery for adenomyosis. Gynecol Obstet Investig. 2004;57:132–8.
4. Nishida M, Takano K, Arai Y, Ozone H, Ichikawa R. Conservative surgical management for diffuse uterine adenomyosis. Fertil Steril. 2010;94:715–9.
5. Osada H. Uterine adenomyosis and adenomyoma: the surgical approach. Fertil Steril. 2018;109:406.
6. Grimbizis GF, Mikos T, Tarlatzis B. Uterus-sparing operative treatment for adenomyosis. Fertil Steril. 2014;101:472–87.
7. Osada H, Onishi M, Yamada Y, Akamine K, Tsubata K, Takagi S. Fiburin secchaku-zai no sosho-chiyu ni oyobosu eikyo, tokuni fibrin kozo no keitaigakuteki-kansatyu nituite (The effect of fibrin adhesive on wound healing, especially the morphological observation of fibrin structure). San-Fujinka No Sekai. 1988;40:801–8.
8. Osada H, Fujii TK, Tanaka H, Tsubata K, Yoshida T, Satoh K. Clinical significance of TachoComb®, a fibrin adhesive in sheet. In: Szabo Z, et al., editors. Surgical technology international VII; 1998. p. 1–5.
9. Osada H, Minai M, Yoshida T, Satoh K. Use of fibrin adhesive to reduce post-surgical adhesion reformation in rabbits. J Int Med Res. 1999;27:242–6.
10. Osada H. Surgical procedure to conserve the uterus for future pregnancy in patients suffering from diffuse adenomyosis: a comprehensive manual and procedure DVD. Tokyo: Medical View; 2006.
11. Osada H, Silber S, Kakinuma T, Nagaishi M, Kato K, Kato O. Surgical procedure to conserve the uterus for future pregnancy in patients suffering from massive adenomyosis. Reprod Biomed Online. 2011;22:94–9.
12. Osada H, Teramoto S, Kato K, Nagaishi M. Triple flap ho niyoru shikyusenkinsho –tekishutsujutsu – Chiryo-seiseki oyobi sanka-gappeisho no bunkenteki kosatsu (Adenomyomectomy by triple-flap method – literature review of treatment outcomes and obstetric complications). J Jpn Soc Endometr. 2018;39:87–97.
13. Osada H. Shujutsu ryoho – triple flap ho niyoru sikyusenkinsho tekishutsujutsu (Operative treatment – adenomyomectomy by triple-flap method). In: Osuga Y, Koga K, editors. Shikyunaimakusho-shikyusenkinsho shindan atlas ando aratana chiryo-senryaku (Endometriosis and adenomyosis of the uterus – diagnostic atlas and new treatment strategies). Tokyo: Nakayama Shoten; 2021.
14. Guise JM, McDonagh MS, Osterweil P, Nygren P, Chan BK, Helfand M. Systematic review of the incidence and consequences of uterine rupture in women with previous caesarean section. BMJ. 2004;329:19.
15. Bujold E, Mehta SH, Bujold C, Gauthier RJ. Interdelivery interval and uterine rupture. Am J Obstet Gynecol. 2002;187:1199–202.
16. Nezhat C, Nezhat F, Bess O, Nezhat CH, Mashiach R. Laparoscopically assisted myomectomy: a report of a new technique in 57 cases. Int J Fertil Menopausal Stud. 1994;39:39–44.
17. Dubuisson JB, Fauconnier A, Deffarges JV, Norgaard C, Kreiker G, Chapron C. Pregnancy outcome and deliveries following laparoscopic myomectomy. Hum Reprod. 2000;15:869–73.
18. Parker WH, Einarsson J, Istre O, Dubuisson JB. Risk factors for uterine rupture after laparoscopic myomectomy. J Minim Invasive Gynecol. 2010;17:551–4.
19. Cobellis L, Pecori E, Cobellis G. Comparison of intramural myomectomy scar after laparotomy or laparoscopy. Int J Gynaecol Obstet. 2004;84:87–8.
20. Kitade M, Kumakiri J, Kuroda K, Jinushi M, Ujihira Y, Ikuma K, et al. Shikyusenkinso gappei-funin ni taishite fukukukyoka shikyu-onzon-ryoho wa yukoka? –jutsugo-ninshinritsu to senko-shujutsu no umu ni yoru shusanki-yogo no kento (Is laparoscopic uterine preservation surgery effective against infertility associated with uterine adenomyosis? – A study of perinatal prognosis by postoperative pregnancy rate and the presence of prior surgery). J Jpn Soc Endometr. 2017;38:70.
21. Morimatsu Y, Matsubara S, Higashiyama N, Kuwata T, Ohkuchi A, Izumi A, et al. Uterine rupture during pregnancy soon after a laparoscopic adenomyomectomy. Reprod Med Biol. 2007;6:175–7.
22. Nezhat C, Li A, Abed S, Balassiano E, Soliemannjad R, Nezhat A, et al. Strong association between endometriosis and symptomatic leiomyomas. JSLS. 2016;20:e2016.00053.
23. Pollio F, Staibano S, Mascolo M, Salvatore G, Persico F, De Falco M, et al. Uterine dehiscence in term pregnant patients with one previous cesarean delivery: growth factor immunoexpression and collagen con-

tent in the scarred lower uterine segment. Am J Obstet Gynecol. 2006;194:527–34.

24. Werner S, Grose R. Regulation of wound healing by growth factors and cytokines. Physiol Rev. 2003;83:835–70.

25. Magyary G. Uber die wundeheilung nach electrischen operationen. Arch Kiln Chir. 1931;169:737–53.

26. Amaral JF. The experimental development of an ultrasonically activated scalpel or laparoscopic use. Surg Laparosc Endosc. 1994;79:555–9.

27. Hauberrisser E. Zur wundeheilung bei wnwendung des hochfrequentzschnittes. unter besonderer berucksichitigung der Mund-, Kiefer-. Und Gesichtchirurgie. Bruns Beit. 1931;153:257–74.

28. Rosin RD, Exarchakos G, Ellis H. An experimental study of gastric healing following scalpel and diathermy incisions. Surgery. 1976;79:555–9.

29. Ghafarnejad M, Akrami M, Davari-Tanha F, Adabi K, Nekuie S. Vasopressin effect on operation time and frequency of electrocauterization during laparoscopic stripping of ovarian endometriomas: a randomized controlled clinical trial. J Reprod Infertil. 2014;15:199–204.

30. Saeki A, Matsumoto T, Ikuma K, Tanase Y, Inaba F, Oku H, et al. The vasopressin injection technique for laparoscopic excision of ovarian endometrioma: a technique to reduce the use of coagulation. J Minim Invasive Gynecol. 2010;17:176–9.

Uterine Transposition

Reitan Ribeiro and Mario M. Leitao Jr

Introduction

Survival rates continue to increase with the evolution of multimodal cancer treatment. Issues related to patients' quality of life have become ever more important, especially those relating to fertility preservation in young individuals [1]. In addition, the increasing incidence of some tumors in young patients, particularly colorectal tumors, [2] and the increase in the average age of first pregnancy [3] make it even more important to develop safe and reproducible options that may allow for preservation of fertility while not compromising oncologic outcomes.

Many pelvic malignancies often require radiotherapy as part of their treatment. The required curative radiation doses will produce ovarian failure, as well as impact the uterus, and lead to permanent infertility. Oocytes are cells that are highly sensitive to radiation, and up to 50% may be destroyed by a 2-Gy radiation dose [4]. The radiotherapy doses required to cause immediate and irreversible ovarian failure are 20.3 Gy at birth, 18.4 Gy at 10 years of age, 16.5 Gy at 20 years of age, and 14.3 Gy at 30 years of age

[4]. The usual therapeutic radiation doses range from 40 Gy to up to 80 Gy, which are obviously significantly higher than the ovarian tolerated doses. Even in tumors relatively distant to the ovaries, such as thigh sarcomas, radiation doses on the ovaries can be significant [5]. The uterus is also negatively affected by pelvic radiotherapy, and these effects include decreased uterine volume, reduced distensibility due to myometrial fibrosis, uterine vascular damage, and endometrial injury [6–10].

To date, no pelvic radiotherapy technique has been able to safely preserve patient fertility. For these patients, the only options are oocyte and/or embryo cryopreservation to have a genetic child and ovarian transposition to maintain ovarian hormonal production. Although ovarian tissue cryopreservation and transplantation are possible, they are still considered experimental [11, 12]. Unfortunately, none of these options and techniques has allowed these women to use their uterus to actually carry a pregnancy to term, thus requiring the use of a gestational carrier, which may not be a readily available option due to religious, legal, social, and/or economic reasons. The only other potential available option for these patients is uterine transplantation [13], which is still considered experimental and has all the disadvantages related to transplantation in general, such as rejection, need for immunosuppressive medication, and surgical complications in the living donor. Moreover, there is a need for

R. Ribeiro (✉)
Department of Surgical Oncology, Erasto Gaertner Hospital, Curitiba, PR, Brazil

M. M. Leitao Jr
Department of Surgery, Memorial Sloan-Kettering Cancer Center, New York, NY, USA
e-mail: leitaom@mskcc.org

further surgery to remove the uterus after the patient has given birth [13].

Uterine transposition (UT) was first described in 2017 [14] and has emerged as a novel potential alternative for preserving the fertility of these patients. In addition, it is an option that may allow for these young women to conceive naturally and spontaneously and then carry a full-term pregnancy.

Indications

- Rectal cancer
- Pelvic sarcomas
- Anal cancer
- Vaginal cancer
- Vulvar cancer
- Cervical cancer (highly selected cases)
- Desire to preserve fertility and carry a child
- Compliant patient

Contraindications

- Tumors infiltrating the body of uterus, tubes, or ovaries.
- Carcinomatosis
- Previous radiotherapy of the pelvis and/or para-aortic area
- Documented infertility
- Previous adnexectomy or any surgery who have damage to the ovarian vessels
- Large leiomyomatous uterus
- Undiagnosed ovarian mass

Preoperative Workup

Evaluation of the ovarian reserve is important to properly advise and select patients for this technique. But even patients with low reserve may desire the surgery. For those patients it is important to understand that their chances of pregnancy are low and that they will probably need fertility assistance such as in vitro fertilization.

Ideally, all patients considering this procedure should have a consultation with a reproductive endocrinologist. However, this may not be possible worldwide but should be given consideration. It is important that all options are presented to these patients including embryo and/or oocyte preservation. Patients should also be informed of surrogacy options as well as adoption. Uterine transposition is a new technique for which we have yet to determine the pregnancy outcomes.

Young patients who develop these pelvic malignancies should undergo a full genetics evaluation. Young patients with colorectal cancers may have Lynch Syndrome and those with certain pelvic sarcomas may have Li-Fraumeni syndrome. Uterine transposition may still be a consideration in patients diagnosed with these syndromes. However, additional discussion is needed as to the need for future prophylactic hysterectomy and/or oophorectomy and timing of such.

Preoperative evaluation of the uterine vessels would be interesting as there is a concern of uterine necrosis after transposition. Unfortunately, the reliable methods to perform such evaluation can be invasive and the risk of uterine necrosis likely cannot be predicted by such preoperative uterine vascular assessments. Uterine transposition also is a two-step technique with one being the transposition from the pelvis to upper abdomen and the second step being the takedown and re-anastomosis to the vagina. It is unlikely that preoperative uterine flow studies prior to the first step would predict future vascular flow or issues from such a two-step technique.

We recommend that young women who are being considered for uterine transposition are made aware of the novelty of this technique and the limitations in our present knowledge. These cases should be carefully and thoughtfully discussed with their oncologic providers to make sure that they are reasonable candidates for this procedure. It is critical that all providers are aware of the plans for the procedure that oncologic outcomes will not be compromised.

Surgery Technique

First Surgery (Uterine Transposition to the Upper Abdomen)

The surgery should be performed with a minimally invasive (MIS) approach via laparoscopy, with or without the robotic platform. We advise against the open approach, due to the necessity of a large midline incision to properly perform the gonadal vessels dissection and uterine attachment to the upper abdomen it may result in more complications. The patient is placed in the modified lithotomy position with the arms along the body (Fig. 17.1). Due to prolonged use of the Trendelenburg position, it is important to ensure that the patient is firmly secured to the table to avoid slipping during surgery. For the pelvic portion of the surgery, the thighs must be slightly flexed and abducted to allow free manipulation of the uterus and access to the rectum, if necessary. This is a novel technique and the presented steps may evolve over time or be modified by others based on their experience.

Standard skin preparation, surgical drape placement, and urinary catheterization are performed. Vaginal antisepsis must be rigorous, as the cervix will be exposed to the abdominal cavity and umbilical region, which may facilitate infection. Standard antibiotic prophylaxis should be given intraoperatively prior to skin incision with choice of drug similar to that for hysterectomy. The use of a uterine manipulator will facili-

tate the procedure. However, it is not required and likely quite difficult to place in very young patients and those who have not been sexually active yet.

Traditional Laparoscopy

For the non-robotic laparoscopic pelvic portion of the surgery, we prefer the surgeon to be positioned on the left side of the patient, the first assistant on the right and the second assistant between the legs, for uterine manipulation (Fig. 17.2). This positioning is very ergonomic and the same trocar placement can be used to the upper abdominal part of the procedure. Uterine manipulation will reduce traction of the uterine vascularization. The monitor is positioned by the patient's legs. The umbilical incision for placement of the first trocar is performed at the base of the umbilicus, since at the end of the procedure this incision will be enlarged and the skin sutured to the aponeurosis along with the cervix, if the cervix is planned to be brought through the umbilicus. Access to abdominal cavity (Veress needle, open or direct entry) and pneumoperitoneum insufflation depends on surgeon preferences.

After achieving pneumoperitoneum, a 10-mm umbilical port is placed. Two 5-mm ports are placed 2 cm medial and cranial to the anterior superior sciatic spine. A third 5-mm port is inserted 8–10 cm below the umbilical port on the midline. A 10-mm suprapubic trocar is used as a camera port to facilitate the retroperitoneal dissection and uterine manipulation in the upper abdomen in accordance with previously described techniques for para-aortic dissection [15].

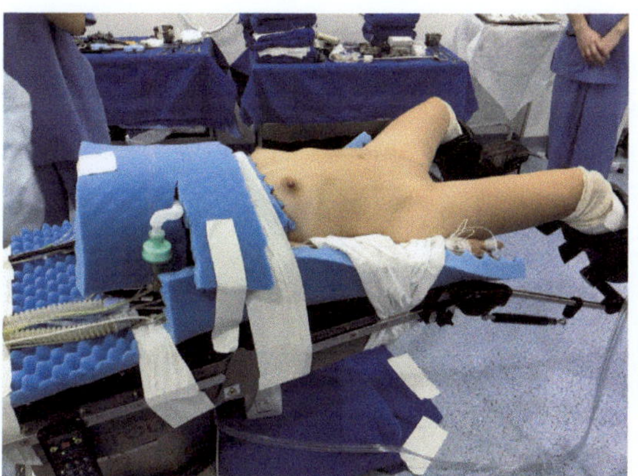

Fig. 17.1 Patient preparation and positioning

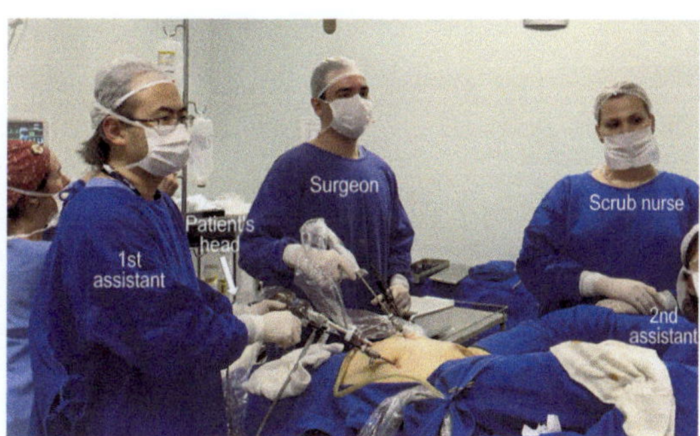

Fig. 17.2 Laparoscopic team positioning

Additional ports should be considered in difficult cases when needed to enhance access and angulation. (Fig. 17.3)

Robotic Assisted Laparoscopy

Entry into the abdomen will be the same as described above if using a robotic platform and should be performed as per surgeon's preferred entry method. The optimal trocar placement may evolve over time. A six-trocar setup seemed to work well to complete both the pelvic and upper abdominal portions of the procedure. (Fig. 17.4) The Xi platform was used and it facilitated the multi-quadrant work without having to move the patient. The described trocar setup should also work with the S or SI platforms, but rotating the patient and moving the platform will be required to move to the upper abdominal portion.

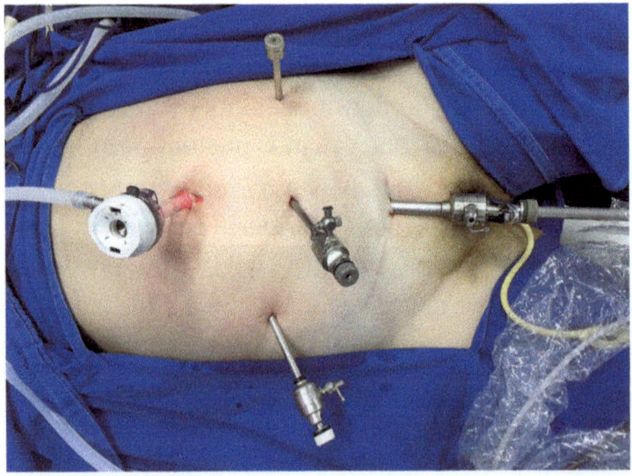

Fig. 17.3 Trocar placement for the non-robotic laparoscopic approach

For the pelvic portion (Fig. 17.4a), the camera trocar is placed at the umbilicus. An assistant port is placed in the LUQ a few centimeters above the camera trocar. A lateral robot instrument trocar for a grasper is placed at the anterior axillary line and in line with the camera trocar. The two operative instruments for the bipolar and monopolar instruments are placed 4–5 cm below the line of the camera trocar and approximately 5–6 cm lateral. This lower placement will optimize range without having to place additional trocar sites when switching to the upper abdomen. Once the pelvic portion is completed, a new camera trocar is placed in midline approximately 4–5 cm from the symphysis (Fig. 17.4b). The other trocars remain the same and instruments can be placed as per surgeon preference. It facilitates visualization of the upper abdominal wall by using a 30-degree robotic scope. The ink marks in Fig. 17.4 show the new location of the transposed uterus and highlights the relation between the trocars (arrows).

A complete and exhaustive evaluation of the abdominal cavity is the first step and cannot be omitted. Any area suspicious for the presence of metastatic disease should be biopsied and sent for frozen section analysis. Uterine transposition should be aborted if there is presence of metastatic disease or if any extension of tumor noted to the vagina, cervix, uterus, and/or ovaries.

The surgery itself can start with transection of the round and broad ligaments. The round and broad ligaments are transected more laterally (Fig. 17.5) than in a simple hysterectomy so that

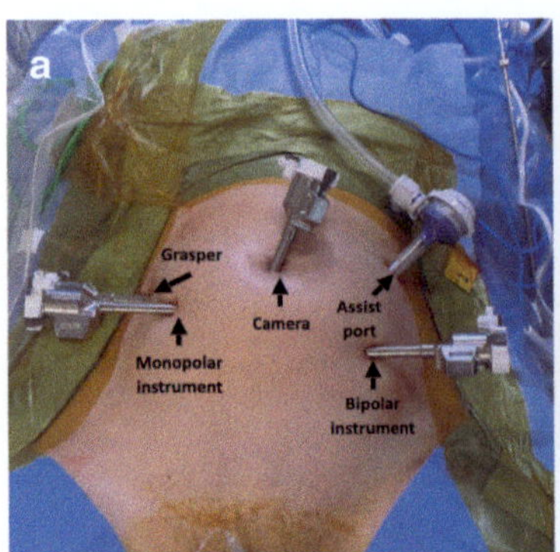

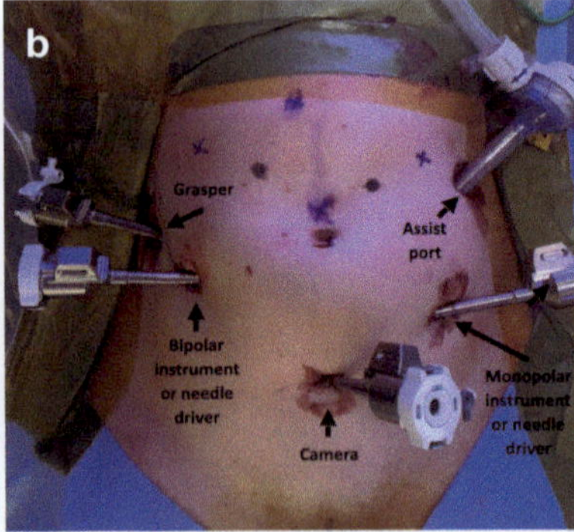

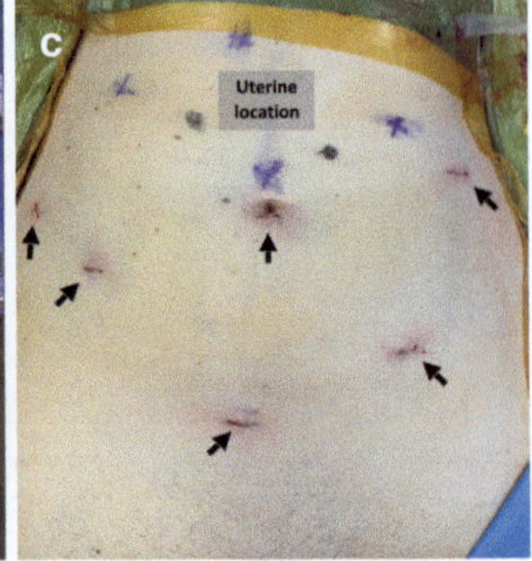

Fig. 17.4 Robotic trocar setup: (**a**) trocar setup for pelvic portion of procedure; (**b**) trocar setup for upper abdominal portion; (**c**) final trocar incisions and marking of transposed uterine location

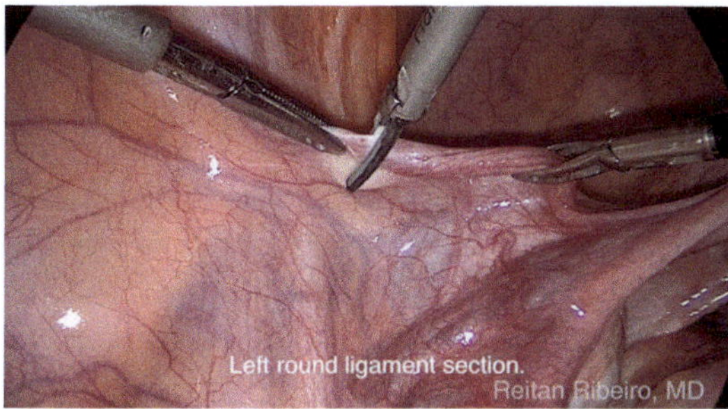

Fig. 17.5 Left young ligament section

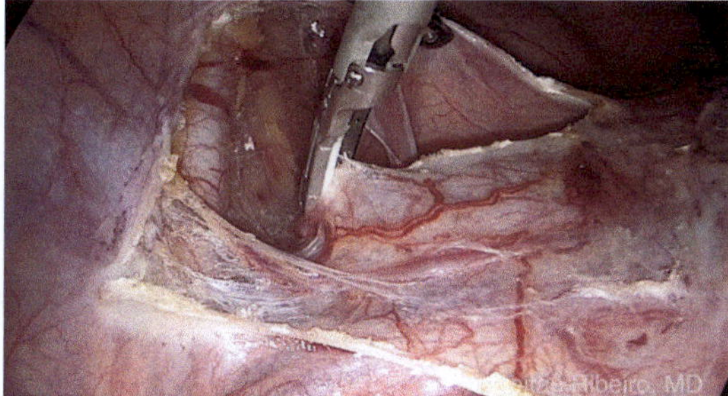

Fig. 17.6 Left lateral "window" creation

these ligaments can be used to attach the uterus and pelvic infundibula to the anterior abdominal wall when the uterus is in the upper abdomen. In addition, a longer round ligament can be reimplanted when repositioned in the pelvis. If the round ligament is sectioned very close to the uterus, most of it will receive radiotherapy, causing its retraction and fibrosis and preventing its reconstruction. The round ligament itself can be transected either before or after isolation of the infundibulopelvic ligament (IP) as per surgeon preference

A "window" is created by opening the two leaves of the broad ligament anterior to the ureter (Fig. 17.6). This window is traditionally opened during a hysterectomy as it ensures that the ureter remains lateral to the dissection of the infundibulopelvic ligaments and away from the dissection that follows. The anterior and posterior leaves can also be transected separately. The anterior leaf can be opened and the pararectal space dissected to identify the ureter clearly and then the posterior leaf entered superior to the ureter to help create more space along the medial pararectal space to help lateralize the ureter. Care is taken to avoid

grasping the fallopian tubes or the IP or utero-ovarian ligaments in order to avoid damaging them or damaging the vascular supply to the uterus, all of which could harm future fertility.

The uterus is then anteverted by manipulation, facilitating transection of the uterosacral ligaments, slightly lateral to their insertion into the uterus. Unlike the round ligament, the choice to transect the uterosacral ligaments near the uterus is made for two reasons. First, their dissection is more morbid and can lead to inferior hypogastric plexus damage, thereby affecting autonomic innervation of the pelvic organs. Second, the uterosacral ligaments are later incorporated during the re-anastomosis of the cervix/uterus to the vagina.

The uterus is then moved posteriorly by manipulation for dissection of the vesicouterine septum. This dissection is performed in the same manner as in any hysterectomy, with the assistant (or the robotic grasper in robotic assisted cases) pulling the bladder anteriorly while the surgeon dissects the vesicouterine septum to within approximately 1 cm of the cervicovaginal junction (Fig. 17.7). This dissection is important and should allow the vaginal suture to be performed on two planes, as described below.

The uterine vessels are then coagulated and ligated just lateral to the cervix, but medial to the ureter (Fig. 17.8), in a fashion similar to an extrafascial hysterectomy. This precaution is important for preventing inadvertent entry into the cervix during transection of the vessels, which can result in ischemia of the distal cervix and its necrosis or atrophy.

The colpotomy is made using monopolar energy in cutting mode to minimize tissue dam-

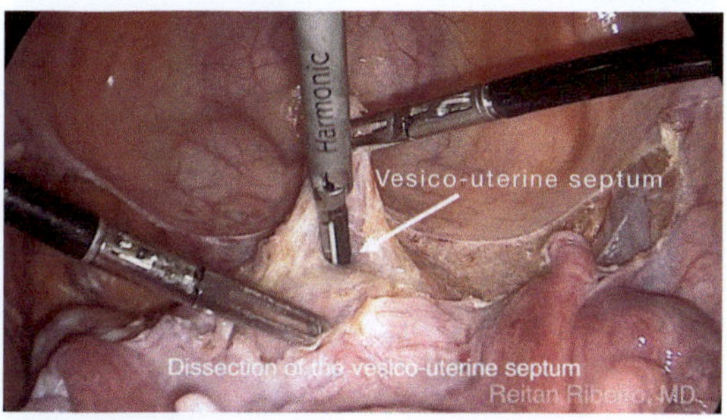

Fig. 17.7 Dissection of the vesico-uterine septum

age and avoid poor vaginal healing. Some surgeons may prefer the use of harmonic energy. A vaginal cup will facilitate this step. The vaginal cuff is then closed (Fig. 17.9) as per surgeon standard using a delayed absorbable suture or barbed

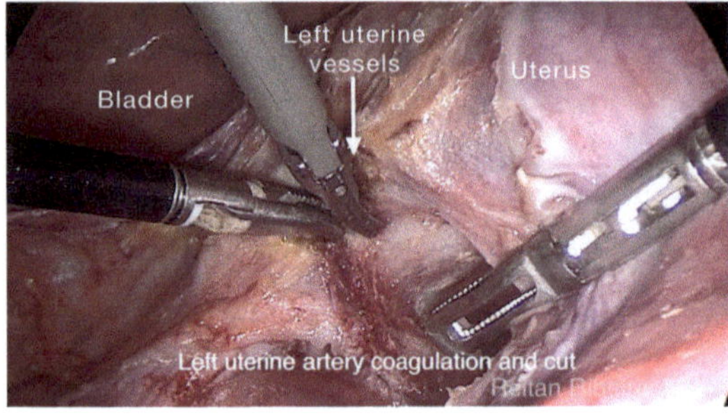

Fig. 17.8 Uterine vessels sealed and transectioned trying to preserve the descending branch of the uterine artery to the cervix

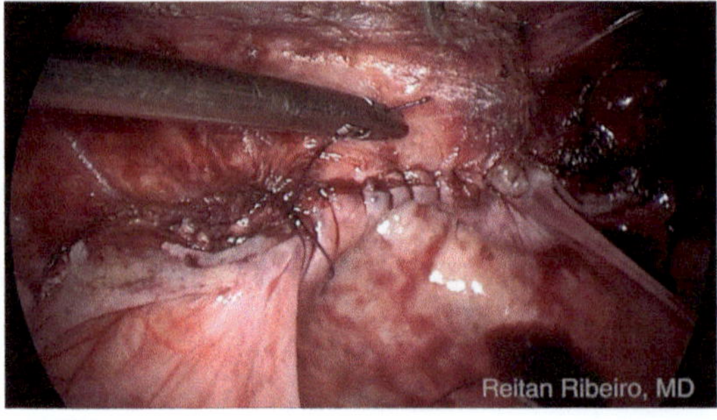

Fig. 17.9 Dual layer closure of vagina

suture. There is no clear evidence that a single or dual layer vaginal closure is best. The IP ligaments are dissected cranially until their intersection with the common iliac artery. At this point, the pelvic portion of the surgery is completed, and the team is repositioned. For robotic-assisted cases, the robot is undocked, the lower abdominal camera trocar is placed, the arms for Xi (or robot and patient for S/Si) are rotated and re-docked.

For the next portion of the surgery, if being done without the robotic platform, the surgeon is on the patient's right side (Fig. 17.10), the first assistant is between the patient's legs, the second assistant is on the left, and the scrub nurse is lateral to the patient's left leg. This positing will allow comfortable full access to the upper abdominal dissection. The surgeon and the first assistant may change positions according to the team preference. The camera is placed in the suprapubic trocar, and the patient is kept in the Trendelenburg position. The screen is located above the patients head.

The omentum is positioned in the supramesocolic region, preferably over the liver. The bowel loops are then placed as far as possible into the upper abdomen. Mobilization of the sigmoid and descending colon is then performed by lateromedial dissection (Fig. 17.11). Cranially, dissection must be carried out to the level of the subcostal margin and medially to the inferior

Fig. 17.10 Team positioning for the proximal gonadal vessels retroperitoneal dissection and uterine placement in the upper abdomen

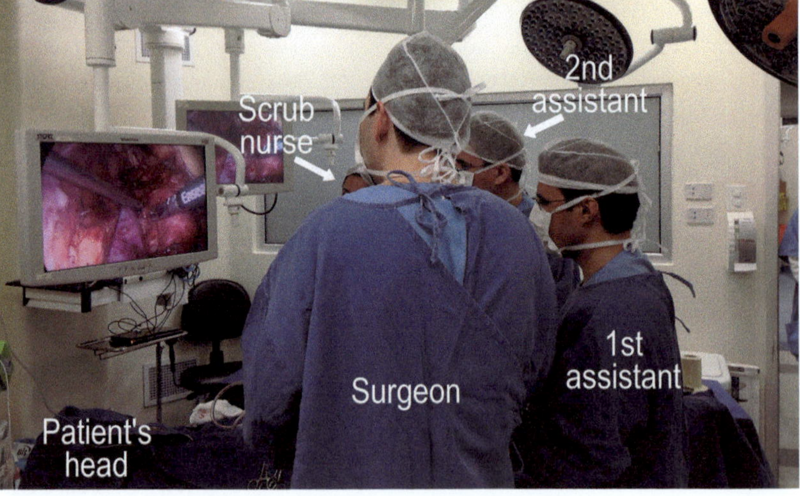

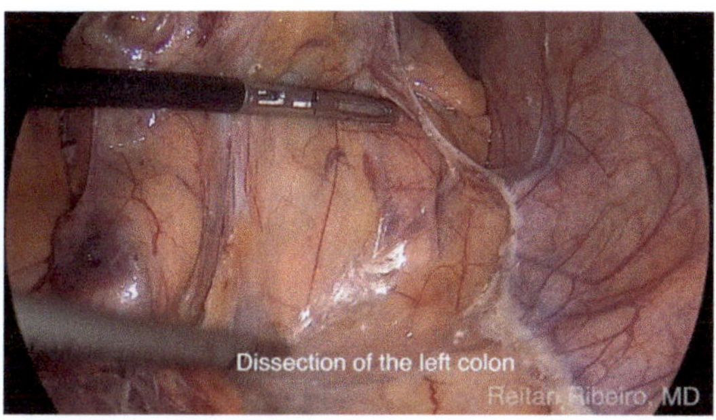

Fig. 17.11 Latero-medial dissection of the left colon

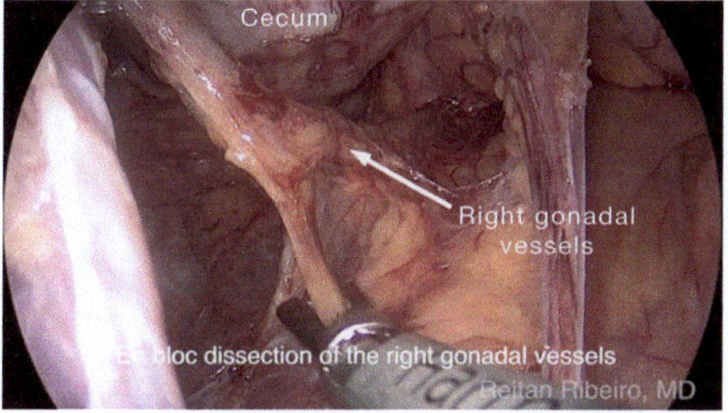

Fig. 17.12 Right gonadal vessels been dissected from distal to proximal while the right colon is lifted-up by the assistant

mesenteric artery. Medial traction of the left colon exposes the gonadal vessels in the retroperitoneal region. The gonadal vessels are then dissected en bloc near to their origin. There should be no effort made to isolate the vessels, which should be dissected while remaining wrapped in the fatty/connective tissue that surrounds them. During this dissection, care should be taken to maintain constant visibility and protection of the left ureter.

Then proceed to the mediolateral dissection of the terminal ileum, cecum, and right colon. Cranially, this dissection is performed to the level of the subcostal margin and medially to the anterior surface of the vena cava. Medial traction of the right colon exposes the ureter on this side and allows its dissection (Fig. 17.12). The same care is taken with the IP ligament dissection on this side.

Extensive dissection of the IP ligaments allows mobilization of the uterus and adnexa to the upper abdomen. While the uterus is pulled by the round ligaments to the upper abdomen, the cecum, ileum, and omentum are gently moved beneath the arch formed by the IP ligaments while the patient is moved from the Trendelenburg position and placed in a neutral position. Care must be taken to avoid rotating the uterus and twisting the IP ligaments. There may be differences in IP ligament length in the same patient, and the uterus can become slightly lateralized at this time. It is important to respect this limitation at the time the uterus is attached to the abdominal wall to prevent traction of the ovarian vessels.

The uterus must be positioned with the distal end of the cervix at the level of the umbilical trocar. At this point the surgeon may choose to attach the uterus and ovaries to the anterior abdominal wall using transabdominal sutures or intraabdominal sutures. This decision depends mostly on how long the gonadal vessels are to allow suturing then to the abdominal wall without tension while the pneumoperitoneum is present. If there is tension during the intraabdominal suture, the best option is to use the transparietal approach and tie the sutures after deflating the abdomen. Intraabominal suturing is facilitated with the robotic platform. 2-0 polypropylene barbed suture can be used to affix the ovaries, broad ligaments, and cervix as described below but intraabdominally with the robotic platform. If there does seem to be some tension, the intrabdominal pressure can be taken down to as low as 6 mm Hg if needed.

Transparietal sutures approach: Two 2–0 polypropylene transparietal stitches are passed approximately 2 cm distally to the costal margins and sutured to the ends of the round ligaments. There should be slight traction to prevent the round ligaments from shortening, but excessive traction may cause ischemia. Then, two additional transparietal stitches are placed to attach the ovaries to the anterior abdominal wall (Fig. 17.13). This modification was introduced after the first case when one ovary migrated close to the radiotherapy field [14], which caused ovarian atrophy. This suture also allows the ovaries to be attached more cranially, and further reduces the incident radiation dose. Usually, these sutures, approximately 2–3 cm lateral to the round liga-

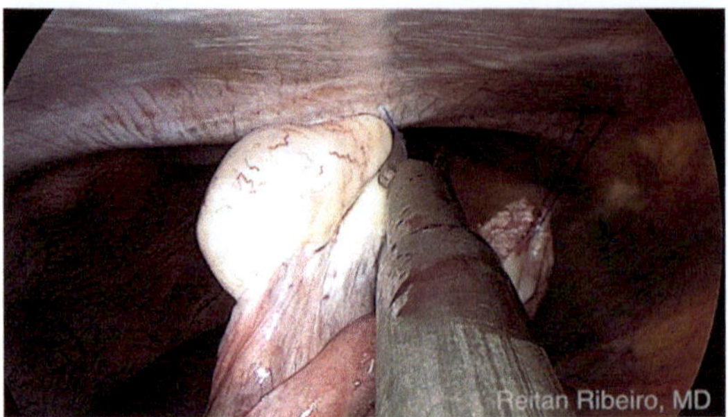

Fig. 17.13 The right ovary is sutured to the anterior abdominal wall, at the level of the subcostal margin. A metallic clip is been placed to help identifying the ovarian position on postoperative imaging

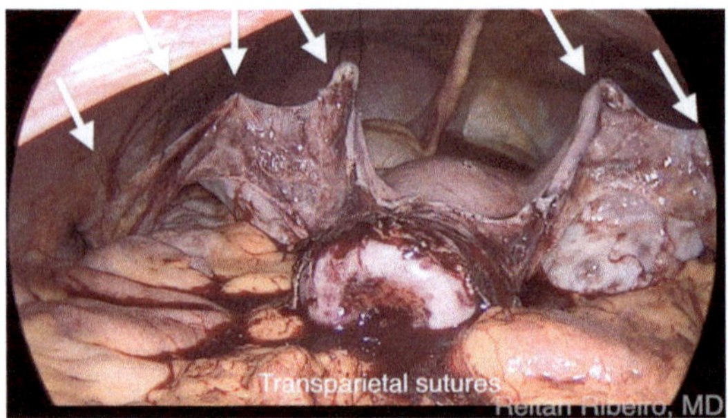

Fig. 17.14 Transparietal sutures of the IP ligaments

ments, are also placed 2 cm below the costal margin. A metal clip can be placed to mark the position of the ovaries (Fig. 17.13). If the surgeon chooses to not use clips, when the patient undergoes planning tomography for radiotherapy, it should be noted below which transfixing suture the ovaries are located so a mark can be made on the patient's skin.

Then, other transparietal sutures are made to secure the IP ligaments to the abdominal wall, with a maximum spacing of 2–3 cm between these sutures (Fig. 17.14), taking care not to puncture or accidentally suture any of the gonadal vessels. These stitches are intended to prevent herniations between the abdominal wall and the IP ligaments. They also prevent the shortening of the gonadal vessels which may difficult the uterine replacement in the pelvis.

An additional stitch on the uterine body is advisable, although we have never observed displacement of the uterus with the sutures described

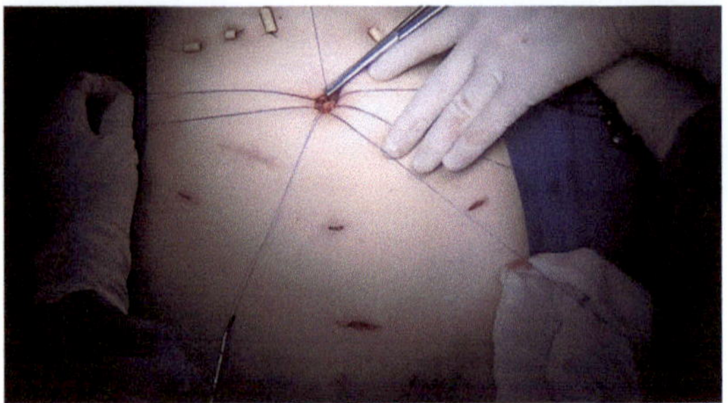

Fig. 17.15 Final aspect of the abdomen using transparietal sutures with skin protection. The sutures used to attach the cervix to the umbilicus are being cut

previously. An external 3-0 polypropylene suture is passed through the umbilical trocar on the posterior face of the cervix and is later used to attach the cervix to the umbilical aponeurosis, if this is planned. The pneumoperitoneum is then released, and only at this time are the transparietal sutures adjusted.

Devices to protect the skin at the suture sites must be used to avoid additional trauma and pain (Fig. 17.15). These sutures cannot be tied with excessive force, and the force applied should be the minimum necessary to keep the ligaments attached to the anterior abdomen without causing ischemia. Some patients have longer gonadal vessels, which makes intracorporeal suture of the ligaments onto the anterior wall possible. In such cases, transparietal sutures can be avoided, as they can cause considerable postoperative pain.

Intracorporeal Approach to Attach the Uterus and Ovaries

The ligaments and ovaries are sutured at the same level as previously mentioned using barbed suture, but non-barbed suture can also be used. Intraabdominal suturing is facilitated by the use of the robotic platform as the non-robotic laparoscopic instruments can be challenging to use for suturing of the uterus in this new position. There are two possible main advantages of this approach: the aesthetic benefit and they cause much less pain than transparietal sutures. An intraabdominal suturing approach is preferred if can be done well and safely as described above. Usually, traditional laparoscopic approach will mean that transabdominal suture will have to be done due to limitations in proper suturing; whereas robotic assisted approach allows the surgeon the opportunity to do intraabdominal suturing.

We have been performing intraoperative assessment of uterine flow using indocyanine green (ICG) given intravenously. This has been mostly for documentation purposes as we are uncertain as to what should be done if no flow is noted. Also, not all centers may be able to perform such assessment and we do not make it a requirement. ICG powder (25 mg) is diluted in 10 ml of sterile water. 4 cc of this is then given intravenously and near infrared imaging (NIR) is used to assess flow. This usually can be noted well within 5 minutes of injection. We would also perform this NIR flow assessment prior to either exteriorizing or suturing up the cervix so that fundal and cervical perfusion can be seen.

Suturing the cervix to the umbilicus and exteriorizing it is certainly the most controversial step of the surgery. There are both advantages and disadvantages. Direct inspection of the cervix, which is the end of the "flap," is important to the procedure's safety, especially if there is no doppler ultrasound or MRI available to evaluate uterine perfusion on the postoperative period, as any necrosis can be seen immediately by clinical examination. For patients who have menstrual cycles during treatment, it can provide an excellent and simple way to evaluate uterine and ovarian function, allow an outlet not just for menses but also mucoid secretion from the cervix. But, on the other hand, it is obviously awkward for patients and adds an additional surgical step and later dissection with a possible increase risk of dehiscence and infection. Also, as described by Baiocchi et al. [16], it may not be possible to attach the cervix in the umbilicus in post-trachelectomy patients, and in this case the surgeon has no option but to leave the cervix inside the abdominal cavity.

For cases in which the cervix will be attached to umbilicus and exteriorized, the pneumoperitoneum is deflated, the umbilical incision is expanded to 2–3 cm, and the posterior wall of the cervix is sutured onto the lower extremity of the aponeurosis incision. An additional five to six 3-0 polypropylene stitches are made to attach the edges of the cervix to the aponeurosis (Fig. 17.15). Then, the skin of the umbilical incision is sutured to the aponeurosis/cervix with absorbable 3-0 polycaprolactone sutures. The skin and the aponeurosis in the suprapubic incision can be sutured according to the surgeon's preference.

In pre-menarchal patients, it is unnecessary to exteriorize the cervix and the cervix is secured to the anterior abdominal wall with single suture. It is also an option to not exteriorize the cervix in women who have menses. A GnRH agonist should be given as soon as possible before the surgery to induce temporary ovarian suppression, since the surgery is usually performed presently to avoid cancer treatment delay. Patients will need to receive appropriate redosing of the GnRH agonist until it is time to re-anastomose the cervix/uterus back to the vagina. The main disadvantage of this approach is that the induced menopausal symptoms may be difficult for some patients. Bone loss is not a true concern as the re-anastomosis is often performed 3–4 months later.

Postoperative Care of the First Surgery

Postoperatively, patients should be placed on a regular diet promptly but try to avoid abdominal distention, which could cause traction of the uterine vessels. Uterine viability can be checked daily using direct vision of the cervix in the umbilicus, if this was done (Fig. 17.16). However, it is not clear at this time as to what should be done if "nonviability" or "ischemia" is noted. We favor the use of extended prophylactic antibiotic therapy, due to cavity contamination from exposure of the cervix inside the abdomen, especially in patients who will not suture the cervix to the umbilicus. This is quite controversial and one could also just follow standard antibiotic prophylaxis as for hysterectomy. Patients should receive thromboprophylaxis with a preoperative dose and then continue for 28 days postoperatively. Obviously, we have no data in such a novel pro-

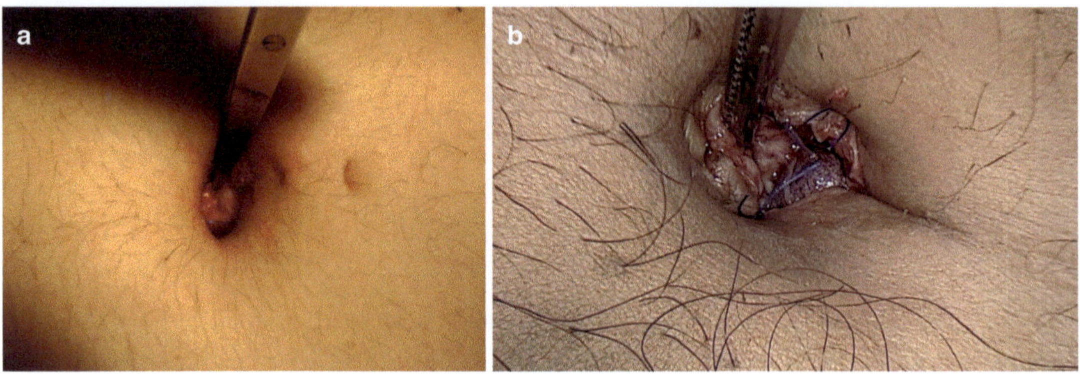

Fig. 17.16 Clinical examination of the cervix to check perfusion on the postoperative period. (**a**) normal perfusion. (**b**) Ischemic cervix

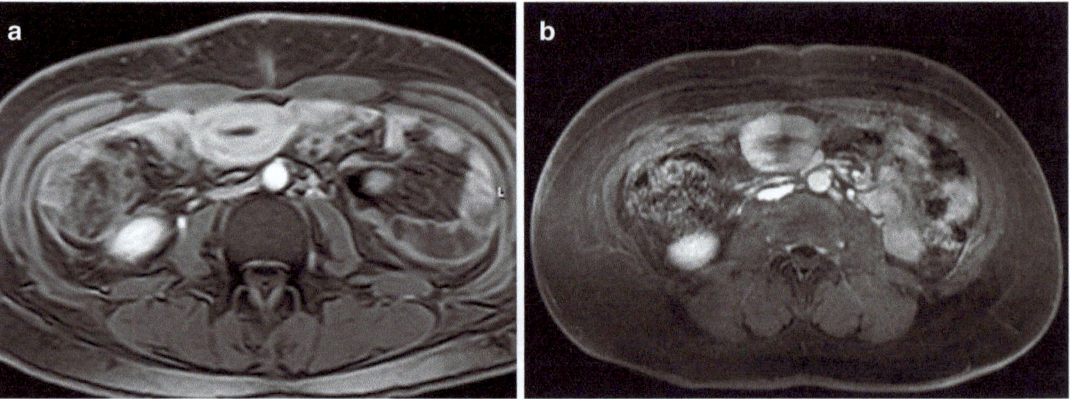

Fig. 17.17 Postoperative MRI showing the uterus in the upper abdomen in two different patients. (**a**) Patient with good uterine perfusion 10 days after surgery. (**b**) Patient with the left side of the uterus without perfusion 4 days after surgery

cedure to test whether this extended thromboprophylaxis is necessary. However, we feel it a reasonable recommendation considering the novelty of this technique and concern for vascular flow and vascular events to uterus.

Length of stay is also unclear and surgeon based at this point. Patients have been typically kept in hospital for 3 days but some have also been sent home the same day or the day after surgery as this is a minimally invasive procedure. The role of ultrasound will remain to be determined, but we do recommend performing a dopplers to assess uterine flow within 2–5 days postoperatively. This is mostly to document flow prior to initiation of radiation therapy. If flow is not documented but patient otherwise feels well then no immediate actions are likely necessary. If there is no flow and concern for symptomatic ischemia then a hysterectomy may be needed. Radiation therapy can be commenced within 7–10 days of the surgery if no complications have developed.

It is important to combine clinical examination with the postoperative doppler or MRI imaging (Fig. 17.17), because some patients can have partial ischemia of the cervix still followed without need of intervention if the uterus is still adequately perfused. In case of uterine necrosis, a hysterectomy has to be performed. If one or both ovaries still have adequate perfusion, the surgery can be converted to a hysterectomy with ovarian transposition.

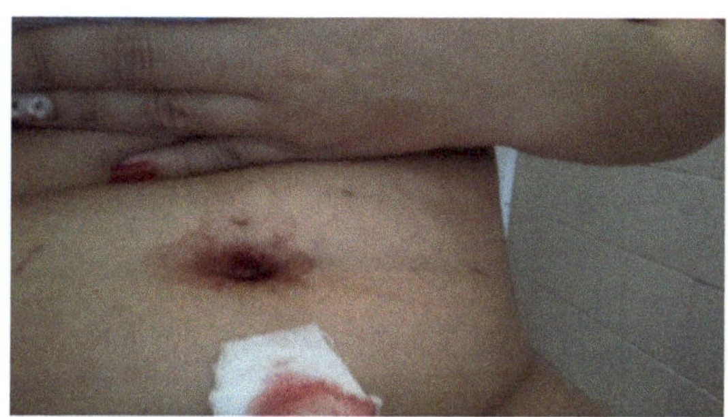

Fig. 17.18 The first umbilical menstruation after uterine transposition

Two weeks after surgery, the transparietal sutures (if used) can be removed, as the resulting fibrosis is already consolidated, and the uterus and adnexa are attached to the abdominal wall. Most patients resume umbilical menses (Fig. 17.18) in a few weeks. Usually, menses is regular and with the same pattern patients had prior to surgery. Some patients report abdominal cramps, despite of the uterus being denervated. The patients will also experience mucoid secretions from the cervix. Despite a theoretical higher risk of infection, the risk of peritonitis is a very rare complication of any stoma. Umbilical endometriosis is a possible complication, but its risk is low and it is relatively simple to treat.

Patients who do not have the cervix attached to the umbilicus should receive continuous gonadotropin-releasing hormone (GnRH) until the time of the second procedure. It is possible that some degree of uterine bleeding and/or mucus secretion may happen inside the abdominal cavity but we have not observed major issues so far.

Second Surgery (Uterine Repositioning in the Pelvis)

Uterine repositioning surgery should be combined with other necessary procedures and performed, in the case of rectal cancer, usually 5–8 weeks after completion of radiotherapy. The preparation and positioning of the patient are the same as in the first surgery. Performing pneumoperitoneum and placing the first trocar requires special attention in these patients. If the cervix has been exteriorized then the cervix is released at the start of the procedure as any other stoma and this then provides a 10-mm entry point for the first trocar. The use of a trocar with a balloon sealing system mechanism is ideal as it prevents the escape of carbon dioxide from the larger defect created from release of the cervix. If the cervix has not been attached to the umbilicus, the first incision should be made using the open technique until there is sufficient experience with the procedure to allow other techniques. For a robotically assisted procedure and in which the cervix has not been exteriorized, it may be possible to use an optical entry at the prior lower midline abdominal camera trocar site.

After placing the umbilical trocar, the other trocars are inserted in the same positions as described for the first procedure, including a 10-mm suprapubic puncture through which the camera is introduced. In addition to the adhesions induced by the transparietal sutures, a few omental adhesions to the uterus and adnexa are usually observed, which are easily released (Fig. 17.19a). After sectioning all adhesions, the uterus and adnexa can be brought to the pelvis. Patients who have had the cervix left inside the abdominal cavity may have the formation of a mucocele / hematocele (Fig. 17.19b).

For patients with rectal cancer, rectosigmoidectomy should be performed in the usual way with the addition of necessary trocars. Following completion of any other necessary abdominal or pelvic surgery, the uterus may then be reanastomosed to the vagina. Expect some adhesion of the IPs to the colon, which must be managed carefully to avoid damaging the vessels and compromising uterine perfusion. These adhesions are the most frequent cause of preventing the uterus in reaching the pelvis.

A vaginal probe is inserted, and the vaginal vault dissected. Care should be taken with the presence of the bladder over the vaginal vault. New dissection of the vesicouterine septum may be necessary, but it should be limited, as bladder injuries are frequent in this type of dissection, especially after radiotherapy. The vaginal apex is then opened using monopolar or harmonic

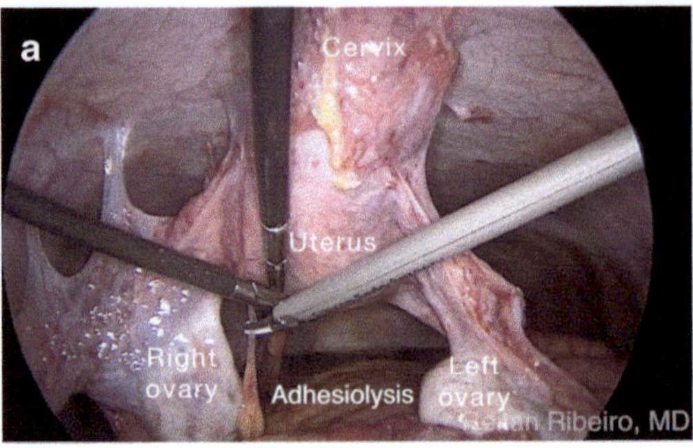

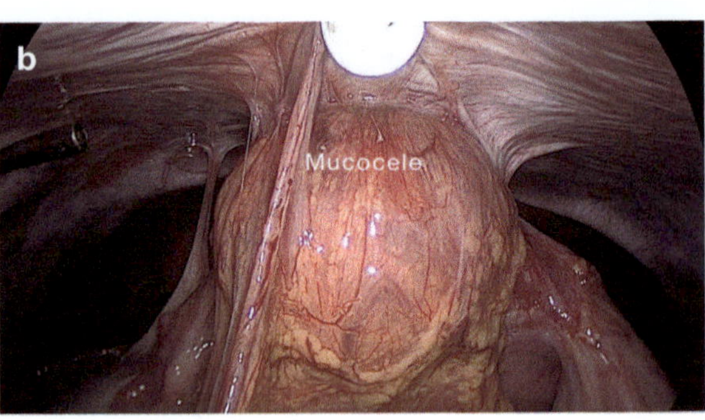

Fig. 17.19 Uterus attached to the anterior abdominal wall. (**a**) Adhesions are expected where the sutures were placed and some omental adhesions are common. (**b**) Cervical mucocele in a patient with the cervix left inside the abdominal cavity

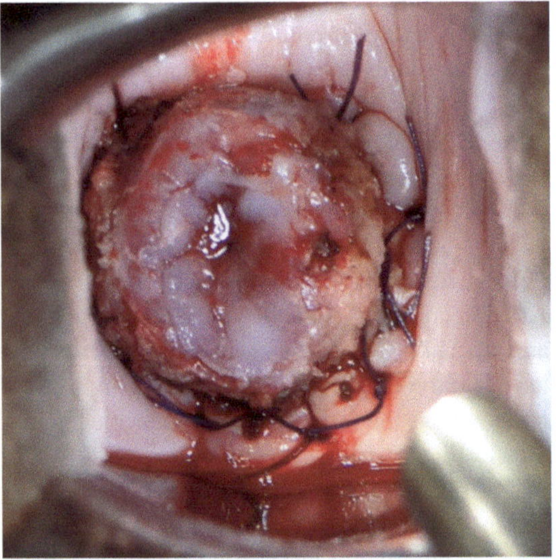

Fig. 17.20 Cervix sutured to the vagina using absorbable sutures

energy, and the cervix is inserted into the vagina. At this point, it is important to ensure that there is no rotation of the uterus that can cause twisting of the gonadal vessels. The cervix is then debrided, removing any fibrotic tissue present, and sutured to the vagina with Vicryl ® 2-0 (Fig. 17.20). This suture can be performed abdominally or vaginally. We prefer the vaginal route as it allows for improved control when positioning the cervix within the vagina and avoids excessive handling of the uterus during suturing, which is ultimately required in the case of transabdominal suturing. The robotic platform facilitates intra-corporeal suturing and this can be done without a vaginal approach, but ultimately it is the surgeon's preference. Whenever the vaginal approach is not possible, such as with pre-menarchal girls and those who have not initiated vaginal intercourse, the utero-vaginal anastomosis needs to be done intra-corporeally. It is preferred to have the cervix placed and projected into vagina and the sutures placed 2–3 cm on the cervical wall beyond the external os. NIR assessment of uterine perfusion using ICG given intravenously as described above is a consideration if available.

One should also consider the risk of dehiscence/poor healing of the cervicovaginal suture after uterine repositioning. A study [17] of patients with IB2 to IIB cervical cancer treated with chemoradiotherapy who underwent consolidation hysterectomy revealed a dehiscence rate of 6%. It is important to note that in the case of uterine transposition where the cervix is sutured to the vagina and is not irradiated, better healing should be observed than in the patients described above.

The round ligaments are then sutured in their remaining lateral portions, and the broad ligament is reconstructed, thereby completing reconstruction. For the ligament reconstruction suture, we prefer polypropylene 2-0, again because it causes less inflammatory reaction and adhesions. The final appearance of the pelvis after complete

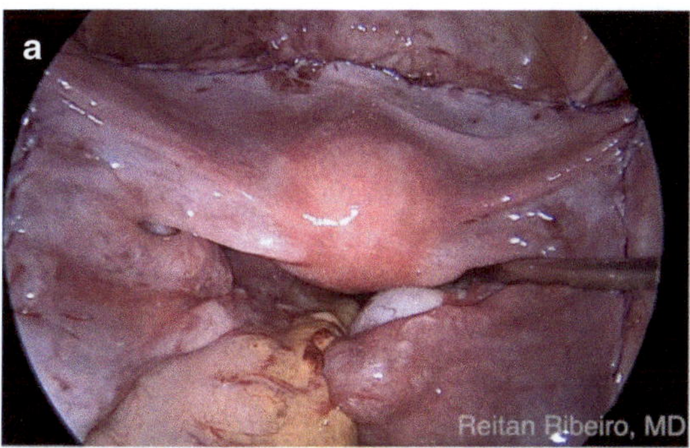
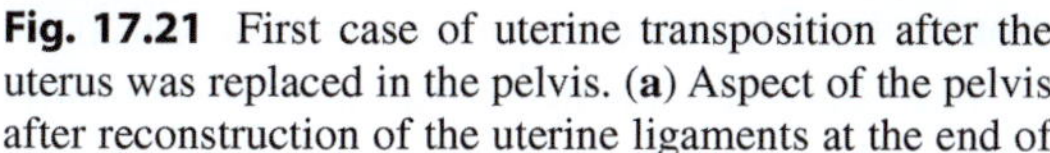

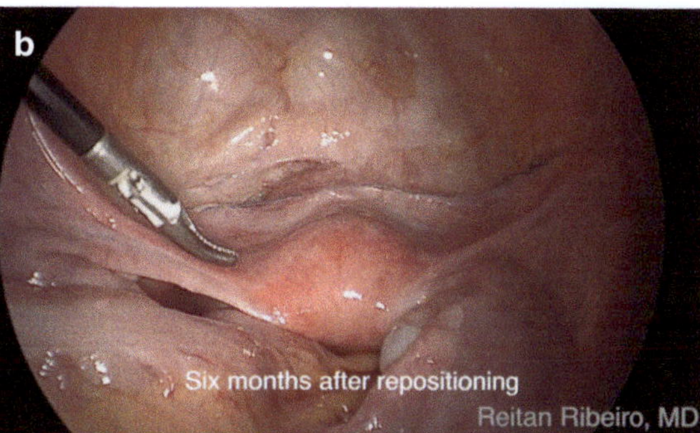

Fig. 17.21 First case of uterine transposition after the uterus was replaced in the pelvis. (**a**) Aspect of the pelvis after reconstruction of the uterine ligaments at the end of the reimplantation. (**b**) Pelvis aspect 6 months after uterine reimplantation

reconstruction is shown in Fig. 17.21a, and the final appearance 6 months after surgery is shown in Fig. 17.21b.

Chromopertubation testing can be performed to assess tubal patency. We do not recommend using a drain unless required by the concomitant surgery, such as in some cases of rectosigmoidectomy. The use of protective colostomy or ileostomy in patients who had concomitant rectosigmoidectomy is a decision of the colorectal team, but we believe the decision should be based on the same criteria used for all patients with rectal cancer.

Postoperative Care of the Second Surgery (Uterine Repositioning)

A patient undergoing uterine repositioning without additional surgery can resume a normal diet soon after surgery and same day or next day discharge is possible. For these patients, antibiotics are restricted to standard recommendations for antibiotic prophylaxis as for a hysterectomy. Antibiotic prophylaxis is determined by the colorectal team if a concurrent colorectal procedure is performed. Typically, patients are discharged on the second postoperative day and are placed on extended thromboprophylaxis if concurrent surgery is performed. We would defer to the colorectal team. If a concurrent procedure is not performed, it may still be reasonable to do extended thromboprophylaxis. We encourage early ambulation and return to normal daily activities as soon as possible. Vaginal intercourse should be avoided for at least 8 weeks after surgery and until clinical examination confirms no vaginal dehiscence and good healing.

Results

To date and to our knowledge, surgeons from nine countries (Argentina, Brasil, Colombia, Germany, Ireland, Saudi Arabia, Peru, and the United States) have reported having performed uterine transposition, but most of these cases have not been published. The results of an initial feasibility trial are about to be published and a second prospective trial to evaluate fertility rate and oncological safety is underway. Therefore, the results we have so far are based on a small series of 15 cases from the authors and mainly extrapolations from the other procedures that have been done to preserve fertility and/or ovarian function: the radical trachelectomy and the ovarian transposition.

Uterine and Gonadal Preservation and Function (Hormonal)

A large number of studies [18–20] of patients undergoing radical trachelectomy have shown viability of the uterus even after ligation of the uterine arteries, while studies of ovarian transposition [21–24] have shown that positioning the ovaries outside the pelvis can preserve their function. It therefore seems logical that combining these procedures may lead to a surgery with complete preservation of reproductive function in these patients.

In radical trachelectomy, a surgery performed in patients with early cervical cancer, the uterine arteries are ligated, the vagina is sectioned, and the remaining cervix is sutured to the vagina. In these patients, uterine necrosis is a rare event reported in less than 1% of cases [19]. Indocyanine green has been used to evaluate uterine perfusion during radical trachelectomy, [18] and it can be used if there is doubt as to uterine viability during this procedure.

Uterine, endometrial and gonadal changes resulting from the removal of the uterus from the pelvis are more difficult to predict. Some data can be extrapolated from ovarian transposition performed on young patients who undergo pelvic radiotherapy. In this procedure, after ligation and section of the utero-ovarian ligaments, the ovaries are dissected together with the gonadal vessels and transposed to the flanks, at the height of the lower kidney pole. Approximately 90% of patients undergoing transposition without additional radiotherapy treatment preserve their hormonal function [24]. This leads us to believe that transposition alone will not completely compromise vascularization of the adnexa and could efficiently nourish the uterus in at least 90% of patients. The success rate for the preservation of ovarian hormonal function varies between 60% and 69% when the patient undergoes further radiotherapy [22, 23, 26]. The factor that seems most important for function preservation is the distance of the ovary from the radiotherapy field, as noted by Hwang et al. [21], where the location of the ovaries more than 1.5 cm above the iliac crest was related to a greater chance of gonadal function preservation. Therefore, we assume that a similar rate of hormonal function preservation would be observed with uterine transposition.

Surgical Complications

Cervical atrophy followed by stenosis is the most common complication and it affected around 30% of the patients. They will need cervical dilatation. One patient had a vaginal cuff dehiscence which did not impact the patient's treatment and outcome. One patient had uterine necrosis and required a hysterectomy. At the same procedure, one of the ovaries was preserved and thus her surgery was converted to an ovarian transposition. Other minor complications were observed, but a larger series of cases is necessary to properly address this issue.

Fertility Rate

In our series, just 1 patient has attempted conception so far. She tried spontaneous conception for 1 year but was unsuccessful and is currently undergoing assisted reproductive options. A second patient has just started attempts at spontaneous conception. As in all fertility sparing surgeries for cancer patients, not all patients are ready to become pregnant immediately, and it may take time in those who are ready. Thus, assessment of fertility rate after uterine transposition will require prolonged surveillance.

Speiser et al. [25] reported that 50 (65%) of 76 women who attempted pregnancy, after radical trachelectomy, became pregnant. It is important to consider that in radical trachelectomy, pelvic lymphadenectomy is performed and the cervix and parametrium are resected, causing a more important anatomical damage than the proposed surgery. However, the uterus is not removed from the pelvis in radical trachelectomy.

Oncological Outcomes and Radiotherapy Delay

Regarding whether uterine transposition might compromise patient prognosis, two issues should be considered: transposition may increase the rate of pelvic recurrence, and surgery and its associated complications may significantly delay treatment. Colorectal cancer patients are probably the ones that can benefit the most from uterine transposition and thus a more detailed discussion is necessary. The first question is the risk of not removing a possible ovarian metastasis not diagnosed in the preoperative work-up. Although the rate of ovarian metastases in cases of colorectal cancer is 3–4%, prophylactic oophorectomy is considered only for postmenopausal women [27], which obviously does not apply to transposition candidates. The rate of local recurrence of rectal cancer has decreased to <10% since the introduction of Total Mesorectal Excision [28]. In the 1990s, neoadjuvant radiotherapy was also demonstrated to be effective in reducing local recurrence. A study by the German Rectal Cancer Study Group [29] consolidated the use of neoadjuvant chemoradiotherapy. An update of this study [30] reported that the 10-year cumulative incidence of local relapse was 7.1% with the use of neoadjuvant chemoradiotherapy.

The primary sites of local recurrence of rectal cancer after radiotherapy and TME are not in the uterus but rather presacral, anastomotic, and lateral [31]. Zhao et al. [32] found that only 23.3% of recurrent tumors were located in the anterior pelvic compartment. Therefore, hysterectomy is not routinely performed during rectosigmoidectomy unless the uterus is infiltrated by the tumor.

The main hindrances to the discussion of fertility preservation with patients are potential delays in the onset of anti-cancer treatment, followed by poor prognosis of disease [33]. Discussion of fertility preservation is cited as a delay in starting cancer treatment by 93% of oncologists [34], and thus, we believe that every effort should be made to demystify fertility preservation procedures to avoid delays to the start of such treatment, as this may increase complications.

Although fertility preservation should not be disregarded in any patient for any reason, including prognosis, age, socioeconomic status, and parity [11], one should bear in mind that fertility preservation might indeed delay the onset of therapy.

On empirical grounds, radiotherapy is usually started 4–6 weeks after hysterectomy so that irradiation does not interfere with vaginal healing. We elected to start radiotherapy 7–10 days after the Uterine Transposition. So far, there has just been 1 case of vaginal cuff dehiscence [14] and it happened on the first day of radiotherapy, suggesting it was related to surgical technical issues and not to the radiation itself.

Finally, it should be considered that there is no standard fertility preservation modality for prepubertal children [11]. This is the first time that such a technique can offer a chance of pregnancy for pediatric patients, as performed by Pareja et al., in Colombia in 2018 [34].

Conclusions

Uterine transposition is an experimental evolving technique. Although the basics are defined, the need for improvement remains. The technique's results are pending and require further study.

References

1. Köhler TS, Kondapalli LA, Shah A, Chan S, Woodruff TK, Brannigan RE. Results from the survey for preservation of adolescent reproduction (SPARE) study: gender disparity in delivery of fertility preservation message to adolescents with cancer. J Assist Reprod Genet. 2011;28:269–77.
2. Meyer JE, Narang T, Schnoll-Sussman FH, Pochapin MB, Christos PJ, Sherr DL. Increasing incidence of rectal cancer in patients aged younger than 40 years: an analysis of the surveillance, epidemiology, and end results database. Cancer. 2010;116(18):4354–9.
3. Mathews TJ, Hamilton BE. Mean age of mothers is on the rise: United States, 2000–2014. NCHS Data Brief. 2016;(232):1–8.
4. Wallace WH, Thomson AB, Saran F, Kelsey TW. Predicting age of ovarian failure after radiation to a field that includes the ovaries. Int J Radiat Oncol Biol Phys. 2005;62:738–44.
5. Kovtun KA, Yeo WP, Phillips CH, Viswanathan A, Baldini EH. Ovary-sparing radiation planning techniques can achieve ovarian dose reduction for soft tissue sarcoma of the buttock and thigh. Sarcoma. 2017;2017:2796925.
6. Larsen EC, Schmiegelow K, Rechnitzer C, Loft A, Müller J, Andersen AN. Radiotherapy at a young age reduces uterine volume of childhood cancer survivors. Acta Obstet Gynecol Scand. 2004;83(1):96–102.
7. Holm K, Nysom K, Brocks V, Hertz H, Jacobsen N, Müller J. Ultrasound B-mode changes in the uterus and ovaries and Doppler changes in the uterus after total body irradiation and allogeneic bone marrow transplantation in childhood. Bone Marrow Transplant. 1999;23(3):259–63.
8. Laursen EM, Holm K, Brocks V, Jarden M, Müller J. Doppler assessment of flow velocity in the uterine artery during pubertal maturation. Ultrasound Obstet Gynecol. 1996;8(5):341–5.
9. Pridjian G, Rich NE, Montag AG. Pregnancy hemoperitoneum and placenta percreta in a patient with previous pelvic irradiation and ovarian failure. Am J Obstet Gynecol. 1990;162(5):1205–6.

10. Li FP, Gimbrere K, Gelber RD, Sallan SE, Flamant F, Green DM, Heyn RM, Meadows AT. Outcome of pregnancy in survivors of Wilms' tumor. JAMA. 1987;257(2):216–9.

11. Loren AW, Mangu PB, Beck LN, et al. Fertility preservation for patients with cancer: American Society of Clinical Oncology clinical practice guideline update. J Clin Oncol. 2013;31(19):2500–10.

12. Jeruss JS, Woodruff TK. Preservation of fertility in patients with cancer. N Engl J Med. 2009;360(9):902–11.

13. Johannesson L, Järvholm S. Uterus transplantation: current progress and future prospects. Int J Women's Health. 2016;8:43–51.

14. Ribeiro R, Rebolho JC, Tsumanuma FK, Brandalize GG, Trippia CH, Saab KA. Uterine transposition: technique and a case report. Fertil Steril. 2017;108(2):320–4.

15. Ribeiro R, Tsunoda A. Laparoscopic approach to gynecologic malignancy. In: Ramirez P, Frumovitz M, Abu-Rustumn N, editors. Principles of gynecologic oncology surgery, vol. 2018. Philadelphia: Elsevier; 2017. p. 344–63.

16. Baiocchi G, Mantoan H, Chen MJ, Faloppa CC. Uterine transposition after radical trachelectomy. Gynecol Oncol. 2018;150(2):387–8.

17. Favero G, Pierobon J, Genta ML, Araújo MP, Miglino G, Diz DCP, M, de Andrade Carvalho H, Fukushima JT, Baracat EC, Carvalho JP. Laparoscopic extrafascial hysterectomy (completion surgery) after primary chemoradiation in patients with locally advanced cervical cancer: technical aspects and operative outcomes. Int J Gynecol Cancer. 2014;24(3):608–14.

18. Escobar PF, Ramirez PT, Garcia Ocasio RE, Pareja R, Zimberg S, Sprague M, Frumovitz M. Utility of indocyanine green (ICG) intra-operative angiography to determine uterine vascular perfusion at the time of radical trachelectomy. Gynecol Oncol. 2016;143(2):357–61.

19. Vieira MA, Rendón GJ, Munsell M, Echeverri L, Frumovitz M, Schmeler KM, Pareja R, Escobar PF, Reis RD, Ramirez PT. Radical trachelectomy in early-stage cervical cancer: a comparison of laparotomy and minimally invasive surgery. Gynecol Oncol. 2015;138(3):585–9.

20. Tang J, Li J, Wang S, Zhang D, Wu X. On what scale does it benefit the patients if uterine arteries were preserved during ART? Gynecol Oncol. 2014;134(1):154–9.

21. Hwang JH, Yoo HJ, Park SH, Lim MC, Seo SS, Kang S, Kim JY, Park SY. Association between the location of transposed ovary and ovarian function in patients with uterine cervical cancer treated with (postoperative or primary) pelvic radiotherapy. Fertil Steril. 2012;97(6):1387–93.

22. Morice P, Juncker L, Rey A, El-Hassan J, Haie-Meder C, Castaigne D. Ovarian transposition for patients with cervical carcinoma treated by radiosurgical combination. Fertil Steril. 2000;74(4):743–8.

23. Shou H, Chen Y, Chen Z, Zhu T, Ni J. Laparoscopic ovarian transposition in young women with cervical squamous cell carcinoma treated by primary pelvic irradiation. Eur J Gynaecol Oncol. 2015;36(1):25–9.

24. Gubbala K, Laios A, Gallos I, Pathiraja P, Haldar K, Ind T. Outcomes of ovarian transposition in gynaecological cancers; a systematic review and meta-analysis. J Ovarian Res. 2014;7:69.

25. Speiser D, Mangler M, Köhler C, Hasenbein K, Hertel H, Chiantera V, Gottschalk E, Lanowska M. Fertility outcome after radical vaginal trachelectomy: a prospective study of 212 patients. Int J Gynecol Cancer. 2011;21(9):1635–9.

26. Pahisa J, Martínez-Román S, Martínez-Zamora MA, Torné A, Caparrós X, Sanjuán A, Lejárcegui JA. Laparoscopic ovarian transposition in patients with early cervical cancer. Int J Gynecol Cancer. 2008;18(3):584–9.

27. Banerjee S, Kapur S, Moran BJ. The role of prophylactic oophorectomy in women undergoing surgery for colorectal cancer. Color Dis. 2005;7:214–7.

28. McNamara DA, Parc R. Methods and results of sphincter-preserving surgery for rectal cancer. Cancer Control. 2003;10:212.

29. Sauer R, Becker H, Hohenberger W, Rödel C, Wittekind C, Fietkau R, et al. Preoperative versus postoperative chemoradiotherapy for rectal cancer. N Engl J Med. 2004;351:1731–40.

30. Sauer R, Liersch T, Merkel S, Fietkau R, Hohenberger W, Hess C, et al. Preoperative versus postoperative chemoradiotherapy for locally advanced rectal cancer: results of the German CAO/ARO/AIO-94 randomized phase III trial after a median follow-up of 11 years. J Clin Oncol. 2012;30:1926–33.

31. Kusters M, Marijnen CA, van de Velde CJ, Rutten HJ, Lahaye MJ, Kim JH, et al. Patterns of local recurrence in rectal cancer; a study of the Dutch TME trial. Eur J Surg Oncol. 2010;36:470–6.

32. Zhao J, Du CZ, Sun YS, Gu J. Patterns and prognosis of locally recurrent rectal cancer following multidisciplinary treatment. World J Gastroenterol. 2012;18:7015–20.

33. Adams E, Hill E, Watson E. Fertility preservation in cancer survivors: a national survey of oncologists' current knowledge, practice and attitudes. Br J Cancer. 2013;108:1602–15.

34. Adams E, Hill E, Watson E. Fertility preservation in cancer survivors: a national survey of oncologists' current knowledge, practice and attitudes. Br J Cancer. 2013;108(8):1602–15.

Recognition and Management of Iatrogenic Injury to the Genitourinary System

18

David Miller and Kathleen Hwang

Introduction

Iatrogenic injuries to the genitourinary system are a rare occurrence but are nonetheless a known risk of intraabdominal surgery. The most common contributing procedures of iatrogenic injury of the genitourinary system are hysterectomy and cesarean section [1]. Every surgeon performing intraabdominal procedures should have a high index of clinical suspicion and a low threshold to evaluate for a potential genitourinary injury. Early recognition and treatment of iatrogenic injuries is paramount for ensuring the best outcome for the patient. Delayed diagnosis of genitourinary injury results in an almost twofold increase in healthcare costs compared to immediately recognized injury [2]. For any recognized injury to the genitourinary system a urologist should be consulted, or should one be unavailable, the patient should be temporized and referred to a center that provides urologic care.

For iatrogenic injuries of the genitourinary system there are both temporizing and definitive treatment options. As a general principle, definitive measures that may have significant downstream effects on quality of life should be deferred until the patient is able to engage in shared decision-making. The selection of treatment method also depends on procedure morbidity, patient condition, effect on quality of life, and later reversibility. It is imperative to understand that ultimately the decision maker at the time of any intraoperative consultation is the consultant.

Iatrogenic Injury to the Bladder

In pelvic surgery, the bladder is the most commonly injured organ due to its close proximity to the other pelvic organs. Predictably, the rate of bladder injury increases as the complexity of procedure increases [3, 4]. Risk factors for bladder injury include anatomic distortions such as congenital anomalies, adhesions, endometriosis, and pelvic organ prolapse as well as reduced exposure resulting in poor visibility of the pelvic organs [4]. Injuries to the bladder are defined as either extraperitoneal or intraperitoneal (Table 18.1).

Mechanisms of Bladder Injury

The most common mechanism of injury to the bladder is laceration either by cold dissection or electrocautery. Injuries to the bladder can also occur via trocar placement or during blunt dissection [4]. Rarely devascularization injury can occur. The grading system for bladder injury is provided below (Table 18.2.). Fairly unique for

D. Miller · K. Hwang (✉)
Department of Urology, University of Pittsburgh
School of Medicine, Pittsburgh, PA, USA
e-mail: millerdt@upmc.edu; hwangky@upmc.edu

S. R. Lindheim, J. C. Petrozza (eds.), *Reproductive Surgery*,
https://doi.org/10.1007/978-3-031-05240-8_18

Table 18.1 Incidence of bladder injury by type of surgery

Surgery	Incidence of bladder injury	References
Transvaginal tape placement	3–9%	Sharp and Adelman [5]
Laparoscopic total hysterectomy	0.75%	Wong et al. [6]
Abdominal hysterectomy	0.58%	Teeluckdharry et al. [7] and Carley et al. [8]
Vaginal hysterectomy	0.51–1.86%	Teeluckdharry et al. [7] and Carley et al. [8]
Cesarean section	0.28–0.47%	Salman et al. [9] and Terry [10]
Laparoscopic supracervical hysterectomy	0.29%	Wong et al. [6]

Table 18.2 American Association for the Surgery of Trauma (AAST) Bladder Injury Grading System [13]

Grade	Description
1	Contusion, intramural hematoma, partial thickness laceration
2	Extraperitoneal bladder wall laceration (<2 cm)
3	Extraperitoneal (>2 cm) or intraperitoneal (<2 cm) or intraperitoneal (<2 cm) bladder wall laceration
4	Intraperitoneal (>2 cm) bladder wall laceration
5	Laceration extending into the trigone, bladder neck, and/or ureteral orifice
6	Nonsalvageable injury

bladder injuries, with the exception of Grade 6 injury, severity has not been shown to correlate with outcomes [1]. Grade of injury does however dictate treatment selection [11, 12].

Diagnosis of Bladder Injury

Iatrogenic injury may be clearly obvious with visible laceration to the bladder, visualization of the foley catheter, or extravasation of urine into the surgical field (Fig. 18.1). Subtle findings include gross hematuria and/or gas distension of the foley catheter bag in laparoscopic cases [1, 14]. Around 5% of injuries are unrecognized at the time of surgery [1, 15]. Signs of bladder

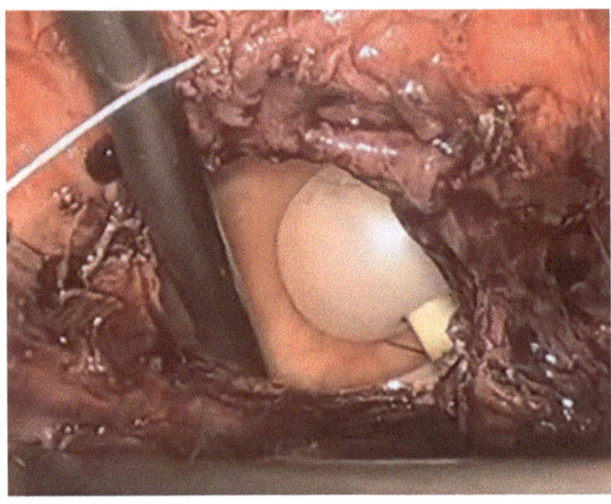

Fig. 18.1 Example of bladder injury. (Image provided by Kathleen Hwang)

injury in the early postoperative period include anuria, oliguria, ileus, new onset ascites, abdominal pain, sepsis, and elevation of blood urea nitrogen to creatinine ratio [14].

Intraoperative use of indigo carmine or methylene blue can help to allow the surgeon to identify an injury not initially seen. Filling can be accomplished through an indwelling urethral catheter either via catheter tip syringe or via gravity using a bag of fluid and irrigation tubing to allow filling to be regulated as needed. Additionally, instillation of these agents can be repeated after repair to assess for watertight closure [16, 17]. As a general principle, when retrograde filling the bladder to evaluate for injury whether it be in the operating room, for plain film cystogram, or for CT cystogram, the bladder must be filled to a volume of at least 300 ml. Lower volumes incompletely distend the bladder which increases the risk of missing an injury [18, 19].

Additionally, cystoscopy should be used if there is concern for possible injury. Detection rates of bladder injuries with cystoscopy are above 95% [7]. It is a procedure that is easy to learn, with low complication rate, and it is inexpensive [20]. Its use has been recommended following both laparoscopic hysterectomy and prolapse/incontinence procedures in several guideline statements [21, 22].

Imaging of the Bladder

Plain film cystogram can be performed in the operating suite and has been shown to identify up to 95% of bladder injuries. Four images are obtained in plain view cystogram (Fig. 18.2). First, a scout image should be taken prior to contrast instillation. Then, 300–400 cc of contrast is instilled via gravity into the bladder. Second, anteroposterior views are taken. Third, an oblique or lateral view should be obtained to evaluate for contrast extravasation behind the bladder. Fourth, an image should be obtained after emptying all the contrast from the bladder [18].

CT cystogram is the gold standard for diagnosing bladder injuries with a sensitivity of 78–95% and specific of 99–100% (Figs. 18.3 and 18.4). Sufficient bladder distention is paramount for the identification of bladder injury, 300–400 ml of dilute contrast (3–5%) should be instilled retrograde into the bladder via gravity. The bag or bottle containing the contrast should be placed no more than 40 cm above the patient's

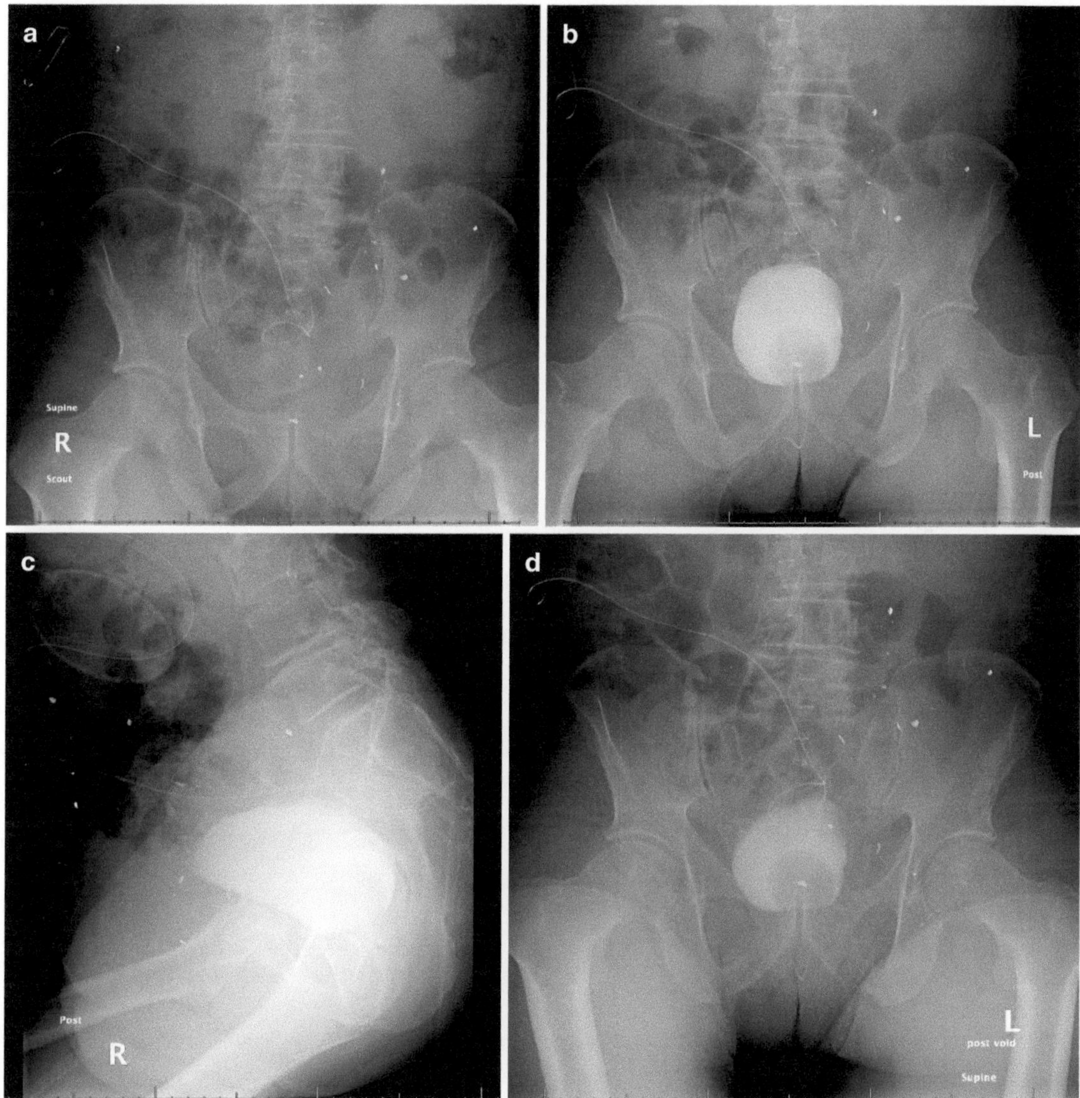

Fig. 18.2 Normal plain view cystogram. (**a**) scout film (**b**) anteroposterior view (**c**) lateral view (**d**) image after contrast has been emptied from the bladder. (Images provided by David Miller)

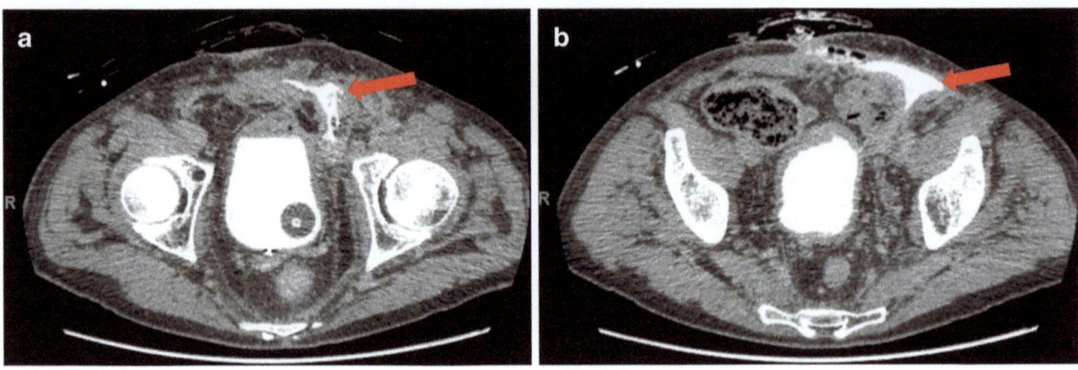

Fig. 18.3 Extraperitoneal perforation with contrast tracking along the abdominal wall (red arrows). (Images courtesy of David Miller)

bladder to minimize the risk of producing vesico-ureteral reflux of contrast which can increase risk of infection [23].

Repair of Bladder Injury: General Principles

First, when a bladder injury has been found, it is key to determine if there has also been ureteral injury as well [12]. The rate of having both a bladder and a ureteral injury is low, around .02% in some series, but should be ruled out nonetheless [24]. Second, if suspicion is high but the injury is not visualized intraoperatively a cystotomy may need to be performed to provide complete visualization of the bladder wall [25]. Third, all recognized intraperitoneal injuries (Grade 3–6) require formal repair and a urologic surgeon should be consulted. Fourth, following repair both a foley catheter and an abdominal drain should be left in place [11, 12].

Extraperitoneal Injury

For uncomplicated Grade 1, Grade 2, and even Grade 3 extraperitoneal injuries the ideal management is conservative with drainage via large lumen urethral catheter (18 or 20F) for 2–3 weeks (Fig. 18.3) [11, 12]. Complicated extraperitoneal injuries include involvement of rectal, vaginal lacerations, and/or foreign bodies in the bladder lumen such as bone. Complicated injuries should be repaired primarily to decrease the risk of fistula formation and facilitate healing [12]. The method of repair is detailed in the following section.

Intraperitoneal Injury

Any intraperitoneal injury should be repaired primarily; this can be done either open or laparoscopically (Fig. 18.4) [26, 27]. The reason for doing so is to prevent peritonitis [11, 12]. The anterior and lateral attachments of the bladder should be mobilized to ensure tension free repair [17]. The injury should be closed with a 2–0 or 3–0 absorbable suture. Permanent sutures have been associated with urinary stone formation, fistulas, and recurrent urinary tract infections [28–30]. The technique of repair is as follows:

1. The first layer: Simple running closure of the mucosa grabbing small bites of muscularis
2. Second Layer: Running imbricating closure of the muscularis and serosa
3. Third Layer: Additional imbricating closure of the serosa

After repair the closure should be tested to ensure it is watertight with instillation of 300 cc of saline, indigo carmine, or methylene blue into the bladder. Finally, a large lumen urethral catheter (18 or 20F) should be left in place to allow for healing [11]. In the case of repairs deemed to have a high risk of breaking down (e.g., repairs in

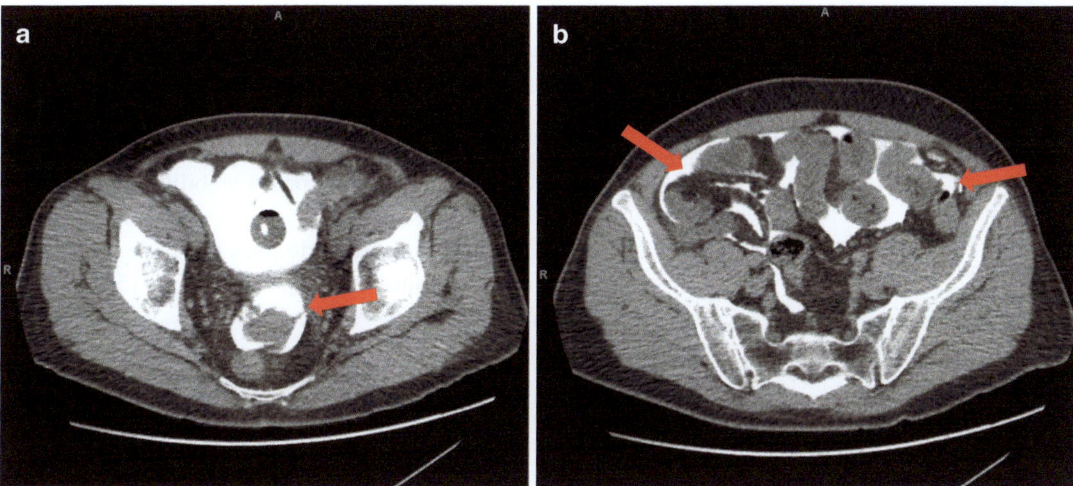

Fig. 18.4 Intraperitoneal perforation (red arrows). (Images courtesy of David Miller)

patients with fistulas, repairs after placenta percreta, and/or repairs involving poor appearing bladder tissue), various flaps can be used to augment the repair [31, 32]. The most common of which is an omental pedicle flap, which is brought down and placed over the bladder repair to isolate it from surrounding tissues. The omentum has unique properties that facilitate wound healing, which include reducing hemorrhage via prothrombic activation, release of polypeptide growth factors resulting in rapid neovascularization, and release of lipids that facilitate vasodilation [33].

Follow-Up

Postoperative antibiotics are not necessary unless there is concern for contaminated surgical field, antibiotics should, however, be given at the time of catheter removal. A drain fluid creatinine level should be checked prior to drain removal to determine if there is continued leakage of urine into the peritoneum and assess the integrity of the repair. The urethral catheter should be left in place for up to 3 weeks following repair. Follow-up plain view cystogram is recommended to ensure integrity of the repair prior to catheter removal [11, 12]. Following catheter removal, a urine analysis should be performed to document resolution of hematuria. Beyond this, no formal cystoscopic surveillance or imaging is recommended [34].

Iatrogenic Ureteral Injury

Iatrogenic injury to the ureter can occur in pelvic or abdominal surgeries with approximately 75% of injuries occurring during gynecologic surgery [35]. Ureteral injury commonly occurs during ligation of the uterine and ovarian vessels, during ureteral mobilization, or when gaining control of bleeding. There is a significantly increased risk of injury to the ureter with laparoscopic hysterectomy compared to open hysterectomy [36, 37] (Table 18.3). Other known risk factors for ureteral injury include large uterine size, endometriosis, pelvic organ prolapse, prior pelvic surgery, and pelvic radiation [38, 39]. The most common site of injury is near the uterosacral ligaments [40]. Preoperative ureteral stent placement has been shown to aid with early recognition of ureteric injury; however, there has been no definitive evidence that shows they decrease the rate of ureteric injury [41, 42]. The use of lighted ureteral stents has also risen in popularity. However, the literature on outcomes of using lighted stents

Table 18.3 Incidence of ureteral injury by type of surgery

Surgery	Incidence of ureteral injury	References
Laparoscopic total hysterectomy	0.35–1.39%	Gilmour et al. [35], Leonard et al. [48], and Härkki-Sirén [36]
Abdominal hysterectomy	0.04–0.35%	Carley et al. [8] and Härkki-Sirén [36]
Vaginal hysterectomy	0.02%	Carley et al. [8] and Härkki-Sirén [36]

Table 18.4 AAST ureteral injury grading scale [52]

Grade	Description
1	Contusion or hematoma
2	<50% transection
3	>50% transection
4	Complete transection with <2 cm devascularization
5	Complete transection with >2 cm devascularization
6	Nonsalvageable injury

is limited to a single report concluding only a theoretical risk reduction in rate or ureteral injury [43]. The most straightforward way to prevent ureteral injury is to identify both ureters intraoperatively and remaining vigilant for potential injury [12, 42, 44]. For laparoscopic and robotic cases, intravenous injection of indocyanine green quickly stains the urothelium and fluorescence is visible through the wall of the ureter. Of note, this requires a near-infrared function on an endoscopic camera but provides excellent visualization to aid in identification of the ureters intraoperatively [45–47].

Mechanism of Ureteral Injury

There are a wide range of mechanisms of injury to the ureter including laceration, ligation, resection, avulsion, devascularization, kinking, and thermal and crush injuries. The selection of treatment for management is affected by both mechanism and grade of injury (Table 18.4). Thermal injuries account for roughly 24% of injuries and

can be especially deceiving [49]. Thermal injuries are deceptive due to difficulty in recognition of the degree of devascularization of the ureter. To date there has been no definitive way of recognizing a devascularized ureter, even presence of peristalsis does not prove viability [50]. This has important implications for eventual repair as the surgeon must debride back to viable ureteral tissue to ensure integrity of the repair [51].

Diagnosis of Ureteral Injury

Ureteral injury differs from bladder injury in that the majority of ureteral injuries are unnoticed at the time of surgery. Only 36% of injuries are recognized intraoperatively during open surgery with the number falling to 12.5% for laparoscopic surgery [25, 53]. When there is concern for possible ureteral injury, a urologist should be consulted for assistance in evaluation. If an injury is unrecognized at the time of surgery, postoperative signs of ureteral injury include flank pain, fever, urinary incontinence, and hematuria [54]. Patients with thermal or partial injuries typically present 10–14 days postoperatively [55].

Intraoperative dye such as indigo carmine or methylene blue also have utility in ureteral injuries. These dyes can be instilled intravenously or in retrograde fashion, and extravasation of the dye into the operative field can help in the identification of an injury. If given intravenously, excretory time is around 10 min for these dyes to enter the urine [34, 56].

Cystoscopy has been shown to drastically improve the intraoperative detection rate of ureteric injuries. Detection of ureteral injuries has been reported to be as high at 97% with use of intraoperative cystoscopy [57]. However, efflux can still be present even with partial ureteral transection, ligation, and/or thermal injury. If clinical concern is high, retrograde pyelogram should be performed via cystoscopic guidance [7, 39].

When injury is suspected, careful and meticulous inspection of the ureters should be performed. This can be done either in an open or laparoscopic fashion. In addition to visualizing any laceration, transection, or ligation, the identification of hematoma and devascularization is important for integrity of repair [44].

Imaging Studies

If the injury is not able to be visualized, an intravenous pyelogram can be performed on the operating table. This study is performed by injecting the patient with 2 cc/kg of intravenous contrast and taking a plain x-ray of the abdomen [58]. Retrograde pyelogram can also be performed on the operating table by injecting contrast through a ureteral catheter into the ureter via cystoscopic guidance (Fig. 18.5).

CT urogram is the recommended modality for assessment of possible ureteral injury should the concern arise postoperatively. This modality includes a delayed phase of usually 10–12 min to allow for contrast to pass into the urine and illuminate any areas of extravasation (Fig. 18.6) [59].

Management

The primary purpose of treating a ureteral injury is to minimize morbidity for the patient and preserve renal function. A repair of the ureter may be performed either open, laparoscopically, or robotically depending on the feasibility and the consulting urologist's skill set [60, 61]. The treatment options for repair are determined by several factors, which include the urologic surgeon's skill set, the timing of recognition of the injury, the grade, and location of injury. To ensure optimal repair, the ureter must be debrided back to viable tissue [51].

Intraoperative Recognition of Ureteral Injury

The following reconstructive principles help to ensure adequate repair: debridement and spatulation of the ends of the ureter, placement of an internal stent, tension-free watertight ureteral closure with interrupted or running absorbable suture, and placement of a drain nearby. Guidelines recommend that partial (grade 2–3) injuries of the ureter be repaired with primary closure over a stent. Repair of grade 4 or 5 injuries depend on the location of the injury and size of the damaged segment. The ureter is stratified into three distinct areas: uppermost is the renal pelvis to the ureteropelvic junction, next is the abdominal ureter from the ureteropelvic junction to the iliac vessels, and finally the pelvic ureter is from iliac vessels to the ureterovesical junction. For injuries to the pelvic ureter, primary ureteral reimplantation should be performed (Fig. 18.7). The length of defect dictates whether a psoas hitch or Boari flap needs to be performed in addition to a tunneled reimplant. For defects of up to 6–10 cm a psoas hitch should be performed (Fig. 18.8). For defects of 12–15 cm length, a Boari flap should be performed (AUA) (Fig. 18.9). A uretero-ureterostomy should be performed for injuries above the iliac vessels, this can safely be performed for loss or ureter up to 3 cm in length [11, 62] (Fig. 18.10). For more complex injuries where the above repairs are not possible, use of bowel or auto-transplantation in the management of an iatrogenic injury is not recommended until the patient can make an informed decision about how to proceed, temporizing interventions such as nephrostomy tube placement should be done [11].

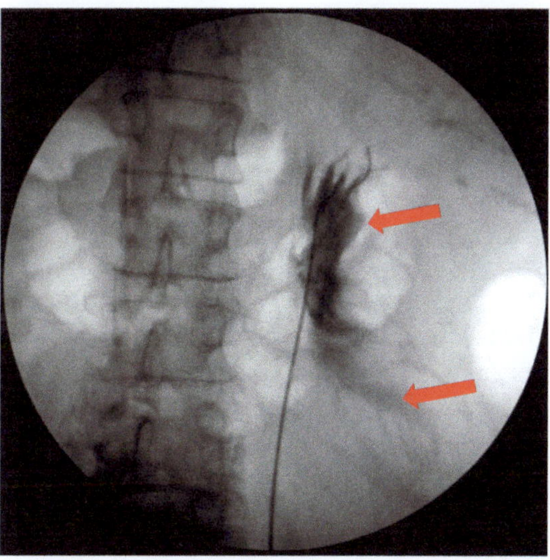

Fig. 18.5 Retrograde pyelogram demonstrating extravasation of contrast (red arrows) into the retroperitoneum consistent with proximal ureteral injury. (Image courtesy of David Miller)

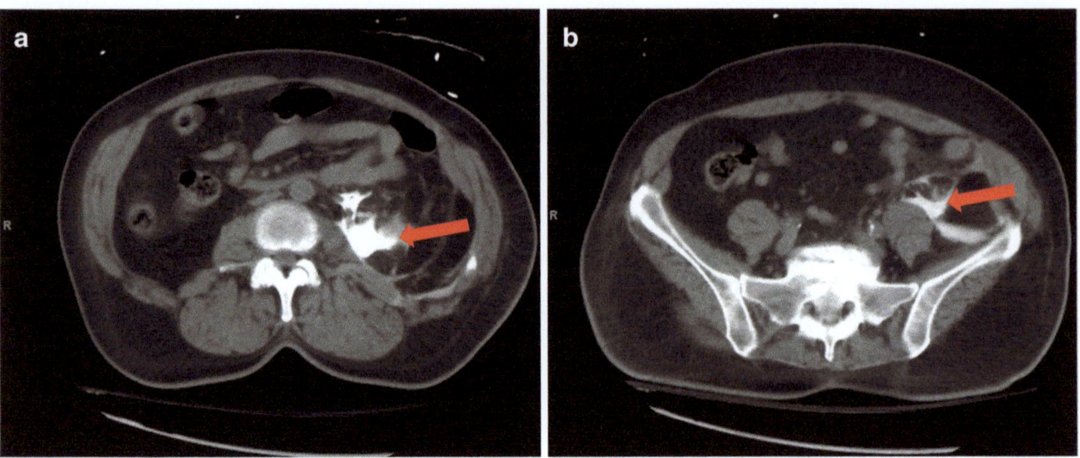

Fig. 18.6 CT urogram demonstrating extravasation of contrast (red arrows) into the retroperitoneum consistent with ureteral injury. (Images courtesy of David Miller)

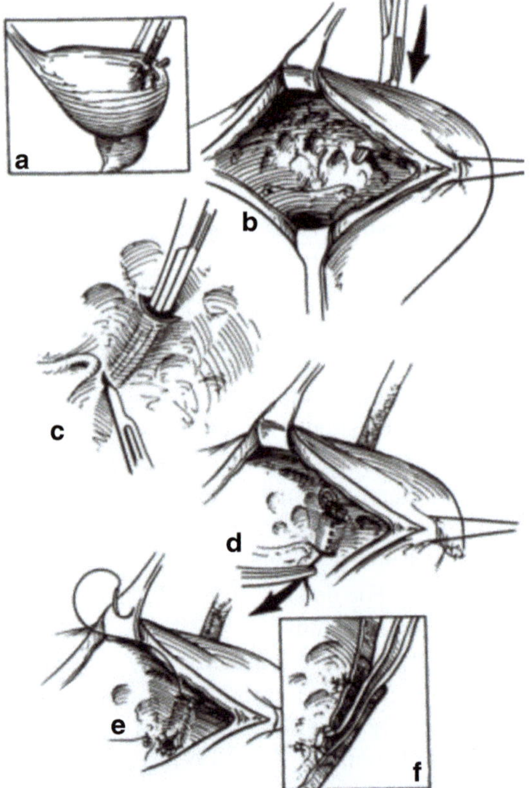

Fig. 18.7 Tunneled ureteroneocystostomy to distal ureteral injury. (Reprinted with permission from Burks and Santucci [51])

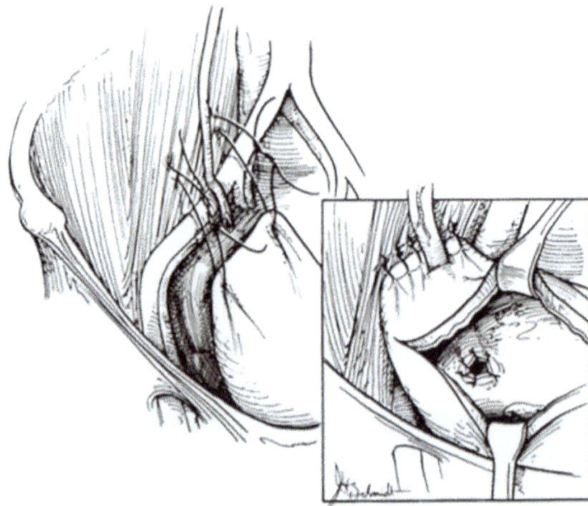

Fig. 18.8 Vesico-psoas hitch for distal ureteral implantation. (Reprinted with permission from Burks and Santucci [51])

Delayed Postoperative Recognized Ureteral Injury

For injuries recognized postoperatively, primary urine diversion with either indwelling ureteral stent placement or nephrostomy tube is recommended [11, 12]. Following which retrograde pyelogram or antegrade nephrostogram can be performed later to assess the need for primary repair of the injury.

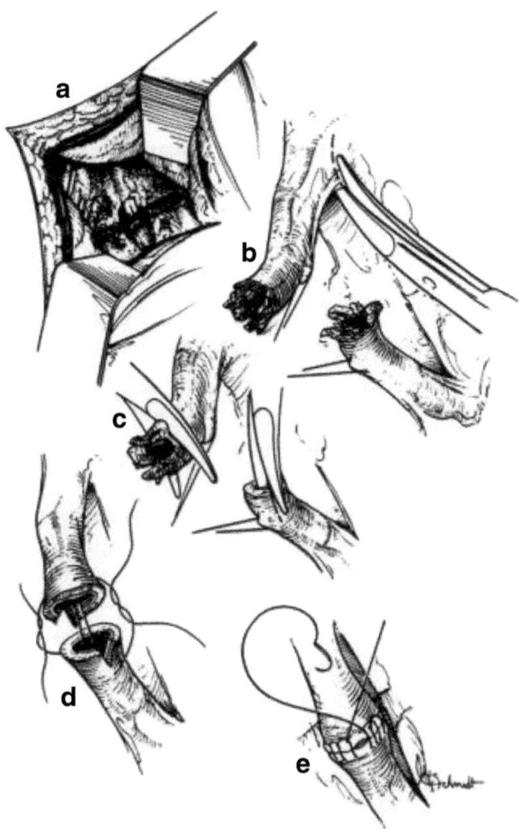

Fig. 18.9 A Boari flap: a flap of bladder is fashioned into a tube and an anastomosis is created between it and the proximal ureter. (Reprinted with permission from Burks and Santucci [51])

Fig. 18.10 Ureteroureterostomy: the ends of the ureters are trimmed and a running anastomosis is performed. (Reprinted with permission from Burks and Santucci [51])

Follow-Up of Ureteral Injuries

The abdominal drain should be removed after checking a drain fluid creatinine to ensure there is no leak. If there is no concomitant bladder injury, bladder drainage with an indwelling urethral catheter is not necessary. The indwelling ureteral stent should be removed in 4–6 weeks. The long-term durability of the repairs detailed is excellent. In a large case series of 181 patients, the success rate of a psoas hitch with ureteral reimplant was 96.7% at a mean follow up of 4.5 years [63]. The durability of ureteroureterostomy is also excellent with another case series reporting no adverse events at a mean follow-up of 33 months postoperatively [62].

Conclusion

Injury to the genitourinary system is a known complication of intraabdominal surgery and occurs regardless of the operating surgeon's expertise. The goal is to prevent these injuries from occurring. To accomplish this, the operating surgeon needs a complete understanding of the anatomy of the pelvis, and preoperative imaging can further define the anatomy identifying distortion from mass effect and congenital anomalies such as duplicated ureters. Preoperative cross-sectional imaging should be obtained to characterize any distortion or congenital anomalies such as duplicated ureters that may be present cross-sectional imaging. When injuries do occur, early recognition and early consultation of urologic surgeons improve patient outcomes. When operating near the bladder or ureters, surgeons should always maintain low threshold for evaluation of possible injury to these structures. When an injury has been recognized, the following principles are key to successful repair: use of absorbable suture, tension-free and watertight closure, urinary drainage with indwelling urethral catheter for all bladder injuries and ureteral stent or nephrostomy tube for ureteral injuries. Though it is humbling to experience this complication, long-term outcomes for patients following repairs are excellent.

References

1. Cordon BH, Fracchia JA, Armenakas NA. Iatrogenic nonendoscopic bladder injuries over 24 years: 127 cases at a single institution. Urology. 2014;84:222–6.
2. Fanning J, Fenton B, Jean GM, Chae C. Cost analysis of prophylactic intraoperative cystoscopic ureteral stents in gynecologic surgery. J Am Osteopath Assoc. 2011;111:667–9.
3. Simson N, Stonier T, Challacombe B, Wheatstone S. When things go wrong: a surgeon's guide to iatrogenic injury (Perspective). Int J Surg. 2019;72:93–5.
4. Ostrzenski A, Ostrzenska KM. Bladder injury during laparoscopic surgery. Obstet Gynecol Surv. 1998;53:175–80.
5. Sharp HT, Adelman MR. Prevention, recognition, and management of urologic injuries during gynecologic surgery. Obstet Gynecol. 2016;127:1085–96.
6. Wong JMK, Bortoletto P, Tolentino J, Jung MJ, Milad MP. Urinary tract injury in gynecologic laparoscopy for benign indication: a systematic review. Obstet Gynecol. 2018;131:100–8.
7. Teeluckdharry B, Gilmour D, Flowerdew G. Urinary tract injury at benign gynecologic surgery and the role of cystoscopy: a systematic review and meta-analysis. Obstet Gynecol. 2015;126:1161–9.
8. Carley ME, McIntire D, Carley JM, Schaffer J. Incidence, risk factors and morbidity of unintended bladder or ureter injury during hysterectomy. Int Urogynecol J Pelvic Floor Dysfunct. 2002;13:18–21.
9. Salman L, et al. Urinary bladder injury during cesarean delivery: maternal outcome from a contemporary large case series. Eur J Obstet Gynecol Reprod Biol. 2017;213:26–30.
10. Tarney CM. Bladder injury during cesarean delivery. Curr Womens Health Rev. 2013;9:70–6.
11. Morey AF, et al. Urotrauma: AUA guideline. J Urol. 2014;192:327–35.
12. Summerton DJ, Kitrey ND, Lumen N, Serafetinidis E, Djakovic N. EAU guidelines on iatrogenic trauma. Eur Urol. 2012;62:628–39.
13. Moore EE, et al. Organ injury scaling III: chest wall, abdominal vascular, ureter, bladder, and urethra. J Trauma Acute Care Surg. 1992;33:337–9.
14. Gomez RG, et al. Consensus statement on bladder injuries. BJU Int. 2004;94:27–32.
15. Eswara JR, Raup VT, Potretzke AM, Hunt SR, Brandes SB. Outcomes of iatrogenic genitourinary injuries during colorectal surgery. Urology. 2015;86:1228–34.
16. Mendez LE. Iatrogenic injuries in gynecologic cancer surgery. Surg Clin N Am. 2001;81:897–923.
17. Partin AW, Dmochowski RR, Kavoussi LR, Peters CA, editors. Campbell-Walsh-Wein urology. 12th ed. Philadelphia: Elsevier; 2020.
18. Quagliano PV, Delair SM, Malhotra AK. Diagnosis of blunt bladder injury: a prospective comparative study of computed tomography cystography and conventional retrograde cystography. J Trauma. 2006;61:410–22.
19. Vaccaro JP, Brody JM. CT cystography in the evaluation of major bladder trauma. Radiographics. 2000;20:1373–81.
20. Ferro A, Byck D, Gallup D. Intraoperative and postoperative morbidity associated with cystoscopy performed in patients undergoing gynecologic surgery. Am J Obstet Gynecol. 2003;189:354–7.
21. AAGL Advancing Minimally Invasive Gynecology Worldwide. AAGL Practice Report: Practice guidelines for intraoperative cystoscopy in laparoscopic hysterectomy. J Minim Invasive Gynecol. 2012;19:407–11.
22. American College of Obstetricians and Gynecologists. ACOG Committee Opinion. Number 372. July 2007. The role of cystourethroscopy in the generalist obstetrician-gynecologist practice. Obstet Gynecol. 2007;110:221–4.
23. Fouladi DF, Shayesteh S, Fishman EK, Chu LC. Imaging of urinary bladder injury: the role of CT cystography. Emerg Radiol. 2020;27:87–95.
24. Benson CR, Thompson S, Li G, Asafu-Adjei D, Brandes SB. Bladder and ureteral injuries during benign hysterectomy: an observational cohort analysis in New York State. World J Urol. 2020;38:2049–54.
25. Esparaz AM, Pearl JA, Herts BR, LeBlanc J, Kapoor B. Iatrogenic urinary tract injuries: etiology, diagnosis, and management. Semin Intervent Radiol. 2015;32:195–208.
26. Nezhat CH, Seidman DS, Farr N, Howard R, Camran N. Laparoscopic management of intentional and unintentional cystotomy. J Urol. 1996;156:1400–2.
27. Poffenberger RJ. Laparoscopic repair of intraperitoneal bladder injury: a simple new technique. Urology. 1996;47:248–9.

28. Seski JC. Iatrogenic intravesical foreign body following Marshall-Marchetti procedure. Am J Obstet Gynecol. 1976;126:514–5.
29. McIntosh LJ, Mallett VT, Richardson DA. Complications from permanent suture in surgery for stress urinary incontinence. A report of two cases. J Reprod Med. 1993;38:823–5.
30. Edlich RF, Rodeheaver GT, Thacker JG. Considerations in the choice of sutures for wound closure of the genitourinary tract. J Urol. 1987;137:373–9.
31. Smith ZL, Sehgal SS, Van Arsdalen KN, Goldstein IS. Placenta percreta with invasion into the urinary bladder. Urol Case Rep. 2014;2:31–2.
32. Kiricuta I, Goldstein AMB. The repair of extensive vesicovaginal fistulas with pedicled omentum: a review of 27 cases. J Urol. 1972;108:724–7.
33. Smith JA, Howards SS, Preminger GM, et al., editors. Hinman's atlas of urologic surgery. 4th ed. Philadelphia: Elsevier; 2018.
34. Corriere JN Jr, Sandler CM. Bladder rupture from external trauma: diagnosis and management. World J Urol. 1999;17:84–9.
35. Gilmour DT, Das S, Flowerdew G. Rates of urinary tract injury from gynecologic surgery and the role of intraoperative cystoscopy. Obstet Gynecol. 2006;107:1366–72.
36. Härkki-Sirén P. Urinary tract injuries after hysterectomy. Obstet Gynecol. 1998;92:113–8.
37. Aarts J, et al. Surgical approach to hysterectomy for benign gynaecological disease. Cochrane Database Syst Rev. 2015. https://doi.org/10.1002/14651858.CD003677.pub5.
38. Vakili B, et al. The incidence of urinary tract injury during hysterectomy: a prospective analysis based on universal cystoscopy. Am J Obstet Gynecol. 2005;192:1599–604.
39. Dandolu V, et al. Accuracy of cystoscopy in the diagnosis of ureteral injury in benign gynecologic surgery. Int Urogynecol J Pelvic Floor Dysfunct. 2003;14:427–31.
40. Grainger DA, et al. Ureteral injuries at laparoscopy: insights into diagnosis, management, and prevention. Obstet Gynecol. 1990;75:839–43.
41. Lee Z, Kaplan J, Giusto L, Eun D. Prevention of iatrogenic ureteral injuries during robotic gynecologic surgery: a review. Am J Obstet Gynecol. 2016;214:566–71.
42. Chou M-T, Wang C-J, Lien R-C. Prophylactic ureteral catheterization in gynecologic surgery: a 12-year randomized trial in a community hospital. Int Urogynecol J Pelvic Floor Dysfunct. 2009;20:689–93.
43. Redan JA, McCarus SD. Protect the ureters. JSLS. 2009;13:139–41.
44. Brandes S, Coburn M, Armenakas N, McAninch J. Diagnosis and management of ureteric injury: an evidence-based analysis. BJU Int. 2004;94:277–89.
45. Kanabur P, Chai C, Taylor J. Use of indocyanine green for intraoperative ureteral identification in non-urologic surgery. JAMA Surg. 2020;155:520.
46. Lee Z, Moore B, Giusto L, Eun DD. Use of indocyanine green during robot-assisted ureteral reconstructions. Eur Urol. 2015;67:291–8.
47. Siddighi S, Yune JJ, Hardesty J. Indocyanine green for intraoperative localization of ureter. Am J Obstet Gynecol. 2014;211:436.e1–2.
48. Léonard F, et al. Ureteral complications from laparoscopic hysterectomy indicated for benign uterine pathologies: a 13-year experience in a continuous series of 1300 patients. Hum Reprod. 2007;22:2006–11.
49. Ostrzenski A, Radolinski B, Ostrzenska KM. A review of laparoscopic ureteral injury in pelvic surgery. Obstet Gynecol Surv. 2003;58:794–9.
50. Drake MJ, Noble JG. Ureteric trauma in gynecologic surgery. Int Urogynecol J. 1998;9:108–17.
51. Burks FN, Santucci RA. Management of iatrogenic ureteral injury. Ther Adv Urol. 2014;6:115–24.
52. Best CD, et al. Traumatic ureteral injuries: a single institution experience validating the American Association for the Surgery of Trauma-Organ Injury Scale grading scale. J Urol. 2005;173:1202–5.
53. Selzman AA, Spirnak JP. Iatrogenic ureteral injuries: a 20-year experience in treating 165 injuries. J Urol. 1996;155:878–81.
54. Bryk DJ, Zhao LC. Guideline of guidelines: a review of urological trauma guidelines. BJU Int. 2016;117:226–34.
55. Wu H-H, et al. The detection of ureteral injuries after hysterectomy. J Minim Invasive Gynecol. 2006;13:403–8.
56. Manoucheri E, Cohen SL, Sandberg EM, Kibel AS, Einarsson J. Ureteral injury in laparoscopic gynecologic surgery. Rev Obstet Gynecol. 2012;5:106–11.
57. Ibeanu OA, et al. Urinary tract injury during hysterectomy based on universal cystoscopy. Obstet Gynecol. 2009;113:6–10.
58. Delacroix S, Winters JC. Urinary tract injures: recognition and management. Clin Colon Rectal Surg. 2010;23:104–12.
59. Patel BN, Gayer G. Imaging of iatrogenic complications of the urinary tract. Radiol Clin N Am. 2014;52:1101–16.
60. Han C-M, et al. Outcome of laparoscopic repair of ureteral injury: follow-up of twelve cases. J Minim Invasive Gynecol. 2012;19:68–75.
61. Tracey AT, et al. Robotic-assisted laparoscopic repair of ureteral injury: an evidence-based review of techniques and outcomes. Minerva Urol Nefrol. 2018;70:231–41.
62. Paick J-S, Hong SK, Park M-S, Kim SW. Management of postoperatively detected iatrogenic lower ureteral injury: should ureteroureterostomy really be abandoned? Urology. 2006;67:237–41.
63. Riedmiller H, Becht E, Hertle L, Jacobi G, Hohenfellner R. Psoas-Hitch ureteroneocystostomy: experience with 181 cases. Eur Urol. 1984;10:145–50.

Retroperitoneal Dissection

19

Leigh A. Humphries, Maria Alejandra Hincapie, and Ceana H. Nezhat

Introduction

The ability to "go retroperitoneal"—to dissect the structures within the retroperitoneum—is an essential skill for the gynecologic surgeon. Entering this space is the starting point for many gynecologic surgeries, from hysterectomy to excision of endometriosis. The primary purpose is to isolate the vital structures of the pelvis: ureters, bladder, rectum, uterus, adnexa, supporting ligaments, iliac vessels, nerves, and lymph nodes. The surgeon uses sharp and blunt techniques to thin and separate the connective tissue, fat, and endopelvic fascia that surround these structures. The secondary purpose is to remove pathology within the retroperitoneum, such as deep infiltrating endometriosis or malignancy. An elegant dissection of the retroperitoneum can be bloodless as long as it follows avascular tissue planes. The complexity of the dissection increases with the extent of pelvic pathology and number of prior surgeries in the space.

Taking a retroperitoneal approach can help simplify an otherwise challenging operation. For example, adhesions and fibrosis due to endometriosis can obscure the adnexa and obliterate the spaces anterior and posterior to the uterus. Beneath this "frozen pelvis," however, the retroperitoneal anatomy is often more predictable and can offer reference points so that the surgeon can restore normal intrapelvic anatomy. When bulky fibroids or other pelvic masses fill the pelvis, opening the retroperitoneum is a logical first step to visualize the ureter and the vessels. Developing the paravesical and pararectal spaces allows the surgeon to control the uterine artery at its origin, providing hemostasis for the rest of the dissection. If unexpected bleeding occurs at the pelvic sidewall, the surgeon can clearly locate retroperitoneal structures before applying thermal energy, suture, or clips to the bleeding site. For deep infiltrating endometriosis, retroperitoneal dissection is necessary to excise the lesions in their entirety, so as to achieve the best pain control, avoid ovarian remnants, and prevent bowel, ureteral, or constriction injuries [1].

Despite the clear importance of these techniques, not all gynecologic surgeons feel comfortable with retroperitoneal dissection. Even surgeons in practice for years may lack the surgical volume or foundational skills to perform ureterolysis, develop the avascular spaces, or resect

L. A. Humphries
Hospital of the University of Pennsylvania,
Philadelphia, PA, USA

Nezhat Medical Center, Atlanta Center for Minimally
Invasive Surgery and Reproductive Medicine,
Atlanta, GA, USA
e-mail: Leigh.Humphries@pennmedicine.upenn.edu

M. A. Hincapie · C. H. Nezhat (✉)
Nezhat Medical Center, Atlanta Center for Minimally
Invasive Surgery and Reproductive Medicine,
Atlanta, GA, USA
e-mail: ceana@nezhat.com

© The Author(s), under exclusive license to Springer Nature Switzerland AG 2022
S. R. Lindheim, J. C. Petrozza (eds.), *Reproductive Surgery*,
https://doi.org/10.1007/978-3-031-05240-8_19

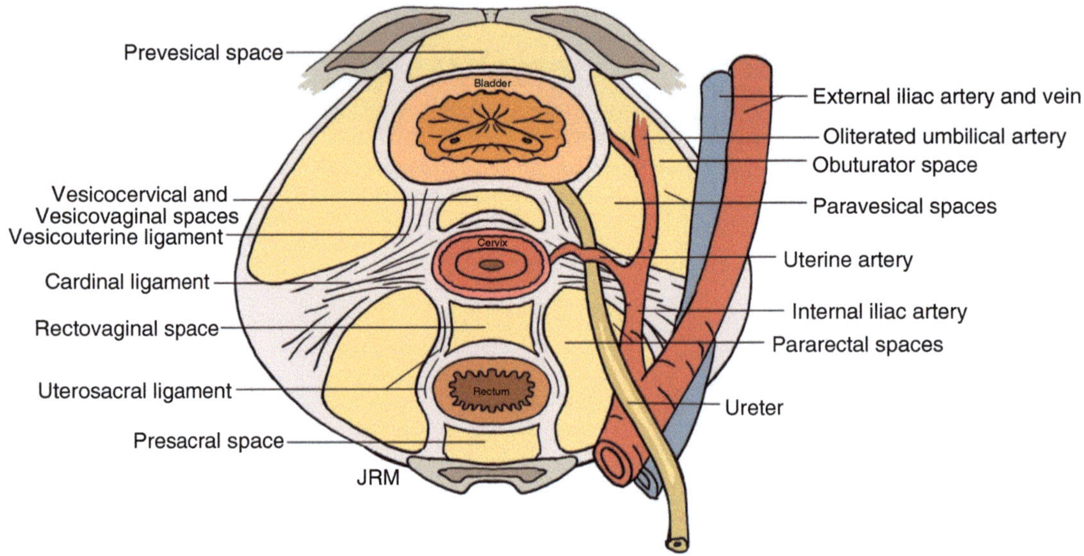

Fig. 19.1 Avascular spaces of the pelvis. The avascular spaces include the paravesical, pararectal, prevesical, vesico-cervical, vesicovaginal, rectovaginal, and presacral spaces

endometriotic lesions. Fertility care has become increasingly nonoperative, with some reproductive endocrinology and infertility fellows graduating without the surgical experience or confidence to operate independently. This chapter can be a resource for novice trainees and seasoned surgeons alike with focus on video laparoscopy approaches with or without robotic assistance.

Retroperitoneal Anatomy

"The eye cannot see what the mind does not know." Strong knowledge of retroperitoneal anatomy is first and foremost. The surgeon must understand the structures and spaces of the pelvis in order to identify them accurately. We therefore begin with a review of clinical anatomy, with a focus on the avascular spaces, ureters, vasculature, and nerves.

Avascular Spaces

The avascular spaces are the basic roadmap for any retroperitoneal dissection. These spaces include the paravesical, pararectal, prevesical, vesicocervical, vesicovaginal, rectovaginal, and presacral spaces (Fig. 19.1). They contain primarily fat and loose areolar tissue and provide access to vessels and nerves. They are potential spaces, meaning they are not naturally present but are created surgically. Endometriotic implants may arise in any of these spaces. Developing the spaces early on in dissection achieves good surgical exposure, makes the procedure safer and faster, and reduces the surgeon's workload and potential for complications.

Paravesical and Pararectal Spaces

A simple line diagram, modified from Rogers and Pasic, shows the paravesical and pararectal spaces, which share a common boundary, the uterine artery (Fig. 19.2). The paravesical and pararectal spaces are bilateral, on either side of the bladder and the rectum, respectively. The paravesical space is bound medially by the vesicouterine ligaments (also called the bladder pillars) and laterally by the obturator internus fascia and pelvic sidewall. Some sources further divide this space into medial and lateral paravesical spaces, separated by the obliterated umbilical artery. The lateral paravesical space, also called

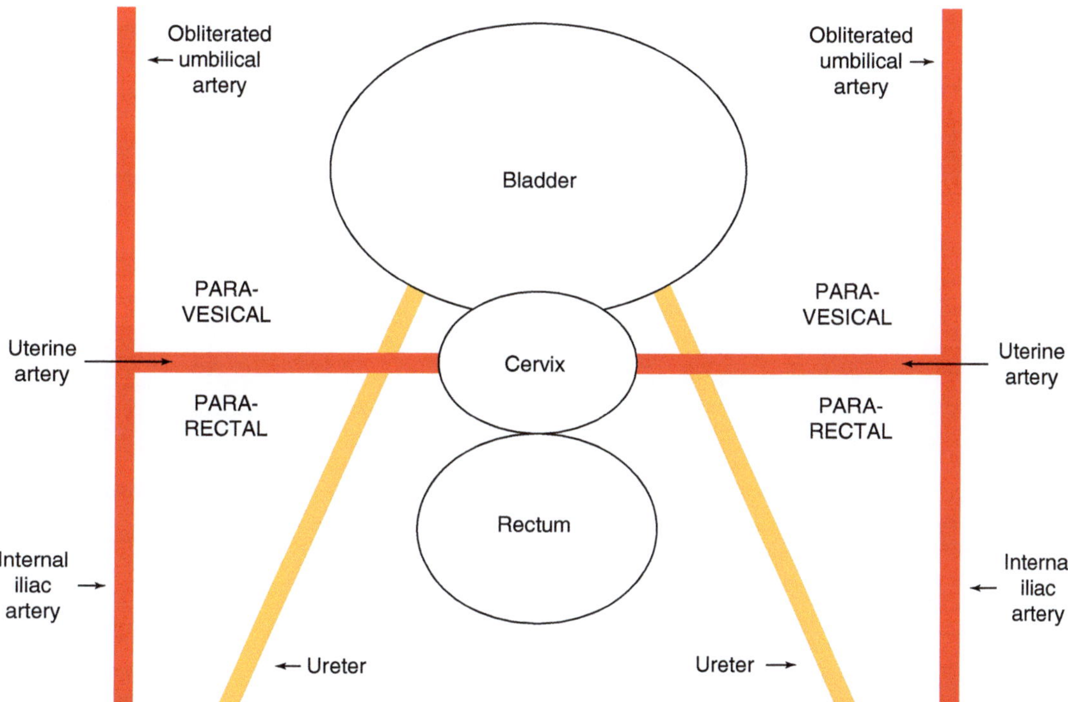

Fig. 19.2 Boundaries of the paravesical and pararectal spaces. The paravesical space is bounded by the bladder medially, obliterated umbilical artery laterally, uterine artery posteriorly, and abdominal wall anteriorly. The pararectal space is bounded by the ureter medially and posteriorly, internal iliac artery laterally, and uterine artery anteriorly. (Modified from Rogers and Pasic [2])

the obturator space, is the site of pelvic lymphadenectomy, as it contains the external iliac and obturator lymph nodes, as well as the obturator nerve and artery.

The pararectal space is posterior to the paravesical space, bounded medially by the rectum and the ureter, laterally by the internal iliac artery and pelvic sidewall, and posteriorly by the sacrum. It can be further divided into the medial pararectal space (also called Okabayashi's space) between ureter and the rectum, and lateral pararectal space (also called Latzko's space) between the ureter and pelvic sidewall.

With a clear view of these spaces, there is good access for managing bladder or ureteric endometriosis. The surgeon can also tackle an obliterated posterior cul-de-sac by starting with this approach, exposing the rectum, ureter, and uterine vessels so the rectum can be dissected from the vagina to open the rectovaginal space. Also, these spaces allow the uterine artery to be clearly visualized at its origin from the internal iliac artery, where it can be occluded permanently or temporarily to reduce intraoperative blood loss (Fig. 19.3).

Prevesical Space

The prevesical space, also called the retropubic space or the space of Retzius, is the most anterior pelvic space, located between the pubic bone and the bladder (Fig. 19.4). Its lateral borders are the arcus tendineus fascia and the ischial spines. This space is continuous with the paravesical spaces and exposes the bladder neck and urethra. In addition to resection of bladder endometriosis, this space is relevant for procedures to treat stress urinary incontinence.

Vesicocervical and Vesicovaginal Spaces

The vesicocervical and vesicovaginal spaces are located in the longitudinal axis between the blad-

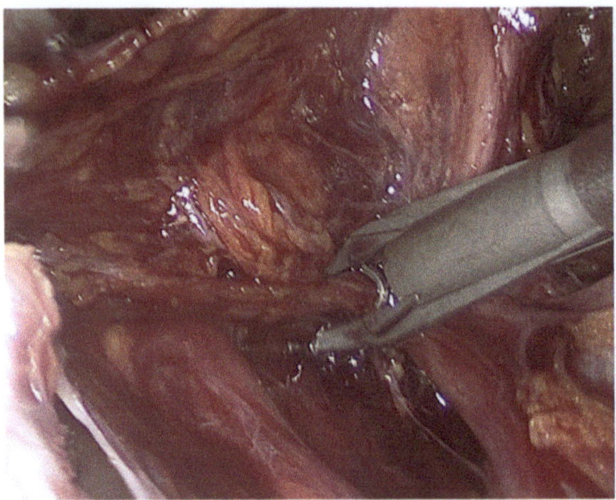

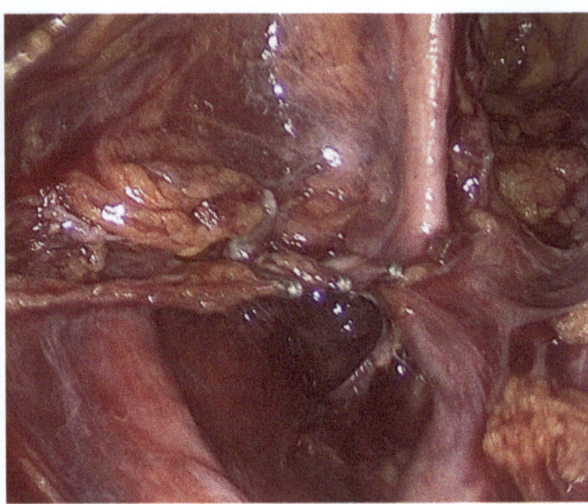

Fig. 19.3 Occlusion of the uterine artery at its origin. The uterine artery can be seen crossing over the ureter ("water under the bridge"). Three vascular clips are applied to the uterine artery at its origin from the internal iliac artery prior to transection

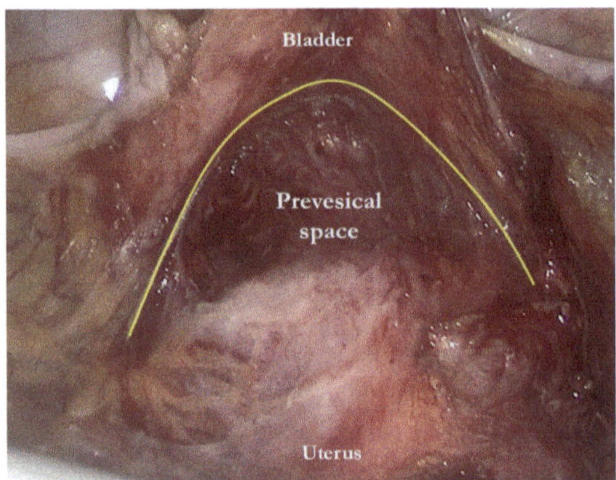

Fig. 19.4 Prevesical Space

der and the cervix and vagina, respectively (Fig. 19.5). They are bounded laterally by the vesicouterine ligaments and paravaginal tissues. The vesicovaginal space ends caudally at the site of fusion between the anterior wall of the vagina and the posterior wall of the urethra. To enter these spaces, the peritoneum may be incised at the anterior cul-de-sac, also called vesicouterine pouch. If the paravesical space has already been developed laterally, the incision in the broad ligament can also be extended anteriorly to open this space. The vesicocervical space is primarily dissected in the midline along the pubocervical fascia, which avoids injury to the vessels or ure-

ters that lie lateral to this space. The bladder is further separated from the vagina during dissection of the vesicovaginal space, which is commonly opened during hysterectomy or resection of vaginal endometriosis.

In cases where anterior cul-de-sac adhesions are encountered, the development of a "New" surgical space lateral and caudal to the vesicocervical space further mitigates genitourinary injuries (Fig. 19.6) [3]. The New space is created by thorough dissection to extend the vesicocervical space bilaterally until both sides connect through the inferior aspect of the vesicouterine adhesions. The vesicocervical ligament is the medial border and the obliterated umbilical arteries lie laterally. The anterior leaf of the broad ligament lies anteriorly and the posterior margin is the parametrium.

Rectovaginal Space

The rectovaginal space is located in the longitudinal axis between the posterior vagina and the rectum, or the rectovaginal septum (Figs. 19.5 and 19.7). This space can be accessed laparoscopically through the peritoneum of the posterior cul-de-sac. However, rectovaginal endometriosis or prior surgeries can cause this cul-de-sac to be obliterated. In these cases, the rectovaginal space is more easily entered with a

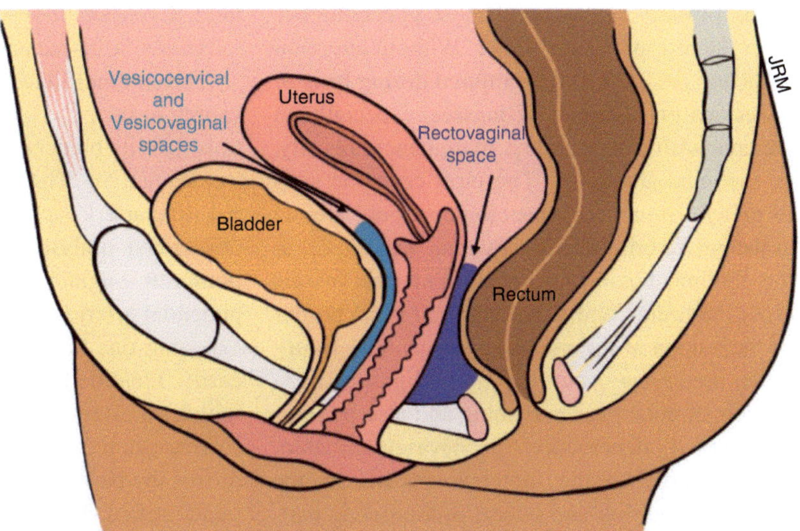

Fig. 19.5 Vesicocervical/vaginal and rectovaginal spaces

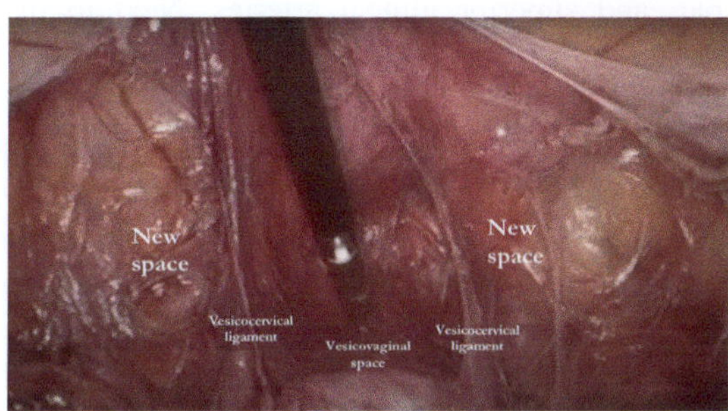

Fig. 19.6 New space. Located slightly caudal and lateral to the vesicocervical space, the New space is developed to isolate anterior adhesions between the bladder and the cervix. It is bordered medially by the vesicocervical ligament (or bladder pillar), caudally by the bladder, anteriorly by the anterior broad ligament, and posteriorly by the parametrium and distal ureter

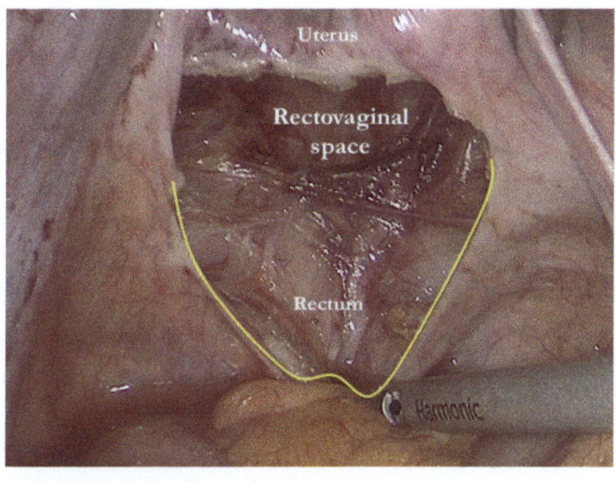

Fig. 19.7 Rectovaginal Space

lateral-to-medial approach, after first opening the bilateral pararectal spaces and isolating the ureters. The middle rectal artery and vein and vaginal veins are also present within this space; disruption of these vessels should be avoided by dissecting within the avascular fascial planes of the rectovaginal septum.

Presacral Space

The presacral space is the retroperitoneal space that lies anterior to the sacrum and the fourth and fifth lumbar vertebrae. It extends up to the bifurcation of the aorta, laterally to the iliac vessels and ureters, caudally to the coccyx and pelvic floor. It contains the median sacral vessels, sacral venous plexus, superior hypogastric plexus, and hypogastric nerves. This space is dissected during excision of endometriosis as well as during sacrocolpopexy for treatment of pelvic organ prolapse. During presacral neurectomy to treat chronic pelvic pain, the visceral nerves of the hypogastric plexus are excised along with the fatty areolar tissue of this space, at the triangle of Cotte.

Ureter

It is prudent for the surgeon to be mindful but not fearful of the ureters. Identification of the ureters is the primary reason why most gynecologists enter the retroperitoneal space. Without attention to the ureters, they may be injured during lysis of adhesions or resection of masses, especially in patients with prior surgery, malignancy, obesity, or anatomic anomalies. The most common sites of ureteral injury in gynecologic surgery are (1) at the pelvic brim near the ovarian vessels, (2) at the cardinal ligament where the uterine vessels cross the ureter, and (3) along the lateral border of the vagina at the uterosacral ligament. Injury to the ureter can occur directly by ligation, transection, angulation, or crushing and also by thermal spread, denervation, or devascularization. Blood supply to the ureter is medial in the abdominal portion and lateral in the pelvic part. Since the blood vessels of the ureter run longitudinally along its outer adventitial layer, this layer should be preserved along with adjacent fatty tissue or "mesoureter," wherever possible. Overall, the best way to avoid ureteral injury is proper dissection technique and awareness of the ureter's location in relation to other organs.

The course of the ureter starts from the renal pelvis at the ureteropelvic junction and descends along the anterior psoas muscle. At the level of the sacral promontory, the ureter crosses the pelvic brim, lateral to medial, over the bifurcation of the common iliac vessels on the right side and medial to the internal iliac on the left in the majority of cases. The ureter runs along the pelvic sidewall in the posterior broad ligament and travels under the uterine artery, hence the phrase "water under the bridge." It then tunnels within the parametrium toward the bladder. On entry into the bladder, it courses within the bladder wall for about 1 to 2 cm and ends at the ureteric orifice in the bladder trigone.

Pelvic Vasculature

Knowledge of the pelvic vessels helps to preserve the blood supply to target organs, avoid vascular injury, and identify landmarks for dissection. The surgeon should focus on maintaining hemostasis throughout the procedure and control bleeding as soon as it enters the surgical field. Even small-vessel bleeding can stain the loose areolar tissue and limit exposure.

The internal iliac artery is the primary blood supply to the pelvis, and it is therefore important to isolate its branches, especially in cases of distorted anatomy. The anterior division of the internal iliac artery includes the following branches: obliterated umbilical, uterine, superior vesical, obturator, vaginal, inferior gluteal, and internal pudendal arteries. Since these are all connected, exposing one branch allows the rest to be more easily identified. For example, the obliterated umbilical artery can be grasped and tugged with a laparoscopic grasper, and this simultaneously moves the base of the uterine artery so that it can be identified. The posterior division of the internal iliac artery includes the lateral sacral, iliolumbar, and superior gluteal arteries. Next to the branches of the internal iliac artery run the corresponding veins.

The external iliac artery, by contrast, produces few branches within the pelvis: the inferior epigastric artery, recurrent obturator artery, and deep circumflex iliac artery. It then descends to the femoral ring below the inguinal ligament, where it becomes the femoral artery and supplies blood to the lower limb. The vascular anastomosis of the external iliac or the inferior epigastric and the obturator vessels is known as the "Corona mortis." It is located behind the superior pubic ramus over the obturator fossa. Attention to these vessels is essential in order to perform a safe dissection.

Pelvic Nerves

Familiarity with the anatomy of the pelvic nerves allows the surgeon to minimize nerve injury during dissection and also appreciate how endometriosis and its surgical treatment can affect the nerves. In severe cases, deep infiltrating endometriosis can infiltrate the sacral plexus or sciatic nerve and cause pain, altered sensation in the legs or pelvis, or even muscle weakness. Chronic pelvic pain (CPP) and bowel or bladder dysfunction in patients with endometriosis has been attributed to chronic inflammation of the nerves. The development of CPP represents a cascade of events initiated at the time of peripheral stimulation or injury. The persistence of pain can result from changes in the nervous system's pathway [4]. Endometriosis resection itself can be extensive, causing nerve disruption that may manifest as short-term bowel or bladder dysfunction.

The pelvis is innervated by networks of nerve fibers that travel primarily within the connective tissue overlying vessels and pelvic viscera. There are various kinds of nerves in the pelvis: somatic, parasympathetic, sympathetic, and mixed autonomic nerves. The superior hypogastric plexus is located in the presacral space over the bifurcation of the aorta and arises from the para-aortic sympathetic trunk. It transmits sympathetic signals from the thoracic/lumbar splanchnic nerves and receives afferent pain signals from the viscera. The superior hypogastric plexus converges into the left and right hypogastric nerves that run along the internal iliac vessels. The hypogastric nerves travel on the pelvic sidewall lateral to the uterosacral ligaments. They merge with the pelvic splanchnic nerves to become the inferior hypogastric plexus, which innervates the parametrium and viscera, including the uterus, vagina, bladder, and rectum. The pelvic splanchnic nerves carry parasympathetic input from S2 to S4 nerve roots and transmit pain sensation from the viscera. The pelvic splanchnic nerves and the inferior hypogastric plexus are the nerves most commonly disrupted during dissection of the pararectal space or parametrium, which can cause urinary retention. Some damage to nerve fibers is unavoidable and has minimal clinical implications; however, if a radical resection is planned, a nerve-sparing technique is generally preferrable.

Other notable retroperitoneal nerves are the genitofemoral nerve and the obturator nerve, both originating from the lumbar plexus. The genitofemoral nerve runs along the surface of the psoas muscle and is responsible for sensation of the medial thigh and lateral labia. The obturator nerve travels along the medial border of the psoas muscle into the obturator space and through the obturator foramen in the pelvis. It provides sensory and motor innervation to the inner thigh.

Dissection Techniques

Knowledge of anatomy and instrumentation combined with judicious microsurgical technique are essential components of a competent reproductive surgeon. Multiple techniques can be used at the same time or in quick succession during the dissection. These techniques are not specific to laparoscopic surgery; rather, they apply to any dissection because they rely on general surgical principles.

Millimeter by Millimeter

The surgeon proceeds through the dissection deliberately millimeter by millimeter or layer by layer. The extra magnification and lighting of laparoscopy is helpful for this technique, especially for handling vessels and nerves. The surgeon confirms the identity of each structure prior to ligating, coagulating, cutting, or retracting. The movements are controlled and make incremental progress. The surgeon avoids quick large movements or blunt dissection in spaces without clear safe boundaries. This steady methodical approach minimizes complications. If an injury does occur, the defect in the structure is limited to 1–2 mm, which can be more easily repaired.

Gentle Teasing and Wiping

A combination of gentle pulling, wiping, and separating of the tissue with soft strokes helps to thin the target area. This technique is useful for "skeletonizing," by which the surgeon strips away any peritoneum, connective tissue, or scarring around a structure, reducing it to its "skeleton" only. The gentle wiping motion can also be used for blunt dissection of areolar tissue and clearing minor bleeding from the surgical field.

Push and Spread

The tip of a blunt grasping instrument is inserted into the area of interest ("push") and then opened to separate the layers of tissue ("spread"). This technique, also called "poke and open," is used in conjunction with gentile teasing and wiping in order to thin connective tissue and isolate underlying structures. It can also be performed with two instruments, both inserted into a window in the peritoneum and spread in opposite directions. Spreading should occur parallel to a delicate structure, such as a vessel or nerve, to avoid shearing.

Traction–Countertraction

"Traction-countertraction" refers to two operators providing traction on tissue in opposite directions, which stretches and thins the tissue. The incision in the tissue should occur between the two instruments, at 90 degrees to the vector of stretching (Fig. 19.8). Countertraction in this way also exposes the ideal avascular plane between opposing surfaces. It is very helpful to have a competent assistant who can arrange tissues at appropriate angles and provide countertraction.

Tenting of the Tissues

The surgeon grasps and "tents" or elevates the tissue away from the underlying structures such as the ureter, bladder, vessels, or nerves. Tenting the peritoneum provides a form of traction that thins the tissue and illuminates anything beneath

it, creating a margin of safety. The grasped layer can then be incised more precisely.

Small Incisions

While blunt dissection is useful in many cases, sometimes dense scarring from endometriosis prevents the blunt separation of tissues. In these cases, various devices can be used to make small deliberate cuts to release the scarring and find the appropriate surgical plane. Generally, these cuts are performed "cold," i.e. without the use of electrosurgery. If electrosurgery is used, the surgeon should pay attention to nearby structures and consider the extent of thermal spread. In certain cases, laser device can be used.

Hydrodissection and Pneumodissection

Hydrodissection refers to the injection of fluid, e.g. saline or diluted vasopressin, into a retroperitoneal potential space, and the pressure of the injection gently separates the connective tissue. This injection develops the potential space, which can be further opened with sharp or blunt dissection. Pneumodissection relies on the same principle. CO_2 gas insufflation creates increased intraperitoneal pressure that opens potential spaces after an initial incision in the peritoneum is made.

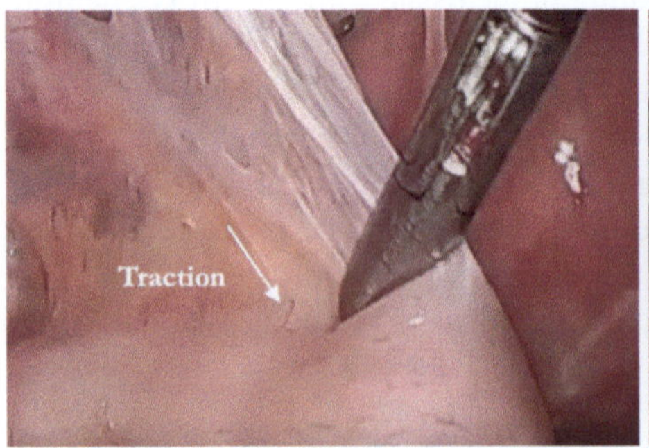
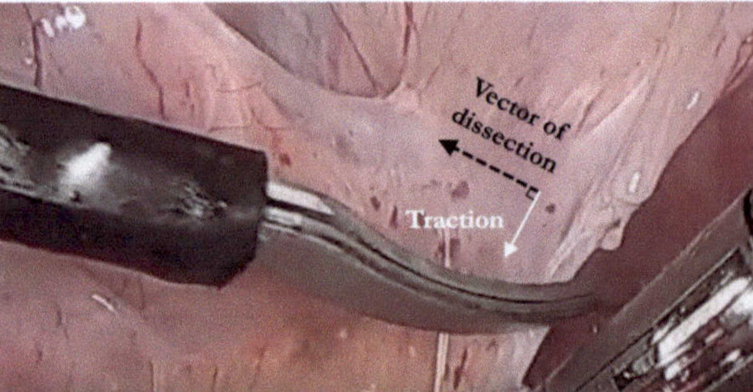

Fig. 19.8 Traction–countertraction. The vector of the dissection should be perpendicular to the direction of the traction or countertraction on the tissue

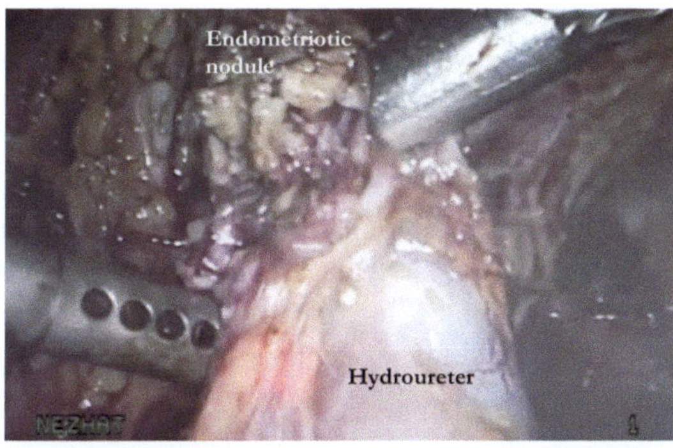

Fig. 19.9 Shaving technique for excising ureteric endometriosis. CO_2 laser is used to shave the endometriotic nodule from the underlying ureter, while the ureter and its blood supply remains intact (full video can be found in *Fertility and Sterility*)

Shaving Techniques

Shaving excision is the preferred technique for removing deep infiltrating endometriosis because it can avoid morbid resections and has good surgical outcomes. It is a microsurgical technique that creates an incision just beneath an endometriotic lesion and proceeds layer-by-layer as superficial as possible. This avoids compromising the integrity of the underlying organ, while still removing the endometriosis in its entirety. It can be successfully performed for lesions in multiple areas, including sigmoid, rectum, bladder, and ureter [5, 6] (Fig. 19.9).

General Tips

Some general tips for making a surgical plan and performing a successful dissection will be discussed in this section.

1. *Take What the Anatomy Gives You.* Be flexible with the surgical plan and willing to switch course based on the patient's anatomy and specific pathology. For example, if dense bladder adhesions are present due to prior cesarean section, myomectomy, or endometriosis, a lateral or posterior approach to develop the vesicovaginal plane may be preferred in order to avoid entering the scar ante-

riorly. This can be done by creating the "New" space, as previously described.

2. *Start with What Is Easy, and What Is Difficult Will Become Easier.* Start by entering an area of peritoneum that is not involved with scar or fibrosis. Work on optimizing exposure and developing the avascular spaces before dissecting areas with increased risk of vascular, bowel, or urinary tract injury. Tackling a large rectovaginal nodule, releasing fibrosis around the ovary, or performing ureterolysis will be easier when the surrounding structures have been identified and retracted away.

3. *Identify the Ureters Early.* Locating the ureters early in the procedure allows the surgeon to dissect the retroperitoneum and excise endometriosis without the risk of inadvertent ureteral injury. The smooth muscles of the ureter undergo intermittent peristalsis, which further aids in its detection. In some cases, placement of preoperative ureteric catheter with or without indocyanine green (ICG) fluorescent-guided surgery is helpful. Catheters transform the ureter into a more rigid tube that can be manipulated during the dissection.

4. *Use the Suction-Irrigator as a Dissection Tool.* The suction-irrigator is a versatile laparoscopic instrument. Its primary purpose is to suction and keep the surgical field clean and dry. When not suctioning, the surgeon should use it to hydrodissect and bluntly separate areolar tissue. If laser is used, the suction-irrigator can also serve as a "backstop" behind the tissue being incised, which prevents the laser from penetrating deeper tissues (Fig. 19.10).

5. *Maintain Hemostasis and Recognize Early Warning Signs of Vascular Injury.* The most common cause of death associated with laparoscopy, apart from anesthetic complications, is injury to major retroperitoneal vessels. Risk of retroperitoneal bleeding can be avoided if the surgeon is vigilant in areas of anatomic distortion and proceeds millimeter by millimeter. Keeping a dry surgical field can facilitate early recognition of vascular injury. If bleeding is suspected, the possibility of a ret-

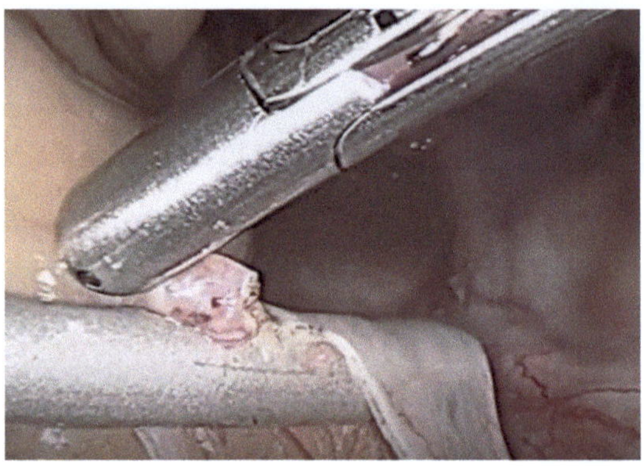

Fig. 19.10 Use of suction-irrigator during laser dissection. The suction-irrigator provides a "backstop" that prevents the laser from incising or causing thermal injury to tissue beneath the target area

roperitoneal hematoma should be considered. Bleeding in the retroperitoneal space should be quickly addressed with pressure by an atraumatic grasper and delineation of the bleeding source and any nearby structures. If bleeding is relatively minor, the surgeon may apply vascular clips, electrosurgery, or hemostatic agents at the site. If hemorrhage from major vessels occurs, the surgeon must isolate the source and apply atraumatic pressure. Repair may be done by laparoscopy or laparotomy depending on the skill and experience of the surgeon, availability of proper instruments, and multidisciplinary support.

Step-by-Step Dissection of the Pelvic Sidewall

Step 1: Perform a Systematic Survey of the Pelvis

With the patient in appropriate degree of Trendelenberg, displace the bowel into the upper abdomen and perform a systematic survey of the pelvis. Start with the sacral promontory where the aorta bifurcates, and continue to the pelvic brim and pelvic sidewalls. Inspect the adnexa, sigmoid, rectum, and posterior cul-de-sac, followed by the bilateral parametria, anterior cul-de-sac, and anterior abdominal wall. Identify all normal landmarks including pelvic organs, ligaments, and any subperitoneal structures that can be visualized transperitoneally, such as the iliac vessels, nerves, and ureters. Note the locations of any endometriotic lesions, adhesions, nodules, and aberrant anatomy. Once the dissection begins, it is harder to locate specific peritoneal lesions due to bleeding or disrupted tissue, so the surgeon should map these areas first.

Step 2: Open the Peritoneum, Ideally at the Pelvic Brim

The ideal site of entry into the retroperitoneum is at the pelvic brim, just lateral and parallel to the ureter after it crosses the bifurcation of the common iliac artery. Entering at this site allows for quick identification of the ureter and iliac vessels and creates a starting point for dissecting the paravesical and pararectal space. It is proximal enough to avoid significant scarring from endometriosis near the adnexa, parametrium, or rectosigmoid. In thin patients, the ureter can often be seen through the peritoneum at the pelvic brim, whereas in obese patients, the ureter may be deeper within fatty tissue. On the left side, it can be helpful to divide the physiologic attachment between the sigmoid mesentery and the sidewall to better expose the pelvic brim.

To make the initial incision, grasp and tent the peritoneum away from any underlying structures, including the ureter and external iliac vessels. Incise the peritoneum with a superficial cut. Extend the incision parallel to the course of the ureter and retract this peritoneal leaf medially, carrying along the ureter.

An alternative entry site into the retroperitoneum, commonly used by gynecologists during hysterectomy, is through an incision in the posterior broad ligament or transection of the round ligament. Identify the ureter deep to this peritoneal opening by dissecting along the medial leaf of the broad ligament and developing the pararectal space. The initial incision in the broad ligament can also be extended cephalad, parallel to the infundibulopelvic ligament toward the pelvic brim, where the ureter is more easily identified.

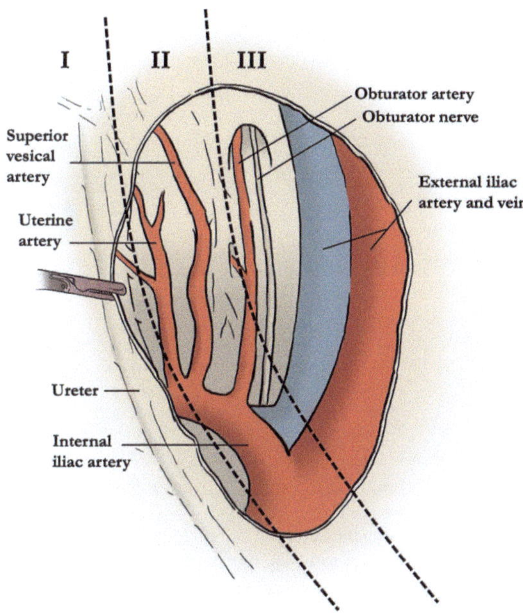

Fig. 19.11 Three layers of the pelvic sidewall. Each of these layers is encountered in succession during pelvic sidewall dissection. Layer I contains the ureter and meso-ureter. Layer II contains the internal iliac vessels and their anterior branches. Layer III contains external iliac vessels and the obturator artery and nerve. (Modified from Rogers and Taylor [7])

Step 3: Identify the Landmarks for the Three Layers of the Pelvic Sidewall

Using push-and-spread, small incisions, and traction-countertraction, separate the loose areolar tissue beneath the peritoneum to expose the initial landmarks of the three layers of the pelvic sidewall (Fig. 19.11). These three layers are identified medial to lateral: (1) the ureter in its parietal peritoneum, (2) the internal iliac vessels and their anterior branches, with associated lymphatics and nerves, and (3) external iliac vessels and the obturator artery and nerve just medial to the psoas muscle.

Step 4: Develop the Avascular Spaces

The sites of endometriosis will dictate which avascular spaces need to be opened, e.g., prevesical space to remove bladder endometriosis, recto-

vaginal and presacral spaces to mobilize the rectosigmoid and remove nodules involving the rectum, and paravesical/pararectal spaces to ligate the uterine artery, perform ureterolysis, or manage parametrial disease with obliterated cul-de-sacs. The steps below constitute a standard approach to developing the avascular spaces of the pelvic sidewall. This should be modified according to the patient's specific pathology.

With medial traction on the peritoneal leaf containing the ureter, develop the pararectal space lateral to the ureter, i.e. between the ureter and the internal iliac artery. This provides the initial exposure to the lateral pelvic sidewall. Dissect this space to the level of the uterine artery and visualize where the uterine artery originates from the internal iliac and crosses the ureter. Next, continue the dissection into the paravesical space, which is continuous with the pararectal space. Any spreading and wiping motions in the paravesical space should be parallel to the uterine artery, to maintain the avascular plane and avoid inadvertent vessel injury. Expose the superior vesical artery and obliterated umbilical artery, the terminal branch of the internal iliac artery. At this point, all of the borders of the paravesical and pararectal spaces can be seen, allowing access to the vesicovaginal or rectovaginal spaces medially (Fig. 19.12). To continue the dissection further laterally, develop the obturator space, where the obturator nerve, artery, and vein as well as obturator lymph nodes can be identified (Fig. 19.13).

Conclusion

Successful dissection of the retroperitoneum gives the surgeon two critical advantages in any pelvic surgery—exposure and mobilization. Even the most challenging surgery becomes easier once the avascular spaces of the pelvis are opened and the critical anatomic structures are identified.

Ultimately, there is no secret to becoming a master of retroperitoneal dissection. A surgeon who possesses strong knowledge of retroperitoneal anatomy and fundamental skills in

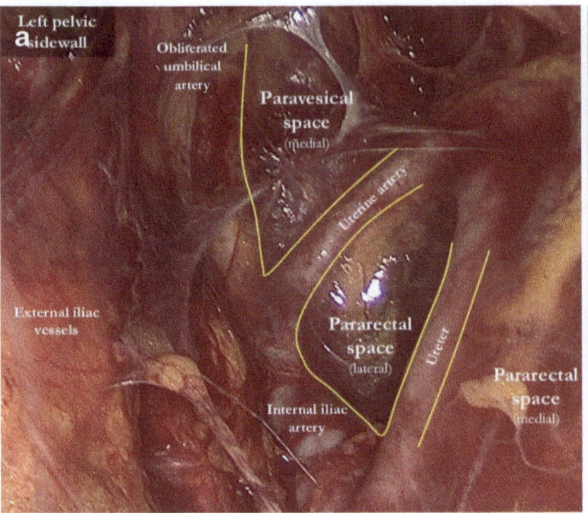

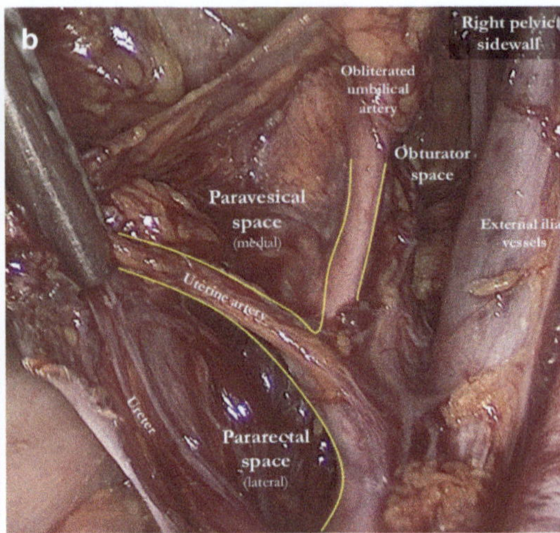

Fig. 19.12 Pelvic sidewall dissection of the paravesical and pararectal spaces, left (**a**) and right (**b**). The medial paravesical space and lateral pararectal space are the spaces most commonly dissected in order to identify the ureter and the uterine artery. The space between the ureter and the rectum is known as the medial pararectal space. The obturator space, also known as the lateral paravesical space, is lateral to the obliterated umbilical artery

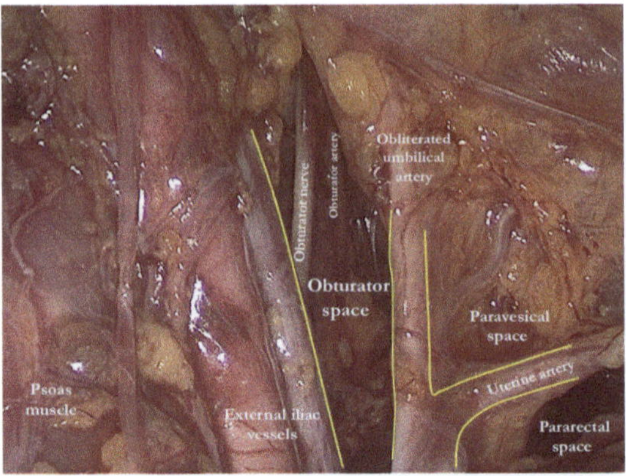

Fig. 19.13 Lateral pelvic side wall, including the obturator space. The obturator space contains the obturator nerve, artery, as well as obturator lymph nodes

laparoscopic dissection can gain proficiency in retroperitoneal dissection simply by practicing. Initially, practice should take place in cadaveric dissections, in simulation, or in cases with relatively straightforward anatomy. Over time, the ability to apply these dissection techniques in cases with highly distorted anatomy, for example, in patients with severe endometriosis, will help to avoid complications, reduce blood loss, and improve surgical outcomes.

References

1. Nezhat C, Nezhat F, Nezhat C, editors. Nezhat's video-assisted and robotic-assisted laparoscopy and hysteroscopy. 4th ed. Cambridge University Press; 2013.
2. Rogers RM, Pasic R. Pelvic retroperitoneal dissection: a hands-on primer. J Minim Invasive Gynecol. 2017;24(4):546–51.
3. Nezhat C, Vu M, Vang N, Tombash E, Nezhat A. Hysterectomy in patients with history of prior cesarean delivery: a reverse dissection technique for vesico-uterine adhesions. OBG Manag. 2019;31(11):38–42.
4. Pinho Oliveira MA, Soares Raymundo T, Lopez-Jaramillo JD, Lopez-Isanoa JD, Villegas-Echeverri JD. Neuroanatomical insights in adolescents with endometriosis and pain. In: Nezhat CH, editor. Endometriosis in adolescents: a comprehensive guide to diagnosis and management. 1st ed. Springer; 2020. p. 227–45.
5. Ananth PK, Humphries LA, Nezhat CH. Use of a shaving technique for surgical management of partial ureteral obstruction due to endometriosis. Fertil Steril. 2020;113(6):1328–9.
6. Lakhi N, Dun EC, Nezhat CH. Hematoureter due to endometriosis. Fertil Steril. 2014;101(6):e37.
7. Rogers RM Jr, Taylor RH. The core of a competent surgeon: a working knowledge of surgical anatomy and safe dissection techniques. Obstet Gynecol Clin N Am. 2011;38(4):777–88.

Deep Infiltrating Endometriosis: Diagnosis and Fertility-Sparing Management in the ART Patient

Salomeh Salari, Kathryn Coyne, and Rebecca Flyckt

Introduction

Definition

Endometriosis is defined as the presence of estrogen-sensitive endometrial glands and stroma outside of the uterine cavity [1]. These ectopic endometrial implants differ molecularly from eutopic endometrium, making the development of medical therapies and treatments significantly more challenging [2].

There are several subcategories of endometriosis based on the location and extent of disease. These include endometriomas, superficial peritoneal endometriosis, and deep infiltrating endometriosis (DIE) [2, 3]. DIE has previously been defined as a nodule extending more than 5 mm beneath the peritoneum and is considered to be the most challenging clinical form of endometriosis [2]. More recently, DIE has also been described as "adenomyosis externa," presenting as a single nodule that is larger than 1 cm in diameter [4]. DIE lesions are most often in the pelvic cavity, and can be found in the anterior compartment (bladder) or more commonly the posterior compartment (vagina, rectum, uterosacral ligaments, ureter) of the pelvis [3]. DIE can be

treated medically, but thus far can only be eliminated through a surgical approach.

Epidemiology

Endometriosis affects 10–15% of all reproductive-aged women, but has also been found in both premenarchal and postmenopausal women [1, 2]. Nearly 40% of women suffering from infertility and 70% of women who suffer from chronic pelvic pain have a diagnosis of endometriosis [4]. It is estimated that the healthcare costs associated with endometriosis are more than $27 billion per year [1]. Many women report the onset of symptoms during adolescence and the average age of diagnosis is approximately 28 years old [2]. Diagnosis of endometriosis is challenging, and is commonly delayed due to misdiagnosis, the widespread use of contraceptives that mask symptoms, and societal normalization of pelvic pain and dysmenorrhea. Gold-standard diagnosis of endometriosis still requires surgical evaluation through direct visualization and biopsy.

Risk Factors

Risk factors associated with endometriosis are mainly related to hormonal factors, and include early menarche, short menstrual cycle intervals, heavy menses, Müllerian anomalies, and nulliparity [1]. Protective factors that can reduce the

S. Salari (✉) · K. Coyne · R. Flyckt
University Hospitals Fertility Center,
Beachwood, OH, USA
e-mail: salomeh.salari@uhhospitals.org;
kathryn.coyne@uhhospitals.org;
rebecca.flyckt2@uhhospitals.org

risk of endometriosis include parity, use of hormonal contraceptives, smoking, exercise, and higher body mass index (BMI) [1].

Pathophysiology

There are several hypotheses regarding the pathophysiology of endometriosis. These include Sampson's theory of retrograde menstruation through the fallopian tubes into the pelvic cavity, as well as theories regarding hematogenous and/or lymphatic circulation, and possible Müllerian remnants that either did not migrate or differentiate (metaplasia) properly during fetal organogenesis [1, 2].

The pathophysiology of DIE is thought to differ between ovarian endometrioma and superficial peritoneal disease. It is believed that both hormonal function (estrogen and progesterone receptors) and immunological factors (i.e. peritoneal macrophages, lymphocytes, natural killer T-cells) are significantly altered in DIE [3]. Decreased apoptosis of nuclear factor kappa-light-chain enhancer of activated B cells (NF-kB), B-cell lymphoma 2 (Blc-2), and anti-Müllerian hormone (AMH), as well as increased proliferation activity related to oxidative stress, may explain the aggressive nature of DIE. There is also increased neuroangiogenesis gene expression (nerve growth factor, vascular endothelial growth factor, and intercellular adhesion molecule) in DIE compared to other phenotypes of endometriosis [3]. A key enzyme for estrogen synthesis, aromatase, is actively expressed within endometriosis lesions, but is not detectable in normal endometrium [5]. Despite the distinct molecular mechanisms of DIE, none of the currently proposed biomarkers has been sufficiently validated for routine use in the diagnosis and workup of DIE [4].

Diagnostic Considerations

Clinical Picture

Though no clinical symptoms are required for the diagnosis of endometriosis, many women with this condition experience chronic pelvic pain, dysmenorrhea, dyschezia, deep dyspareunia, adnexal masses, and infertility due to chronic and inflammatory changes, which can significantly and chronically diminish quality of life [2]. Pelvic pain is the most commonly associated symptom of endometriosis, and often worsens in the premenstrual period. Though the stages of endometriosis and pain do not correlate well, there is a well-documented relationship between the severity of DIE and intensity of pain [6]. The location of patients' pain caused by DIE are often specific to the anatomical location of involvement (Fig. 20.1). Lesions can create a mass-like effect with evidence of fibrosis, particularly when located near the bowel, uterine ligaments, or even on the ovarian cortex [2]. Deep dyspareunia might indicate lesions in the pouch of Douglas or uterosacral ligaments. Dyschezia correlates with gastrointestinal/bowel involvement. Flank pain, dysuria, or hematuria can be associated with bladder or ureteral involvement. Studies have shown that the presence of posterior compartment lesions (rectal or vaginal) and the extent of adnexal adhesions are related to the severity of dysmenorrhea (Fig. 20.1) [6]. Postsurgically, patients with DIE have better improvements in pain scores compared to those with superficial endometriosis and chronic pain.

Infertility is of particular concern with severe adhesive disease, though debate remains as to whether minimal/mild peritoneal disease is also associated with non-idiopathic infertility [2]. There are several possible mechanisms of infertility including: sperm DNA damage or abnormal oocyte cytoskeleton (resulting in impaired quality of the ovum) due to the abnormal peritoneal environment, endometrial lining defects affecting implantation, adhesions or scarred fallopian tubes, and accelerated depletion of follicles from increased granulosa cell activity causing oocyte maturation and apoptosis [2]. Furthermore, studies have shown that women with endometriosis without a surgical history have lower AMH levels compared to those without disease [2, 7]. While the predominant mechanism remains unclear, studies have shown that patients pursuing in vitro fertilization (IVF) with ovarian

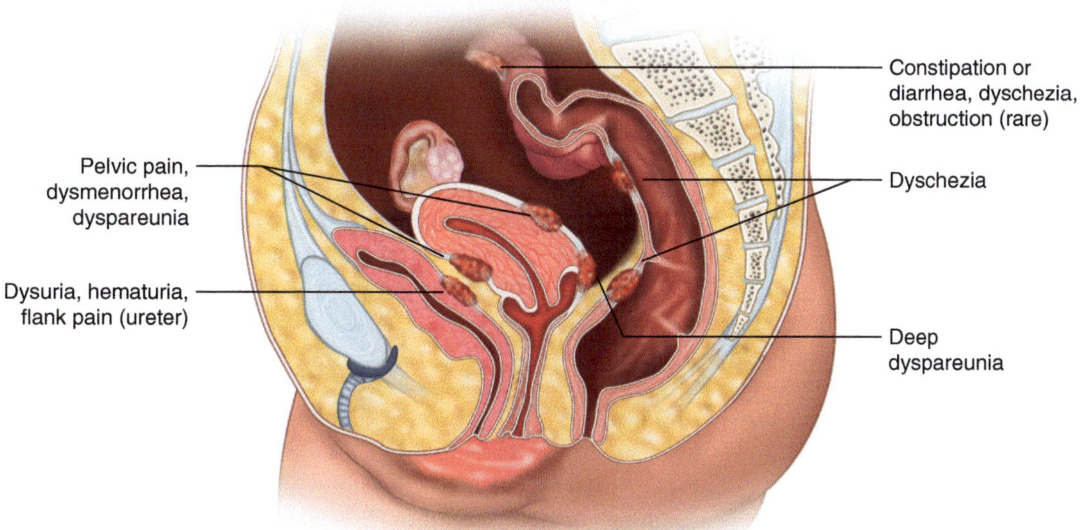

Fig. 20.1 Sagittal view of the pelvis, displaying typical endometriosis symptoms in relation to the location of DIE lesions; these symptoms often overlap

endometrioma-associated DIE have lower cumulative pregnancy rates compared to those with isolated ovarian endometrioma [8]. However, it remains unclear whether DIE is independently associated with infertility [2]. Furthermore, in the absence of pelvic anatomy distortion, the mechanisms whereby endometriosis relates to secondary infertility are less well understood.

Surgery can be used to stage the severity of disease. There are several methods of classification of endometriosis. The American Society for Reproductive Medicine (ASRM) has a staging classification system that categorizes disease as minimal, mild, moderate, or severe. This system was updated and renamed the revised ASRM (rASRM) classification where Stage I and II are designated for minimal or mild disease, and Stage III-IV indicates moderate or severe disease. This staging system was initially created for the assessment of fertility but is now often used to quantify the burden of disease despite not being validated or taking DIE specifically into account. Additionally, there is poor correlation with effects on quality of life [9]. Other classification systems include the ENZIAN-score (reports the depth of DIE and localization/expan-

sion) and the Endometriosis Fertility Index (predicts fertility outcomes based on surgical findings and the rASRM classification) [2].

Diagnosis

Surgery with pathology confirmation remains the gold standard for diagnosis of endometriosis. Histologically, one will identify endometrial glands, stroma, and hemosiderin-laden macrophages [2]. Clinically, endometriosis is most often diagnosed based on history and physical exam as well as imaging. On pelvic exam, clinicians may palpate for nodules or masses, a fixed uterus (often retroverted), or uterine and adnexal tenderness [1]. Of note, it is important to also rule out other disease processes including myofascial pain, and pelvic (adhesions, adenomyosis, pelvic inflammatory disease), gastrointestinal (irritable bowel syndrome, hemorrhoids), urologic (painful bladder syndrome, interstitial cystitis), or psychologic (depression, sexual abuse) disorders. Imaging, such as ultrasonography or magnetic resonance imaging (MRI), can also be utilized to identify and localize endometriosis.

Interventions

Though medical management such as ovulation-suppressing hormonal treatments is a reasonable first-line option for pain relief, this is not recommended for patients seeking fertility treatment and pregnancy. Further, medical management should be considered suppressive rather than curative and will not resolve DIE [2]. Surgical management has been associated with improvements in both spontaneous pregnancy rates and pregnancies resulting from fertility treatments, as discussed later in this chapter (see "Postoperative Considerations" section). While postoperative hormonal suppression does not improve fecundability and should not be used postoperatively in women seeking pregnancy, it is recommended when a patient has completed child-bearing or wishes to delay child-bearing; medical treatment in this setting may prevent recurrence of disease and symptoms as well as the need for reoperation. Without hormonal suppression, pain symptoms have a recurrence risk of 50% at five years postoperatively [10].

Controversy exists regarding the use of ART prior to planned surgical management of DIE. Similarly, in the setting of known or suspected DIE, there is debate regarding whether and when to operate if fertility (rather than pain management) is the goal. Though there continues to be debate regarding the usefulness and timing of surgical management in an ART population, once agreed upon with the patient, the following recommendations in this chapter may be used to guide decision-making on identifying the appropriate surgical candidate, fertility-sparing operative approaches based on location of the endometriosis, and possible complications and recovery.

Preoperative Considerations

Surgical Candidacy

When assessing the surgical candidacy of a patient, particular attention should be paid to patients with comorbidities that could increase the patient's risk of anesthesia (i.e. cardiac or pulmonary) and post-anesthesia complications (i.e. obstructive sleep apnea), increase wound healing time (i.e. diabetes mellitus) or make optimal patient positioning (steep Trendelenburg) difficult (i.e. morbid obesity). When in doubt, referral for presurgical evaluation by an anesthesia team is appropriate. Urine pregnancy tests are always recommended in reproductive-aged patients to ensure a current pregnancy is not potentially disrupted during surgery.

Workup

Specific diagnostic markers reliable for clinical use in the diagnosis of endometriosis have yet to be identified. BCL6 is a putative maker for endometriosis; however, its use has not been widely validated for DIE detection or surveillance for recurrence of disease after medical treatment or excisional surgery. The CA-125 test can be mildly elevated in women with endometriosis compared to those without; however, it has poor diagnostic accuracy and has low specificity and should not be used to monitor for either detection, severity, or recurrence of endometriosis. Preoperative laboratory tests can be ordered if clinically indicated, including a blood count to assess starting hemoglobin, metabolic panel to assess the kidney function with a creatinine level, and a type and screen in the event of blood transfusion. Further labs/preoperative testing should be based on a patient's medical history, such as a hemoglobin A1c for those with diabetes or pre-diabetes, or an electrocardiogram or echocardiogram for those with heart disease.

Imaging

Imaging can be useful for preoperative assessment and surgical mapping, including determining whether there is a potential need for bowel or bladder resection. This allows for more appropriate counseling of the patient on risks of surgery and the ability to coordinate with colorectal or urological surgeons.

Ultrasound remains the modality of choice for pelvic pain; however, it can be challenging for evaluation of DIE without the appropriate institutional expertise. For standardization, there exists a four-step process for identifying and characterizing endometriosis on dynamic ultrasound. The first step is evaluation of the uterus and adnexa, including cysts/endometriomas and adenomyosis, which is often found concurrently with DIE [2, 11]. The second step involves using the transvaginal probe to localize areas of tenderness in the pelvis that might correlate with areas of DIE. The third step focuses on the pouch of Douglas (posterior cul de sac) where the probe is used to apply pressure on the cervix to see if the anterior rectum moves freely across the vagina near the posterior fornix (also known as the "sliding sign"). The last and fourth step of ultrasonographic evaluation is evaluating the anterior (bladder) and posterior (uterosacral ligaments, rectovaginal septum, vaginal wall, rectum) compartments for nodules [11].

Ultrasonography is highly operator-dependent; however, studies at experienced centers have shown sensitivity and specificity higher than 95% in the rectocervical and rectosigmoid spaces and approximately 75% in the uterosacral ligaments [12, 13]. The sensitivity for DIE specifically is less, at 80% [13].

Another useful preoperative imaging modality is magnetic resonance imaging (MRI), which has a similar sensitivity and specificity to ultrasound in the diagnosis of DIE in the uterosacral ligaments (85%, 88%) and colorectal endometriosis (88%, 92%) [14]. MRI has also been shown to have similar sensitivity and specificity to ultrasound for rectosigmoid endometriosis (greater than 90%) [2, 14]. Thus, MRI is a reasonable option for presurgical imaging in place of ultrasound or if ultrasound findings are equivocal (Figs. 20.2, 20.3, 20.4, 20.5, and 20.6). Despite these benefits, MRI is more expensive,

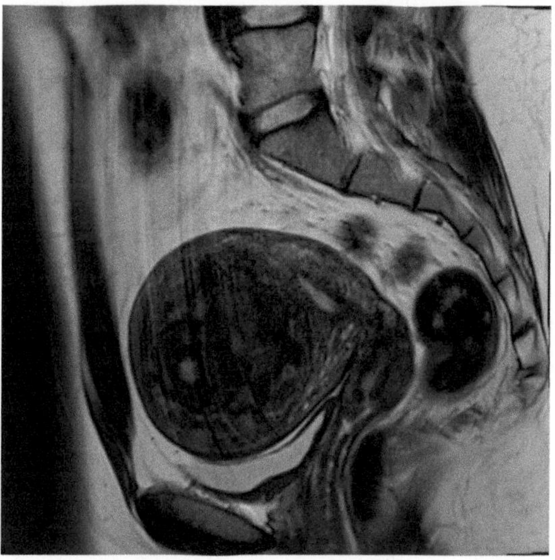

Fig. 20.2 Normal cul de sac on MRI, sagittal view

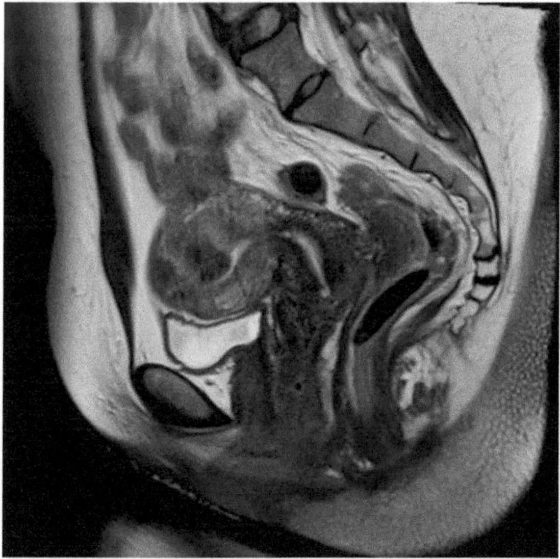

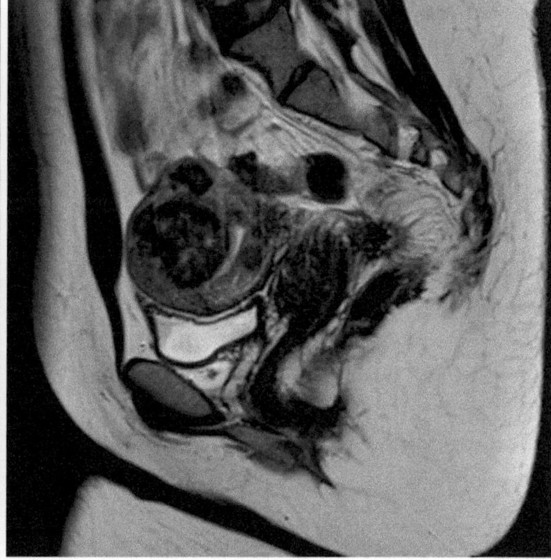

Figs. 20.3 and 20.4 Obliterated cul de sac on MRI, sagittal view

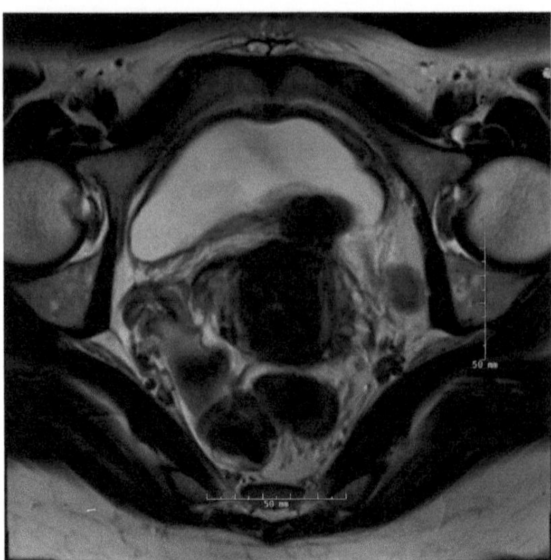

Fig. 20.5 Genitourinary endometriosis (bladder) on MRI, axial view

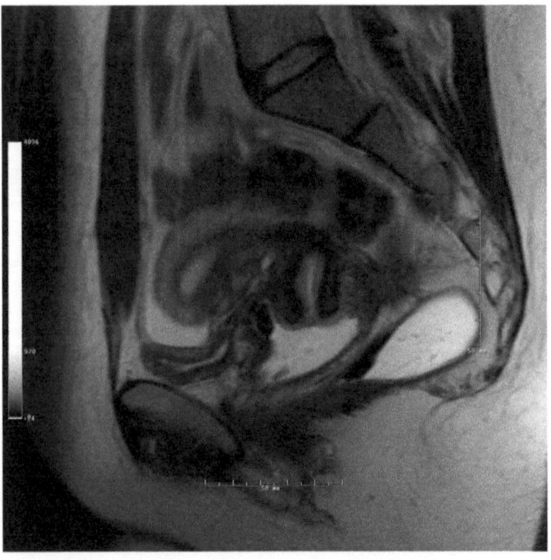

Fig. 20.6 Rectovaginal endometriosis on MRI, sagittal view

takes longer to perform, and necessitates appropriate equipment and staff. In our experience, an institutional radiology "champion" may be helpful in establishing structured reporting on MRIs performed for presurgical endometriosis evaluation.

Operative Approach

Prior to Surgery

Fertility planning and indications for surgery should be considered prior to the surgical procedure as depicted in the flowchart below [15, 16]. Choices for surgery and/or in vitro fertilization (IVF) for treatment of infertility in the setting of DIE should be discussed. For example, in patients who have previously undergone surgery for endometriosis or who have known low ovarian reserve, IVF could be proposed as the first step [17]. Additionally, oocyte freezing may be considered prior to ovarian surgery if fertility preservation is desired [18] (Table 20.1).

Other presurgical considerations to ensure adequate preparation include planning for the use of a uterine manipulator and rectal probe, as well as possible ureteral stenting and bowel preparation based on surgeon preference [19]. A uterine manipulator allows for improved visualization and facilitates dissection in the posterior compartment. A rectal probe aids in identifying and avoiding the rectum, particularly when the posterior cul de sac is densely adhered. Ureteral stents can be considered when ureteral endometriosis is suspected, most notably when hydronephrosis is present preoperatively or when large excision of bladder lesions is planned, in order to visualize the ureters and their insertion into the bladder trigone. Though there is no consensus regarding the utility of bowel preparation, it can be considered to minimize the risk of contamination of bowel contents in the abdominal cavity with planned entry into the bowel.

Intraoperative Evaluation

To ensure no lesion is missed during surgery, it is best to have a systematic approach to the pelvis when performing DIE surgery. Typically, a survey of the upper abdomen including liver and diaphragm is performed at the start of the case.

Table 20.1 Fertility planning and indications for surgery in patients with DIE [16]

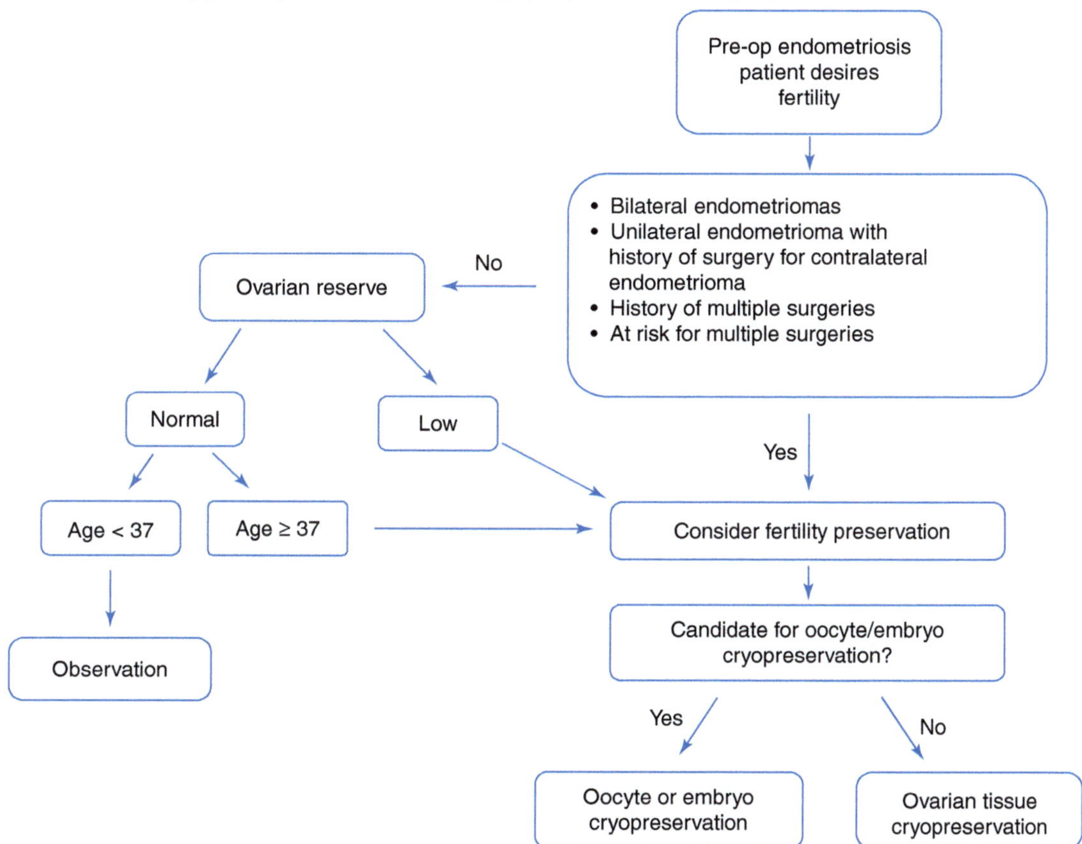

Important anatomical structures should be identified, including uterus, adnexa, ureters, bladder, colon, small bowel, diaphragm, major vessels, and nerves. When surveying these structures, lesions should be identified and ideally documented. Signs of DIE lesions include but are not limited to fibrosis (with or without characteristic dark spots), dense adhesions, distortion of anatomical structures, reduced tissue elasticity, and hemorrhagic cystic structures [19]. An important principle when performing excision of endometriosis is to perform the less complex steps first. Initially, restoration of pelvic anatomy and adhesiolysis are undertaken. This can be performed with a combination of blunt and sharp dissection. With DIE, this process can take more than an hour or two. Restoration of normal anatomy can make subsequent excision easier as it helps to isolate and separate the lesions from nearby structures. Identification and mobilization of the ureter to a safe position are also part of the pre-excision setup. It may be necessary to place accessory port sites to optimize exposure and surgeon positioning. Our laparoscopic setup routinely uses 4–5 trocars, including the port for the camera in the base of the umbilicus. Depending on availability, one or two surgical assistants or trainees may be helpful in obtaining optimal positioning and exposure. Some surgeons prefer a robotic approach, although the benefits of this beyond personal preference have not been established [20].

The most common locations of endometriosis include the ovaries, peritoneum (particularly the broad ligament and cul de sac), and the uterosacral ligaments [2]. Urogenital lesions have been reported to have a prevalence of only 1–2% of those diagnosed with endometriosis, ureteric lesions 0.1–0.4%, and gastrointestinal tract lesions have a prevalence of 5–15% [4]. However more recent studies indicate that the prevalence of urogenital lesions may be much higher [21]. Within the gastrointestinal tract, the most common locations are the rectosigmoid colon, the sigmoid colon, and the rectum, with the ileum, appendix, and cecum being less likely [4, 22]. Although the majority of lesions are superficial, over time some can become transmural.

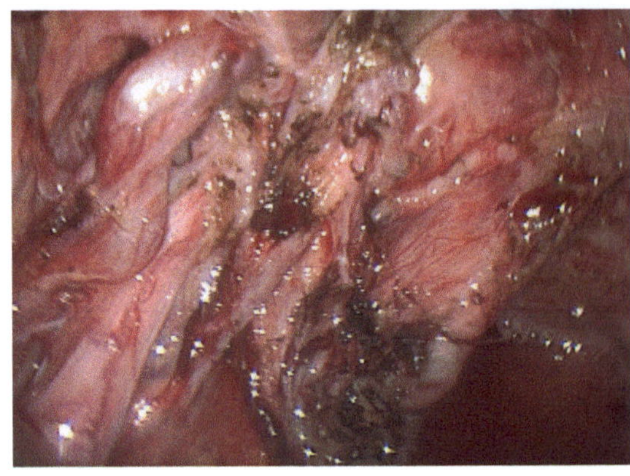

Fig. 20.7 Intraoperative image of pararectal space, showing the uterine artery in relation to the ureter

General Surgical Management

Superficial endometriosis implants that are positioned safely away from underlying structures may be removed via simple excision; however, the full extent of the disease may often be larger than the visible lesion [23]. With ovarian endometriomas that are commonly found with DIE, excision may be performed via a stripping technique, which has been demonstrated to be superior to cyst drainage and ablation in improving spontaneous pregnancy rates 9–12 months postoperatively [24].

Surgical management of DIE and more extensive extragenital endometriotic lesions is often more complex than that of superficial peritoneal disease and endometriomas. DIE may involve risky sites such as the uterosacral ligaments, the rectovaginal septum, the posterior vaginal wall, the bowel, the urinary tract, and the diaphragm.

Rectovaginal Endometriosis

Rectovaginal digital examination should be performed prior to resection in order to assess the extent of the lesion and involvement in surrounding structures. Once in the abdominal cavity for laparoscopic excision, ureterolysis can be performed by making a peritoneal incision between the ipsilateral ureter and the infundibulopelvic ligament; this mobilizes the peritoneum medially away from the ureter. Next the pararectal space should be entered and developed. The boundaries of the pararectal space are classically described

as the hypogastric artery, uterine artery, and the ureter (Fig. 20.7). Our primary approach is to develop this area via peritoneal dissection with ureterolysis, though one can also open the broad ligament from above, which is also known as "the superior approach" [23]. With peritoneal dissection, the rectum can be retracted to the contralateral side with the assistance of a rectal probe or end-to-end anastomosis (EEA) sizer to avoid injury. When the rectum is adhered to the posterior uterus, dissection should start laterally. After identification of major vessels and the ureters, dissection can then be carried toward the midline to open the rectovaginal space.

In addition to mobilizing the rectum away from the area of excision, care should also be taken to avoid the middle rectal vessels and intramesenteric nerve bundles during excision, as the lesion may commonly be in close proximity to the rectal wall and extend all the way to the muscles of the pelvic floor. We routinely perform procto-insufflation after excision of DIE, using a "bubble test" to inject air into the rectum after the pelvis is generously lavaged with irrigation fluid. Absence of bubbles while the bowel lumen above the dissection is compressed with atraumatic graspers ensure there is no leakage. Other techniques such as use of intraoperative procto-sigmoidoscopy may also be helpful to evaluate the integrity of the rectum after excision, particularly if electrosurgical instruments were used [25].

Gastrointestinal Tract Endometriosis

The rectum, as described above, and the sigmoid are the most commonly affected sites of the gastrointestinal tract (76%). Other areas where endometriosis may be found are the appendix (18%), the cecum (5%), and the ileum, jejunum, or other parts of small intestine (3%) [25, 26]. There are various techniques used for excision of gastrointestinal DIE, including shaving, discoid, and segmental resection [27]. Shaving may be employed for lesions involving bowel mesentery, serosa, or superficial muscularis (less than 2–3 mm) [28]. Discoid excision may be performed for single infiltrative lesions with depth more than 5 mm and no more than one-third invasion of the bowel wall [27, 29]. Finally, segmental resection may be performed for lesions larger than 3 cm, multifocal lesions, or when there is narrowing of the lumen [29]. Lesion size can be assessed preoperatively with MRI. Colorectal surgeon colleagues can perform endoscopy as well to determine bowel lumen size. These can be confirmed with an intraoperative survey prior to removal of DIE lesions. These techniques are discussed further below.

Advanced Operative Techniques for Bowel DIE

Choosing the optimal technique involves considering a patient's pain level, the number of nodules, the size of the nodule(s), distance from anal verge, and depth of involvement of the muscularis (Fig. 20.8) [30]. For example, patients with severe pain and involvement of the inner layer of the muscularis or deeper would be good candidates for segmental resection. Furthermore, patients with only involvement of the outer layer of the muscularis but who have multiple nodules causing severe pain may also be good candidates for segmental resection. Shaving technique may

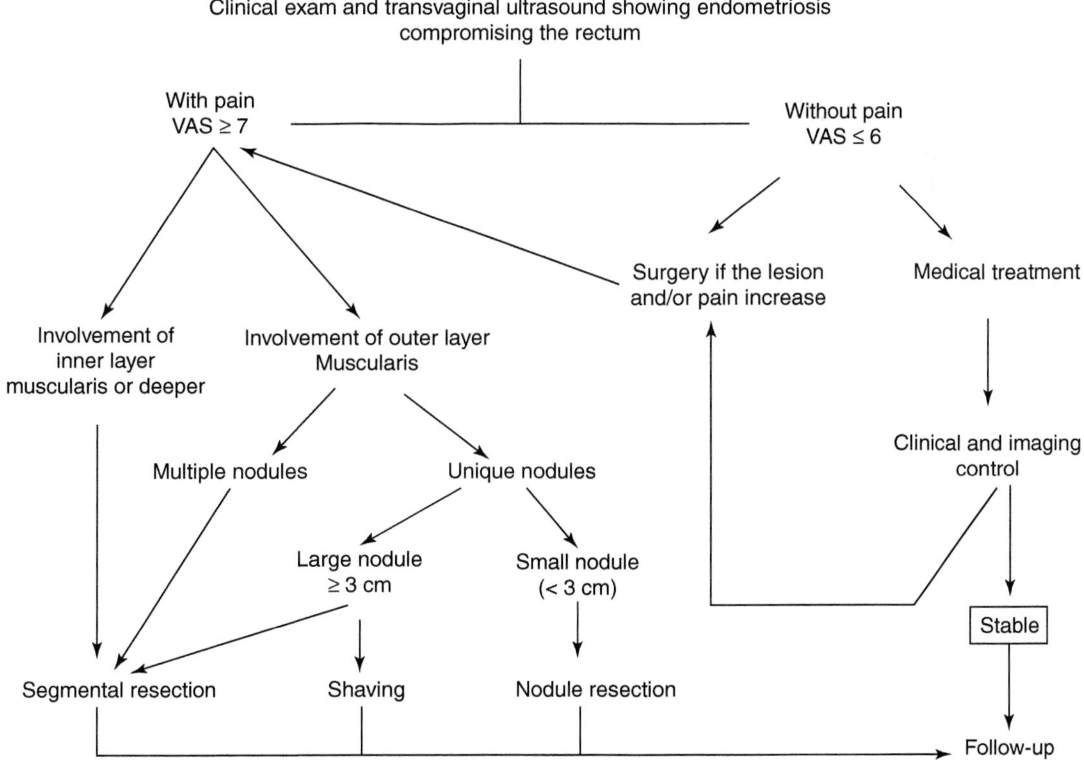

Fig. 20.8 Flow chart of when and how to operate on bowel DIE based on VAS-visual analogic scale. (From Ref. [30])

be best implemented when DIE involvement is only to the outer layer of the muscularis and there is a single large nodule (greater than or equal to 3 cm), though segmental resection may also be considered for large nodules. Discoid resection, where the bowel lumen is entered, can be performed for small singular nodules (less than 3 cm) with involvement only of the outer layer of the muscularis. Shaving and discoid techniques should not be utilized if more than 50–60% of the circumference of the rectum or sigmoid wall is involved [30].

Shaving Technique

For superficial lesions that are not circumferential involving a structure or constricted lumen of bowel, shaving may be used to remove lesions. With this technique, the bowel wall is not opened. It is important to first develop any retroperitoneal spaces in close proximity just as with the resection technique in order to identify the ureters and other structures such as nerves or blood vessels prior to resection [31]. Once that has been accomplished, the next step is to grasp the lesion with grasping forceps and place it on traction. Then, from the proximal to distal end of the lesion, full-thickness shaving is performed with laparoscopic scissors or other common instruments including electrosurgery, harmonic energy, plasma energy, or carbon dioxide laser.

When the bowel is involved, the surgeon should follow the contour of the bowel around the lesion, taking care to identify healthy tissue and completely dissect the lesion off the bowel (Figs. 20.9, 20.10, and 20.11). Several interrupted stitches of 3-0 Vicryl or PDS can be used to reapproximate the muscularis. Electrocautery should generally be avoided when working on the bowel to prevent thermal injury. For those without significant experience in surgical management of DIE, this can be performed in collaboration with general or colorectal surgery. If a small entry into the bowel lumen occurs inadvertently during shaving, the defect may be repaired with several single interrupted stitches of delayed absorbable suture in a plane parallel to the long axis of the bowel to avoid strictures forming. If there is uncertainty regarding entry into the

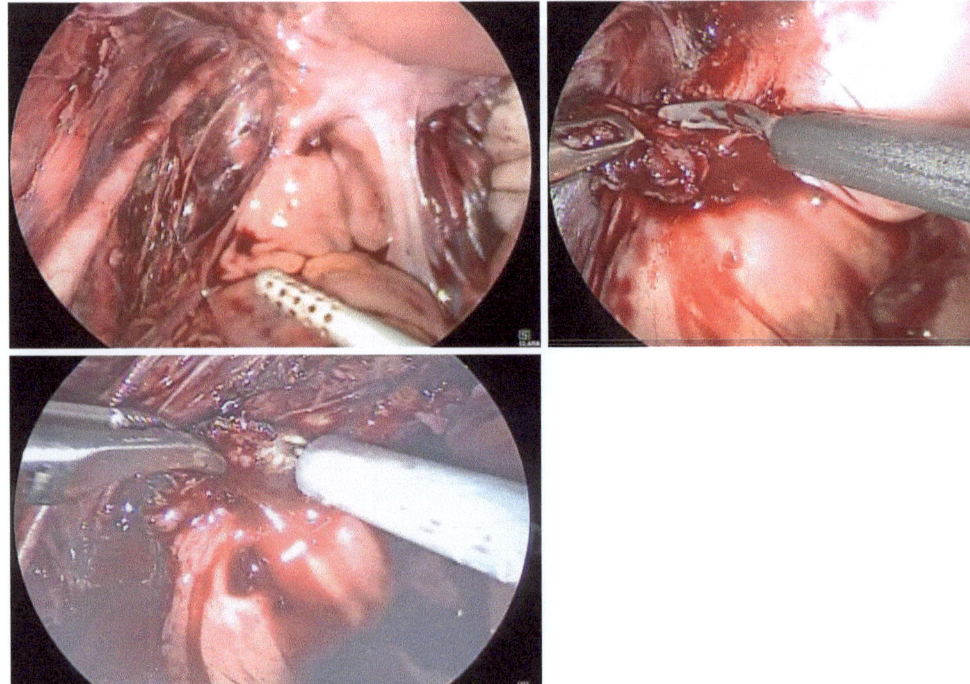

Figs. 20.9, 20.10, and 20.11 Shaving of rectal nodule

lumen, procto-insufflation may be utilized, as previously described.

Discoid Resection

When the anterior wall of the rectum is affected by endometriosis, discoid resection may be performed [32]. This involves resection of the anterior wall of the rectum, and can be accomplished by resection of the nodule followed by closure with either suture repair or stapler repair [28]. Stapler repair can be performed transabdominally with a linear stapler or trans-anally with a circular stapler [33, 34]. In most cases, this technique is performed either solely by general or colorectal surgery colleagues, or in close collaboration with them.

Resection begins as previously described, first with lysis of adhesions, ureterolysis, and development of retroperitoneal and pararectal spaces. Then, the lesion is surrounded by dissecting the lateral and anterior wall of the bowel. The lesion may next be freed from the posterior aspect of the uterus and/or vagina via laparoscopic cutting. In order to more clearly identify areas of excision, stay sutures may be placed bilaterally around the lesion. The lesion is then sharply dissected. Repair may follow as above either via suture or stapler. Again, examination may be performed with air insufflation from the rectum under fluid-emersion to assess for leakage and ensure complete closure.

Segmental Resection

Segmental resection should be considered if there are endometriotic lesions greater than 3 cm, if there are several lesions in close proximity, or if there is narrowing of bowel lumen [35, 36]. When a segment of bowel is excised, end-to-end anastomosis is performed via a circular stapling device. Once again, care should be taken to first isolate the affected area by adhesiolysis, developing spaces, and identifying surrounding structures. Usually when resecting bowel, the sigmoid should be released from the left lateral abdominal wall and the retroperitoneal space opened. The ureter should be dissected on both side walls and freed and laterally displaced to develop the pararectal space (Fig. 20.7). Probes are placed in the

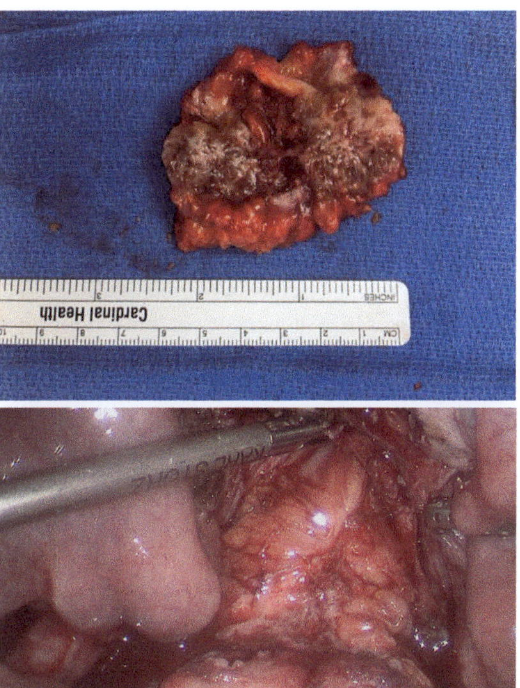

Figs. 20.12 and 20.13 Segmental resection of a bowel nodule

vagina and the rectum to identify the area in which the rectum is fused to the vagina at the level of the cervix. Dissection starts laterally and towards the midline. The recto-vaginal septum below the lesion is dissected. Then the lesion is taken off the vagina and remains on the bowel (Figs. 20.12 and 20.13) [37]. Adequate dissection of the recto-vaginal space below the lesion allows a stapling device to be applied. The diseased portion of bowel is then exteriorized through a mini-laparotomy and subsequently transected just proximally to the diseased area.

At this point, the anvil of the circular stapler is placed inside the stump, followed by placing purse-string suture, and then the bowel is reintroduced into the abdominal cavity. An EEA circular stapler is then introduced through the anus, connected to the anvil, and activated. To decrease the risk of anastomotic leaks, care should be taken with resection of low rectal lesions, defined as less than 5–8 cm from the anal verge [30]. To ensure adequate closure and assess for leaks, a rigid sigmoidoscope may be placed to directly visualize the anastomosis. The pelvis is filled with irrigation fluid, and then while compressing the bowel proximal to the anastomosis, air may be insufflated through the sigmoidoscope to assess for appropriate distention as well as monitor for bubbles of air in the pool of fluid. If there is a stream of bubbles, care must be taken to identify and over sew the area of leakage. Rarely, revision of the anastomosis is indicated.

In cases where a portion of the vagina has been excised along with the rectum, we suggest creating a diverting loop ostomy that can later be reversed after the vagina has been allowed to heal. When the anastomosis is less than 5 cm from the anal verge, a loop is also brought up.

If the appendix is grossly affected by endometriosis, appendectomy may be performed. Given the relatively high incidence rate of microscopic disease of the appendix in DIE patients, it also may be reasonable to routinely perform appendectomy at the time of laparoscopy, but there is no formal guidance on this topic [38]. Dissection is begun by following the tenia of the cecum to the base of the appendix, at which point the mesoappendix is divided, which can be accomplished with electrocautery. The appendiceal artery runs through the mesoappendix, and care should be taken to ensure the artery is adequately sealed and divided in this step. The base of the appendix may then be ligated between endoloops using laparoscopic scissors, or divided with an endoscopic linear cutting stapler. The base of the cecum should be inspected and the appendix should be removed via a sterile endoscopic bag.

The choice for surgical treatment of intestinal endometriosis may be guided by the location, size and depth of the lesion, as well as the surgical expertise of the surgeon and availability for intraoperative consults if indicated. As previously discussed, imaging such as MRI can be of particular value for preoperative planning to avoid urgent intraoperative consults. Surgical excision may be indicated when the small bowel is affected due to the risk of small bowel obstruction. The benefit for surgical resection of gastrointestinal lesions with the goal of improving fertility outcomes appears limited.

Genitourinary Endometriosis

Genitourinary endometriosis most commonly involves the bladder and ureters (25–85% and 15–75% of the cases, respectively), and rarely may involve the kidneys and urethra (5%) [39–42].

Ureteral endometriosis is strongly associated with endometriosis of the uterosacral ligaments, and may be the result of pelvic sidewall endometriotic lesions. The two histologic subtypes of ureteral endometriosis are extrinsic and intrinsic. Extrinsic ureteral endometriosis involves infiltrating endometriosis and inflammatory reactions that lead to ureteral obstruction from the outside and not involving the muscular layer of the ureter. Intrinsic ureteral endometriosis invades the ureter wall and muscular layer with or without reaching the lumen [43]. Either extrinsic or intrinsic ureteral endometriosis may incur hydronephrosis, which could lead to ipsilateral renal dysfunction. If hydronephrosis is identified preoperatively, ureteral stenting is recommended; however, hydronephrosis often goes undetected due to nonspecific complaints [44].

Extrinsic ureteral endometriosis may be managed with ureterolysis and subsequent excision of the surrounding fibrotic tissue. Ureterolysis should be initiated in areas of healthy tissue and progressively advancing toward the affected location. If ureterolysis fails or if an intrinsic ureteral lesion is identified distant to the bladder, segmental resection with end-to-end anastomosis (EEA) may be indicated if possible. Successful anastomosis is dependent upon complete mobilization of the ends, and aided by ureteral stents. Intrinsic lesions within close proximity to the bladder may require resection and reimplantation of the ureter into the bladder via either the psoas hitch technique or a Boari procedure (tubularization of a flap of bladder when the diseased ureteric segment is too long and direct reimplantation is not feasible), depending on surgeon preference. It is beneficial to coordinate with urologic colleagues prior to planned ureterolysis for assistance with difficult resections or possible complications. If ureteral surgery is performed for either intrinsic or extrinsic endometriosis, serial kidney ultrasound should be performed every 6 months to monitor for hydronephrosis [45].

Bladder endometriosis commonly involves the detrusor muscle, but can also involve the mucosa in rare cases [21, 39, 41, 46]. Cystoscopy may be performed to evaluate for bladder endometriosis and ureteral stents may be introduced at that time if indicated. Bladder lesions are typically easily identified on cystoscopy; however, if the round ligaments are pulled medially, the ventral compartment may be obliterated secondary to fibrosis. When a nodule is identified, dissection starts in the healthy peritoneum adjacent to the lesion when possible. It is important to develop the vesico-vaginal space to dissect the dorsal wall of the bladder away from the uterus and the ventral wall of the vagina to fully mobilize the bladder away from surrounding structures, taking care when scar tissue is present particularly with prior history of Cesarean section. Dissection should continue until a soft plane of connective tissue has been reached distal to the lesion. Once the lesion is isolated, it is grasped, the tissue is placed on traction, and the lesion excised with grossly free margins. Closure of the bladder defect is accomplished with running suture of absorbable monofilament material in either a mono- or double-layer fashion, avoiding the mucosa and only including the detrusor muscle. Barbed suture is also acceptable and safe. Upon completion, the bladder may be retrograde filled with normal saline to assess for leakages, which are managed by single interrupted stitches of the same suture.

Resection of larger lesions may be limited when the uterus is involved and must be preserved for fertility. If larger lesions are not involving the uterus and able to safely be resected, in order to allow healing of the defect, a transurethral Foley catheter should remain in place for 8–10 days and a cystogram should be performed prior to removal [19]. With smaller resections and repairs, the catheter may be removed earlier.

Diaphragm Endometriosis

Diaphragmatic endometriosis may be superficial or more deeply infiltrating. With intraabdominal laparoscopy, superficial lesions may be coagulated or ablated with low-energy electrocautery. When laparoscopy is performed in the dorsal lithotomy position, only the ventral part of the diaphragm is able to be visualized. Larger lesions may be associated with diaphragmatic fenestrations and resection can prove complicated, possibly leading to pneumothorax or bloody pleural effusions, thus must be managed by a multidisciplinary team [47].

Postsurgical Considerations

Postsurgical Complications

There are multiple possible complications that should be discussed with patients prior to surgical management of DIE. As such, caution should be taken in young and otherwise healthy women whose primary purpose for surgery is to improve fertility outcomes. Immediately postoperatively, the short-term complications include bleeding, postoperative fever, anastomotic leak, and infection/abscess. Other complications with potentially more long-term sequelae include rectovaginal fistulas, strictures, and effects on ongoing bowel function.

Though every institution and surgeon has different rates of complications, multiple studies have estimated the frequency of rectovaginal fistula to be anywhere from 0% to 14% and the likelihood of abscess/infection 1% to 5% [30, 48]. Studies of patients several years postsurgery have found that segmental bowel resection of DIE is associated with a higher rate of symptoms including abdominal pain or incomplete bowel movements; however, there was no significant increase in constipation or fecal incontinence compared to those who underwent surgery without bowel resection [49]. Furthermore, these patients did not show decreased patient satisfaction and a similar proportion of these patients compared to those who did not undergo bowel resection stated they would elect for the same surgery again. There was no statistical significance between the two groups regarding improved symptoms of dysmenorrhea, non-menstrual pelvic pain, dyschezia, or lower back pain [49]. At the time of surgery, if there is full thickness resection of vaginal implants, concern for bowel injury, or if low segmental bowel resection is necessary for full excision of endometriosis lesions, patients may benefit from an ostomy for diversion during healing of anastomoses.

Postsurgical ART Outcomes

Once a patient has reached a point in their fertility treatment that ART is recommended, the question often arises (for those with known or suspected DIE) whether surgery for DIE should be performed prior to ART for the purpose of improving their chance of success. *In our experience, surgery can be considered in patients with refractory pain, large endometriomas (i.e. greater than 4 cm), or significant and bothersome bowel symptoms.* In the absence of these signs and symptoms, our practice is to reserve DIE surgery for patients with more than one failed implantation of high-quality embryos. This practice pattern arises from the complex and risky nature of surgical excision of DIE, the overall favorable prognosis of patients undertaking IVF and embryo transfer, and the potential to decrease ovarian reserve with endometrioma excision or adhesiolysis that often accompanies DIE surgery. Long-term complications of DIE (especially in the setting of bowel resection) may be especially poorly tolerated in fertility patients who were otherwise previously healthy and without significant pain symptoms.

It is important to note that studies suggest that extensive excision of peritoneal endometriosis lesions does not negatively impact ovarian reserve or function when ovarian disease does not exist; however, if ovarian lesions are removed or if extensive ovariolysis is undertaken, ovarian responses are expected to be poorer, as seen by decrease in AMH levels. However, even in cases with ovarian involvement, overall pregnancy rates are higher in those who underwent surgery versus those who did not [50]. For patients with recurrence of a large endometrioma who intend to undergo IVF, repeat surgeries would not be recommended given the anticipated continued decrease in AMH levels. However, aspiration of endometriomas is a minimally invasive alternative approach that would improve oocyte retrieval and ovarian response compared to expectant management [51].

Pregnancies via IVF have been shown to occur anywhere from 3 to 18 months postoperatively, suggesting that the benefits of surgery on fertility outcomes begin shortly after surgery and persist for an extensive period of time [50]. While there is benefit to waiting for patients to heal postoperatively and to ensure no surgical complications arise prior to beginning ART protocols, there is debate as to how long a woman should wait postoperatively prior to undergoing ART. Some studies have shown that no difference occurs in fertility outcomes when ART is pursued either less than or greater than 6 months after surgery [50, 52]. However, other studies note that the immediate postoperative period (less than 6 months after surgery) is significantly more favorable for conception, particularly for women with more advanced disease [53]. The theory is that since endometriosis is a progressive disease, time can have a detrimental effect on fertility if there is disease recurrence or incomplete excision of disease. Based on this, our practice has been to perform ART 1–2 months after DIE surgery and recovery.

Conclusion

DIE lesions are most often found in the pelvic cavity, either in the anterior compartment or more commonly in the posterior compartment involving the posterior vagina, rectum, uterosacral ligaments, and ureters. Many women experience chronic pelvic pain and genitourinary or gastrointestinal symptoms. However, symptoms are not required for the diagnosis of DIE. In patients who do report symptoms, DIE lesion location correlates well with the severity of patient discomfort and pain. Though DIE can be treated medically with hormonal suppression, this is not definitive management and should not be used in patients who desire pregnancy. Hormonal suppression both acts as a contraceptive and has not shown an increase in pregnancy rates when used prior to ART. Surgery can be utilized to stage the severity of disease and definitively diagnose the disease via pathology.

Prior to surgery, imaging (ultrasound, MRI) can be of high value for preoperative assessment and surgical mapping. In particular, it can be determined if bowel or bladder resection is needed and preoperative consultations can be performed with other surgical specialty colleagues. Choice of imaging modality can be institution-dependent, based on the experience and comfort level of sonographers/technicians and radiographic interpreters.

Surgically, it is important to take a systematic approach to the pelvis so as to not miss any lesions. First, all important structures are identified, including the uterus, adnexa, ureters, bladder, colon, small bowel, diaphragm, and major vessels and nerves. Lesions are most commonly located on the ovaries, peritoneum (particularly the broad ligament and cul de sac), and the uterosacral ligaments. After identifying and documenting DIE lesions, removal of lesions may be performed via shaving, discoid resection, or segmental resection depending on the size, depth of invasion, and number of nodules.

Postoperatively, short-term complications include bleeding and infection while long-term complications include fistula, strictures, leakage of anastomosis, and changes in bowel function. It is recommended that patients begin ART soon after surgery, as early as 1–2 months postoperatively. Both rates of spontaneous conception and success rates of ART have been shown to be increased after surgical excision of DIE; however, routine excision of suspected DIE is not recommended given the complex and invasive nature of DIE excision and the overall favorable pregnancy rates achieved via IVF in this population.

Pain symptoms in patients with endometriosis have a recurrence risk of up to 50% at 5 years postoperatively [10]. This is most likely due to incomplete excision of endometriosis given the technical challenges that require surgical expertise. Some studies show that patients with complete excision of DIE lesions have a recurrence rate of only 2% at 5 years postoperatively [22].

There is a role for medical management (hormonal therapy) after a patient has completed child-bearing in order to suppress symptoms and decrease the likelihood of repeat surgeries.

Overall, surgical management of DIE is reasonable to consider in patients who have failed more than one implantation of high-quality embryos or who have significant symptoms including chronic pelvic pain, large ovarian cysts, and/or bowel symptoms. This chapter reviewed the diagnosis and clinical picture of DIE as well as best operative approaches to fully excise DIE lesions in patients seeking improved fertility outcomes.

References

1. Parasar P, Ozcan P, Terry KL. Endometriosis: epidemiology, diagnosis and clinical management. Curr Obstet Gynecol Rep. 2017;6:34–41.
2. Falcone T, Flyckt R. Clinical management of endometriosis. Obstet Gynecol. 2018;131:557–71.
3. Tosti C, Pinzauti S, Santulli P, Chapron C, Petraglia F. Pathogenetic mechanisms of deep infiltrating endometriosis. Reprod Sci. 2015;22:1053–9.
4. Lindheim SR, Glenn T, Gagneux P, Maxwell RA, Jl Y, Findley AD, Bhagavath B. Current challenges in the diagnosis of deep infiltrating endometriosis. Androl Gynecol Curr Res. 2018; https://doi.org/10.4172/2327-4360.1000162.
5. Bulun SE, Yang S, Fang Z, Gurates B, Tamura M, Zhou J, Sebastian S. Role of aromatase in endometrial disease. J Steroid Biochem Mol Biol. 2001;79(1–5):19–25. https://doi.org/10.1016/s0960-0760(01)00134-0.
6. Chapron C. Deep infiltrating endometriosis: relation between severity of dysmenorrhoea and extent of disease. Hum Reprod. 2003;18:760–6.
7. Kitajima M, Dolmans M-M, Donnez O, Masuzaki H, Soares M, Donnez J. Enhanced follicular recruitment and atresia in cortex derived from ovaries with endometriomas. Fertil Steril. 2014;101:1031–7.
8. Ballester M, Oppenheimer A, Mathieu d'Argent E, Touboul C, Antoine J-M, Nisolle M, Daraï E. Deep infiltrating endometriosis is a determinant factor of cumulative pregnancy rate after intracytoplasmic sperm injection/in vitro fertilization cycles in patients with endometriomas. Fertil Steril. 2012;97:367–72.
9. Practice bulletin no. 114: management of endometriosis. Obstet Gynecol. 2010;116:223–36.
10. Guo S-W. Recurrence of endometriosis and its control. Hum Reprod Update. 2009;15:441–61.
11. Guerriero S, Condous G, van den Bosch T, et al. Systematic approach to sonographic evaluation of

the pelvis in women with suspected endometriosis, including terms, definitions and measurements: a consensus opinion from the International Deep Endometriosis Analysis (IDEA) group. Ultrasound Obstet Gynecol. 2016;48:318–32.

12. Abrao MS, Gonçalves MO d C, Dias JA, Podgaec S, Chamie LP, Blasbalg R. Comparison between clinical examination, transvaginal sonography and magnetic resonance imaging for the diagnosis of deep endometriosis. Hum Reprod. 2007;22:3092–7.

13. Bazot M, Malzy P, Cortez A, Roseau G, Amouyal P, Daraï E. Accuracy of transvaginal sonography and rectal endoscopic sonography in the diagnosis of deep infiltrating endometriosis. Ultrasound Obstet Gynecol. 2007;30:994–1001.

14. Bazot M, Bornier C, Dubernard G, Roseau G, Cortez A, Daraï E. Accuracy of magnetic resonance imaging and rectal endoscopic sonography for the prediction of location of deep pelvic endometriosis. Hum Reprod. 2007;22:1457–63.

15. Adamson GD, Kennedy S, Hummelshoj L. Creating solutions in endometriosis: global collaboration through the world endometriosis research foundation. J Endometr. 2010;2:3–6.

16. Llarena NC, et al. Fertility preservation in women with endometriosis. Clin Med Insights Reprod Health. 2019;13:1179558119873386. https://doi.org/10.1177/1179558119873386.

17. Dunselman GAJ, Vermeulen N, Becker C, et al. ESHRE guideline: management of women with endometriosis. Hum Reprod. 2014;29:400–12.

18. Working group of ESGE, ESHRE, and WES, Saridogan E, Becker CM, et al. Recommendations for the surgical treatment of endometriosis—part 1: ovarian endometrioma. Gynecol Surg. 2017;14:27.

19. Working group of ESGE, ESHRE, and WES, Keckstein J, Becker CM, et al. Recommendations for the surgical treatment of endometriosis. Part 2: deep endometriosis †‡¶. Facts Views Vis Obgyn. 2020;11(4):269–97.

20. Hickman LC, Kotlyar A, Luu TH, Falcone T. Do we need a robot in endometriosis surgery? Minerva Ginecol. 2016;68(3):380–7. Epub 2015 Dec 11. PMID: 26658115.

21. Knabben L, Imboden S, Fellmann B, Nirgianakis K, Kuhn A, Mueller MD. Urinary tract endometriosis in patients with deep infiltrating endometriosis: prevalence, symptoms, management, and proposal for a new clinical classification. Fertil Steril. 2015;103:147–52.

22. Dousset B, Leconte M, Borghese B, Millischer A-E, Roseau G, Arkwright S, Chapron C. Complete surgery for low rectal endometriosis: long-term results of a 100-case prospective study. Ann Surg. 2010;251:887–95.

23. Morozov V, Lakhi N, Nezhat C. Chapter 9: Laparoscopic surgery for the management of endometriosis. Reproductive surgery. Cambridge University Press, Cambridge, UK; 2018.

24. Brown J, Farquhar C. Endometriosis: an overview of Cochrane reviews. Cochrane Database Syst Rev. 2014; https://doi.org/10.1002/14651858.CD009590.pub2.

25. Nezhat C, Pennington E, Nezhat F, Silfen SL. Laparoscopically assisted anterior rectal wall resection and reanastomosis for deeply infiltrating endometriosis. Surg Laparosc Endosc Percutan Tech. 1991;1:106–8.

26. Nezhat F, Nezhat C, Pennington E. Laparoscopic proctectomy for infiltrating endometriosis of the rectum. Fertil Steril. 1992;57:1129–32.

27. Nezhat F, Nezhat C, Pennington E, Ambroze W. Laparoscopic segmental resection for infiltrating endometriosis of the rectosigmoid colon: a preliminary report. Surg Laparosc Endosc. 1992;2:212–6.

28. Messori P, Faller E, Albornoz J, Leroy J, Wattiez A. Laparoscopic sigmoidectomy for endometriosis with transanal specimen extraction. J Minim Invasive Gynecol. 2013;20:412.

29. Nezhat C, Nezhat F, Pennington E. Laparoscopic treatment of infiltrative rectosigmoid colon and rectovaginal septum endometriosis by the technique of videolaparoscopy and the CO2 laser. Br J Obstet Gynaecol . 1992;99:664–7.

30. Abrao MS, Petraglia F, Falcone T, Keckstein J, Osuga Y, Chapron C. Deep endometriosis infiltrating the recto-sigmoid: critical factors to consider before management. Hum Reprod Update. 2015;21:329–39.

31. Gingold JA, Falcone T. The retroperitoneal approach to endometriosis. J Minim Invasive Gynecol. 2017;24(6):896. www.jmig.org. https://doi.org/10.1016/j.jmig.2017.02.019.

32. Malzoni M, et al. Laparoscopic technique for discoid resection of rectal endometriotic nodules. J Minim Invasive Gynecol. 2021;28(1):16–7. www.jmig.org. https://doi.org/10.1016/j.jmig.2020.05.016.

33. Faller E, Albornoz J, Messori P, Leroy J, Wattiez A. A new technique of laparoscopic intracorporeal anastomosis for transrectal bowel resection with transvaginal specimen extraction. J Minim Invasive Gynecol. 2013;20:333.

34. de Almeida A, Fernandes LF, Averbach M, Abrão MS. Disc resection is the first option in the management of rectal endometriosis for unifocal lesions with less than 3 centimeters of longitudinal diameter. Surg Technol Int. 2014;24:243–8.

35. Haggag H, Solomayer E, Juhasz-Böss I. The treatment of rectal endometriosis and the role of laparoscopic surgery. Curr Opin Obstet Gynecol. 2011;23:278–82.

36. Jatan AK, Solomon MJ, Young J, Cooper M, Pathma-Nathan N. Laparoscopic management of rectal endometriosis. Dis Colon Rectum. 2006;49:169–74.

37. Malzoni M, et al. Surgical principles of segmental rectosigmoid resection and reanastomosis for deep infiltrating endometriosis. J Minim Invasive Gynecol. 2020;27(2):258. www.jmig.org. https://doi.org/10.1016/j.jmig.2019.06.018.

38. Ribeiro DM, Ribeiro GP, Santos TP, Chamie L, Cretella CM, Serafini P. Incidental appendectomy in the surgical treatment of deep endometriosis infiltrating the bowel: anatomopathological findings in a series of 109 patients. J Minim Invasive Gynecol. 2015;22:S30–1.
39. Acker O, Robert Y, Carpentier F, Vinatier D, Cosson M. [Symptomatic bladder or ureteral endometriosis: report of 8 cases and review of the literature]. Ann Chir. 2003;128:34–9.
40. Carmignani L, Ronchetti A, Amicarelli F, Vercellini P, Spinelli M, Fedele L. Bladder psoas hitch in hydronephrosis due to pelvic endometriosis: outcome of urodynamic parameters. Fertil Steril. 2009;92:35–40.
41. Fadhlaoui A, Gillon T, Lebbi I, Bouquet de Jolinière J, Feki A. Endometriosis and vesico-sphincteral disorders. Front Surg. 2015; https://doi.org/10.3389/fsurg.2015.00023.
42. Badri AV, Jennings R, Patel P, Eun DD. Renal endometriosis: the case of an endometrial implant mimicking a renal mass. J Endourol Case Rep. 2018;4:176–8.
43. Lakhi N, Dun EC, Nezhat CH. Hematoureter due to endometriosis. Fertil Steril. 2014;101:e37.
44. Miranda-Mendoza I, Kovoor E, Nassif J, Ferreira H, Wattiez A. Laparoscopic surgery for severe ureteric endometriosis. Eur J Obstet Gynecol Reprod Biol. 2012;165:275–9.
45. Ulrich U, Buchweitz O, Greb R, et al. National German Guideline (S2k): guideline for the diagnosis and treatment of endometriosis. Geburtshilfe Frauenheilkd. 2014;74:1104–18.
46. Le Tohic A, Chis C, Yazbeck C, Koskas M, Madelenat P, Panel P. [Bladder endometriosis: diagnosis and treatment. A series of 24 patients]. Gynecol Obstet Fertil. 2009;37:216–21.
47. Roman H, Chanavaz-Lacheray I, Scotté M, Marpeau L. Laparoscopic management of diaphragm endometriosis. J Minim Invasive Gynecol. 2008;15:151S.
48. Roman H, FRIENDS group (French coloRectal Infiltrating ENDometriosis Study group). A national snapshot of the surgical management of deep infiltrating endometriosis of the rectum and colon in France in 2015: a multicenter series of 1135 cases. J Gynecol Obstet Hum Reprod. 2017;46:159–65.
49. Soto E, Catenacci M, Bedient C, Jelovsek JE, Falcone T. Assessment of long-term bowel symptoms after segmental resection of deeply infiltrating endometriosis: a matched cohort study. J Minim Invasive Gynecol. 2016;23:753–9.
50. Bianchi PHM, Pereira RMA, Zanatta A, Alegretti JR, Motta ELA, Serafini PC. Extensive excision of deep infiltrative endometriosis before in vitro fertilization significantly improves pregnancy rates. J Minim Invasive Gynecol. 2009;16:174–80.
51. Petrozza JC. Transvaginal ethanol sclerosis versus saline aspiration of endometriomas prior to IVF: a randomized controlled trial. Obstet Gynecol Int J. 2018. (Crossref).;9(1) https://doi.org/10.15406/ogij.2018.09.00293.
52. Surrey ES, Schoolcraft WB. Does surgical management of endometriosis within 6 months of an in vitro fertilization–embryo transfer cycle improve outcome? J Assist Reprod Genet. 2003;20:365–70.
53. Coccia ME, Rizzello F, Cammilli F, Bracco GL, Scarselli G. Endometriosis and infertility surgery and ART: an integrated approach for successful management. Eur J Obstet Gynecol Reprod Biol. 2008;138:54–9.

Crisis Management in the Office Setting

21

Robert A. Roman, Carey Camille Roberts, Rachel Booth, and Steven R. Lindheim

Introduction

Surgical training is often focused on the development of surgical skills that prevent complications from occurring and are reinforced in the operating room daily. For many surgeons, managing a crisis is often out of their comfort zone – with strategies based on anecdotal experience from personally managing an intraoperative complication or from seeing mentors manage a crisis in the past [1]. This process is often passive, random, and can lead to inconsistent learning experiences across trainees. Lack of training is further compounded by the shift of certain hospital-based procedures to the office setting, where the same providers are expected to deliver the same high-quality and safe patient care with less available resources than are available in the inpatient setting.

Reproductive surgery remains an indispensable treatment to restore normal anatomy to the uterus, ovaries, and/or fallopian tubes to facilitate conception. While reproductive surgery has been primarily performed in a hospital setting, diagnostic and operative hysteroscopic procedures have expanded into the realm of office-based procedures. The American College of Obstetricians and Gynecologists (ACOG) defines an office procedure as a short interventional technique involving non-incisional diagnostic/therapeutic procedures including excisional intervention [2]. With advances in hysteroscopic technology, this has further facilitated its transition to the office setting. This has included intrauterine device removals, polypectomy, myomectomy, lysis of adhesions, septoplasty, and proximal tubal cannulation [3]. This shift towards office-based procedures has been well documented within the past two decades, with at least 10–12% of hysteroscopies being performed in the outpatient setting [4–6]. This continues to enhance patient satisfaction and provide improved continuity of care, higher reimbursements, convenient office scheduling, and avoidance of general anesthesia.

In the United States (US), outpatient surgeries are regulated by the Joint Commission

R. A. Roman (✉)
Medical College of Georgia at Augusta University, Section of Reproductive Endocrinology, Infertility, and Genetics, Augusta, GA, USA
e-mail: rroman@augusta.edu

C. C. Roberts
Weill Cornell Medicine, Department of Anesthesiology, New York, NY, USA

R. Booth
Wright State University Boonshoft School of Medicine, Dayton, OH, USA
e-mail: Rachel.booth@wright.edu

S. R. Lindheim
Wright State University Boonshoft School of Medicine, Dayton, OH, USA

Center for Reproductive Medicine, Ren Ji Hospital, School of Medicine, Shanghai Jiao Tong University, Shanghai, People's Republic of China
e-mail: lindheim@wright.edu

© The Author(s), under exclusive license to Springer Nature Switzerland AG 2022
S. R. Lindheim, J. C. Petrozza (eds.), *Reproductive Surgery*,
https://doi.org/10.1007/978-3-031-05240-8_21

guidelines, though there is no equivalent organization for office procedures. ACOG released a Task Force emphasizing the lack of office patient safety guidelines and provides guidance for gynecologists to improve patient safety measures, mainly in part due to lack of standardization across gynecologists performing office-based procedures and for maintaining safe office practices [7]. Furthermore, despite the increase in office-based procedures, there remains an overall lack of training where residency training programs' surgical volume largely resides in the inpatient setting. Surprisingly, 97% of US medical residents and fellows graduate without performing gynecologic procedures in the office setting and even less likely to be equipped to effectively manage emergent complications [8].

With smaller instruments and increasing comfort, surgeons continue to push the boundaries for the types of procedures that are performed in the office setting, including patients with higher American Society of Anesthesiologists (ASA) Physical Status classification and subsequently higher perioperative risk. Even with the most meticulous patient selection criteria, patients can still present with challenging airways, difficulty achieving adequate sedation or pain control, or even vasovagal reactions during office procedures [9]. Fortunately, procedural complications are rare, with the most frequent hysteroscopic complication (uterine perforation) occurring in 0.76% of cases [9]. However, since providers will need to manage the unexpected, a paradigm shift is necessary in the event of a crisis. This chapter seeks to provide guidance, algorithms, and examples to aid in preparation for a crisis in reproductive surgery. We will take readers through three specific crises using the reported STOP (*Stop, Think, Observe, Plan*) framework to effectively manage such scenarios [10, 11].

Crisis Management

A crisis is a catastrophic event that is characterized by an element of surprise, a short decision time, and a perceived threat to the patient [12].

These events can lead to significant morbidity and mortality, though, fortunately, many can be averted and mitigated. The steps taken to deal with catastrophic events before, during, and after they occur is referred to as Crisis Management (CM) [12]. CM principles were initially developed in the business and aviation industry as a reaction to the large-scale industrial and environmental disasters in the 1980s [13]. These principles have become increasingly relevant in the surgical setting, allowing for the development of strategies that better equip physicians with the skills to manage a complication and its potential adverse outcomes. How one handles a crisis will often determine the patient's ultimate outcome. Four components of CM can improve overall results: understanding and managing human behavior, team leadership, simulation training, and panic control [14].

Understanding and Managing Human Behavior During a Crisis

Given that humans react unpredictably and differently in a crisis, appreciating the human element is critical in any surgical team's CM approach given its disorienting nature. When faced with a crisis, surgeons will naturally activate their hypothalamic-pituitary-adrenal axis which leads to several physiologic and behavioral changes in response to stress. Traditionally known as the "fight-or-flight" response, sympathetic activation leads to acute cortisol, epinephrine, and norepinephrine release and has many physiologic functions including increased heart rate, increased blood pressure, increased respiratory rate, increased muscle strength, and increased mental activity [15]. The goal of the fight-or-flight response is to first ensure one's own personal safety then secondarily followed by the safety of others. Providers should be cognizant of this initial stress response, reassure themselves that they are indeed personally safe, and then focus on how to take care of their patient in a crisis. While sympathetic activation is meant to be productive, this response can also lead to maladaptive behaviors in a crisis including decreased recall of short-term memory, frustration, or panic which can decrease efficiency in CM [15].

Human behavior was previously thought to be personal, with mistakes being attributed to poor physician training or insight. Modern approaches to address human behavior by approaching it from a systems-based perspective minimize personal blame while prioritizing patient safety [16]. System-based changes began to include things such as alarms, checklists, or safety triggers, while protective measures attempted to curtail the error from continuing once it happened, which will be detailed under simulation training [17].

Team Leadership

Physicians are often seen as the team leader in the moment of a crisis. However, when a crisis occurs, most physicians have little experience in CM, managing themselves as well as their surgical teams through a crisis. This is seen even in those with the longest of medical careers.

Interestingly, surgeons often regard their own ability to lead their surgical team with higher confidence than their nursing colleagues. In a study by Makary et al., surgeons rated that 85% of other surgeon colleagues have "high" or "very high" surgical teamwork. In contrast, nurses rated their collaboration with surgeons "high" or "very high" only 48% of the time [18]. Team leadership is essential to effectively communicate, define roles, and assign tasks for health care team members during a crisis.

Applying experience from cardiac arrest resuscitation "codes," ideal team leaders are individuals that can keep the health care team organized, clearly define team member roles, utilize both verbal and nonverbal communication, use closed-loop communication, and have situational awareness [19, 20]. Closed-loop communication should involve the sender giving a message and the receiver repeating this back to avoid any misunderstandings during a crisis. The role of team leader should be decided in advance so that the health care team can be organized promptly, and resuscitative measures be initiated effectively.

Simulation Training

Few studies have explored the impact of simulation and CM, though there is data to suggest it positively impacts a physician's future behavior during a crisis and improves patient outcomes [21]. Previous exposure, even in the simulation setting, allows providers to be "proactive instead of reactive" when crises arise. The efficacy of simulation training in medical education relies on active preparation, design of clinical scenarios with differing levels of difficulty, as well as debriefing after the session and providing feedback.

Health care teams should implement procedure drills on a regular basis with the entire health care team (including physicians, nursing staff, assistants, anesthesia) to discuss pre-, intra-, and postoperative considerations to prevent unanticipated events from leading to an adverse event, assigning each team member with specific tasks to perform and message repetition to improve communication during a crisis [2, 22].

ACOG has recommended several practice guidelines that should be incorporated into the office setting prior to performing office procedures. These include written guidelines that should be established with periodic staff training on policies and procedures associated with CM [2]. Policies should be developed detailing who will be checking equipment functioning and managing medication inventory and at what intervals they will be performed. A designated person should confirm that practicing physicians have continued proficiency in performing office-based procedures. At least one other provider, in addition to the operating physician, should be certified in basic life support (BLS) to assist the primary surgeon as needed [2]. From a systems perspective, practices can also preemptively develop protocols for hospital transfer and a good relationship with a nearby admitting hospital [2].

Furthermore, ACOG specifically recommends that checklists be developed for the management of a clinical scenario that applies to most patients (i.e., checklist for management of uterine perforation) and that physicians should clearly document that they followed the protocol and the reasoning behind any deviations [17]. Physicians should work closely with their office staff including nurses and other staff members to develop and update protocols as necessary.

Panic Control

Finally, the most important concept in CM is panic control—as it is the one factor that providers can directly influence and control during a crisis. Given the rarity of these events, it has been reported that at most 10–20% of providers remain calm when faced with a crisis [23]. A STOP framework (*Stop, Think, Observe, Plan*) was developed to illustrate a mental checklist that providers could refer to during a crisis [10, 11].

After recognizing a crisis, providers should first *stop* to transition their mindset from autopilot to manual gear. By interrupting all activity, the provider mitigates the immediate, but avoidable sympathetic response that can lead to panic [10]. Providers should use this time to assess the patient's stability and check their airway, breathing, and circulation (ABC). Next, they should concomitantly *think* through the differential diagnosis and *observe* findings that can help narrow their differential diagnosis to form a *plan* of management. We apply the "panic control" STOP (*Stop, Think, Observe, Plan*) mental framework to different clinical scenarios to highlight the application of it to enhance physician preparation for handling potentially life-threatening emergencies. To aid in the application of crisis management to reproductive surgery, three potential sentinel scenarios outlining its application are discussed.

Patient Case [1]

1. *History*:

A 33-year-old nulligravid female with unexplained infertility was diagnosed with an endometrial polyp and was scheduled for office hysteroscopy prior to proceeding with in vitro fertilization (IVF). She received ibuprofen and diazepam preoperatively and is comfortable with minimal anxiety. A speculum was placed, followed by the administration of paracervical block using a total of 10 mL of lidocaine without epinephrine. Next, a 5 mm operative hysteroscope was placed through the cervix with some degree of difficulty. After entry into the uterine cavity, a fundal broad-based polyp was identified. During the resection with a morcellating blade, the sedated patient began to move on the table. The surgeon pulled the hysteroscope back and visualized a midline uterine perforation.

2. *Risk Factors*:

Uterine perforation most commonly occurs using blunt devices such as a suction cannula (51.3% cases) or Hegar dilator (24.4%) but can also occur with sharp instrumentation such as an endometrial curette (16.2%) [24]. Uterine perforation can occur anteriorly (40%), in the cervical canal (36%), laterally (38%), posteriorly (13%), or at the fundus (13%) [25]. Risk factors for uterine perforation include cervical stenosis, Asherman syndrome, Mullerian anomalies, uterine fibroids, acutely anteflexed/retroflexed uterus, postmenopausal status, parous uterus, retained products of conception, and previous uterine surgery. Providers should triage patients for the office or inpatient setting based on these risk factors to mitigate the risk for potential uterine perforation and its sequelae.

3. *Management*:

The provider should apply the STOP mnemonic.

Stop: The polypectomy should be immediately terminated.

Think: Signs of uterine perforation include loss of resistance during uterine instrumentation, difficulty with visualization during hysteroscopy due to increased bleeding or difficulty distending the uterine cavity, large fluid deficit, visualization of abdominal contents including bowel or omentum inside the uterine cavity. At the time of a suspected uterine perforation, the provider should call for assistance.

Observe: Assess the patient's airway, breathing, and circulation. Next, attempt to identify the location of uterine perforation (midline, anterior, posterior, or lateral). In lateral perforations, uterine vessels may be injured, resulting in broad ligament hematoma or hemodynamic instability secondary to acute blood loss anemia [26]. If the patient is hemodynamically unstable, has excessive vaginal bleeding, or abdominal pain, transferring to an inpatient setting should immediately be considered.

Plan: If the patient is hemodynamically stable, further assessment of the perforation should be performed to decide if management in an inpatient setting is warranted. If a fundal perforation occurred with blunt instrumentation, the risk of intraabdominal injury is low, and the patient may be observed in the office and managed as an outpatient. This includes strict precautions to notify their physician with the development of severe abdominal pain, abdominal distension, heavy vaginal bleeding, hematuria, or fever [26]. Anterior uterine perforation has a higher risk of bladder perforation, especially in patients with multiple prior cesarean deliveries, and a cystoscopy may be warranted to rule out bladder injury. If the patient is at low risk for complications due to the location of uterine perforation with no active bleeding, monitoring as an outpatient can be considered.

Perforations that occur at the level of the cervix or laterally have a higher likelihood of injury to the broad ligament and uterine vessels. These patients can present with broad ligament hematoma or intraabdominal hemorrhage and should be transferred to an inpatient setting for urgent laparoscopic evaluation. Uterine perforation after sharp instrumentation or energy devices presents a higher risk of bowel or bladder injury and diagnostic laparoscopy should be considered [26].

In patients with any possible bowel or bladder injury, excessive uterine or vaginal bleeding, or broad ligament hematoma, transfer and observation as an inpatient is the most conservative approach. If a large fluid deficit has been identified, physicians should evalu-ate for possible fluid overload and pulmonary edema.

4. *Prevention*:

Patient selection for the office setting should be based on patient risk factors for uterine perforation. Patients with cervical stenosis or extensive intrauterine pathology such as large, International Federation of Gynecology and Obstetrics (FIGO) type 0–2 leiomyomas, Mullerian anomalies, or Asherman syndrome should only be done in office by the most experienced hands and strongly considered for the hospital setting due to prolonged duration of the procedure and the possible need for energy devices [5].

Patient Case [2]

1. *History*:

A 30-year-old G2P0020 female with a history of Asherman syndrome status post hysteroscopic lysis of adhesions presented for a second-look diagnostic office hysteroscopy. The patient arrived 20 min prior to her procedure where she was consented, received ibuprofen orally, and underwent a paracervical block with 8 mL of 1% lidocaine. Shortly thereafter, she complained of circumoral paresthesia, a metallic taste, and then quickly became disoriented.

2. *Presentation*:

Local anesthetic systemic toxicity (LAST) is a complication of regional or neuraxial anesthesia. It occurs when local anesthetic is either absorbed or injected intravenously causing neurological or cardiovascular symptoms.

The severity of LAST is determined by multiple factors including the type and dosage of local anesthetic given and the degree of tissue absorption. Tissues with greater perfusion or injections near blood vessels have higher rates of local anesthetic systemic absorption [27]. For example, a paracervical block is more likely to have systemic absorption than a neuraxial block under a spinal or epidural.

Table 21.1 Maximum doses of local anesthetics. For reference, 1% lidocaine has 10 mg/mL and 2% has 20 mg/mL. To calculate the correct dosage, the provider should decide on the percentage of lidocaine dosage used and the total number of mL used to determine total dose administered [29]

Local anesthetic	Maximum dose without epinephrine (mg/kg)	Maximum dose with epinephrine (mg/kg)
Lidocaine	5	7
Bupivicaine	2.5	3
Mepivicaine	7	8

The type of local anesthetic can also influence the timing and nature of the initial symptoms. Lidocaine is more likely to initially present with neurologic symptoms such as tinnitus, dizziness, and seizures followed by more severe cardiovascular symptoms. In contrast, bupivacaine is a longer-acting local anesthetic that presents first with cardiovascular collapse, making an early diagnosis of LAST more difficult [28].

Table 21.1 illustrates maximum doses of local anesthetic with and without epinephrine. For example, lidocaine 2% contains 20 mg/mL lidocaine. Thus, for a 60 kg patient, the maximum dose of lidocaine 2% without epinephrine is 15 mL and lidocaine 2% with epinephrine is 21 mL.

3. *Treatment*:

   The provider should apply the STOP mnemonic.

   Stop: Immediate management is to stop the injection of local anesthetic and call for help.

   Think: In patients with LAST, early neurologic manifestations present as agitation, dizziness, circumoral numbness, metallic taste, tinnitus, muscle fasciculations, and paresthesias. With worsening toxicity, central nervous system depression can occur, and patients can present with coma and tonic-clonic seizures. Signs of cardiovascular involvement may present initially with hypertension and tachycardia followed by hypotension and conduction defects evident with bradycardia, arrhythmias, and EKG changes, and eventually cardiac arrest.

Observe: In this scenario, signs of worsening neurologic depression should alert the provider that the patient may have difficulty maintaining her airway. The following steps need to occur simultaneously to provide the best patient care in the setting of LAST.

Plan: Secure the patient's airway and ventilate with 100% oxygen. The rapid deterioration of patient consciousness compromises the respiratory system leading to apnea, hypercarbia, and hypoxia.

To prevent seizures, administer an antiepileptic such as a benzodiazepine (consider midazolam 2 mg IV if immediately available). Literature suggests a small dose of propofol may be used; however, it will worsen cardiovascular collapse in patients with cardiovascular instability. A 20% lipid emulsion (Intralipid ®) bolus of 1.5 mL/kg over 1 min should be administered followed by an infusion of 0.25 ml/kg/min. If the patient remains hypotensive or hemodynamically unstable, a bolus dose may be repeated twice more as well as doubling the infusion rate. Continue infusion for 10 min after achieving cardiovascular stability. Maximum recommended dose of lipid emulsion is 12 ml/kg.

In treating hypotension and bradycardia, traditional therapies are used for the management of hemodynamic instability. If ACLS is required, a lower dose of epinephrine (less than 1 mcg/kg) should be used. Given that cardiovascular collapse is secondary to cardiac effects of local anesthetic toxicity (not cardiogenic in nature), typical code drugs that may further depress nodal conduction, cardiac contractility or exacerbate arrhythmias such as beta blockers, calcium channel blockers, and local anesthetics, should be avoided.

4. *Prevention*:

   American Society of Regional Anesthesia and Pain Medicine (ASRA) provides multimodal suggestions on the prevention of LAST [29]. Concerning patient selection particularly in the office setting, practitioners should be aware of preexisting cardiovascular and neurologic conditions to aid in the detection of symptoms. Patients with certain conditions such as advanced age, ischemic heart disease, underlying cardiac conduction abnormalities, metabolic disease, or those currently on sodium channel blocking agents are at increased risk for LAST [28].

With respect to drug delivery, one should consider the discussion of local anesthetic dose as part of a pre-procedural "time out" with goals to use the lowest effective dose. Aspirate prior to injection to observe for blood in the syringe; and if there is no concern of intraarterial or intravenous injection, proceed with incremental injection while monitoring for patient symptoms. With injection, ask patients about possible symptoms such as tinnitus, circumoral numbness, or metallic taste.

Patient Case [3]

1. *History*:

A 37-year-old G1P0010 with secondary amenorrhea after previous suction dilation and curettage for septic abortion and imaging consistent with mild to moderate intrauterine adhesions presented for surgical management. She was scheduled for an outpatient hysteroscopic adhesiolysis and was classified as ASA Class I. An anesthesiologist administered deep sedation under monitored anesthesia care. After she was adequately anesthetized, a 5 mm rigid hysteroscope was inserted into the cervical canal, but the view of the uterine cavity was obstructed by blood. After removing and reinserting the hysteroscope three times and placing the patient in significant Trendelenburg, the endometrial cavity was visualized and adhesions were easily resected. At the end of the case, the anesthesiologist noted that the patient became hypotensive with a blood pressure 80/42 mmHg accompanied by a decrease in oxygen saturation.

2. *Pathophysiology*:

Venous embolus is a complication of hysteroscopy associated with the entrapment of room air (venous air embolism, VAE) or gas from either insufflated carbon dioxide or smoke produced from electrosurgery (venous gas embolism, VGE) in the venous system. Air or gas in the venous system enters the right heart then flows into the vessels of the pulmonary circulation. In this circumstance, the venous gas bubbles are removed by the lung at a rate that mainly depends on the compensatory rise in pulmonary artery pressure. However, when the amount of entrained gas or air exceeds the rate of pulmonary clearance, pulmonary artery pressure progressively rises. The rise in pulmonary artery pressure or pulmonary hypertension causes right heart strain and clinically significant hypotension. Blockages in these pulmonary vessels lead to dead space with decreased oxygenation and ventilation evidenced by hypercarbia and hypoxia [28].

Larger gas or air emboli entrained in the right heart create a mechanical obstruction thus preventing flow into the pulmonary circulation leading to pulmonary hypertension. Massive right ventricular failure and cardiovascular collapse may ensue. Of note, microvascular emboli have also been associated with an inflammatory response leading to pulmonary edema and bronchoconstriction secondary to activation of endothelial mediators from damaged vasculature [30].

3. *Risk factors*:

A number of factors associated with hysteroscopy predispose patients to VAE/VGE.

Equipment and procedural factors leading to VAE/VGE are the use of high flow and pressurized intrauterine gas, unpurged fluid in-flow line, piston-like action of repetitive insertions of the hysteroscope into the uterine cavity and inadequate uterine flushing of bubbles. Trendelenburg position also elevates the uterus above the level of the heart, increasing the risk for air entrapment. Disruption of vasculature, particularly in patients with large venous channels such as in pregnancy or vascular myoma, increases the risk of atmospheric pressure exceeding venous pressure, entrapping air in the venous system, and creating a venous air embolism [31].

4. *Treatment*:

The provider should apply the STOP mnemonic.

Stop: When concern for VAE/VGE arises from either an anesthesiologist or surgeon, immediate communication is imperative. Firstly, call for assistance and arrange ambulance transportation to an inpatient facility. If the patient is already inpatient, then the surgeon should notify the code team.

Think: Symptoms of VAE/VGE reported by the patient may include shortness of breath, chest pain, or chest tightness.

Observe: You may observe hypoxia with decreased oxygen saturation, hypercarbia (though end-tidal carbon dioxide may be increased or decreased), hypotension, tachycardia or bradycardia, arrhythmias, and tachypnea [32]. A "mill-wheel" murmur is observed if air is entrained in the right heart.

Plan: The mainstay of treatment for VAE/VGE is supportive.

Patients should be placed on supplemental oxygen if available and the field (in this case, the cervix) flooded with saline or occluded with wet gauze to prevent further air entrapment [31]. Additionally, they should be placed in neutral position (uterus no longer above the level of the heart) and left lateral decubitus position (Durant's maneuver) to assist with air movement away from the right ventricular outflow tract. Intravenous fluids should run open to increase central venous pressure (CVP). If available, inotropic and vasopressor support (such as norepinephrine) can maintain hemodynamic stability and organ perfusion [33].

Further management of VAE would clearly need to take place in the inpatient setting. If hemodynamic instability persists and air lock of the right ventricular outflow tract is suspected, one should consider right-sided central line placement to aspirate air from the right ventricle. Lastly, if nitrous oxide is being administered, it should be discontinued to prevent further increase in size of VAE/VGE.

5. *Prevention*:

The prevention of clinically significant room and gas emboli during hysteroscopic surgery depends upon an educated awareness of contributing factors by the surgeon, anesthesiologist, and nursing personnel. Office personnel must be trained to purge air from the fluid lines prior to surgery, avoid entry of air into fluid lines, turn off pumps during bag changes, use a Y-connector on the fluid inflow line in order to reduce air entrainment during bag changes, and provide continuous careful attention to fluid deficit. Basic equipment must be available to fulfill the requirements for monitoring of fluid deficit, assessment and control of intrauterine pressure, and anesthesia monitoring [34].

The surgeon should always employ good judgment in patient selection taking into consideration the size, number, FIGO type, and location of myomas. The minimum amount of intrauterine pressure for good visualization should be utilized. If the cervix is dilated, prevention of exposure to air through packing with wet gauze may be considered [32]. Fluid hydration to assure adequate CVP intraoperatively and use of pneumatic calf compression devices to minimize venous capacitance are appropriate measures of prevention.

In the office setting, one must have an emergency cart with medications in the event of advanced cardiac life support (ACLS), LAST, venous air embolism, over-sedation, or anaphylaxis. The emergency cart may include epinephrine, norepinephrine, atropine, naloxone, diphenhydramine, hydrocortisone, and Intralipid®. There are currently no guidelines regarding whether supplemental oxygen should be required in the office setting for these scenarios but can be considered. Consultation with your anesthesiologist prior to performing these office procedures can be beneficial and discussion with the office surgical staff to maintain an adequate supply of these medications.

Conclusion

Inevitably, errors and adverse events will occur in medicine. CM will always have importance in both office and operating room settings for the reproductive surgeon and these cases have served as an example in select scenarios. However, there are other scenarios that providers will need to be prepared for. Health care providers should discuss CM with their health care team and create an office culture that embraces human error and emphasizes team leadership, simulation training, and panic control. Providers should emphasize the importance of effective communication during a crisis, define goals for health care team members, and employ message repetition strategies to improve team communication. Procedural drills with the entire health care team discussing preoperative, intraoperative, and postoperative considerations can reinforce key elements of CM. The STOP mental framework will arm providers with a panic control strategy as they maneuver through a crisis. Finally, the awareness that human error occurs more often from systems errors than from personal faults will allow health care teams to shift their focus on developing system-based changes such as alarms, checklists, treatment guidelines, and root-cause analyses to prevent errors from occurring again. Health care teams should be cognizant of CM strategies to optimize patient safety and it is critically important that we, as a team, discuss how CM can be applied to our individual practices.

References

1. Moorthy K, Munz Y, Forrest D, Pandey V, Undre S, Vincent C, Darzi A. Surgical crisis management skills training and assessment: a simulation-based approach to enhancing operating room performance. Ann Surg. 2006;244(1):139–47.
2. Levy BS, Ness DL, Weinberger SE. Consensus guidelines for facilities performing outpatient procedures: evidence over ideology. Obstet Gynecol. 2019;133(2):255–60. https://doi.org/10.1097/AOG.0000000000003058.
3. Wortman M, Daggett A, Ball C. Operative hysteroscopy in an office-based surgical setting: review of patient safety and satisfaction in 414 cases. J Minim Invasive Gynecol. 2013;20(1):56–63. https://doi.org/10.1016/j.jmig.2012.08.778.
4. Cullen K, Hall M, Golosinskiy A. Ambulatory surgery in the United States, 2006. Natl Health Stat Rep. 2009;11:1–27.
5. Hysteroscopy. ACOG technology assessment in obstetrics and gynecology no. 13. American College of Obstetricians and Gynecologists. Obstet Gynecol. 2018;131:e151–6.
6. Urman RD, Ba P, Shapiro FE. Office-based surgical and medical procedures: educational gaps. Ochsner J. 2012;12:383–8.
7. Erickson TB, Kirkpatrick DH, DeFrancesco MS, Lawrence HCI. Executive summary of the American College of Obstetricians and Gynecologists Presidential Task Force on patient safety in the office setting: reinvigorating safety in office-based gynecologic surgery. Obstet Gynecol. 2010;115(1):147–51. https://doi.org/10.1097/AOG.0b013e3181c4f966.
8. Wortman M, Carroll K. Office-based gynecologic surgery (OBGS): past, present, and future: part I. Surg Technol Int. 2019;35:173–84.
9. Jansen FW, Vredevoogd CB, van Ulzen K, Hermans J, Trimbos JB, Trimbos-Kemper TC. Complications of hysteroscopy: a prospective, multicenter study. Obstet Gynecol. 2000;96(2):266–70. https://doi.org/10.1016/s0029-7844(00)00865-6.
10. Lipshy KA, LaPorta A. Operating room crisis management leadership training: guidance for surgical team education. Bull Am Coll Surg. 2013;98(10):24–33.
11. Lipshy KA. Crisis management leadership in the operating room: have you prepared your team to handle any crisis they might encounter in the OR, or are they destined to fail? San Diego: Creative Team Publishing; 2013.
12. Bundy J, Pfarrer MD, Short CE, Coombs WT. Crises and crisis management: integration, interpretation, and research development. J Manag. 2016;43(6):1661–92. https://doi.org/10.1177/0149206316680030.
13. Shrivastava P, et al. Understanding industrial crises. J Manag Stud. 1988;25:285–304.
14. Operating room crisis management leadership training: guidance for surgical team education. The Bulletin. https://bulletin.facs.org/2013/10/or-crisis-management/. Accessed 6 Apr 2020.
15. Chu B, Marwaha K, Sanvictores T, et al. Physiology, stress reaction. [Updated 2020 Oct 10]. In: StatPearls [Internet]. Treasure Island (FL): StatPearls Publishing.
16. Donaldson MS. An overview of to err is human: re-emphasizing the message of patient safety. In: Hughes RG, editor. Patient safety and quality: an evidence-based handbook for nurses. Rockville: Agency for Healthcare Research and Quality (US); 2008. Chapter 3.
17. Clinical guidelines and standardization of practice to improve outcomes: ACOG Committee Opinion,

Number 792. Obstet Gynecol. 2019;134(4):e122–5. https://doi.org/10.1097/aog.0000000000003454.

18. Makary MA, Sexton JB, Freischlag JA, et al. Operating room teamwork among physicians and nurses: teamwork in the eye of the beholder. J Am Coll Surg. 2006;202(5):746–52. https://doi.org/10.1016/j.jamcollsurg.2006.01.017.

19. Saiboon IM, Apoo FN, Jamal SM, et al. Improving the position of resuscitation team leader with simulation (IMPORTS); a pilot cross-sectional randomized intervention study. Medicine (Baltimore). 2019;98(49):e18201. https://doi.org/10.1097/md.0000000000018201.

20. Zern SC, Marshall WJ, Shewokis PA, Vest MT. Use of simulation as a needs assessment to develop a focused team leader training curriculum for resuscitation teams. Adv Simul (Lond). 2020;5:6. https://doi.org/10.1186/s41077-020-00124-2.

21. Boet S, Bould MD, Fung L, et al. Transfer of learning and patient outcome in simulated crisis resource management: a systematic review. Can J Anaesth. 2014;61(6):571–82. https://doi.org/10.1007/s12630-014-0143-8.

22. Edworthy J, Hellier E, Newbold L, Titchener K. Passing crisis and emergency risk communications: the effects of communication channel, information type, and repetition. Appl Ergon. 2015;48:252–62. https://doi.org/10.1016/j.apergo.2014.12.009.

23. Runciman WB, Merry AF. Crises in clinical care: an approach to management. Qual Saf Health Care. 2005;14(3):156–63. https://doi.org/10.1136/qshc.2004.012856.

24. Shakir F, Diab Y. The perforated uterus. Obstet Gynaecol. 2013;15:256–61.

25. Grimes DA, Schulz KF, Cates WJ Jr. Prevention of uterine perforation during curettage abortion. JAMA. 1984;251(16):2108–11.

26. Nezhat C, Nezhat F, Nezhat C. Nezhat's textbook of minimally invasive surgery: including hysteroscopy, vaginoscopy, and robotic-assisted procedures. Cambridge University Press; 2014.

27. Christie LE, Picard J, Weinberg GL. Local anaesthetic systemic toxicity. BJA Educ. 2014;15(3):136–42. https://doi.org/10.1093/bjaceaccp/mku027.

28. Miller RD, Pardo M, Stoelting RK. Basics of anesthesia. Philadelphia: Elsevier/Saunders; 2011.

29. Neal JM, Barrington MJ, Fettiplace MR, et al. The Third American Society of Regional Anesthesia and Pain Medicine Practice Advisory on Local Anesthetic Systemic Toxicity: executive summary 2017. Reg Anesth Pain Med. 2018;43(2):113–23. https://doi.org/10.1097/aap.0000000000000720.

30. Eisenach JC, Zornow MH. Yao & Artusio's anesthesiology: problem-oriented patient management, 4th edition. Anesthesiology. 1999;91:1562. https://doi.org/10.1097/00000542-199911000-00069.

31. Verma A, Singh MP. Venous gas embolism in operative hysteroscopy: a devastating complication in a relatively simple surgery. J Anaesthesiol Clin Pharmacol. 2018;34(1):103–6. https://doi.org/10.4103/joacp.JOACP_235_15.

32. Rademaker BM, Groenman FA, van der Wouw PA, Bakkum EA. Paradoxical gas embolism by transpulmonary passage of venous emboli during hysteroscopic surgery: a case report and discussion. Br J Anaesth. 2008;101(2):230–3. https://doi.org/10.1093/bja/aen138.

33. Van Dijck C, Rex S, Verguts J, Timmerman D, Van de Velde M, Teunkens A. Venous air embolism during hysteroscopic myomectomy: an analysis of 7 cases. Gynecol Obstet Investig. 2017;82(6):569–74. https://doi.org/10.1159/000455044.

34. Groenman FA, Peters LW, Rademaker BM, Bakkum EA. Embolism of air and gas in hysteroscopic procedures: pathophysiology and implication for daily practice. J Minim Invasive Gynecol. 2008;15(2):241–7. https://doi.org/10.1016/j.jmig.2007.10.010.

Risk Mitigation Strategies for Physicians

22

Jody Lyneé Madeira and Jerry A. Lindheim

Introduction

In a medical malpractice lawsuit, a patient or client claims that they were harmed when a hospital, doctor, or medical professional through a negligent act or omission to act causes an injury. The negligence may be the result of errors in diagnosis, treatment, aftercare, or health management [1]. According to a 2019 Medscape Malpractice Report, more than half of physicians are sued over the course of their careers, regardless of whether they did or did not make a medical error [2] and are understandably interested in learning how to avoid this outcome. Evading malpractice lawsuits is difficult and depends on many complex factors. But physicians can do a lot to reduce the risk of medical malpractice. This chapter describes the legal history of medical malpractice, describe its elements; discuss the current landscape of medical malpractice (focusing on obstetrics and gynecology); examine why patients sue and how medical and health care providers can mitigate risks;

and explore how to cope with Medical Malpractice Stress Syndrome.

Historical Perspectives on Medical Malpractice

Efforts to hold physicians responsible for their actions date back to one of the oldest legal writings, Hammurabi's Code, best known for the principle of justice through an "eye for an eye." The Code [3] used this Draconian principle to hold physicians directly physical or financial accountable through several uncompromising provisions:

- If a physician shall make a large incision with a bronze operating-knife and kill him or shall open a growth with a bronze operating-knife and destroy the eye, his hands shall be cut off. Code Law #218
- If a physician shall make a severe wound with a bronze operating-knife on the slave of a freed man and kill him, he shall replace the slave with another slave. Code Law #219
- If a physician shall open an abscess (growth, tumor, cavity) with a bronze operating-knife and destroy the eye, he shall pay the half of the value of the slave. Code Law #220

Some believe that these strict provisions mean that physicians have always had to practice

J. L. Madeira
Indiana University Maurer School of Law, Bloomington, IN, USA
e-mail: jmadeira@indiana.edu

J. A. Lindheim (✉)
Lindheim Law, Cherry Hill, NJ, USA
e-mail: jlindheim@lockslaw.com

S. R. Lindheim, J. C. Petrozza (eds.), *Reproductive Surgery*,
https://doi.org/10.1007/978-3-031-05240-8_22

"defensive medicine" [4]. But for over a millennia, there were little to no accountability mechanisms other than physicians' oaths. Around the fifth century B.C., physicians who took the Oath of Hippocrates pledged they would act for the good of their patients according to their ability and judgment and never do harm to anyone [3]. More updated tools for holding physicians responsible for harms to patients did not evolve until nearly 1600 years later in 1164 A.D., when a physician was sued for practicing "unwholesome medicine" in *Everad v. Hoskins*, the first recorded case of medical malpractice.

An established medical malpractice framework came in the 1374 case of *Stratton v. Swanlond*, where a highly regarded surgeon by the name of John Swanlond promised to surgically repair a woman's injured hand, but the patient's hand was still deformed afterwards. The patient then sued for breach of contract based on the physician's promise that he could fix her hand. Although the lawsuit was dismissed for technical reasons, the judge issued the following comment in his written opinion: "If a smith undertakes to cure my horse, and the horse is harmed by his negligence or failure to cure in a reasonable time, it is just that he should be liable."

Although *Stratton v. Swanlond* set the framework for subsequent claims against physicians, it was not until 1768 that the eminent English jurist Sir William Blackstone elaborated upon the concept of medical "malpractice" and tied it to physicians, applying the term "mala praxis" to describe "neglect of unskillful [sic] management of [a person's] physician, surgeon, or apothecary…because it breaks the trust which the party had placed in his physician and tends to the patient's destruction" [5].

Britain's legal system emigrated to America with its colonies, and the first reported American medical malpractice case was the 1794 Connecticut case of *Cross v. Guthery*, where, as in *Stratton v. Swanlond*, the husband sued the physician after his wife died several hours after surgery. Notably this lawsuit was for breach of contract—promising to skillfully give care and obtain a good result—not for the physician's inability to comply with professional standards of care. Apparently, Dr. Guthery had expressed his regrets to her husband, and then sent him a bill for 15 pounds. Cross hired a lawyer, who persuaded a jury to dismiss Dr. Guthery's bill and award Cross 40 pounds as compensation for the loss of his wife's companionship.

Legal Elements of a Medical Malpractice Claim

In the United States, a patient alleging medical malpractice must generally prove four elements: (1) that the physician had a legal duty to provide care or treatment to the patient; (2) that the physician breached this duty by failing to adhere to the standards of the profession; (3) that the breach of duty caused injury to the patient; and (4) that the patient suffered damages from the injury that the legal system can redress through money or other means.

A physician owes a legal duty to a patient whenever a professional relationship is established between them. The general idea of a legal duty is that, in civilized society, each person owes a duty of reasonable care to others. Thus, where a doctor treats a patient, the doctor is said to owe the patient a duty of reasonable professional care.

Once a physician owes a patient a legal duty, the question is whether that duty was breached. To prove a physician breached a professional duty, a patient must establish what standard of care the physician should have followed. The precise definition of "standard of care" differs from state to state, but it generally refers to that care which a reasonable, similarly situated healthcare professional would have provided to the patient. Each medical professional and subspecialty have defined standards of practice. It is rarely obvious that the standard of care has been breached; common examples are when a surgical instrument is left in a patient's body, or when a physician operates on the wrong limb. Otherwise, expert witness testimony is usually essential to establishing that the standard of care has been breached since a jury of lay persons cannot understand the nuances of medical care

To have legal relevance, a breach of the medical standard of care must have caused injury to the patient. To prove causation, an injured plaintiff must show that the alleged breach is directly related to a subsequent injury. The patient must also show that there is no policy reason why the physician should not be held liable for the breached standard of care, or that the injury cannot be attributed to other factors. In defending physicians from this element, defense counsel typically argue "no harm, no foul." For instance, if a physician delays in performing a test but this delay does not harm the patient, then defense counsel will argue there is no "causal harm" and thus no medical negligence. For example, a child falls from a tree, injures her hand, and is taken to the emergency room where Dr. Smith examines and discharges her without performing any tests or either taking x-rays. If a week passes and the child is taken back to the emergency room where Dr. Jones takes an x-ray that reveals a fracture, the plaintiff would argue that Dr. Smith breached the medical standard of care in not taking an x-ray. But if the child's hand is casted and heals properly without any deformity, defense counsel would argue that the child was not harmed by the delay in diagnosis, so that any deviation in treatment was "no harm and thus no foul."

Damages, the fourth and final element of medical malpractice lawsuits, are decided at the end of litigation. Damages are discretionary; juries may award monetary damages to compensate the injured patient and/or their family members. Punitive damages are rarely awarded in medical malpractice cases and are reserved for especially egregious conduct, including deliberately altering or destroying medical records or sexual misconduct towards a patient. A plaintiff that cannot show damages loses their medical malpractice lawsuit. For instance, using the example above, if an undiagnosed fractured hand was treated using a splint instead of a closed reduction and/or a cast when the fracture pattern clearly called for open fixation and casting, the treating physician may have committed malpractice if the fracture did not heal or healed incorrectly, requiring the patient to undergo multiple operations and incur increased expenses. But a fracture that heals correctly despite a breach of standard of care and the patient sued for medical malpractice but could not show actual damages, a jury would only award limited damages.

The Current Landscape of Physician Medical Malpractice in the United States

Medical mistakes are a major problem and are an increasing cause of patient mortality. In a 2016 study from Johns Hopkins concerning medical death rates in the United States over an eight-year period, researchers estimated that medical mistakes resulted in more than 250,000 American deaths—the third leading cause of death, behind only cancer and heart disease [6].

A 2016 American Medical Association (AMA) survey found that more than half of all physicians will be named in a lawsuit during their career, regardless of whether they did or did not make a medical error [2]. On average, 68 liability claims were filed per every 100 physicians [7]. According to a 2019 Medscape Malpractice Report [8] of over 4300 physicians in 29+ specialties, physicians claimed that their lawsuit was a terrible experience; yet, only a small percentage of lawsuits are decided against the physician. The Medscape Malpractice report found that 59% of physicians had been sued; specialists (62%) were sued more often than primary care physicians (52%), with the top four most frequently sued specialties being general surgeons (85%); urologists (84%); otolaryngologists (83%); and OB/GYN & Women's Health practitioners (83%). Consistent with prior surveys, 33% of claims alleged physicians failed to diagnose or delayed diagnosis; 29% involved complications from treatment or surgery; and 26% of claims alleged poor outcome or disease progression. More than half of physicians reported experiencing shock at being sued, while 13% were not surprised at all and 29% of physicians who were sued could identify the incident that triggered the suit.

Common Categories of Malpractice Claims

Several common errors that may lead to medical malpractice lawsuit. These include but are not limited to failure to diagnose, failure to identify a treatment complication, inadequate follow-up, medication errors, and communication factors.

Failure to diagnose is the most common malpractice claim. Whether from a physician's inattentiveness or outright incompetence, failure to diagnose can lead to an undiscovered condition or produce misdiagnosis. Delayed diagnosis can affect patients' health and well-being, and can result in no treatment, ineffective treatment, or treatment that is downright harmful. Physicians can also *fail to identify treatment complications.* Surgical errors account for roughly one-third of all medical malpractice claims. These errors might occur during surgery, when the surgeon inadvertently injures an organ or blood vessel, causing internal bleeding, sepsis, or death. Postoperative management, including immediate and follow-up care, is also critical; if a patient becomes seriously ill or dies due to negligent follow-up care from medical staff, the physician and hospital can be held liable. A similar category of claims stem from *inadequate follow-up,* such as when physicians do not follow through with testing or test results are not received in a timely fashion. Physicians and their staff must track order status to ensure that all are reviewed and considered when creating treatment plans. At the same time, physicians should conserve medical and patient resources by only ordering necessary tests and interventions, avoiding *defensive medicine.*

Medication errors affect an estimated 1.5 million people in the United States each year and can result from physician or pharmacy error. Physicians should be aware of all patient medications and educate patients on the importance of taking medications only as prescribed and immediately contacting the physician's office if medications are not having intended effects. Using electronic prescribing helps lower malpractice risks.

Several malpractice claims stem from inadequate physician–patient communication. It is imperative to take time to ensure patients understand their diagnosis, treatment, and medication plans, and assure their understanding. Although constrained by institutional policies, physicians must allocate enough time to examine and converse with patients. Allowing patients to fully explain their concerns demonstrates the physician's concern, empathy, and likeability. The more quality time a physician spends with a patient, the less likely the physician will be sued.

Research suggests that malpractice suits are not fueled by substandard care but by communication breakdowns [9], increasing chances that patients will sue regardless of whether there has actually been medical error [10, 11]. Vincent et al. demonstrated that patients' decisions to take legal action depend on the original injury *and* a secondary injury, insensitive communication, failure to provide information, and lack of apology. Furthermore, liability or exposure by the medical provider to a lawsuit can be predicted by the medical provider's inability to effectively communicate and develop and maintain rapport with their patients, especially when an adverse event occurs [10].

Minimizing Medical Malpractice Risk

Although the prospect of being sued is enough to inject trepidation into the boldest of physicians, there are several tactics that can be used to mitigate that risk, including adopting a conscientious self-awareness, refraining from blaming others, following applicable policies, keeping thorough records, practicing good communication skills, and exhibiting appropriate emotions in interactions with patients and caregivers.

A conscientious attitude and self-awareness can prevent medical errors, improve the quality of care, and encourage physicians to take responsibility when needed. Blaming others for adverse outcomes increases the risk of poor communication and an unapologetic stance.

Though it might seem common sense, adherence to clinical guidelines and hospital policies is an effective way to improve quality care and reduce variation in care. National and international clinical guidelines have been systematically developed to assist evidence-based clinical decision making. Comparing deviations to normative guidelines can help determine the degree to which a particular physician's conduct adhered to accepted standards. These guidelines, however, may change from time to time. To maintain licensure, physicians must fulfill continuing medical education requirements. Taking programs that are most relevant to care specializations will ensure that physicians stay informed of current scientific and technological developments.

One of the most practical risk mitigation strategies is maintaining thorough patient records. If the treating doctor does not document something happened, it is difficult to prove it occurred. Accurate and thorough charting preserves the chain of decisions and events leading up to an alleged patient injury. In addition, this information is essential to answer questions about duty of care in a deposition or other proceeding months or years after an alleged injury occurs. Documentation has legal credibility when it is contemporaneous, accurate, truthful, and appropriate.

Many strategies for mitigating risk affect the doctor–patient relationship itself. Excellent communication skills play a key role in decreasing the risk of malpractice lawsuits; "patients who like their doctors don't sue, no matter what their lawyer says. . . . Patients sue when their feelings are ignored or when they are angered by lack of genuine concern for their welfare…Though it provides no guarantee, a sound physician–patient relationship is a powerful antidote to frivolous lawsuits" [9]. Furthermore, one study details that almost one-third of lawsuits related to some form of communication, whether inattentiveness, discourtesy or rudeness, a general breakdown, and inadequate information [12].

Poor physician communication practices can prompt patients to suspect that physicians are being deceptive or concealing information—and that it is necessary to sue to obtain information

[13]. In reviewing how many patients filed malpractice claims following perinatal injuries, Hickson et al. evaluated claims in Florida between 1986 and 1989. Questionnaires were completed by 127 (35%) of a total of 368 such families. The authors found that the number of patients who reporting suing because they doubted a physician's honesty was identical to the percentage who reported filing because they wanted remuneration [13].

In examining what kinds of breakdowns in communication contribute to malpractice claims, one study reviewed malpractice deposition transcripts and concluded that several types of communication problems existed in over 70% of cases, including: (1) deserting the patient, (2) devaluing patients' views, and (3) delivering information poorly [14].

Other studies on malpractice also conclude that providing adequate explanations about diagnosis and treatment and developing a trusting, respectful relationship with patients are important to reducing exposure to litigation [15]. Research shows that those medical providers who have difficulty in communicating effectively have a greater likelihood of being sued [16].

Transparent communication is particularly essential when patients have bad outcomes. Physicians should maintain eye contact while addressing the patient and feel comfortable making appropriate compassionate expressions and gestures. Though some physicians may avoid visiting the patient when relatives are present, it is important to let patients and caregivers know that the treating doctor understands their problems.

Closely related to open and transparent communication are situationally appropriate emotional statements and expressions that demonstrate the doctor's engagement when interacting with patients. Patients especially appreciate empathic care providers who take time to put themselves in patients' situations and try to understand the condition from their perspectives. Behaviors such as eye contact, nodding, or brief responsive utterances can encourage patients to share difficult or intimate details, build rapport, and strengthen physician–patient relationships.

The most controversial aspect of communication and emotional engagement is the apology. The act of apologizing, the thinking goes, restores dignity and respect to the patient and adds humanity and credibility to the physician, draining away the anger that often motivates lawsuits and high settlements. In 2014, National Public Radio reported on a Johns Hopkins study of 236 patients who completed questionnaires, which revealed that only 9% of patients stated that a doctor's office or medical facility openly admitted causing harm and that physicians rarely apologized for medical or hospital errors, particularly those resulting in injury or infection. The report further explained that most healthcare professionals were inclined to withhold information concerning medical mistakes and errors and only disclosed harm under pressure (including from litigation) and only 11% apologized to patients or their families [16].

Although the concern of practitioners is that an apology may prompt litigation, to provide a balance with the effectiveness of transparency and communication and concerns with its impact with litigation, 39 states and the District of Columbia have passed laws permitting physicians to apologize, express sympathy, or share condolences without those statements being used as evidence against them in court.

Attorneys understand that medical providers are human and that errors are inevitable. Taking responsibility does not mean admitting negligence, but rather acknowledging that a complication has occurred and trying to minimize the consequences. The worst thing a medical provider can do is attempt to conceal or lie about a medical error. Medical and legal professionals as well as ethicists and members of the public all believe that physicians are obligated to disclose medical errors [17]. Ethically, disclosure is in the patient's best interest; legally, it is part of the physician's duty to the patient. Patients benefit from knowing about medical errors to make timely treatment decisions to minimize or correct related complications and avoid future misdiagnosis. Moreover, patients who are injured by a physician's negligence deserve compensation.

The Experience of Being Sued

Physicians who face medical malpractice lawsuits find that they do not conclude quickly and can take years to resolve. A malpractice case entails lengthy process, including discovery and investigation. Physicians who are sued find this experience enormously time-consuming and taxing. According to the 2019 Medscape Malpractice Report [2], 42% of physicians spent more than 40 hours preparing for their defense, including getting records, meeting with counsel, and preparing for depositions and discussions (this excluded the trial itself). Forty percent of physicians reported that lawsuits lasted for 1–2 years; but 27% reported that litigation lasted 3–5 years. Most suits do not proceed to trial. The Medscape report indicated that as many as 33% of lawsuits were settled before trial; 3% were settled at trial, 11% went to trial and returned a verdict for the physician; 3% went to trial and returned a verdict for the plaintiff; and 44% of the cases were dismissed by the plaintiff or court [2].

Physicians defending a malpractice case need to stay focused and avoid obsessing over the case or its potential outcome. Some can experience Medical Malpractice Stress Syndrome (MMSS) due to the trauma of being sued. Those experiencing MMSS endure feelings of isolation, negative self-image, feelings of helplessness and hopelessness, and depression [18]. Physical syndromes may also appear or intensify. The prolonged nature of a medical malpractice case can aggravate preexisting emotional and physical symptoms. Physicians with MMSS exhibit physical symptoms that hamper their ability to practice medicine; some try to cope by working longer hours, while others become insecure in their abilities and avoid work altogether. Still others lose focus and have difficulty concentrating [19]. Physicians with MMSS commonly exhibit irritability and anger with patients and staff, further increasing malpractice litigation risk.

Left unrecognized and untreated, MMSS can have a similar outcome to clinical depression and anxiety: physician suicide [19]. There are several ways to cope with litigation trauma and MMSS. The most extreme option is to cease practicing medicine, which is not viable or desirable for most physicians. A more productive choice is to take control of the situation and regain physical and emotional health by strengthening social support systems, learning more about the case instead of regarding it as a mystery, and seeking the appropriate medical and psychiatric help to treat emotional and physical symptoms of MMSS [20].

Conclusion

This chapter provides some historical perspectives on the origins of medical malpractice, reviews legal elements related to medical malpractice, discusses the current litigation landscape, and explores the driving forces behind litigation. It also provides useful strategies for mitigating legal risk, including open communication. Given the enormous strain on health care providers, preserving emotional wellness is paramount to overcome the stresses that a medical malpractice lawsuit can create.

References

1. American Board of Professional Liability Attorney.
2. Medscape malpractice report 2019.
3. Powis Smith JM. Origin & history of Hebrew law. Chicago: University of Chicago Press; 1931.
4. Faria MA Jr. Orig Publ J Med Assoc Ga. Mar 1995.
5. Austin Wallace R. Brief history of medical liability litigation and insurance. W V Med J. 2017;113(5). West Virginia State Medical Association.
6. Makary MA, Daniel M. Medical error-the third leading cause of death. BMJ. 2016;353:i2139.
7. Guardado JR. Policy research perspectives-medical liability claims frequency among U.S. physicians. Chicago: American Medical Association; 2017.
8. Verghese A. Hard cures: doctors themselves could take several steps to reduce malpractice suits. New York Times. 16 Mar 2003. Quoted by Roter D. The patient-physician relationship and its implications for malpractice litigation. J Health Care Law Policy. 2006;9:304–14.
9. Hickson GB, Jenkins DA. Identifying and addressing communication failures as a means of reducing unnecessary malpractice claims. N C Med J. 2007;68(5):362–4.
10. Vincent C, Young M, Phillips A. Why do people sue doctors? A study of patients and relatives taking legal action. Lancet. 1994;343:1609–13.
11. Roter D. The patient-physician relationship and its implications for malpractice litigation. J Health Care Law Policy. 2006;9:304–14.
12. Hickson GB, Wright Clayton E, Githens PB, Sloan FA. Factors that prompted families to file medical malpractice claims following perinatal injuries. JAMA. 1992;267(10):1359–63.
13. Beckman HB, Markaksi KM, Suchman AL, Frankel RM. The doctor-patient relationship: lessons from plaintiff depositions. Arch Intern Med. 1994;154:1365–70.
14. Shapiro RS, Simpson DE, Lawrence SL, et al. A survey of sued and nonsued physicians and suing patients. Arch Intern Med. 1989;149:2190–6.
15. NPR, 21 Nov 2014.
16. Falkner ES. The medical malpractice in obstetrics: a gestalt approach to reform. Cardoza Women's Law J. 1997;4:1–32.
17. Wu AW, Cavanaugh TA, McPhee SJ, Lo B, Micco GP. To tell the truth: ethical and practical issues in disclosing medical mistakes to patients. J Gen Intern Med. 1997;12:770–5.
18. AANA News Bulletin. July 2007. http://bit.ly/2iLgzd4.
19. Medical Malpractice Stress Syndrome, ACEP.org. http://bit.ly/2ivZlHg.
20. Reyes R, Reyes C. Medical malpractice stress syndrome takes its toll. Emergency Medicine News. Feb 2017.

Nigel Pereira and Victoria W. Fitz

Introduction

The birth of the first baby resulting from in vitro fertilization (IVF) in 1978 marked an important milestone in the inception of assisted reproductive technologies (ART). Since then, at least nine million babies have been born worldwide through IVF [1]. Efficient ovarian stimulation protocols and successful laboratory techniques have often been recognized as the main causes of accelerated ART utilization; however, the standardization of a simple outpatient oocyte retrieval technique has played an equally important role in increasing the safety and efficacy of ART. In this chapter, we outline the history of oocyte retrieval techniques, summarize current standards for oocyte retrieval, and appraise the existing medical literature pertaining to complications associated with oocyte retrieval.

N. Pereira (✉)
The Ronald O. Perelman and Claudia Cohen Center for Reproductive Medicine, Weill Cornell Medical College, New York, NY, USA
e-mail: nip9060@med.cornell.edu

V. W. Fitz
Division of Reproductive Endocrinology and Infertility, Massachusetts General Fertility Center, Boston, MA, USA
e-mail: vfitz@mgh.harvard.edu

A Brief History of Oocyte Retrieval Techniques

The earliest description of oocyte retrieval in humans appeared in two successive manuscripts published by Rock and Menkin in 1944 and 1948, respectively [2]. In their 1944 manuscript [2], the authors presented their experience of retrieving a single oocyte from a 38-year-old para 4 woman undergoing laparotomy on cycle day 10 and another 31-year-old para 6 woman undergoing laparotomy on cycle day 11. Their subsequent publication in 1948 [3] summarized their experience of retrieving 800 oocytes via laparotomy from women undergoing various gynecologic surgeries. However, the invasiveness and morbidity associated with laparotomy necessitated a better oocyte retrieval technique.

In the late 1950s and early 1960s, Patrick C. Steptoe, a British gynecologist, published several important manuscripts describing the use of laparoscopy for various gynecologic pathologies. Steptoe's 1968 publication in *The Lancet* detailed his technique of retrieving oocytes via laparoscopy during the natural menstrual cycle [4]. This publication prompted a successful scientific collaboration between Robert Edwards and Patrick Steptoe who further refined their surgical and laboratory techniques for IVF [5]. This collaboration eventually resulted in the birth of the first IVF baby in 1978 [6]. Louise Brown, the first IVF baby, was born to a mother who underwent laparoscopic oocyte retrieval during the natural menstrual cycle and had a history of severe tubal disease requiring at least two prior laparotomies [6]. Despite the early novelty of IVF, it soon became evident that the retrieval of single oocytes via laparoscopy during the natural menstrual cycle limited IVF success rates [7]. The addition of ovulation induction agents and gonadotropins, in combination with laparoscopic oocyte retrieval, increased IVF success rates over the next several years, owing to the availability of multiple embryos for transfer [8].

The technical limitations of laparoscopic oocyte retrieval, specifically the need for general anesthesia, operating room setting, and longer procedural time, resulted in further refinement of oocyte retrieval technique. Lenz and colleagues were the first to demonstrate the feasibility of ultrasound-guided follicular puncture [9, 10]. Their technique required localization of ovarian follicles with a transabdominal probe and passage of a needle through the abdominal wall and bladder into the ovarian follicles [9, 10]. This type of oocyte retrieval could be performed with local or general anesthesia. In their initial study of 30 infertile patients, oocytes were retrieved in 17 (57%) of the patients [10]. The authors noted that extensive pelvic adhesions did not impede the procedure and that the technique was atraumatic, inexpensive, and time efficient for retrieving oocytes [10]. Gleicher and colleagues [11] as well as Dellenbach and colleagues advanced the work of Lenz and developed a transvaginal ultrasound-guided oocyte retrieval (TVOR) technique [12, 13]. In this technique, ovarian follicles were aspirated under local anesthesia by passing the retrieval needle through the posterior fornix into the cul-de-sac and the ovary [13]. Furthermore, this technique could be performed in an outpatient setting without general anesthesia. Following a report of at least 100 oocyte retrievals using this technique and subsequent live births [13], there was an almost immediate shift from the laparoscopic route to the transvaginal ultrasound-guided route. As of 2021, TVOR is considered the standard of care across IVF centers worldwide. Most centers use a high-frequency transvaginal ultrasonographic trans-

ducer laden with a needle sheath that is used to visualize the ovaries. A 30-cm, 16-G, single-lumen or double-lumen aspiration needle is used to puncture the ovarian follicles using the needle sheath as a guide [14, 15]. A constant pressure of 80–100 mm Hg assists in the collection follicular fluid [14, 15].

Complications of Oocyte Retrieval

Complications associated with early oocyte retrieval attempts, especially via laparotomy or laparoscopy, were due to underlying pelvic adhesive pathology. However, developments in ultrasound technology, anesthetics, anti-microbial prophylaxis, and retrieval needles have simplified the technique for TVOR. Furthermore, these advancements have improved the overall safety and efficacy of oocyte retrieval for IVF. For example, a retrospective study of almost six million ART cycles occurring in Europe between 1997 and 2011 reported a complication rate of less than 0.5% associated with TVOR [16]. Despite the reassuring safety profile of oocyte retrievals, occasional complications may occur and are discussed in the following sections and summarized in Table 23.1.

Most complications associated with TVOR are caused by iatrogenic trauma to ovarian vessels, pelvic organs, or vasculature from the oocyte aspiration needle [17]. One of the earliest retrospective studies of 647 patients undergoing TVOR reported that 10 (1.5%) patients required hospital admission due to perioperative complications [18]. Specifically, nine patients required intravenous (IV) antibiotic therapy, and one required inpatient observation for an expanding broad ligament hematoma [18]. The study concluded that a history of prior pelvic inflammatory disease and/or adnexal adhesions predisposes patients to TVOR-associated perioperative complications. A subsequent larger study of 23,827 oocyte retrievals [17] supported the overall safety of TVOR with a total of 96 complications associated with the procedure. Patients with complications were more likely to be younger, have a lower body mass index (BMI), have a longer pro-

Table 23.1 Summary of common complications associated with oocyte retrieval as reported in the medical literature

Complication type	Incidence	Management/treatment
Bleeding complications		
Vaginal bleeding	0.008–18.1%	Local compression of the laceration site or an interrupted suture
Intra-abdominal bleeding	0.06–0.36%	Expectant management for mild-to-moderate hemoperitoneum Laparoscopy, laparotomy, and/or blood product replacement for severe hemoperitoneum
Injuries to urinary tract		
Bladder injuries	0.008%	Managed expectantly or occasionally with bladder irrigation and cystoscopy
Ureteral injuries	Limited to case reports	Early ureteral stenting
Infectious complications		
Pelvic inflammatory disease/tubo-ovarian abscess	0.003–0.04%	Intravenous antibiotics or surgical drainage
Pain and anesthesia complications		
Pain	0.03–6.9%	Oral analgesia or intravenous analgesia should be considered in patients with high oocyte yield
Anesthesia complications	0.05–0.36%	Intraoperative conversion to laryngeal mask airway or an oral/nasal airway

cedural time, and have a higher number of oocytes retrieved when compared to patients without complications. Surgeon experience was also identified as a possible risk factor for TVOR-related complications, with the incidence of complications being significantly reduced after 250 procedures.

Bleeding Associated with Oocyte Retrieval

Bleeding Complications

Bleeding due to TVOR could be at the vaginal puncture site or within the abdomen. Isolated vaginal lacerations or vaginal bleeding without concomitant abdominal bleeding may occur in 0.008–18.1% of patients [17, 19–21]. The wide range is likely due to the difference in the definition of clinically pertinent vaginal bleeding after TVOR at different centers. In most cases, local compression of the laceration site or an interrupted suture is sufficient to achieve hemostasis. Large vaginal hematomas can occur very rarely after TVOR [23].

In contrast, intra-abdominal bleeding after TVOR occurs in approximately 0.06–0.36% of cases but can be a more serious complication [21, 24]. Such bleeding usually occurs due to puncture of the ovarian follicles and ovarian vessels or, more rarely, due to direct injury to the pelvic organs [17]. In a study of 10,251 retrieval cycles, Zhen and colleagues [24] identified 22 (0.2%) patients with intraperitoneal bleeding. Five (0.05%) patients with severe bleeding required laparotomy or laparoscopy, while the remaining 17 patients were managed conservatively. Independent studies [17, 22] have confirmed that mild-to-moderate hemoperitoneum (<200 mL blood), especially in clinically stable patients, can be managed expectantly. Figures 23.1 and 23.2 show mild-to-moderate hemoperitoneum within 24–48 h of an oocyte retrieval.

Studies have suggested that severe hemoperitoneum can be identified in 30% of patients within 1 h and 90% of patients within 24 h of TVOR [25]. Patients with severe hemoperitoneum or those with clinical symptoms such as abdominal distention, guarding, or orthostatic hypotension require prompt surgical evaluation and blood product replacement [26–28]. A longer

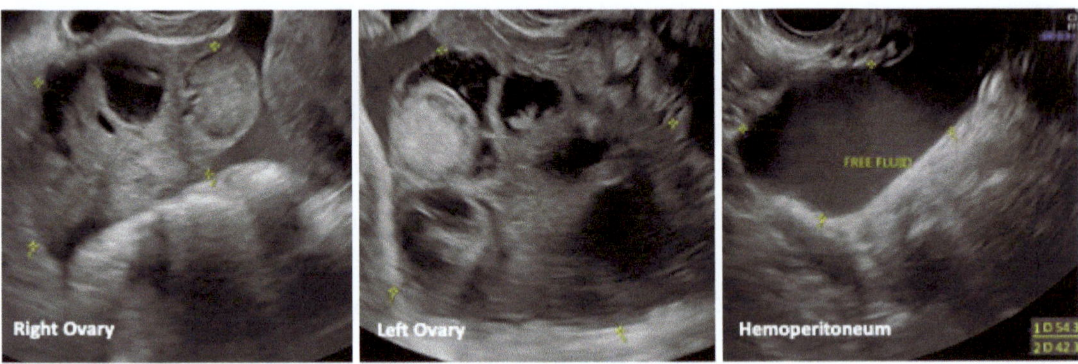

Fig. 23.1 Mild-to-moderate hemoperitoneum, especially pronounced in the posterior cul-de-sac 48 h after TVOR. A total of 13 oocytes were retrieved in this patient

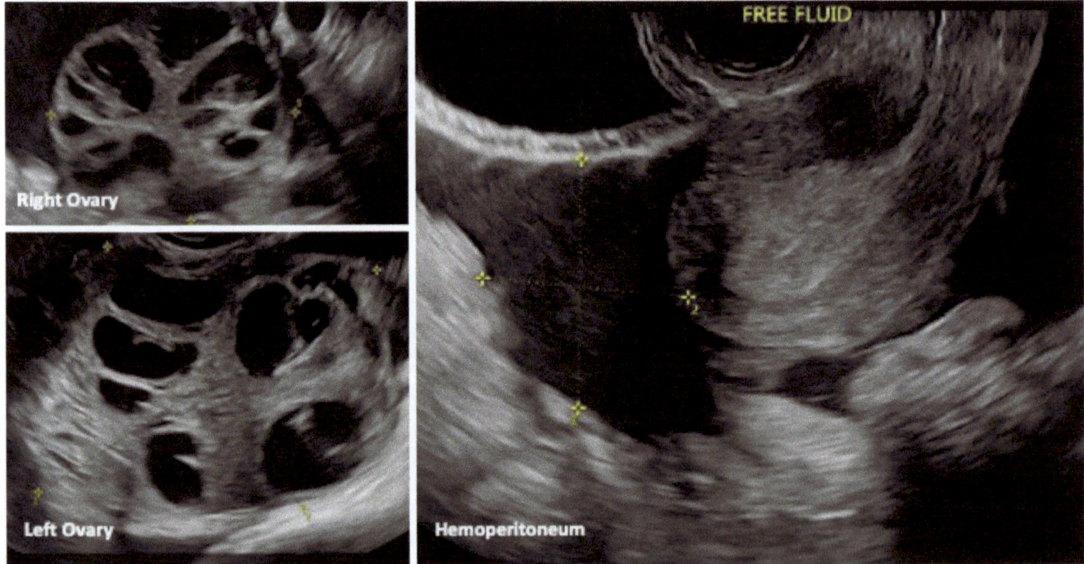

Fig. 23.2 Mild-to-moderate hemoperitoneum in the anterior and posterior cul-de-sac 24 h after TVOR. A total of 16 oocytes were retrieved in this patient

time interval between TVOR and surgical intervention has been associated with an increased risk of oophorectomy [25]. Angiographic embolization has been utilized for the management of some cases of severe hemoperitoneum after oocyte retrieval [29]. Patients with underlying coagulation disorders can have a higher risk of intra-abdominal bleeding with TVOR [30–32], and such patients may present with delayed hemoperitoneum [31].

Direct vascular injury to the iliac blood vessels is exceptionally rare during TVOR, despite its close proximity to the ovaries. Levi-Setti and colleagues reported only 1 patient out of 23,827 oocyte retrievals requiring emergent laparotomy to repair a small laceration of the iliac vein [17]. Direct injury to the iliac blood vessels may result in pseudoaneurysms when extravasated blood is walled off by the surrounding layers of the connective tissue [33, 34].

Minimizing Bleeding Complications

Experts have suggested that the transvaginal ultrasonographic probe should be well applied to the vaginal wall in order to reduce the space between the ovarian cortex and vaginal walls [35]. This avoids any intervening bowel loops or blood vessels, thereby reducing the risk of bleeding. They also recommend maintaining the needle within the ovary to avoid repetitive vaginal and ovarian punctures [35]. Aspiration of multiple follicles through the same ovarian cortex puncture should also be attempted [35]. Finally, manipulation of the retrieval needle should be performed in a steady and gentle manner, avoiding abrupt movements as much as possible [35].

Urinary Tract Injuries

Bladder Injuries

The anatomical location of the bladder and its close relationship to the vaginal puncture sight increases the risk of needle-associated injury, especially when the pressure exerted by the transvaginal ultrasound probe causes the walls of the bladder to collapse, thereby limiting visualization of the bladder [36]. With an estimated incidence of appoximately 0.008%, bladder injuries during TVOR occur less often than bleeding complications do [17]. Needle injuries to the bladder may result in transient macroscopic hematuria [36, 37] or bladder hematoma formation [38, 39], which can be managed expectantly or occasionally with bladder irrigation and cystoscopy. Massive hematuria with hemodynamic instability [40] or vesicovaginal fistula formation [41] may occur in exceptionally rare cases after TVOR.

Ureteral Injuries

Injuries to the ureters occur less frequently than bladder injuries and are mostly limited to case reports [42–48]. A history of endometriosis, prior abdominal surgery, pelvic inflammatory disease (PID), or anatomical anomalies of the urinary tract may increase the risk of iatrogenic ureteral injury during TVOR [43]. Ureteral injuries may present with immediate or delayed clinical symptoms such as abdominal, suprapubic, or flank pain, urinary retention or urgency, fevers, chills, nausea, and vomiting [43]. Early diagnosis of ureteral injury is imperative. In such cases, ureteral stenting serves as an effective therapeutic option, thereby avoiding the formation of a fistulous tract [43, 49, 50]. A delay in the recognition of ureteral injuries may result in urinary obstruction or renal dysfunction, ultimately requiring nephrostomy, ureteric re-implantation, or even nephrectomy [43, 44].

Minimizing Injuries to the Urinary Tract

A full bladder can distort uterine anatomy and may increase the distance between the ovaries and vaginal fornices [35]. Thus, patients should be encouraged to empty their bladders completely prior to TVOR to minimize urinary injuries [35]. Drainage of urine with a straight catheter is reasonable if the bladder does not appear empty at the time of placement of the transvaginal ultrasonographic probe.

Infectious Complications

Pelvic Infections

In principle, pelvic infections due to TVOR occur due to the inoculation of pathogenic bacteria into the intraperitoneal space. This may occur due to the introduction of vaginal bacteria during vaginal puncture or due to the un-intentional puncture of a bowel loop, hydrosalpinx, or endometrioma during TVOR [35, 51]. Re-activation of latent pelvic infections may also occur [35]. Several prior studies have noted that pelvic infections after TVOR are most likely to occur in women with prior history of pelvic inflammatory disease (PID), history of endometriosis, or history of pelvic surgery [17–22].

Levi-Setti and colleagues reported ten (0.04%) cases of infectious complications in their large study of 23,827 oocyte retrievals [17]. Six patients required inpatient hospitalization for

TVOR-related PID, while three with tubo-ovarian abscess (TOA) required surgical treatment [17]. Of note, the hospital stay was the longest for these six patients with PID, when compared to all other complications in this large study. In a different study, Aragona and colleagues reported two (0.003%) cases of ovarian abscess in a cohort of 7098 IVF cycles [24]. Both patients were treated with surgery – one required oophorectomy, and the other was treated with drainage of the abscess. Most data suggest that the majority of patients with TVOR-related PID have indolent symptoms and can be treated with IV antibiotics [17, 18, 35]; however, occasionally patients can present with persistently high fevers or tachycardia, peritonitis, and septic shock, which warrants immediate surgical attention [18, 52]. Rare cases of PID due to pelvic tuberculosis or actinomycosis after TVOR have been reported [53–55]. Even rarer cases of spondylodiscitis or vertebral osteomyelitis due to TVOR have been published in the medical literature [56, 57].

At least one study has suggested that pelvic infection after TVOR may have a detrimental effect on IVF implantation rates [58]. Thus, postponement of embryo transfer should be considered when post-TVOR PID is suspected [58]. PID and TOA have been reported well after embryo transfer and the establishment of an early pregnancy [59–65]. In such cases, TOAs may rupture [59, 60], necessitating urgent treatment in order to avoid adverse perinatal outcomes. It is interesting to note that the incidence of PID and TOA is much lower in the oocyte donors when compared to the infertile patient population, likely due to the lack of risk factors such as PID, endometriosis, or pelvic surgery [26].

Endometriomas and Pelvic Infections

The excision of endometriomas prior to IVF remains controversial [66, 67]. It is postulated that the contents of an endometrioma may serve as an excellent culture medium for the inoculation of bacteria and the spread of a pelvic infection [68]. Furthermore, the presence of an endometrioma may be detrimental to developing oocytes and distort ovarian anatomy, thereby impeding access to ovarian follicles during TVOR and increasing the risks of un-intentional endometrioma puncture. These concerns have been exemplified by independent investigators who have reported an increased risk of PID or TOA after TVOR in patients with endometriomas [69–71]. However, more recent data have assuaged these concerns pertaining to endometriomas. First, TOAs can occur spontaneously in women with endometriomas and no prior history TVOR or IVF [72]. Therefore, it is possible that the perceived increased risk of infectious complications in women with endometriomas undergoing IVF is not linked to IVF per se but rather sporadic occurrences related to endometriomas themselves [72]. Second, oocytes exposed to endometrioma fluid have similar fertilization, early embryo development, and pregnancy rates when compared to control oocytes [73, 74]. Finally, while TVOR may be technically challenging in patients with multiple or large endometriomas, the magnitude of these difficulties is modest at best [75]. Figure 23.3 shows an intrauterine pregnancy at 9 weeks after transfer of a single fresh blastocyst in a patient with a 4-cm left ovarian endometrioma.

Hydrosalpinges and Pelvic Infections

The presence of hydrosalpinges can have a detrimental effect of IVF outcomes due to the suspected embryotoxicity of the hydrosalpinx fluid [76, 77]. Thus, treatment of hydrosalpinges prior to IVF and embryo transfer is generally recommended [76–79]. Management via salpingectomy [79, 80], ultrasonographic fluid aspiration [78, 80], or ultrasonographic sclerotherapy has been described [81]. Some data have suggested that ultrasonographic aspiration or sclerotherapy may be associated with rapid re-accumulation of hydrosalpinx fluid and therefore negates any beneficial effects [80]. Hydrosalpinges resulting from prior PID or pelvic surgeries confer a higher risk of post-TVOR pelvic infections, especially when un-intentional rupture of a hydrosalpinx occurs [17, 35].

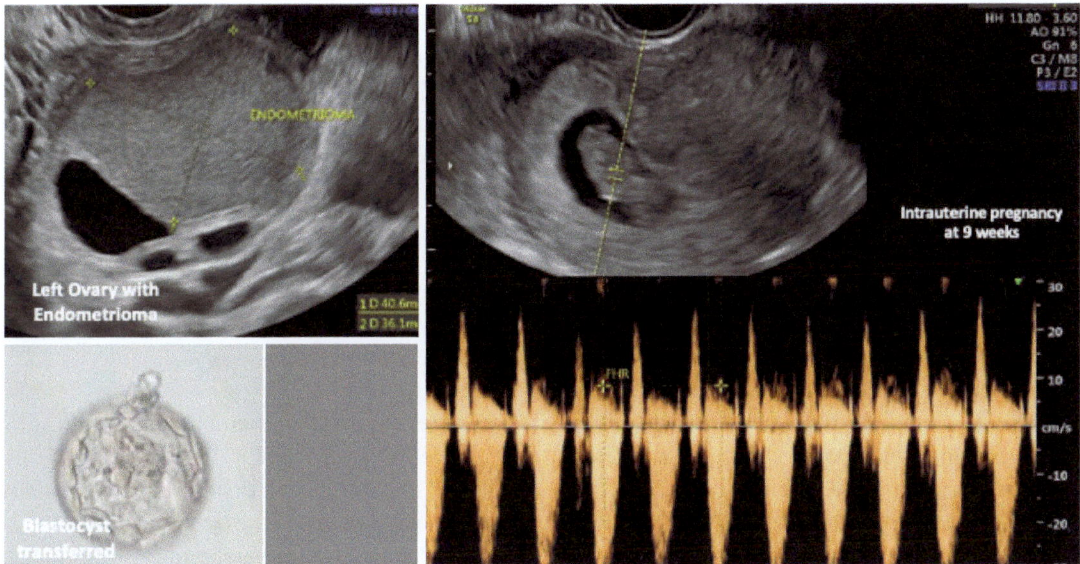

Fig. 23.3 An early intrauterine pregnancy at 9 weeks of gestational age after transfer of a single blastocyst in a patient with left ovarian endometrioma

Minimizing Infectious Complications

Prepping of the vagina, cervix, and perineum should be considered prior to TVOR with povidone-iodine or hexachlorophene solution and copious irrigation with sterile saline solution [14, 15, 35]. This approach minimizes bacterial contamination of the vagina [35]. Patients with history of endometriosis, PID, pelvic adhesions, previous pelvic surgery, or ruptured appendicitis can be considered at high risk for pelvic infection [14, 15, 35]. Administration of IV antibiotics should be considered shortly before or during TVOR in such patients and can include IV cephalosporins or oral doxycycline [35]. It is important to note that prospective trials are currently lacking to validate the generalizability or superiority of prophylactic antibiotic regimens in patients considered high risk for pelvic infection [15]. Pelvic infections after TVOR may still occur despite adequate antibiotic prophylaxis [70].

Pain and Anesthesia Complications

One of the major advantages of TVOR over earlier retrieval techniques was that the former resulted in less pain, especially when combined with conscious sedation or local anesthesia [82]. Despite adequate anesthesia, women undergoing TVOR may still experience pain. For example, 51 (6.9%) of women undergoing their first IVF cycle reported the oocyte retrieval to be very or extremely painful [83]. Bodri and colleagues reported two (0.05%) cases of severe pain in a cohort of oocyte donors undergoing 4052 oocyte retrievals [26]. In a prospective study of 1058 oocyte retrievals, Ludwig and colleagues reported that 3% of all patients experienced severe to very severe pain after TVOR, which continued in 2% of patients 2 days after TVOR [19]. Approximately, 0.7% patients required inpatient hospitalization of the management of this pain [19]. Levi-Setti and colleagues reported six (0.03%) cases of isolated pelvic pain in their study, all of whom required hospitalization [17]. Most studies suggest that pain after TVOR is increased with the number of oocytes retrieved [17, 19]. Other studies have proposed that prior negative gynecological experiences or ongoing side effects during ovarian stimulation may be predictors of pain after oocyte retrieval [83].

A wide variety of anesthesia and analgesia protocols are available to women undergoing TVOR [82, 84–86]. There is no current evidence to recommend the avoidance of any technique or drug for TVOR, especially given the high degree of patient satisfaction with most protocols [82, 86]. Recent data indicate that 84% and 95% of clinics in the UK and USA, respectively, utilize conscious sedation [82]. Currently, most centers may use a combination of propofol, fentanyl, and midazolam for TVOR [87]. This combination is easy to administer and safe in cooperative and healthy individuals [87]. However, anesthesia and analgesia protocols should be individualized to a woman's preference and local availability of certain medications [82, 86]. Anesthesia complications are relatively infrequent and may include bronchospasm (0.36%) [21] or circulatory shock and nausea (0.05%) [17]. Serious complications such as atrial fibrillation, or cardiorespiratory insufficiency, agitation, and confusion may occur rarely [17]. Obese patients generally require higher doses of propofol and fentanyl and may have longer oocyte retrievals [88, 89]. They may also require intraoperative conversion to laryngeal mask airway or an oral/nasal airway [88, 89]. However, serious intraoperative and postoperative anesthesia complications remain uncommon even in obese individuals [88, 89].

Minimizing Pain and Anesthesia Complications

Gentle manipulation of the retrieval needle should be performed during TVOR, with avoidance of sudden lateral movements [33]. Multiple punctures of the vaginal wall and ovaries should be avoided [33]. Post-TVOR oral analgesia or IV analgesia should be considered in patients with high oocyte yield [33]. Recent studies have also demonstrated that adjuncts such as music or acupuncture may reduce the risk of pain after TVOR [90, 91]. The use of an aspiration needle with smaller gauge can also result in significantly lower pain scores during oocyte retrieval [92]. Postoperative IV ketorolac has been found to decrease the amount of postoperative opioid use following TVOR [93]. This retrospective study found no increase in complication rates, includ-

ing bleeding, in the group that received ketorolac though the overall prevalence of complication was low. This agrees with prior investigations which demonstrated lower pain scores in those who receive ketorolac and no significant difference in pregnancy rates or live birth outcomes with its use [94].

Special Circumstances

At times, the stimulated ovaries may not be accessible via the transvaginal route. This may occur due to the distortion of pelvic anatomy by enlarged myomatous uteri or pelvic adhesions [95, 96]. Women with ovarian transposition surgery, Müllerian anomalies, or obesity may also have ovaries that are difficult to access transvaginally [95, 96]. In such cases, transabdominal oocyte retrieval or a combined transvaginal and transabdominal route may be used, yielding good oocyte numbers [96]. Transabdominal oocyte retrieval may be the route of choice in transgender patient or virginal women. A study by Roman-Rodriguez and colleagues [95] compared 95 cases of transabdominal oocyte retrieval with 278 cases of transvaginal oocyte retrieval and found no statistical difference in pregnancy rates or complications between the two modalities. Furthermore, there was no difference in intraoperative complications, postoperative pain, hospital admissions, or post-retrieval infections requiring antibiotics. There was no evidence for increased abdominal pain, pelvic inflammatory disease, hemoperitoneum, urinary tract infections, or transient macroscopic hematuria. Despite the noted safety of transabdominal oocyte retrieval, providers should account for increased procedure and anesthesia time associated with transabdominal oocyte retrieval. Ex vivo or extracorporeal retrieval of mature oocytes from oophorectomized specimens has been described in patients with ovarian cancer [97, 98]. By avoiding follicular puncture within the pelvic cavity, ex vivo oocyte retrieval minimizes the risk of malignant cell spillage and cancer upstaging [97].

Conclusion

TVOR remains a vital step in the IVF process. While most oocyte retrievals are performed without event, occasional minor and major complications may occur. Most complications can be managed in the outpatient setting; however, certain potentially life-threatening complications require inpatient treatment or immediate surgical treatment. The European Society of Human Reproduction and Embryology (ESHRE) has provided several good practice recommendations to avoid complications during TVOR [35]. While most strategies to prevent complications have focused on technical considerations and infection prevention, future efforts are aimed at surgical training and achieving adequate competence [35].

References

1. ART Fact Sheet 2020 – ESHRE.
2. Rock J, Menkin MF. In vitro fertilization and cleavage of human ovarian eggs. Science. 1944;100(2588):105–7.
3. Menkin MF, Rock J. In vitro fertilization and cleavage of human ovarian eggs. Am J Obstet Gynecol. 1948;55(3):440–52.
4. Steptoe PC. Laparoscopy and ovulation. Lancet. 1968;2(7574):913.
5. Edwards RG. Tribute to Patrick Steptoe: beginnings of laparoscopy. Hum Reprod. 1989;4(8 Suppl):1–9.
6. Steptoe PC, Edwards RG. Birth after the reimplantation of a human embryo. Lancet. 1978;2(8085):366.
7. Edwards RG, Steptoe PC, Purdy JM. Establishing full-term human pregnancies using cleaving embryos grown in vitro. Br J Obstet Gynaecol. 1980;87(9):737–56.
8. Fishel SB, Edwards RG, Purdy JM, Steptoe PC, Webster J, Walters E, Cohen J, Fehilly C, Hewitt J, Rowland G. Implantation, abortion, and birth after in vitro fertilization using the natural menstrual cycle or follicular stimulation with clomiphene citrate and human menopausal gonadotropin. J In Vitro Fert Embryo Transf. 1985;2(3):123–31.
9. Lenz S, Lauritsen JG, Kjellow M. Collection of human oocytes for in vitro fertilisation by ultrasonically guided follicular puncture. Lancet. 1981;1(8230):1163–4.
10. Lenz S, Lauritsen JG. Ultrasonically guided percutaneous aspiration of human follicles under local anesthesia: a new method of collecting oocytes for in vitro fertilization. Fertil Steril. 1982;38(6):673–7.
11. Gleicher N, Friberg J, Fullan N, Giglia RV, Mayden K, Kesky T, Siegel I. EGG retrieval for in vitro fertilisation by sonographically controlled vaginal culdocentesis. Lancet. 1983;2(8348):508–9.
12. Dellenbach P, Nisand I, Moreau L, Feger B, Plumere C, Gerlinger P, Brun B, Rumpler Y. Transvaginal, sonographically controlled ovarian follicle puncture for egg retrieval. Lancet. 1984;1(8392):1467.
13. Dellenbach P, Nisand I, Moreau L, Feger B, Plumere C, Gerlinger P. Transvaginal sonographically controlled follicle puncture for oocyte retrieval. Fertil Steril. 1985;44(5):656–62.
14. Huang JY, Rosenwaks Z. Assisted reproductive techniques. Methods Mol Biol. 2014;1154:171–231.
15. Pereira N, Hutchinson AP, Lekovich JP, Hobeika E, Elias RT. Antibiotic prophylaxis for gynecologic procedures prior to and during the utilization of assisted reproductive technologies: a systematic review. J Pathog. 2016;2016:4698314.
16. Ferraretti AP, Nygren K, Andersen AN, de Mouzon J, Kupka M, Calhaz-Jorge C, Wyns C, Gianaroli L, Goossens V, European IVF-Monitoring Consortium (EIM), for the European Society of Human Reproduction and Embryology (ESHRE). Trends over 15 years in ART in Europe: an analysis of 6 million cycles. Hum Reprod Open. 2017;2017(2):hox012.
17. Levi-Setti PE, Cirillo F, Scolaro V, Morenghi E, Heilbron F, Girardello D, Zannoni E, Patrizio P. Appraisal of clinical complications after 23,827 oocyte retrievals in a large assisted reproductive technology program. Fertil Steril. 2018;109(6):1038–1043.e1.
18. Tureck RW, García CR, Blasco L, Mastroianni L Jr. Perioperative complications arising after transvaginal oocyte retrieval. Obstet Gynecol. 1993;81(4):590–3.
19. Ludwig AK, Glawatz M, Griesinger G, Diedrich K, Ludwig M. Perioperative and post-operative complications of transvaginal ultrasound-guided oocyte retrieval: prospective study of >1000 oocyte retrievals. Hum Reprod. 2006;21(12):3235–40.
20. Bennett SJ, Waterstone JJ, Cheng WC, Parsons J. Complications of transvaginal ultrasound-directed follicle aspiration: a review of 2670 consecutive procedures. J Assist Reprod Genet. 1993;10(1):72–7.
21. Siristatidis C, Chrelias C, Alexiou A, Kassanos D. Clinical complications after transvaginal oocyte retrieval: a retrospective analysis. J Obstet Gynaecol. 2013;33(1):64–6.
22. Aragona C, Mohamed MA, Espinola MS, Linari A, Pecorini F, Micara G, Sbracia M. Clinical complications after transvaginal oocyte retrieval in 7,098 IVF cycles. Fertil Steril. 2011;95(1):293–4.
23. Wais M, Chan C. Massive vaginal hematoma – a complication of in vitro fertilization. J Obstet Gynaecol Can. 2018;40(1):72–4.
24. Zhen X, Qiao J, Ma C, Fan Y, Liu P. Intraperitoneal bleeding following transvaginal oocyte retrieval. Int J Gynaecol Obstet. 2010;108(1):31–4.
25. Nouri K, Walch K, Promberger R, Kurz C, Tempfer CB, Ott J. Severe haematoperitoneum caused by

ovarian bleeding after transvaginal oocyte retrieval: a retrospective analysis and systematic literature review. Reprod Biomed Online. 2014;29(6):699–707.

26. Bodri D, Guillén JJ, Polo A, Trullenque M, Esteve C, Coll O. Complications related to ovarian stimulation and oocyte retrieval in 4052 oocyte donor cycles. Reprod Biomed Online. 2008;17(2):237–43.

27. Bandyopadhyay S, Kay V. A rare case of rupture of ovary causing haemorrhagic shock following uncomplicated oocyte retrieval--a case report. Hum Fertil (Camb). 2010;13(2):105–6.

28. Ragni G, Scarduelli C, Calanna G, Santi G, Benaglia L, Somigliana E. Blood loss during transvaginal oocyte retrieval. Gynecol Obstet Investig. 2009;67(1):32–5.

29. Kart C, Guven S, Aran T, Dinc H. Life-threatening intraabdominal bleeding after oocyte retrieval successfully managed with angiographic embolization. Fertil Steril. 2011;96(2):e99–e102.

30. Revel A, Schejter-Dinur Y, Yahalomi SZ, Simon A, Zelig O, Revel-Vilk S. Is routine screening needed for coagulation abnormalities before oocyte retrieval? Fertil Steril. 2011;95(3):1182–4.

31. Mashiach R, Stockheim D, Zolti M, Orvieto R. Delayed intra-abdominal bleeding following trans-vaginal ultrasonography guided oocyte retrieval for in vitro fertilization in patients at risk for thrombo-embolic events under anticoagulant therapy. F1000Res. 2013;2:189.

32. El-Shawarby SA, Margara RA, Trew GH, Laffan MA, Lavery SA. Thrombocythemia and hemoperitoneum after transvaginal oocyte retrieval for in vitro fertilization. Fertil Steril. 2004;82(3):735–7.

33. Pappin C, Plant G. A pelvic pseudoaneurysm (a rare complication of oocyte retrieval for IVF) treated by arterial embolization. Hum Fertil (Camb). 2006;9(3):153–5.

34. Bozdag G, Basaran A, Cil B, Esinler I, Yarali H. An oocyte pick-up procedure complicated with pseudoaneurysm of the internal iliac artery. Fertil Steril. 2008;90(5):2004.e11–3.

35. ESHRE Working Group on Ultrasound in ART, D'Angelo A, Panayotidis C, Amso N, Marci R, Matorras R, Onofriescu M, Turp AB, Vandekerckhove F, Veleva Z, Vermeulen N, Vlaisavljevic V. Recommendations for good practice in ultrasound: oocyte pick up †. Hum Reprod Open. 2019;2019(4):hoz025.

36. Souza MDCB, Souza MM, Antunes RA, Tamm MA, Silva JBD, Mancebo ACA. Bladder hematoma: a complication from an oocyte retrieval procedure. JBRA Assist Reprod. 2019;23(1):75–8.

37. Ashkenazi J, Ben David M, Feldberg D, Shelef M, Dicker D, Goldman JA. Abdominal complications following ultrasonically guided percutaneous transvesical collection of oocytes for in vitro fertilization. J In Vitro Fert Embryo Transf. 1987;4(6):316–8.

38. Modder J, Kettel LM, Sakamoto K. Hematuria and clot retention after transvaginal oocyte aspiration: a case report. Fertil Steril. 2006;86(3):720.e1–2.

39. Su YT, Huang KH, Chuang FC, Lan KC. Use of an Ellik evacuator to remove tenacious bladder clots resulting from transvaginal oocyte retrieval: 2 cases and a literature review. Taiwan J Obstet Gynecol. 2019;58(6):880–4.

40. Jayakrishnan K, Raman VK, Vijayalakshmi VK, Baheti S, Nambiar D. Massive hematuria with hemodynamic instability--complication of oocyte retrieval. Fertil Steril. 2011;96(1):e22–4.

41. Al-Shaikh GK, Abotalib ZM. Vesicovaginal fistula formation after oocyte retrieval. Taiwan J Obstet Gynecol. 2013;52(4):597–8.

42. Burnik Papler T, Vrtačnik Bokal E, Šalamun V, Galič D, Smrkolj T, Jančar N. Ureteral injury with delayed massive hematuria after transvaginal ultrasound-guided oocyte retrieval. Case Rep Obstet Gynecol. 2015;2015:760805.

43. Vilos AG, Feyles V, Vilos GA, Oraif A, Abdul-Jabbar H, Power N. Ureteric injury during transvaginal ultrasound guided oocyte retrieval. J Obstet Gynaecol Can. 2015;37(1):52–5.

44. Grynberg M, Berwanger AL, Toledano M, Frydman R, Deffieux X, Fanchin R. Ureteral injury after transvaginal ultrasound-guided oocyte retrieval: a complication of in vitro fertilization-embryo transfer that may lurk undetected in women presenting with severe ovarian hyperstimulation syndrome. Fertil Steril. 2011;96(4):869–71.

45. Miller PB, Price T, Nichols JE Jr, Hill L. Acute ureteral obstruction following transvaginal oocyte retrieval for IVF. Hum Reprod. 2002;17(1):137–8.

46. Catanzarite T, Bernardi LA, Confino E, Kenton K. Ureteral trauma during transvaginal ultrasound-guided oocyte retrieval: a case report. Female Pelvic Med Reconstr Surg. 2015;21(5):e44–5.

47. Fugita OE, Kavoussi L. Laparoscopic ureteral reimplantation for ureteral lesion secondary to transvaginal ultrasonography for oocyte retrieval. Urology. 2001;58(2):281.

48. Coroleu B, Lopez Mourelle F, Hereter L, Veiga A, Calderón G, Martinez F, Carreras O, Barri PN. Ureteral lesion secondary to vaginal ultrasound follicular puncture for oocyte recovery in in-vitro fertilization. Hum Reprod. 1997;12(5):948–50.

49. Spencer ES, Hoff HS, Steiner AZ, Coward RM. Immediate ureterovaginal fistula following oocyte retrieval: a case and systematic review of the literature. Urol Ann. 2017;9(2):125–30.

50. Mongiu AK, Helfand BT, Kielb SJ. Ureterovaginal fistula formation after oocyte retrieval. Urology. 2009;73(2):444.e1–3.

51. Van Hoorde GJ, Verhoeff A, Zeilmaker GH. Perforated appendicitis following transvaginal oocyte retrieval for in-vitro fertilization and embryo transfer. Hum Reprod. 1992;7(6):850–1.

52. Nikkhah-Abyaneh Z, Khulpateea N, Aslam MF. Pyometra after ovum retrieval for in vitro fertilization resulting in hysterectomy. Fertil Steril. 2010;93(1):268.e1–2.

53. Annamraju H, Ganapathy R, Webb B. Pelvic tuberculosis reactivated by in vitro fertilization egg collection? Fertil Steril. 2008;90(5):2003.e1–3.
54. Asemota OA, Girda E, Dueñas O, Neal-Perry G, Pollack SE. Actinomycosis pelvic abscess after in vitro fertilization. Fertil Steril. 2013;100(2):408–11.
55. Van Hoecke F, Beuckelaers E, Lissens P, Boudewijns M. Actinomyces urogenitalis bacteremia and tuboovarian abscess after an in vitro fertilization (IVF) procedure. J Clin Microbiol. 2013;51(12):4252–4.
56. Debusscher F, Troussel S, Van Innis F, Holemans X. Spondylodiscitis after transvaginal oocyte retrieval for in vitro fertilisation. Acta Orthop Belg. 2005;71(2):249–51.
57. Almog B, Rimon E, Yovel I, Bar-Am A, Amit A, Azem F. Vertebral osteomyelitis: a rare complication of transvaginal ultrasound-guided oocyte retrieval. Fertil Steril. 2000;73(6):1250–2.
58. Ashkenazi J, Farhi J, Dicker D, Feldberg D, Shalev J, Ben-Rafael Z. Acute pelvic inflammatory disease after oocyte retrieval: adverse effects on the results of implantation. Fertil Steril. 1994;61(3):526–8.
59. Han C, Wang C, Liu XJ, Geng N, Wang YM, Fan AP, Yuan BB, Xue FX. In vitro fertilization complicated by rupture of tubo-ovarian abscess during pregnancy. Taiwan J Obstet Gynecol. 2015;54(5):612–6.
60. Varras M, Polyzos D, Tsikini A, Antypa E, Apessou D, Tsouroulas M. Ruptured tubo-ovarian abscess as a complication of IVF treatment: clinical, ultrasonographic and histopathologic findings. A case report. Clin Exp Obstet Gynecol. 2003;30(2–3):164–8.
61. den Boon J, Kimmel CE, Nagel HT, van Roosmalen J. Pelvic abscess in the second half of pregnancy after oocyte retrieval for in-vitro fertilization: case report. Hum Reprod. 1999;14(9):2402–3.
62. Matsunaga Y, Fukushima K, Nozaki M, Nakanami N, Kawano Y, Shigematsu T, Satoh S, Nakano H. A case of pregnancy complicated by the development of a tubo-ovarian abscess following in vitro fertilization and embryo transfer. Am J Perinatol. 2003;20(6):277–82.
63. Yalcinkaya TM, Erman-Akar M, Jennell J. Term delivery following transvaginal drainage of bilateral ovarian abscesses after oocyte retrieval: a case report. J Reprod Med. 2011;56(1–2):87–90.
64. Patounakis G, Krauss K, Nicholas SS, Baxter JK, Rosenblum NG, Berghella V. Development of pelvic abscess during pregnancy following transvaginal oocyte retrieval and in vitro fertilization. Eur J Obstet Gynecol Reprod Biol. 2012;164(1):116–7.
65. Sharpe K, Karovitch AJ, Claman P, Suh KN. Transvaginal oocyte retrieval for in vitro fertilization complicated by ovarian abscess during pregnancy. Fertil Steril. 2006;86(1):219.e11–3.
66. Somigliana E, Vercellini P, Viganó P, Ragni G, Crosignani PG. Should endometriomas be treated before IVF-ICSI cycles? Hum Reprod Update. 2006;12(1):57–64.
67. Practice Committee of the American Society for Reproductive Medicine. Endometriosis and infertility: a committee opinion. Fertil Steril. 2012;98(3):591–8.
68. Benaglia L, Somigliana E, Iemmello R, Colpi E, Nicolosi AE, Ragni G. Endometrioma and oocyte retrieval-induced pelvic abscess: a clinical concern or an exceptional complication? Fertil Steril. 2008;89(5):1263–6.
69. Moini A, Riazi K, Amid V, Ashrafi M, Tehraninejad E, Madani T, Owj M. Endometriosis may contribute to oocyte retrieval-induced pelvic inflammatory disease: report of eight cases. J Assist Reprod Genet. 2005;22(7–8):307–9.
70. Romero B, Aibar L, Martínez Navarro L, Fontes J, Calderón MA, Mozas J. Pelvic abscess after oocyte retrieval in women with endometriosis: a case series. Iran J Reprod Med. 2013;11(8):677–80.
71. Padilla SL. Ovarian abscess following puncture of an endometrioma during ultrasound-guided oocyte retrieval. Hum Reprod. 1993;8(8):1282–3.
72. Villette C, Bourret A, Santulli P, Gayet V, Chapron C, de Ziegler D. Risks of tubo-ovarian abscess in cases of endometrioma and assisted reproductive technologies are both under- and overreported. Fertil Steril. 2016;106(2):410–5.
73. Khamsi F, Yavas Y, Lacanna IC, Roberge S, Endman M, Wong JC. Exposure of human oocytes to endometrioma fluid does not alter fertilization or early embryo development. J Assist Reprod Genet. 2001;18(2):106–9.
74. Suzuki T, Izumi S, Matsubayashi H, Awaji H, Yoshikata K, Makino T. Impact of ovarian endometrioma on oocytes and pregnancy outcome in in vitro fertilization. Fertil Steril. 2005;83(4):908–13.
75. Benaglia L, Busnelli A, Biancardi R, Vegetti W, Reschini M, Vercellini P, Somigliana E. Oocyte retrieval difficulties in women with ovarian endometriomas. Reprod Biomed Online. 2018;37(1):77–84.
76. Nackley AC, Muasher SJ. The significance of hydrosalpinx in in vitro fertilization. Fertil Steril. 1998;69(3):373–84.
77. Vandromme J, Chasse E, Lejeune B, Van Rysselberge M, Delvigne A, Leroy F. Hydrosalpinges in in-vitro fertilization: an unfavourable prognostic feature. Hum Reprod. 1995;10(3):576–9.
78. Van Voorhis BJ, Sparks AE, Syrop CH, Stovall DW. Ultrasound-guided aspiration of hydrosalpinges is associated with improved pregnancy and implantation rates after in-vitro fertilization cycles. Hum Reprod. 1998;13(3):736–9.
79. Murray DL, Sagoskin AW, Widra EA, Levy MJ. The adverse effect of hydrosalpinges on in vitro fertilization pregnancy rates and the benefit of surgical correction. Fertil Steril. 1998;69(1):41–5.
80. Fouda UM, Sayed AM, Abdelmoty HI, Elsetohy KA. Ultrasound guided aspiration of hydrosalpinx fluid versus salpingectomy in the management of patients with ultrasound visible hydrosalpinx under-

going IVF-ET: a randomized controlled trial. BMC Womens Health. 2015;15:21.

81. Jiang H, Pei H, Zhang WX, Wang XM. A prospective clinical study of interventional ultrasound sclerotherapy on women with hydrosalpinx before in vitro fertilization and embryo transfer. Fertil Steril. 2010;94(7):2854–6.

82. Kwan I, Wang R, Pearce E, Bhattacharya S. Pain relief for women undergoing oocyte retrieval for assisted reproduction. Cochrane Database Syst Rev. 2018;5(5):CD004829.

83. Frederiksen Y, Mehlsen MY, Matthiesen SM, Zachariae R, Ingerslev HJ. Predictors of pain during oocyte retrieval. J Psychosom Obstet Gynaecol. 2017;38(1):21–9.

84. Roest I, Buisman ETIA, van der Steeg JW, Koks CAM. Different methods of pain relief for IVF and ICSI oocyte retrieval – a Dutch survey. Eur J Obstet Gynecol Reprod Biol X. 2019;4:100065.

85. Rolland L, Perrin J, Villes V, Pellegrin V, Boubli L, Courbiere B. IVF oocyte retrieval: prospective evaluation of the type of anesthesia on live birth rate, pain, and patient satisfaction. J Assist Reprod Genet. 2017;34(11):1523–8.

86. Guasch E, Gómez R, Brogly N, Gilsanz F. Anesthesia and analgesia for transvaginal oocyte retrieval. Should we recommend or avoid any anesthetic drug or technique? Curr Opin Anaesthesiol. 2019;32(3):285–90.

87. Vlahos NF, Giannakikou I, Vlachos A, Vitoratos N. Analgesia and anesthesia for assisted reproductive technologies. Int J Gynaecol Obstet. 2009;105(3):201–5.

88. Egan B, Racowsky C, Hornstein MD, Martin R, Tsen LC. Anesthetic impact of body mass index in patients undergoing assisted reproductive technologies. J Clin Anesth. 2008;20(5):356–63.

89. Romanski PA, Farland LV, Tsen LC, Ginsburg ES, Lewis EI. Effect of class III and class IV obesity on oocyte retrieval complications and outcomes. Fertil Steril. 2019;111(2):294–301.e1.

90. Stener-Victorin E. The pain-relieving effect of electro-acupuncture and conventional medical analgesic methods during oocyte retrieval: a systematic review of randomized controlled trials. Hum Reprod. 2005;20(2):339–49.

91. Cheung CWC, Yee AWW, Chan PS, Saravelos SH, Chung JPW, Cheung LP, Kong GWS, Li TC. The impact of music therapy on pain and stress reduction during oocyte retrieval – a randomized controlled trial. Reprod Biomed Online. 2018;37(2):145–52.

92. Iduna Antigoni Buisman ET, de Bruin JP, Maria Braat DD, van der Steeg JW. Effect of needle diameter on pain during oocyte retrieval-a randomized controlled trial. Fertil Steril. 2021;115(3):683–91.

93. Seidler EA, Vaughan DA, Leung AQ, Sakkas D, Ryley DA, Penzias AS. Routine ketorolac at oocyte retrieval decreases postoperative narcotic use by more than 50%. Fertil Steril Rep. 2021;2(2):156–60. https://doi.org/10.1016/j.xfre.2021.02.003.

94. Mesen TB, Kacemi-Bourhim L, Marshburn PB, Usadi RS, Matthews M, Norton HJ, Hurst BS. The effect of ketorolac on pregnancy rates when used immediately after oocyte retrieval. Fertil Steril. 2013;100(3):725–8.

95. Roman-Rodriguez CF, Weissbrot E, Hsu CD, Wong A, Siefert C, Sung L. Comparing transabdominal and transvaginal ultrasound-guided follicular aspiration: a risk assessment formula. Taiwan J Obstet Gynecol. 2015;54(6):693–9.

96. Barton SE, Politch JA, Benson CB, Ginsburg ES, Gargiulo AR. Transabdominal follicular aspiration for oocyte retrieval in patients with ovaries inaccessible by transvaginal ultrasound. Fertil Steril. 2011;95(5):1773–6.

97. Pereira N, Hubschmann AG, Lekovich JP, Schattman GL, Rosenwaks Z. Ex vivo retrieval and cryopreservation of oocytes from oophorectomized specimens for fertility preservation in a BRCA1 mutation carrier with ovarian cancer. Fertil Steril. 2017;108(2):357–60.

98. Fatemi HM, Kyrou D, Al-Azemi M, Stoop D, De Sutter P, Bourgain C, Devroey P. Ex-vivo oocyte retrieval for fertility preservation. Fertil Steril. 2011;95(5):1787.e15–7.

Reproductive Surgery in Austere Settings

Alfred Murage, Timona Obura, and Joseph Njagi

Introduction

The provision of optimal reproductive health relies on adequate healthcare investments. This must be coupled with relevant healthcare infrastructure, skilled healthcare workers, appropriate medical equipment and supplies and much more. Unfortunately, multiple elements that feed into optimal healthcare are usually lacking in resource-limited settings. This often translates into lack of key health services to deserving poor populations. Minimally invasive reproductive surgery (MIRS) is one such example, which is largely lacking in many resource-poor African countries. Appropriate strategies can be put in place to address gaps in MIRS in resource-poor settings.

A. Murage (✉)
Harley Street Fertility Centre, Nairobi, Kenya
e-mail: amurage@mygyno.co.ke

T. Obura
Department of Obstetrics and Gynecology, Aga Khan University Hospital, Nairobi, Kenya
e-mail: timona.obura@aku.edu

J. Njagi
Department of Obstetrics and Gynecology, PCEA Tumutumu Hospital, Nyeri, Kenya

Kenya as a Case Study in MIRS in Low-Resource Settings

Kenya is located on the eastern coast of Africa. It is categorized by the World Bank as a lower-middle-income country. It has a population of about 51.4 million, a gross national income (GNI) per capita of USD 1620 and a GDP of USD 87.9 billion [1]. Healthcare is poorly funded, with an allocation of 5.1% of the national government budget [2]. This level of healthcare funding is way below the WHO target of 15% budgetary allocation as recommended in 2001 [3]. This translates into poor overall public healthcare systems, as partly evidenced by a very low physician ratio per 1000 people of 0.157 [4]. Public healthcare is supplemented by private healthcare, which is only accessible to a minority of people due to higher out-of-pocket costs and limited health insurance coverage [5].

The fertility rate in Kenya remains high at 3.5 children per woman, as compared to worldwide rates of 2.4 [1]. But there is a high infertility rate as mirrored in other developing countries in Africa and Asia. There are high rates of tubal disease, with some studies reporting rates of up to 50% [6]. This immediately points to preventable factors and accompanying needs for appropriate skills in reproductive tubal surgery. The burden of other pelvic pathologies that requires skills in reproductive surgery includes high prevalence of symptomatic uterine fibroids and endometrial disease (Fig. 24.1a–e showing examples of common pelvic pathology amenable to MIRS). This is in addition to the potential for MIRS in other benign gynaecological conditions.

The availability of MIRS in the public healthcare system in Kenya is dismal. Secondary and tertiary healthcare facilities (Fig. 24.2) have the potential to provide MIRS. Current data suggests

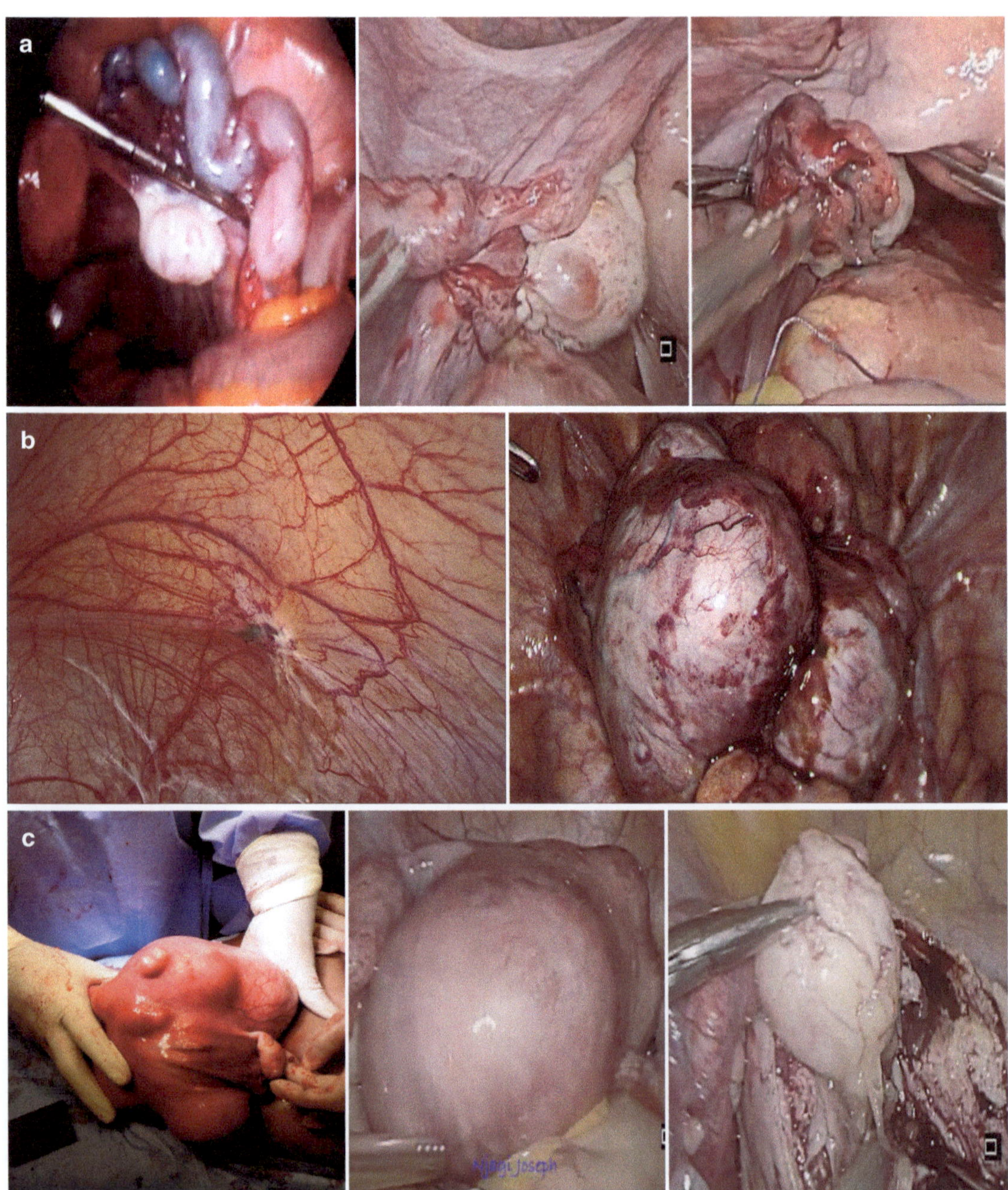

Fig. 24.1 Common pelvic pathologies amenable to MIS in low-resource settings. (**a**) Tubal disease related to infertility (hyrosalpinges, tuboplasty). (**b**) Endometriosis related to infertility/severe pelvic symptoms. (**c**) Symptomatic fibroids. (**d**) Endometrial synechie related to infertility. (**e**) Endometrial polyps and sub-mucus fibroids related to abnormal uterine bleeding/infertility

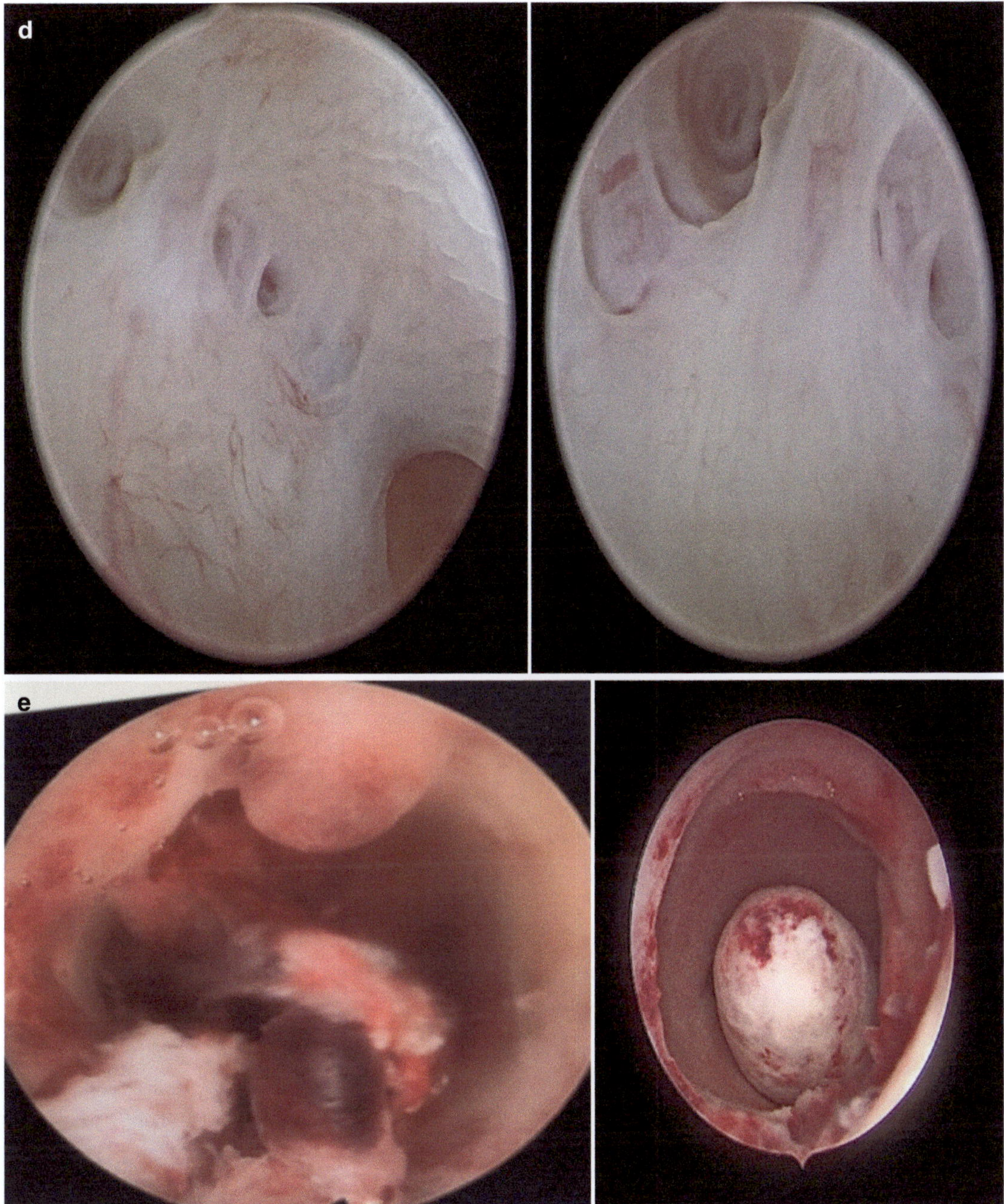

Fig. 24.1 (continued)

that only about 4% of such public healthcare facilities offer some sort of MIRS, though this figure has been reported to be improving ("Personal Communication", Head Division of Referral Services, Ministry of Health Kenya, and Table 24.1) [7]. In comparison, private healthcare facilities are mostly located in urban centres [5], providing up to 10% MIRS procedures ("Personal Communication", Head Division of Referral Services, Ministry of Health Kenya). However

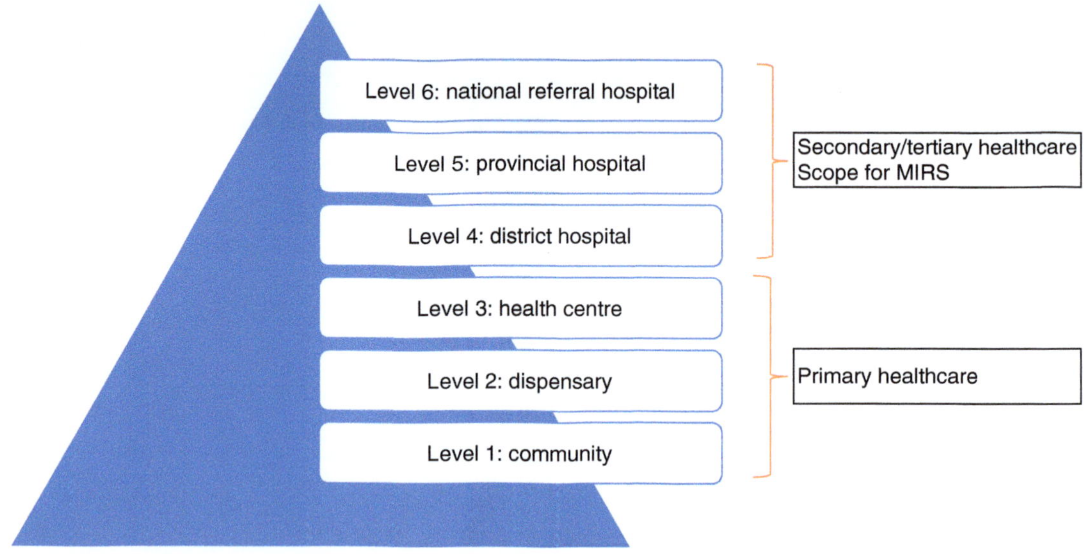

Fig. 24.2 Hierarchy of healthcare delivery in Kenya. (Adapted from Ministry of Health Kenya)

Table 24.1 Status of MIRS in public healthcare in Kenya

Level of service delivery	Number of facilities	MIS availability
Level 4	73	0
Level 5	12	0
Level 6	4	4
Total	89	4.5%

Data analysis from Ref. [7]

private healthcare can only be accessed by a minority of the population, mostly due to higher costs.

Why is there a lower MIRS provision in the public sector? The answer lies partly with overall public healthcare investments. The general infrastructure in public healthcare facilities is lacking. The operating theatres are basic, and the availability of skilled MIRS teams is largely lacking. Surgical operating spaces are constrained, which furthermore must be shared with all other surgical workload within the facilities. MIRS surgical equipment is largely lacking, mandating improvisation and repeated re-use of disposable equipment (Figs. 24.3 and 24.4) including limited access to haemostats for high blood loss procedures such as myomectomy. Additionally, post-surgical recovery areas are not suitable for a high throughput of MIRS workload (Fig. 24.5).

Furthermore, supportive surgical care systems such as haematological services are limited, where severe anaemia is rampant pre-, intra- and post-operatively [8]. Thus, this limits a focus on MIRS.

Currently, the Kenya Society for Endoscopic Specialties (KESES) has about 150 members, and only about 15% are formally trained or skilled in MIRS ("Personal Communication", KESES President). Most of such MIRS experts work primarily in the private sector, leaving the public sector devoid of MIRS expertise. All these factors feed into poor provision of MIRS in the public health sector. Comparatively, the private sector has MIRS multi-disciplinary teams, dedicated MIRS surgical spaces and appropriate availability of MIRS equipment (Fig. 24.6). This opens up the possibilities of partnerships and scales up MIRS skills in the public sector to model the private set-up.

To circumvent the MIRS issues long term, strategies must be identified to remedy the prevailing status of MIRS in low-resource settings. To some extent, this is occurring and includes the ongoing project supported by KESES which is trying to widen the availability of MIRS to rural health facilities and to the wider public sector.

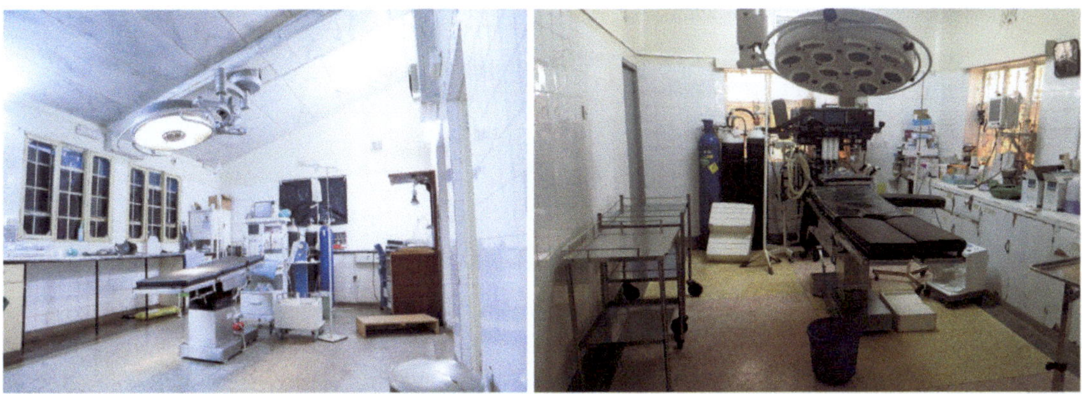

Fig. 24.3 An example of basic operating theatre in public healthcare facilities. Spaces are constrained, and such theatres serve all surgical disciplines within the facilities, negating specific focus on MIRS

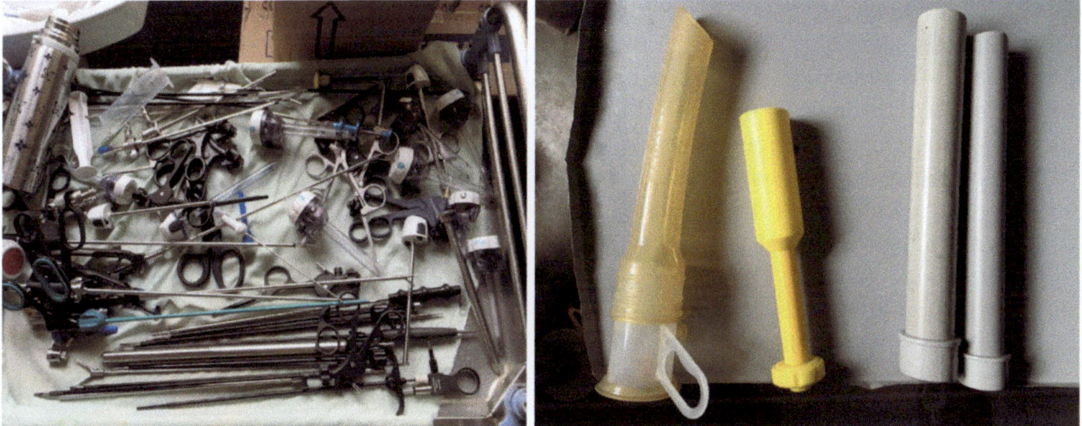

Fig. 24.4 Example of MIRS equipment in a public health facility. Some of the equipment is disposable but often gets re-used, and some equipment is improvised from locally available cheap material

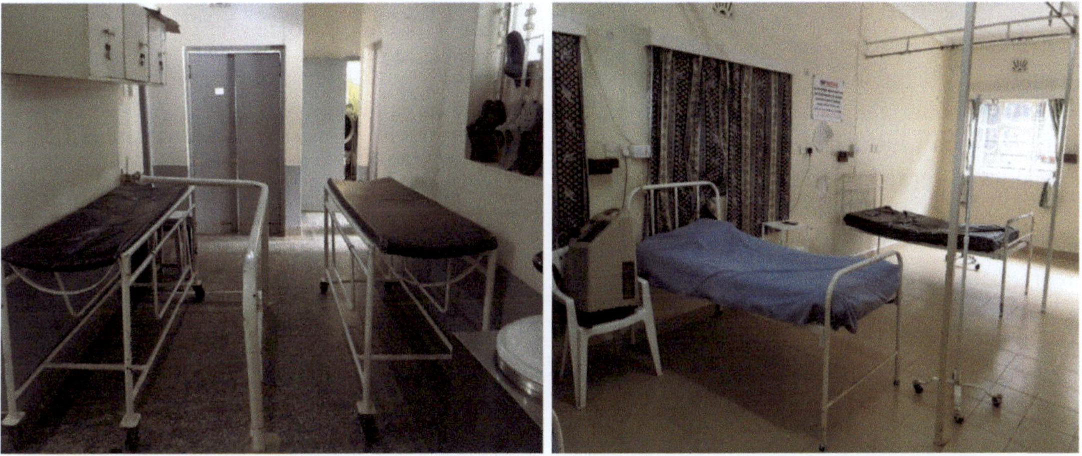

Fig. 24.5 An example of a post-operative recovery section with limited monitoring in a public health facility

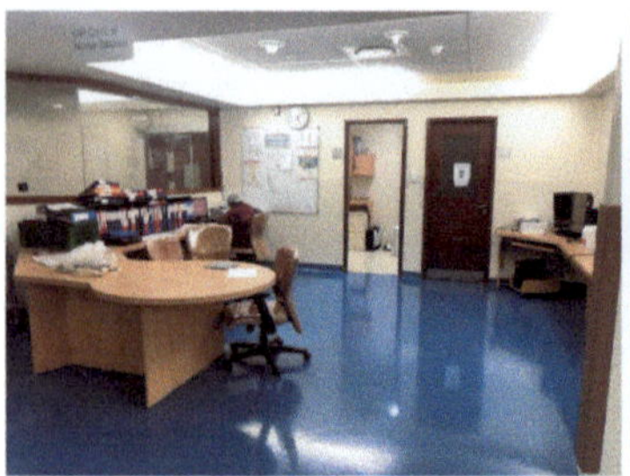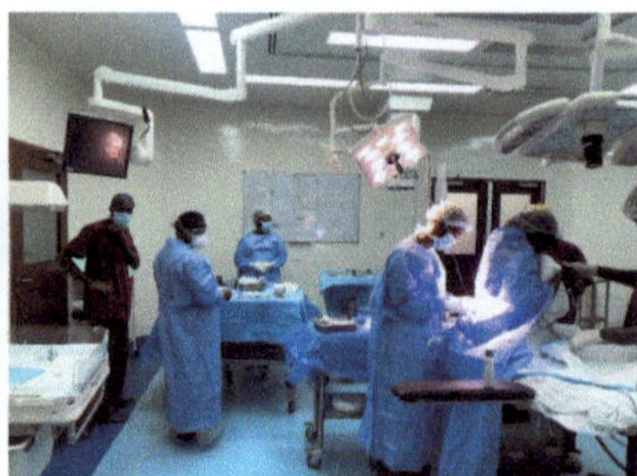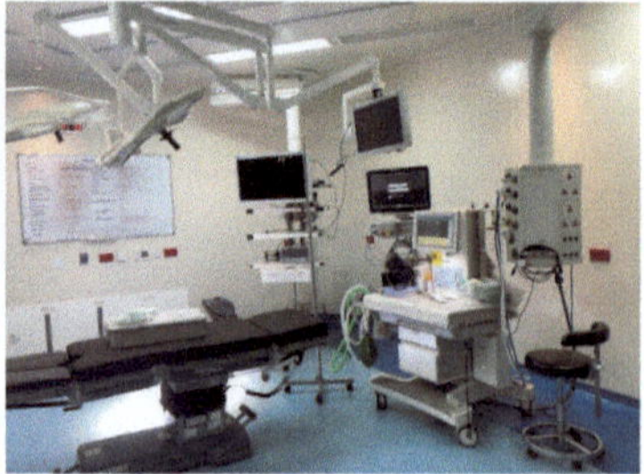

Fig. 24.6 An example of a dedicated and appropriately structured MIRS operating theatre in a private facility

This project relies on volunteers and donated surgical equipment. Appropriate MIRS cases are batched together in specific regions in the country, where procedures are usually conducted over 2–3 days, with a locally identified lead surgeon facilitating the whole program. The project has a large emphasis on training and transfer of skills. Sustainability is pegged on identifying regional MIRS centres and ongoing funding. However, the long-term solution for routine provision of MIRS in Kenya and other countries is strengthening of the public healthcare system, with increased governmental budgetary allocation to healthcare funding. This would improve the current healthcare infrastructure, including staffing and equipment. There must be a consequent focus on reproductive health and appropriate investments to upscale reproductive surgery.

Collaborations can address immediate reproductive surgical needs in the meantime. Public-private partnerships (PPPs) can play a vital role, as already demonstrated by the KESES project in Kenya. Other stakeholders, including local fertility societies, can advocate and facilitate relevant training. Collaborations with western institutions, including the Society for Reproductive Surgeons, an affiliate society of the American Society for Reproductive Medicine, can accelerate transfer of skills and technology. Such collaborations would include locally based reproductive research opportunities providing platforms for local solutions. Surgical equipment manufacturers may also help bridge current gaps

with availability of MIRS equipment in low-resource settings. Re-looking at the possibilities of re-usable equipment at lesser costs remains a viable option. Such networked efforts could yield desirable reproductive surgical outcomes in the immediate term, with deliberate efforts to assure sustainability for the long term.

References

1. https://databank.worldbank.org/source/world-development-indicators. Accessed 15 May 2020.
2. National and County health budget analysis Kenya (Financial Year 2018/19). http://www.healthpolicyplus.com/ns/pubs/11306-11563_NationalandCountyBudgetAnalysis.pdf. Accessed 12 Aug 2020.
3. WHO Abuja Declaration 2001. https://www.who.int/healthsystems/publications/Abuja10.pdf. Accessed 12 Aug 2020.
4. The 2018 update, global health workforce statistics. Geneva: World Health Organization. https://www.who.int/hrh/statistics/hwfstats/en/. Accessed 15 May 2020.
5. Pharmaccess, October 2016. https://www.pharmaccess.org/wp-content/uploads/2018/01/The-healthcare-system-in-Kenya.pdf. Accessed 10 Jun 2020.
6. Murage A, Muteshi M, Githae F. Assisted reproduction services provision in a developing country: time to act? Fertil Steril. 2011;96(4):966–8.
7. Kenya Master Health Facility List. http://kmhfl.health.go.ke/#/home. Accessed 10 Aug 2020.
8. Ngichabe S, Obura T, Stones W. Intravenous tranexamic acid as an adjunct haemostat to ornipressin during open myomectomy. A randomized double blind placebo controlled trial. Ann Surg Innov Res. 2015;9:10.

Index

O

P

Q

R

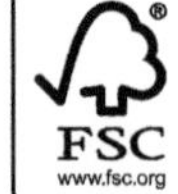

MIX
Papier aus verantwortungsvollen Quellen
Paper from responsible sources
FSC® C105338

If you have any concerns about our products,
you can contact us on
ProductSafety@springernature.com

In case Publisher is established outside the EU,
the EU authorized representative is:
**Springer Nature Customer Service Center GmbH
Europaplatz 3, 69115 Heidelberg, Germany**

Printed by Libri Plureos GmbH
in Hamburg, Germany